Affective Computing and Interaction:
Psychological, Cognitive and Neuroscientific Perspectives

Didem Gökçay
Middle East Technical University, Turkey

Gülsen Yildirim
Middle East Technical University, Turkey

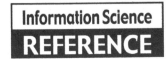

INFORMATION SCIENCE REFERENCE

Hershey · New York

Director of Editorial Content:	Kristin Klinger
Director of Book Publications:	Julia Mosemann
Acquisitions Editor:	Lindsay Johnston
Development Editor:	Dave DeRicco
Publishing Assistant:	Milan Vracarich Jr.
Typesetter:	Milan Vracarich Jr., Casey Conapitski
Production Editor:	Jamie Snavely
Cover Design:	Lisa Tosheff

Published in the United States of America by
Information Science Reference (an imprint of IGI Global)
701 E. Chocolate Avenue
Hershey PA 17033
Tel: 717-533-8845
Fax: 717-533-8661
E-mail: cust@igi-global.com
Web site: http://www.igi-global.com

Library of Congress Cataloging-in-Publication Data

Affective computing and interaction : psychological, cognitive, and
neuroscientific perspectives / Didem Gokcay and Gulsen Yildirim, editors.
     p. cm.
  Includes bibliographical references and index.
   ISBN 978-1-61692-892-6 (hardcover) -- ISBN 978-1-61692-894-0 (ebook) 1.
Human-computer interaction. 2. Human-machine systems. 3. Affect
(Psychology)--Computer simulation. I. Gokcay, Didem, 1966- II. Yildirim,
Gulsen, 1978-
  QA76.9.H85A485 2011
  004.01'9--dc22
                              2010041639

British Cataloguing in Publication Data
A Cataloguing in Publication record for this book is available from the British Library.

All work contributed to this book is new, previously-unpublished material. The views expressed in this book are those of the authors, but not necessarily of the publisher.

Table of Contents

Section 1
Foundations

Chapter 1

Aysen Erdem, Hacettepe University, Turkey
Serkan Karaismailoğlu, Hacettepe University, Turkey

Chapter 2

Mark Ashton Smith, Girne American University, Turkey

Chapter 3

Didem Gökçay, Middle East Technical University, Turkey

Section 2
Emotional Frameworks and Models

Chapter 4

Matthias Scheutz, Tufts University, USA

Section 3
Affect in Non-Verbal Communication

Section 4
Affect in Language-Based Communication

Section 5
Emotions in Human-Computer Interaction

Epilogue
A Philosophical Perspective on Incorporating Emotions in Human-Computer Interaction 359
  Zeynep Başgöze, Middle East Technical University, Turkey
  Ahmet Inam, Middle East Technical University, Turkey

Detailed Table of Contents

Section 1
Foundations

Chapter 1

Aysen Erdem, Hacettepe University, Turkey
Serkan Karaismailoğlu, Hacettepe University, Turkey

Emotions embody goal-directed behavior for survival and adaptation through the perception of variations in the environment. At a physiological level, emotions consist of three complementary components: Physical sensation, emotional expression and subjective experience. At the level of anatomical structures though, trying to segregate distinct components is impossible. Our emotions are resulting products of compatible and coordinated cortical and sub-cortical neural mechanisms originating from several anatomical structures. In this chapter, an overview of the three physiological components and underlying anatomical constructs will be presented.

Chapter 2

Mark Ashton Smith, Girne American University, Turkey

In this chapter the objective is to taxonomize unconscious and conscious affective and emotional processes and provide an account of their functional role in cognition and behavior in the context of a review of the relevant literature. The position adopted is that human affect and emotion evolved to function in motivational-cognitive systems and that emotion, motivation and cognition should be understood within a single explanatory framework. A 'dual process' that integrates emotion, motivation and cognition, is put forward in which emotion plays different functional roles in implicit motivations and explicit motivations.

Chapter 3

Didem Gökçay, Middle East Technical University, Turkey

The dimensional account of emotions has gained impetus over the last decade. The quantitative representation provided by the dimensional view of emotions is very valuable for applications in affective computing. The two principal axes, valence and arousal, obtained from semantic maps through factor analysis differentially modulate the psychophysiology measures and event related potentials. In addition, there exists distict localizations for valence/arousal-related emotional evaluation processes. Our current knowledge regarding these differences are reviewed in this chapter. Two different models (circumplex, PANA) have been coined to account for the distribution of data clustered within emotional categories. In this chapter, these models are also discussed comparatively in detail.

Section 2
Emotional Frameworks and Models

Chapter 4

Matthias Scheutz, Tufts University, USA

This chapter examines the utilization of affective control to support the survival of agents in competitive multi-agent environments. The author introduces simple affective control mechanisms for simple agents which result in high performance both in ordinary foraging tasks (e.g., searching for food) and in social encounters (e.g., competition for mates). In the proposed case, affective control via the transmission of simple signals can lead to social coordination. Therefore, this case prevents the need for more complex forms of communication like symbolic communication based on systematic representational schemata.

Chapter 5

N Korsten, Kings College London, UK
JG Taylor, Kings College London, UK

In order to achieve 'affective computing' it is necessary to know what is being computed. That is, in order to compute with what would pass for human emotions, it is necessary to have a computational basis for the emotions themselves. What does it mean quantitatively if a human is sad or angry? How is this affective state computed in their brain? It is this question, on the very core of the computational nature of the human emotions, which is addressed in this chapter. A proposal will be made as to this computational basis based on the well established approach to emotions as arising from an appraisal of a given situation or event by a specific human being.

Human emotions are based on typical configurations of beliefs, goals, expectations etc. In order to understand the complexity of affective processing in humans, reactions to stimuli, perception of our bodily reaction to events or just the feeling related to something should be considered but this is not adequate. Besides, our body does not respond just to external stimuli (events); it reacts to our interpretation of the stimulus, to the meaning of the event as well. In order to build affective architectures we also have to model the body, and its perception. In this chapter, with the help of these facts, the author will analyze the cognitive anatomies of simple anticipation-based emotions in addition to some complex social emotions.

Section 3
Affect in Non-Verbal Communication

Nonverbal communication is the main channel through which we experience inner life of others, including their emotions, feelings, moods, social attitudes, etc. This attracts the interest of the computing community because nonverbal communication is based on cues like facial expressions, vocalizations, gestures, postures, etc. that we can perceive with our senses and can be (and often are) detected, analyzed and synthesized with automatic approaches. In other words, nonverbal communication can be used as a viable interface between computers and some of the most important aspects of human psychology such as emotions and social attitudes. As a result, a new computing domain seems to emerge that we can define "technology of nonverbal communication". This chapter outlines some of the most salient aspects of such a potentially new domain and outlines some of its most important perspectives for the future.

Chapter 8

The objective of this chapter is to introduce the reader to the recent advances in computer processing of facial expressions and communicated affect. Human facial expressions have evolved in tandem with human face recognition abilities, and show remarkable consistency across cultures. Consequently, it is rewarding to review the main traits of face recognition in humans, as well as consolidated research on the categorization of facial expressions. The bulk of the chapter focuses on the main trends in computer analysis of facial expressions, sketching out the main algorithms and exposing computational considerations for different settings. The authors then look at some recent applications and promising new projects to give the reader a realistic view of what to expect from this technology now and in near future.

Chapter 9

Living in a computer era, the synergy between man and machine is a must, as the computers are integrated into our everyday life. The computers are surrounding us but their interfaces are far from being friendly. One possible approach to create a friendlier human-computer interface is to build an emotion-sensitive machine that should be able to recognize a human facial expression with a satisfactory classification rate and, eventually, to synthesize an artificial facial expression onto embodied conversational agents (ECAs), defined as friendly and intelligent user interfaces built to mimic human gestures, speech or facial expressions. Computer scientists working in computer interfaces (HCI) put up impressive efforts to create a fully automatic system capable to identifying and generating photo - realistic human facial expressions through animation. This chapter aims at presenting current state-of-the-art techniques and approaches developed over time to deal with facial expression synthesis and animation. The topic's importance will be further highlighted through modern applications including multimedia applications. The chapter ends up with discussions and open problems.

Section 4
Affect in Language-Based Communication

Chapter 10

Living in a computer era, the synergy between man and machine is a must, as the computers are integrated into our everyday life. The computers are surrounding us but their interfaces are far from being friendly. One possible approach to create a friendlier human-computer interface is to build an emotion-sensitive machine that should be able to recognize a human facial expression with a satisfactory classification rate and, eventually, to synthesize an artificial facial expression onto embodied conversational agents (ECAs), defined as friendly and intelligent user interfaces built to mimic human gestures, speech or facial expressions. Computer scientists working in computer interfaces (HCI) put up impressive efforts to create a fully automatic system capable to identifying and generating photo - realistic human facial expressions through animation. This chapter aims at presenting current state-of-the-art techniques and approaches developed over time to deal with facial expression synthesis and animation. The topic's importance will be further highlighted through modern applications including multimedia applications. The chapter ends up with discussions and open problems.

Chapter 11

Gülsen Yıldırım, Informatics Institute, METU, Turkey
Didem Gökçay, Informatics Institute, METU, Turkey

In this chapter, the authors examine some of behavioral problems frequently observed in computer-mediated communication and point out that a subset of these behavioral problems is similar to those of patients with brain lesions. The authors try to draw an analogy between the lack of affective features in text-based computer-mediated communication (CMC) versus the functional deficits brought along by regional brain damage. In addition, they review the social psychological studies that identify behavioral problems in CMC, and merge the literature in these different domains to propose some requirements for initiating conceptual changes in text-based CMC applications.

Chapter 12

Yuuki Kato, Tokyo University of Social Welfare, Japan
Douglass J. Scott, Waseda University, Japan
Shogo Kato, Tokyo Woman's Christian University, Japan

This chapter focuses on the roles of interpersonal closeness and gender on the interpretation and sending of emotions in mobile phone email messages. 91 Japanese college students were shown scenarios involving either a friend or an acquaintance describing situations intended to evoke one of four emotions: Happiness, sadness, anger, or guilt. The participants' rated their emotions and composed replies for each scenario. Analysis revealed that in the happy and guilt scenarios, emotions experienced by the participants were conveyed to their partners almost without change. However, in the sad and angry scenarios, the emotions sent to the partners were weaker than the actual emotions experienced. Gender analysis showed that men were more likely to experience and express anger in the anger scenario, while women were more likely to experience and express sadness in the anger scenario. In addition, more women's replies contained emotional expressions than did the men's messages.

Section 5
Emotions in Human-Computer Interaction

Chapter 13

Magy Seif El-Nasr, Simon Fraser University, Canada
Jacquelyn Ford Morie, University of Southern California, USA
Anders Drachen, Dragon Consulting, Copenhagen

The interactive entertainment industry has become a multi-billion dollar industry with revenues overcoming those of the movie industry (ESA, 2009). Beyond the demand for high fidelity graphics or stylized imagery, participants in these environments have come to expect certain aesthetic and artistic qualities that engage them at a very deep emotional level. These qualities pertain to the visual aesthetic, dramatic structure, pacing, and sensory systems embedded within the experience. All these qualities are carefully crafted by the creator of the interactive experience to evoke affect. In this book chapter, we will attempt to discuss the design techniques developed by artists to craft such emotionally engaging experiences. In addition, we take a scientific approach whereby we discuss case studies of the use of these design techniques and experiments that attempt to validate their use in stimulating emotions.

    Mahir Akgün, Pennsylvania State University, USA
    Göknur Kaplan Akıllı, Middle East Technical University, Turkey
    Kürşat Çağıltay, Middle East Technical University, Turkey

The current chapter focuses on affective issues that impact the success of human computer interaction. Since everybody is a computer user now and interaction is not only a technical activity, users' affective processes cannot be ignored anymore. Therefore, the issues related to these affective processes that enable efficient, effective and satisfactory interaction with computers are explored. An extensive literature review is conducted and studies related with affective aspects of human computer interaction are synthesized. It is observed that there is a need to adapt computers to people and affect is an important aspect of this trend. Likewise, human characteristics have to be reflected to the interaction. The findings of this chapter are especially important for those people who are planning to bring affect into the computerized environments.

    Karla Conn Welch, University of Louisville, USA
    Uttama Lahiri, Vanderbilt University, USA
    Nilanjan Sarkar, Vanderbilt University, USA
    Zachary Warren, Vanderbilt University, USA
    Wendy Stone, Vanderbilt University, USA
    Changchun Liu, The MathWorks, USA

This chapter covers the application of affective computing using a physiological approach to children with Autism Spectrum Disorders (ASD) during human-computer interaction (HCI) and human-robot interaction (HRI). Investigation into technology-assisted intervention for children with ASD has gained momentum in recent years. Clinicians involved in interventions must overcome the communication impairments generally exhibited by children with ASD by adeptly inferring the affective cues of the children to adjust the intervention accordingly. Similarly, an intelligent system, such as a computer or robot, must also be able to understand the affective needs of these children - an ability that the current technology-assisted ASD intervention systems lack - to achieve effective interaction that addresses the role of affective states in HCI, HRI, and intervention practice.

Video-games, like movies, music and storybooks are emotional artifacts. We buy media to alter our affective state. Through consumption they impact our physiology and thus alter our affective world. In this chapter we review the ways in which playing games can elicit emotion. This chapter will discuss the increased power of video-game technology to elicit affect, and show how the mash-up of traditional and interactive techniques have delivered a richness of emotion that competes with film and television. We then conclude by looking forward to a time when video-games become the dominant medium, and the preferred choice when seeking that emotional fix.

Foreword

"Some emotions don't make a lot of noise. It's hard to hear pride. Caring is real faint - like a heartbeat. And pure love why, some days it's so quiet, you don't even know it's there."- E. Bombeck

Real life affective states felt by *real people* are complex. It would be so much easier for us, scientists, if they were describable simply by the six prototypical categories of Ekman (anger, disgust, fear, happiness, sadness, and surprise), but they are not. For instance, the first and simplest affective state, which we discover in childhood, is *curiosity*. When does an automatic affect recogniser need to model *curiosity*, and how? The affective state *regret* lacks immediacy, and mostly comes upon reflection. Should affect interfaces model *regret*? More specifically, *why* do we researchers feel the need to sense affect at all, *what* models, expressions and affective states should we focus on, in *which* context, and *how* can we do all these?

The best way to seek answers to these questions, and provide an insight as to where affective computing field stands today, is to look at its past and present, and carry forward the knowledge and experience acquired into the future. One of the more recent answers to the question of *why we need to sense affect* came in the early 1990s, when Mayer and Salovey published a series of papers on emotional intelligence suggesting that the capacity to perceive and understand emotions define a new variable in personality. Goleman introduced the notion of emotional intelligence or Emotional Quotient (EQ) in his 1995 best-selling book by discussing why EQ mattered more than Intelligence Quotient (IQ). Goleman drew together research in neurophysiology, psychology and cognitive science. Other scientist also provided evidence that emotions were tightly coupled with all functions we, humans, are engaged with: attention, perception, learning, reasoning, decision making, planning, action selection, memory storage and retrieval. Following these, Rosalind Picard's award-winning book, Affective Computing, was published in 1997, laying the groundwork for giving machines the skills of EQ. The book triggered an explosion of interest in the emotional side of computers and their users, and a new research area called affective computing emerged.

When it comes to *what to model and sense* (*which* affective states, in *which* context), affective computing has advocated the idea that it might not be essential for machines to posses all the emotional intelligence and skills humans do. Humans need to operate in all possible situations and develop an adaptive behaviour; machines instead can be highly profiled for a specific purpose, scenario, user, etc. For example, the computer inside an automatic teller machine probably does not need to recognize the affective states of a human. However, in other applications (e.g., effective tutoring systems, clinical settings, and monitoring user's stress level) where computers take on a social role such as an instructor or helper, recognizing users' affective states may enhance the computers' functionality.

In order to achieve such level of functionality, the initial focus of affective computing was on the recognition of prototypical emotions from acted (posed) data and a single sensorial source (modality). However, as natural human-human interaction is multimodal, the single sensory observations are often ambiguous, uncertain, and incomplete. Therefore, in the late 1990s computer scientists started using multiple modalities for recognition of affective states. The initial interest was on fusing visual (facial expressions) and audio (acoustic signals) data. The results were promising, using multiple modalities improved the overall recognition accuracy helping the systems function in a more efficient and reliable way. Starting from the work of Picard in the late 1990s, interest in detecting emotions from physiological (bio) signals emerged.

The final stage affective computing has reached today is, combining multiple cues and modalities for sensing and recognition, and moving from acted (posed) data, idealised conditions and users towards real data, real life, and real people. The attempt of making affect technology tangible for the real world and the real people is closely linked to Ray Kurzweil's prophecy. Kurzweil predicted that by 2030 we can purchase for 1000 USD the equivalent information processing capacity of one human brain, and by 2060 digital computing will equal the processing capacity of all the human brains on the earth. If computing capacity continues to increase; further advances in high resolution digital imaging, compression algorithms and random access mass storage is achieved; broadband/wired/wireless communication is available worldwide; size, cost, and power consumption of computational/communications hardware continue to decrease; portable power generation/storage advancement continue, then computers will become much more connected to people (and vice versa) than they already are today.

Coupling the new horizons reached in technology and cognitive sciences, the focus of affective computing research is gradually moving from *just* developing more efficient and effective automated techniques to concentrating on more context-/culture-/user-related aspects (*who* the user is, *where* she is, *what* her current task is, and *when* the observed behaviour has been shown). In this transitional process, affective computing research is constantly attempting to bridge technology and humans not only for more natural human-computer interaction (HCI) but also for improved human-human interaction by becoming *curious* on *how* real-life conditions, tasks, and relationships affect humans, and *whether* and *how* the field can positively impact these (e.g., affect sensing for autism).

This book contributes to answering such *why, what, and how questions* by providing an overview of frameworks and models of affect, highlighting the present and future of affect sensing and recognition, and looking at affect in HCI context. Each section explores the give and take of various aspects, from foundations and background of affect in cognition (Section 1) to theoretical models of affect (Section 2), and how these are used in order to create automatic affect recognisers based on verbal and nonverbal signals (Sections 3 & 4), and how created automatic systems have influenced HCI to date (Section 5). The book concludes with an extremely interesting philosophical discussion on whether it is possible and desirable to create *machines that work exactly like humans do*.

Evolutionary theory hypothesises that specific expressive behaviours were selected over the course of human evolution because they had adaptive value in social relationships. This hypothesis suggest that the evolution and future of affective computing is, indeed, an *ongoing* wondrous journey where machines (computers) meet humans, and where key issues and themes of affective communication, such as context, emotion colouring, multimodality, back-channelling, intensity, duration, continuity, and sustainability, evolve over the course of time, and over the course of that encounter. The authors and readers of this book thus become a part of this wondrous journey.

Hatice Gunes
Imperial College, UK & University of Technology, Australia

Preface

For many years, researchers in computer science have focused on rational thinking but discarded the contribution of emotions in machine learning, artificial intelligence and decision making. Similarly in cognitive science, emotions have been considered as exclusive processes for the survival instincts of animals. After the evolution of mankind from hominoids, the limbic system, which sustained all the emotional processing has been thought to be downplayed by a superior system centered in the prefrontal cortex, which sustained all the high-level executive functions involving monitoring, attention, conflict resolution, working memory. However in the last decade, through astonishing progress in cognitive neuroscience, our understanding of the sub-processes in emotion and cognition have progressed. Nowadays, emotion and cognition are viewed as complementary counterparts, interacting through complex top-down and bottom-up systems.

In the light of recent findings from neuroscience research, the emotional experience of the end-users in human-computer interaction may be thought over. Particularly, creating, triggering, sustaining and detecting emotions at the site of the end-user as well as the capability to imitate emotions will prevail as active research areas of our times. Designing interfaces considering affective tools as well as aesthetics; handling game designs in such a way that the user engagement is managed via emotional experiences; greeting/rehabilitating users with affective agents; creating agents with beliefs, desires and intentions are the most promising examples of this new trendy approach.

In the current literature, affective interactions most often refer to the involvement of affect in the interaction between a user and a system. In this type of interaction, usually psychophysiological measures such as skin conductance, eye-blink, heart rate, or electrophysiological measures such as eeg, or behavioral measures such as facial expressions, speech prosody, gestures are input to an automated system. This system then tries to classify the psychological state of the user through machine learning or pattern recognition techniques. After inferring the psychological state of the human, the machine can adapt or manipulate its 'behavior' or more technically its outputs for communicating more efficiently with its user. Although this is an exciting and still unraveled endeavor, there exists a bigger challenge. Rather than inferring a psychological state from the user inputs by choosing from a set of predefined classes, an affective computing system can instead model the actual affective internal world or an affective internal representation as it exists in a human. This allows for a time-varying continuum of emotions, similar to that of the human. If we want the human-computer interaction to occur in a domain similar to the phenomenal world, this new approach seems to be indispensable. Unfortunately, there are two major obstacles that hinder us from implementing such systems in the near-term: 1. The neuroanatomical underpinnings of the affective processes in the human brain are extremely complex and far from being well-understood, hence the field is not quite ready for developing affective models 2. A dynamical platform to model such a system is hard to implement and validate because affective inputs/outputs should be produced and tested in several different temporal scales, while the affective representations across these temporal scales also overlap.

In this book, we humbly aimed at serving two purposes: First, capturing the current state of art in affective computing within the context of affective interactions. And second, providing fundamental knowledge to facilitate development of future affective systems which dynamically interact using affective internal representations. Sections 1 and 2 serve the second purpose, while sections 3, 4, and 5 serve the first purpose.

In section 1, the foundations of affect are reviewed according to the cognitive science, psychology and neuroscience perspectives. Chapter 1 describes the neuroanatomy and neurophysiology of the limbic and prefrontal systems which participate in the sensation, expression, and subjective feeling of emotions in detail. Chapter 2 presents a dual processing approach within the emotional network of the human brain. According to this approach, dual processing occurs based on implicit and explicit motivations; the implicit part is rooted on the low-level limbic areas whereas the explicit system, which is also normative is centered within the pre-frontal areas. Chapter 3 summarizes the widely accepted emotional axes, valence and arousal, and their emergence from cognitive evaluations, as well as psychophysiological measures.

Section 2 contains remarkable examples of theoretical emotional frameworks or models, mostly built by using subsets of knowledge provided in section 1. In chapter 4, design of affective agents is discussed. Based on evolutionary demands, how to change the behavior of these agents is also highlighted. In chapter 5, neural networks are utilized to model six basic emotions and a subset of social emotions, using current, standard, expected, and predicted values of a situational signal. Chapter 6 models complex social emotions using logic, by replacing expectation and predictions with Belief and Goals.

Sections 3 and 4 focus on the expression of emotion in affective interactions. In section 3, up to date reviews of the current work in the technology of nonverbal communication are provided. More specifically, chapter 7 focuses on vocalizations, gestures, postures, while chapter 8 focuses on automatically decoding facial expressions and chapter 9 focuses on facial expression synthesis with computers. Currently, these are the most popular research areas in affective computing. In section 4, a collection of chapters addressing affect in verbal communication is presented. Unfortunately, applications of affective computing in verbal interactions are scarce. This is why we included chapter 10 on the role of affect in human language development. Understanding the primary roles affect plays in language development might aid in the development of affective language learning systems. Chapter 11 highlights the behavioral problems that emerge in text-based computer mediated communication such as email and chat environments. The viewpoint of chapter 11 is centered more towards western populations. In chapter 12, a case study on mobile phone messages is provided in a Japanese population. From here, we learn that affective messages are modulated differently in a non-western population when text-based environments are used.

Finally section 5 brings together fascinating discussions on affective computing in human-computer interaction as well as current trends and promising technologies for designing interactive environments based on affective interactions. In chapter 13, manipulation of affect in interactive environments such as films and games is discussed in detail. This chapter also presents development of adaptive games based on the user's psychophysiological measures. In chapter 14, a general overview of affective aspects in human-computer-interaction is provided, especially for designing efficient affective interfaces and feedback messages. In chapter 15, a wonderful case study is summarized for utilizing adaptive artificial agents such as avatars, for the rehabilitation of autistic patients who are known to have affective deficits. The behavior of the machine (a robot arm, or an avatar), can be manipulated during the training of the patient by using the patient's psychophysiological signals in a feedback loop. Finally in chapter 16, an innovative approach to the presence of emotions in game technologies is provided: 'How can games elicit emotions in the user?', and 'How does this compare to the emotions elicited in films?' are the main questions tackled.

The selected chapters end with an Epilogue, which contains a brief philosophical discussion on the possibility and plausibility of creating affective machines.

We would like to conclude by saying that in this collection, we tried to assemble several aspects of affective interactions in an interdisciplinary and pleasant reading format so that the literature in neuroscience, psychology and computing fields can be merged lucidly. We hope that this book will reach out to communities associated with computer science, cognitive science or cognitive neuroscience and help in uncovering and representing the elusive interplay between emotion and cognition in affective interactions.

Didem Gökçay
Middle East Technical University, Turkey

Gülsen Yıldırım
Middle East Technical University, Turkey

Acknowledgment

Assembling this book in its current form was a challenging collaborative effort.

We would like to express our gratitude to the editorial advisory board members who helped during the review phase, contributed to the foreword and chapters. Our editorial advisory board consisted of experts in the fields of neuroscience, computational neuroscience, psychology, affective interaction design, affective computing, affect recognition, affective social computing, human-computer interaction and emotion modeling. Many thanks to Nadia Bianchi-Berthouze, Emrah Duzel, Hatice Gunes, Magy Seif El-Nasr, Mark Ashton Smith and John Taylor.

We invited our colleagues to review chapters during the review phase to obtain impartial perspectives and to enhance the interdisciplinary content. We would like to applaud our external reviewers: Umut Baysan, Murat Perit Çakır, Uğur Halıcı, Annette Hohenberger, Buciu Ioan, Albert Ali Salah and Bilge Say for their valuable input regarding how to improve the individual chapters.

We used the existing infrastructure, computational facilities and Internet services of Middle East Technical University while working on several aspects of this book. We appreciate the efforts of the system administrators and staff who have participated in this production behind the scenes.

Finally, we would like to express our sincere thanks to our development editors, Elizabeth Ardner, Dave de Ricco and Myla Harty for their continuous support throughout the production phase.

Didem Gökçay
Middle East Technical University, Turkey

Gülsen Yildirim
Middle East Technical University, Turkey

Section 1
Foundations

Chapter 1
Neurophysiology of Emotions

Ayşen Erdem
Hacettepe University, Turkey

Serkan Karaismailoğlu
Hacettepe University, Turkey

ABSTRACT

Emotions embody goal-directed behavior for survival and adaptation through the perception of variations in the environment. At a physiological level, emotions consist of three complementary components: Physical sensation, emotional expression and subjective experience. At the level of anatomical structures though, trying to segregate distinct components is impossible. Our emotions are resulting products of compatible and coordinated cortical and sub-cortical neural mechanisms originating from several anatomical structures. In this chapter, an overview of the three physiological components and underlying anatomical constructs will be presented.

INTRODUCTION

Complex organisms must not only perceive and evaluate changes in their internal and external environment, but also generate appropriate responses to survive. In general, emotions help an organism to survive by embodying a multitude of nervous system functions for perception of the valuable components of the external environment. At the same time, emotions are a way for directly communicating our internal world to others through non-verbal means (Öztürk et al., 2005). Emotions aid an individual to interact with his/her external –or more specifically social- environment in a flexible way, while also helping in the regulation of an individual's internal world.

Emotional information is used for personal, as well as social decision making of an individual with

DOI: 10.4018/978-1-61692-892-6.ch001

respect to the surrounding dynamical processes. Briefly, we can say that an emotion is an evaluative response. These responses are physiological and behavioral impulses that prepare the organisms for escaping or approaching dangerous versus safe objects. Actually, emotions consist of not a single but a multitude of responses in presence of a stimulus (Öztürk et al., 2005).

In summary, we can say that 'emotions may be characterized as a response to an environmental event that allow for goal-directed behavior in the adaptation of the organism to changing environmental demands. This response involves cognitive, affective, behavioral, and autonomic sub-systems' (Oatley & Jenkins, 1996; Hagemann et al., 2003). At a physiological level, most of the recent research in affective neuroscience strive to elucidate the prominent components of neural networks of emotion. When considered from this perspective, there are three distinct but complementary components of emotions (Bownds, 1999):

1. **Physical sensation**: Consists of the components within the autonomic nervous system which we call physiological arousal.
2. **Emotional expression**: Consists of our behaviours such as facial expressions, gestures and posture for reflecting our feelings such as sadness, anger, happiness.
3. **Subjective experience**: Consists of the personal feeling of our current emotion such as fear, anger, and happiness.

It is extremely difficult to identify all emotional states that we go through. Because of this, emotions can be simply categorized as basic (primary) and social (secondary). The basic emotions are innate and related to the anatomical structures in the limbic system (for ex. Amygdala). They consist of organized automatic and stereotypical behaviours (Izard, 2009), that are consistent across cultures. These basic emotions are essential for survival, evolution and development. There are six basic emotions that are widely accepted: happiness,

sadness, anger, fear, disgust, and surprise. These emotions can further be grouped as pleasant (happiness, surprise) and unpleasant (sadness, anger, fear, disgust). The pleasant emotions consist of positive affect causing approach to stimuli whereas the unpleasant emotions consist of negative affect that is repellant (Izard, 2009). On the other hand, social emotions differ from the basic emotions primarily because they are learned through social interaction as the individual grows. Social emotions embody personal experiences such as guilt, embarrassment/shame, and pride (Damasio, 1994). Other than these, it is also necessary to consider background emotional processes such as mood, which are elicited in a totally different way.

PHYSICAL SENSATION AND AUTONOMIC NERVOUS SYSTEM

When we investigate areas that are responsible of the complementary components of emotions, we would have to say that the hypothalamus, brain stem, and medulla spinalis are specifically responsible from the physical sensations which include physiologic components of the autonomic nervous system (see Figure 1).

Hypothalamus and the Autonomic Nervous System

Although small in physical size, hypothalamus is an extremely important structure. It acts as a relay station conjoining incoming signals from a lot of different areas. It consists of different cell groups and its basic responsibility is in the homeostatic ogranization of the internal environment (maintenance of internal stability). Hypothalamus controls most of the endocrinal, vegetative and emotional behaviour of the body. Several nuclei contained within the hypothalamus play different roles: For example the excitation of lateral and posterior areas increases blood pressure and heart rate while the excitation of the preoptic area

Figure 1. Main structures those are responsible from the physical sensation of emotion

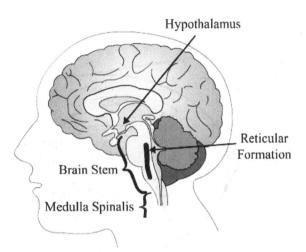

reduces these. Similarly, while the frontal areas activate mechanisms responsible from decrease of the body temperature, the posterior areas activate heat preserving mechanisms. The side areas of hypothalamus are known as the centers for thirst and hunger. The area close to the medial part of the hypothalamus serves as the satiety center. In addition, hypothalamus controls excretion of water from kidneys, and birth through the release of oxytocine hormone (Guyton & Hall, 2006).

With the inclusion of a multitude of centers in the brain stem and medulla spinalis, the hypothalamus is incharge of the activation of the autonomic nervous system and the regulation of reflex responses. Under any emotional stimulus, the signals incoming to the hypothalamus induce and effect on the autonomic nervous system. What is the importance of the autonomic nervous system then? What is its duty?

As mentioned earlier, the autonomic nervous system maintains the homeostasis of our internal envionment. It works without our conscious will. There are two main parts of the autonomic nervous system: sympathetic and parasympathetic. Other than a few exceptions, these two systems counteract. While one system increases activity in and organ, the other supresses it. The parasympathetic

system is active under resting or peaceful conditions, maintains energy storage and preservation. Its effects are local. Sympathetic system on the other hand, is also named as the system for 'fight or flight'. It prepares the individual for a fleeing or fighting response.

What are the main effects imposed by the sympathetic system? In case of danger, our heart rate and blood pressure increases, because blood and oxygen consumption by our vital organs has increased. Respiratory rate and depth also increases to satisfy the increased oxygen demand. Bronchi in the respiratory tract widen. On the contrary, the digestive tract's blood demands decrease. The digestive functions slow down, or even stop the blood demand in this area. The muscles which provide motor movements in this area are relaxed, prohibiting defecation and micturation. Production of urine slows down. All other secretions such as saliva are decreased. Glucose in the bloodstream increases, because our vital organs and muscles are in need of energy. Our pupils are dilated to be able to immerse more light. Muscle tone increases and reflexes speed up. We became more alert. The effects of the neurotransmitters (adrenalin ve noradrenalin) that induce these changes, especially those that effect the heart, start late and end late.

Figure 2. Limbic lobe

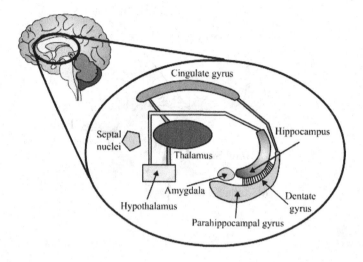

This is why our heart still keeps pounding for a while even when the danger is over. On the other hand, by the induction of the neurotransmitter acetylcholine, the parasympathetic system induces chages that counteract with these. Heart rate and blood pressure decreases. Respiratory rate decreases, causing the bronchi to constrict. Digestion and absorption speed up, causing increased blood delivery to this area. Secretions are increased, the pupils constrict. In short, it becomes important to restore the consumed energy (Guyton & Hall, 2006; Hagemann et al., 2003; for an overview, see Lovallo & Sollers, 2000).

EMOTIONAL EXPRESSION AND THE LIMBIC SYSTEM

When we say that there are three complementary components in the physiology of emotions, we also have to specify that it is extremely difficult to isolate the underlying areas exclusively according to the functionality of these components. This is because many areas in the brain have assumed responsibility for a multitude of differing tasks. Hypothalamus is an outstanding example for this. Hypothalamus not only effects physical

sensation, but also has many effects on emotional expressions and behaviours. For example, if we stimulate lateral hypothalamus, we cause the animal to exhibit agressive, fighting behaviour. When we remember that this same area is implicated in thirst and hunger related behaviour, we can find an answer to why animals become nervous when they are hungry. On the contrary, when a medial nucleus of the hytpothalamus is activated, the animal becomes relaxed, eats less and feels nutritional satisfaction causing satiety. In a normal animal, the rage feeling is held under control by the inhibiting signals that come from the medial nuclei of hypothalamus (Guyton & Hall, 2006).

Historically, it was Paul Broca who first indicated that there is a specific area in the medial aspect of the brain, around corpus callosum and brain stem, which is separated from the surrounding cortex with clear borders. Broca named this area as the limbic lobe (limbus: border), because of its distinct borders around the brain stem. Limbic lobe embodies the cingulate gyrus, parahippocampal gyrus and the hippocampal formation consisting of dentate gyrus and subiculum (see Figure 2). Broca thought that this area was prominent for the olfactory sense having its major inputs from the olfactory bulb, without foreseeing the importance of this region for emotional processes. It was James Papez (Papez, 1937) who coined the first idea about the relationship of the limbic lobe and emotion.

Based on the existing knowledge regarding organization of emotional expressions by hypothalamus, identification of emotions by cortex and manipulations of emotions by cognitive processes, Papez defined a new pathway called the 'Papez circuit'. According to this, hippocampal formation processes the incoming information from the cingulate gyrus and forwards it to the mammillary body of the hypothalamus through fornix. The projections going through the mammillary body run through the posterior part of the thalamus and loop back to the cingulate gyrus. In Papez circuit, the interaction between the hypothalamus and cingulate gyrus is bidirectional, providing cortical control for the emotional expression (through cingulate to hypothalamus), as well as emotional experience (through hypothalamus to cingulate).

The initial definitions of the limbic system started out with the Papez circuit. Due to the consequential similarity between the structures involved in Broca's limbic lobe and Papez circuit, this region of the brain which is involved in emotions is named as the 'limbic system'. Interestingly, the person who made the limbic system popular was neither Broca nor Papez. By extending the limbic system to include the septal area, nucleus accumbens, amygdala and orbitofrontal cortex, it was the physiologist Paul McLean who accentuated the limbic system.

Advancing research showed later that some of the main structures within the Papez circuit such as hippokampus were not actually related to emotions. Papez had included hippocampus in the circuit because rabies cases were characterized by the Rabies virus' attacks to the hippocampus and the symptoms associated with Rabies were related to emotional changes such as terror and rage. As a matter of fact, Papez was being misled by thinking that hippocampus was coordinating

hypothalamus' actions; although we now know that it is the amygdala which coordinates the activities of hypothalamus.

Heinrich Kluver and Paul Bucy (1939) conducted some experiments on monkeys after the proposal of the Papez circuit for emotions. They observed abnormal behaviour which they later named as 'Kluver-Bucy syndrome' in animals that underwent bilateral temporal lobectomy (removal of the temporal lobe in both hemispheres). One of the most important behavioral changes was visual agnosia: although the visual perception was good, visual recognition was mediocre. These animals would put everything within their visual area into their mouth, unlike other animals (Sometimes, similar behaviour is also observed in human patients with temporal lobe lesions). The lobectomized monkeys were trying to contract everything around them physically, showed hyperactivity and hypersexuality. In addition, they also exhibited differences in their emotional behaviour. While they were agressive, wild and fearful towards humans beforehands, they became extremely tame after the surgery. No agressive displays were observed when they ware handled. Furthermore, while normal monkeys became fearful when they saw a snake, their natural predator, the lobectomized ones did not display any signs of fear. In short, the lobectomized monkeys were void of fear and agression. Later research proved that similar sypotoms are observed even when amygdala is removed exclusively. Therefore a rather specific region, amygdala, started to receive all the attention regarding the control of emotional behaviour.

The Amygdala and Its Outputs for Emotional Expression

Amygdala was first identified at the beginning of the 19th century as a structure resembling almond in the medial temporal lobe. Amygdala is a complex structure consisting of approximately 10 nuclei, and it participates in most behavioral functions (LeDoux, 2007). Although the term 'amygdaloid complex' better reflects the complexity of this structure, we will keep using the term amygdala for the remaining parts of this text.

Around the end of 1930's researchers have noticed that after damage to the amygdala, fear response, as well as feeding and sexual responses are altered (Klüver & Bucy, 1939). Downer (1961) proved the important contribution of amygdala to agressive behaviour through an interesting experiment. He removed the amygdala of Rhesus monkeys unilaterally. At the same time, he disconnected the two hemispheres by severing the connections that carried information through the corresponding areas of the brain on both sides. During the experiments alternatingly, one eye was closed while the animal was exposed to the sight of natural predators. This way, he was able to form an animal model such that the intact amygdala only receives visual input from the seeing eye which is co-located inside the same hemisphere. According to Downer, the emotional behaviour of the animal should be determined by the seeing eye. When the animal saw the predator with the eye on the same side with the lesioned amygdala, he presented symptoms similar to Kluver-Bucy syndrome. But when the animal saw the predator with the eye on the same side with the intact amygdala, it showed natural emotional behaviour consisting of aggression and fear.

More interestingly, amygdala also takes part in the regulation of acquired (or learned) emotional responses. The best example regarding classical fear conditioning response is probably the experiment done by Joseph LeDoux and his colleagues. In this experiment, rats are trained using a specific sound such that after the sound is presented, the animal receives an electrical shock to its foot. The fear response of the animals is recorded in terms of their blood pressure and duration of freezing behavior. While the animals showed no specific response to this sound before training, they showed increased blood pressure and freezing behavior after training. By the help of this paradigm LeDoux (1995; 2000) was able

to isolate the neural circuitry between the sound and fear, which implicated that the the medial geniculate nucleus (MGN) of the Thalamus is the key player. The incoming auditory information is carried from Thalamus to the amygdala through direct connections. Furthermore, when these direct connections are severed, this fear response is no longer observed. Continuing studies of LeDoux showed that amygdala's nuclei confined to the central area project directly to the reticular nucleus of the mid-brain, which plays an important role in the formation of the freezing response. In a similar way, the projections from the reticular nucleus enter the hypothalamus causing increased blood pressure (LeDoux, 2000).

Amygdala exhibits its manipulatory presence in several cognitive and behavioral functions including attention, perception, and explicit memory. It is a general belief that the amygdala manages the processes in the evaluation of the emotional meaning of an external stimulus, which in turn helps in the organization of cognitive functions. Amygdala exhibits its modulatory role on a wide area in the brain, including STS (superior temporal sulcus) (Amaral et al., 2003), primary visual cortex, fusiform face area, orbitofrontal kortex (e.g., Davidson et al., 1990; Schmidt & Fox, 1999) and anterior cingulate cortex (see Figure 3). Outputs from the amygdala alter the cognitive processes within cortical areas by causing release of hormones and neurotransmitters (please see the appendix for a brief overview of the neurotransmitters related to emotions). For example, by modulating the activity of superior temporal sulcus, amygdala may contribute to the perception of motion (Amaral et al., 2003; Chouchourelou et al., 2006): such as perceiving slow movements performed by sad people and fast pacing by angry people (Pollick et al., 2001). Furthermore, explicit memories regarding the emotional situations are enforced through amygdalar outputs leading to the hippocampus (LeDoux, 2007).

Although fear and mechanisms related to fear constitute the most prominent areas in current

Figure 3. Main amygdalar outputs for emotional expressions

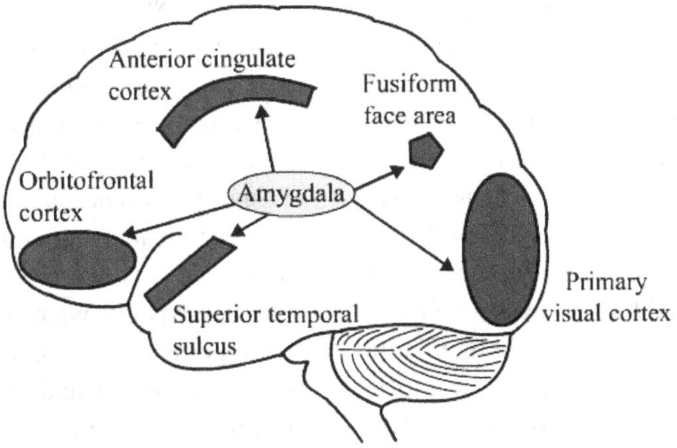

research, amygdala preserves its importance in pleasure-related or appetitive positive emotions as well. When damages are induced to other areas of the amygdala, conditioned response to food reward disappears (Holland & Gallagher, 2003). In quite a few studies, amygdala activity in response to positive affective stimuli such as music (Blood & Zatorre, 2001), male orgasm (Holstege et al., 2003) decreases amygdalar activity. In general it can be said that when compared to positive emotional stimuli, negative emotional stimuli are more effective to create amygdalar activity (Zald, 2003).

Amygdala is in charge of the regulation of both unconscious emotional state and conscious feeling. Amygdala contains 2 projections with respect to its dual-functionality in emotion. Through its many interconnections with the hypothalamus and the autonomous nervous system, the amygdala participates in the autonomic expression of the emotional state. Through its connections of the cingulate gyrus and prefrontal cortex, it participates in the conscious feeling of emotions, which is described in the next section on 'subjective experience of emotions'.

Frontal Lobe

The importance of human frontal lobe in terms of social and emotional behaviors is shown in famous Phineas Gage, the railway man. In 1848, USA, while Phineas Gage was working on the railroad as usual, suddenly the dynamites, which they were utilizing for breaking the rocks, exploded by accident and the iron pipe Gage was holding in hand pierced the left side of his skull. This accident caused a serious impairment on his frontal cortex. However, Gage was luckily healed, except his left eye was blind, which is great luck on such a serious accident. He was touching, hearing, seeing, using his hands skillfully, walking etc. There was no significant impairment on his speech and language abilities. However, in time, people around him realized that Gage's character had changed drastically. The man, who was dignified, adaptable, energetic, hard working and responsible before the accident, became another human being after the accident. He was rude, immoral, abusive and intolerant when his wills were frustrated. He had no future plans and he was no longer taking advices. As he was no longer productive on his job, he was fired. His life was ruined more and more and he probably died because of status epilepticus[1] eventually.

At first this incident was not assessed as it deserved, since Gage's abilities such as attention, sensation, memory, language and intelligence were not impaired. The degeneration which arouse in his character and social life did not attract attention at that time, because the most widely accepted view was that if speech, sensation and memory were not impaired then social life and executive functions could not be impaired. This conflict could very lately strike the attention of the scientific community. In 1935, John, Fulton and Carlyle reported that chimpanzees were calmed when their frontal cortex is removed (lobotomy) and called this effect as the "calming effect of frontal lobectomy" (Horwitz, 1998). After a few months of this report, a Portuguese neuropsychiatrist, Egas Moinz conducted the first prefrontal lobotomy in humans. In order to cure an emotional illness which accompanies an acute mental illness, he removed the orbital frontal cortex, cutting the limbic association link.

After many years, the researchers, who inquired Gage incident again, displayed that the iron pipe did not harm the regions responsible for motor and language functions, but it did affect both hemisphere's ventro-medial prefrontal cortex, but especially the left one. Some other incidents got into the literature where frontal lobe is damaged. The fact that these patients showed similar impairments to Gage's, made it clear that especially the prefrontal cortex has a crucial role in planning the future, behaving according to social codes, deciding appropriately in order to survive and acting appropriately.

In recent years, countless studies demonstrated that the prefrontal region is very closely related to positive and negative emotions.

Frontal lobe has an important role on the development of any kind of spontaneous behaviors, such as facial expression and speech. It is also crucial in controlling the processes necessary to perceiving the emotion from the other lobes (un-

derstanding the facial expressions, in particular) (Lane & Nadel, 2006). Similarly, frontal lobe rectifies the behaviors depending on the internal and external information. If the information is not processed properly, then the behaviors are corrupted. For example, the mammalians' primary visual cortex sends information both to the visual association area and to the prefrontal cortex and amygdala (Lane & Nadel, 2006). We know that the visual pathways reaching to amygdala have an important role in regulating the fear response. For instance in a study conducted on cats, when encountered with a cat shaped as a "Halloween profile", the cats respond with similar postures and approach the perineal or head region of the stimulus cat. A piloerection on the back and tail region, slowed respiration, perspiration on the paws and dilatation on the pupil are observed on these cats. This affective response to the Halloween configuration is typical; however no such response is seen when the Picasso cat (a cat profile which does not resemble to a regular cat) is used as stimulus. The cats pay little attention to the Picasso cat. The "Halloween profile" cat threatens the cats, while Picasso cat does not. If there is a lesion in cats' visual cortex naturally they do not respond to the stimulus ("Halloween profile" cat), because their perception is seriously impaired. The cats with impaired amygdala are oriented to the stimulus and approaches to it; however they do not respond affectively (no piloerection, no autonomic response). The cats with frontal lesions, however, are oriented to the stimulus, but rather than approaching to it, they avoid it (nor an autonomic response).

All of these examples show that the visual pathways reaching amygdala are very crucial for the formation of fear response to the species specific visual stimulus. The visual pathways to the prefrontal cortex, on the other hand, have a role on the formation of the behavior pattern appropriate to the species specific typical stimulus. Moreover, the primates, whose amygdala or frontal lobe is impaired, are incompetent in perceiving the species specific stimuli (e.g. facial expressions or vocalization) (Lane & Nadel, 2006).

All emotions are expressed with stereotypical somatic motor responses (especially the motor movements of facial muscles) and visceral motor system. This necessitates the activity of the central nervous structures which govern the preganglionic autonomic neurons located in the brain stem and the spinal cord. It is interesting that the more the voluntary facial expressions reflect the real emotions (e.g. fear, anger, happiness), the more the autonomic response gets stronger. Furthermore, physiological responses may start with the stimuli coming from the forebrain: for instance with odor, music, watching a movie. This neuronal activity that started on the forebrain reaches the visceral and somatic motor nuclei which coordinate the emotional behaviors through hypothalamus and brainstem reticular formation. Among these structures hypothalamus is the central structure which regulates both the visceral and the somatic motor components. Hypothalamus functions like this, through the synapses it forms with reticular formation.

Reticular Formation

Rete means "web" in Latin. In fact, when this formation is examined histologically, it seems as a structure which is located on the inner regions of the brain stem with cells extending to everywhere and as a web-like structure formed from those cells' bundles. The main jobs of reticular formation are visceral and motor control, sensory control and control of consciousness.

The short neurons located in RF have important role on the regulation of stereotypical or coordinated movements (e.g. cardiovascular functions, respiration, eye movements, chewing, swallowing). RF provides the coordinated activation of autonomic and somatic effector systems which are in charge during these activities. For example, RF is crucial in regulating the movements during the chewing action (the chin gets open and closed

rapidly) in order to prevent biting of the tongue or the cheeks; or in providing the emotional face expression in accordance with the stimuli coming from the superior centers (limbic system, cerebral cortex and cerebellum). Hence, facial expressions are not only started with the voluntary motor activity beginning from the motor cortex on the posterior frontal lobe, but it also starts with the stimuli coming from forebrain regions in order to provide emotional expression.

RF does not only get information from hypothalamus, but also from the fibers descending from the limbic system on the forebrain region. Affecting the somatic and motor behaviors, these fibers elicit the emotion expression, independent from the motor cortex which sends stimuli in order to carry out voluntary motor movements. Therefore, there are two parallel ways which provide us to accomplish the emotional expressions voluntarily or involuntarily.

The first one is the pathway descending from the motor cortex on the posterior frontal lobe which provides the voluntary motor contractions. The other one is the involuntary pathway which reaches to the brain stem and reticular system from medial and ventral forebrain and hypothalamus, and which stimulates the visceral and somatic motor neurons around here (see Figure 4).

Best example for this is the facial paralysis that is built up because of damage on the pathway between primary motor cortex and facial nerve (corticobulbar tractus)[2]. The motor nucleus of the facial nerve is located in Pons and the fibers coming from this nucleus innervate all the mimic muscles on the superior and inferior parts of the face. If there is damage on this motor nerve's nucleus or on it until it reaches the mimic muscles, a motor function loss occurs on the same half of the face and no muscle can be used. However, if damage occurs before the facial nerve leaves the brain stem, i.e. somewhere between the motor cortex and the motor nucleus located on the brain stem, the manifestation will be different. The upper parts of the face are stimulated by motor

Figure 4. Voluntary and involuntary motor innervations of facial nerve

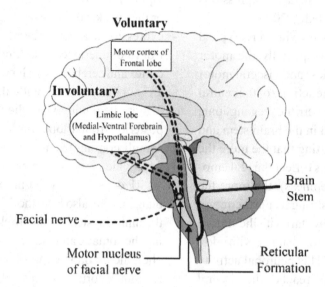

Figure 5. Different aspect of upper and lower motor neuron lesion of facial nevre. Smooth shaded area represents the lower motor neuron lesion of facial nevre which causes whole plegia of right side of face and <u>dotted</u> shaded are area represents the upper motor neuron lesion of facial nevre which causes semi-plegia of left side of face

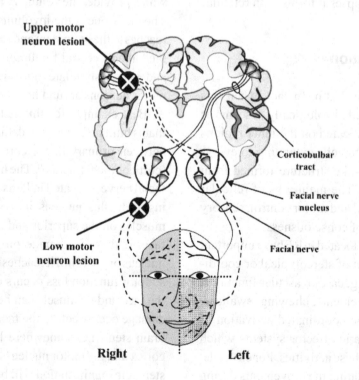

cortex bilaterally. The lower face, on the other hand, is stimulated only by contralateral motor cortex. Thus, if damage occurs somewhere between the motor cortex and the motor nucleus located on the brain stem, only the opposite lower part of the face will lose motor functions. However, it is very interesting that although these patients cannot perform voluntary motor activity on the paralyzed part of the face, they can still perform facial expressions responding to the emotional stimuli. This situation, which is called volintary-emotional dissociation, is actually the proof of the fact that the stimuli which elicit the emotional expression are not coming from motor cortex, but they are coming directly from the brain's emotional systems to the facial nucleus. This pathway is mediated by the reticular formation. On the contrary, in the emotional facial paresis, patients can move their mimic muscles voluntarily; but they cannot perform spontaneous emotional expressions on the muscles of the opposite side of the face (see Figure 5).

SUBJECTIVE EXPERIENCE OF EMOTIONS

The Amygdala and Its Inputs for Emotional Subjective Evaluations

As mentioned earlier, many regions of the brain participate in a multitude of tasks. Because of this, it is not surprising that the structures involved in the expression of emotion also participate in emotional subjective evaluation. For example, while amygdala participates in emotional expression through its outputs, it is also responsible in the subjective evaluation of emotions through its inputs. For the processing of inputs, it wouldn't be wrong to say that the lateral amygdala acts as a door-keeper. This region is the main area receiving major inputs from all sensory systems –visual, auditory, somatosensory (including pain), olfactory and taste. The information coming from the

olfactory and taste systems is forwarded to other amydaloid nuclei. The amygdala also receives inputs from the other areas of the brain, facilitating processing of an array of different types of information. For example, auditory input comes from two resources: auditory part of the thalamus and auditory cortex. The auditory information coming from the Thalamus is weakly encoded with respect to frequency characteristics, generating a signal which has less precision but allows faster processing. On the other hand, the imcoming cortical inputs arrive from not primary but higher association cortices, providing much more detailed (already processed) information in comparison to thalamic inputs. However the processing associated with these signals is slow due to the large number of underlying synaptic connections. For several emotions, especially fear, accurate and fast processing of the arriving information to the amygdala is of ultimate importance. Forming fast, primitive emotional responses are indispensable for emergencies. In other words, amygdala facilitates responding to sudden, unexpected stimuli impulsively. For example, we can generate an emotional response to a snake that we see in a meadow. This kind of fast response is preparatory for the amygdala before the arrival of slow inputs from upstream cortices (LeDoux, 1995; LeDoux, 2000). Later, when they project into the lateral amygdala, these sensory inputs establish connections with the other nuclei inside the amygdala. In order for these sensory inputs to have an effect on the behavioral response, they must go through inter-maygdalar connections.

Amygdala is the most critical structure to perceive and analyse facial expressions such as fear and anger (Adolphs et al., 1994; Adolphs et al., 1999; Young et al., 1996). For example, just catching a glimpse of the white part in the eyes of a fearful person is adequate to stimulate the amygdala (Whalen et al., 2004). Therefore we can say that even hints of danger are sufficient to trigger this system (Amaral et al., 2003; Sato et al., 2004). Amygdala, also receives inputs from the visual cortex, especially from the fusiform face area, which allows its participation in facial expression recognition in a very complex way. When subjects are shown angry faces subliminally (30 msec) versus neutral faces for 170 msec, they consciously recollect only seeing neutral faces. However, PET studies indicate amygdalar activity for this type of subliminal presentation of emotional faces, while amygdalar activation is absent for similar subliminal presentation of neutral faces (Pitkanen et al., 1997). In addition, when amygdala is severed bi-laterally, it is known that fear, anger and disgust expressions can not be recognized correctly (Morris et al., 1996).

Prefrontal Cortex

The lower part of prefrontal cortex which is close to the eyes is named as orbitofrontal cortex (OFC), and the activity therein allows evaluation of positive or negative emotions (for reviews, see Bechara et al., 2000). In several fMRI experiments, it has been shown that the OFC activation is associated with affective content of positive stimuli in many domains such as sampling food (Kringelbach et al., 2003), vision (Rolls, 2000), exposure to odors (Rolls et al., 2003a), hearing music (Blood & Zatorre, 2001), or even for somatosensory stimuli (Rolls et al., 2003b). Still, it is not clear how OFC effects the formation of positive affective reactions. Prefrontal cortex sends massive projections to the nucleus accumbens in subcortex (Zahm, 2000). And the stimulation of the nucleus accumbens causes positive affective reactions (Peciña & Berridge, 2000). Due to the projections of OFC to nucleus accumbens (Davidson et al., 2000), it is possible that OFC is indirectly participating in the regulation of positive affective reactions, or OFC may also directly be in charge of the formation of positive affective states. It is interesting that damages inflicted upon the prefrontal cortex result only in subtle affective deficits but not an entire loss in positive affective reactions (Berridge, 2003). Due to this probably it can be inferred that OFC

mainly participates in the regulation of voluntary emotions and associated emotional strategies.

Studies performed in non-human primates indicate that OFC responds to emotional stimuli, but does not participate in decisions regarding the response itself (Wallis & Miller, 2003; Padoa-Schioppa & Assad, 2006). This brings up the question 'Which area then performs the decisions for emotional behaviour?' For example, consider a woman hearing some sounds coming from the entrance in the middle of the night. She may panic at first, but then when she hears her husband's voice at the door, she relaxes. In this scenario, due to input from the auditory stream to the amygdala, the woman initially believes there is danger. In the danger situation, OFC considers the information received and sends inputs to the amygdala to remove its inhibition. The uninhibited amygdala alerts the autonomic nervous system for alarm due to emotional arousal. But when the woman understands she is not in danger, by hearing her spouse's voice, the same cycle beginning with the auditory input is repeated with this new emotional information. However, this time, using a different pathway directed from the OFC to the amygdala's central nuclei, the hypothalamic autonomic center is inhibited, which in turn triggers autonomic homeostasis and the woman relaxes. Therefore OFC does not directly embark in the planning of action (Barbas, 2007). However, the lateral prefrontal cortex (LPFC) may assume an executive role for deciding how to act. Because the LPFC obtains many signals from the visual and auditory association cortices, for considering detailed environmental situations. In addition, there are bidirectional connections between the lateral and orbitofrontal cortices (Barbas, 2007). Shortly, many areas within the prefrontal cortex have critical importance for the perception of the current and varying emotional situation. While lateral prefrontal cortex is responsible from the basic goal-states which are directed by emotions, medial prefrontal cortex is responsible from the cognitive presentation of the primary emotional situation (Esslen et al., 2004).

Cingulate Cortex

The segregation of emotion and cognition in the prefrontal cortex is also found in the cingulate cortex of the limbic system. Cingulate cortex can be divided into two part based upon cytoarchitecture and function: Anterior cingulate cortex (ACC) and Posterior cingulate cortex (PCC) (Bush et al., 2000; Esslen et al., 2004). The dorsal part of ACC is responsible from cognitive functions, complex motor control, motivation and participates in working memory whereas the ventral part is responsible from the evaluation of motivational information and meaning of emotions such as happiness, sadness, and disgust as well as arrangement of emotional responses. While ACC exhibits executive features, PCC embarks in evaluative roles. PCC activates in happiness and sadness (Esslen et al., 2004), but just like the prefrontal cortex, ACC activates for both positive and negative stimulants (Breiter et al., 1997; Firestone et al., 1996; Mathew et al., 1997). Although the cingulate cortex assumes multitude of functions, it is especially considered as the neuronal marker of positive affective reactions. More importantly, it is considered essential for the formation of positive affective reactions (Esslen et al., 2004). In humans, when cingulate gyrus is damaged operatively to cure pain, the patients develop depression). In rats, damage to the cingulate cortex induces ignorance with respect to reward versus punishment (Bussey et al., 1997).

Ventral Striatum Systems

Ventral striatum is an area where lots of affective states such as reward are reflected. Nucleus accumbens, which is a sub-component of ventral striatum, is primarily activated by anticipation of monetary reward (Knutson et al., 2001). The reward system, overlaps with emotions but it is a complex system itself, consisting of many sub-components with duties commissioned to a wide range of brain areas including medial temporal cortex, orbitofrontal cortex, dopaminergic neurons and amygdala, as well as ventral striatum. Major cognitive components of the reward system consist of 'the detection of past rewards, the prediction and expectation of future rewards and the use of information about future rewards to control goal-directed behaviour' (Schultz, 2000). Ventral striatum plays a central role in the reward system especially in reward detection and goal representation. (For an overview, see Schultz, 2000).

Also stimulants such as cocaine or amphetamines generate a positive affective state which correlates with increased dopamine levels in ventral striatum, especially in nucleus accumbens (Di Chiara & Imperato, 1988; Esslen et al., 2004). In addition, electrical stimulation of nucleus accumbens causes smiling laughter and euphoria (Okun et al., 2004; Esslen et al., 2004).

Empathy and Mirror Neurons

Empathy can be defined as putting ourselves in someone else's place and considering feeling and thinking like this other person. The term 'empathy' comes from Greek, the 'em' prefix means 'in' or 'at' and 'pathos' means feeling. Empathy is specifically important in establishing relationships and socialization. The mirror neurons which are first discovered by accident in macaque monkeys are thought to be related to empathy as well. In the early studies of Rizzolatti and his colleagues, while collecting single cell neuron recordings from the premotor cortex of monkeys for studying the hand and mouth movements, neurons are observed to fire when the monkeys handled food. Interestingly, the same set of neurons fired, also when someone else in the room handled food just as if the monkey itself was handling it. The mirror neurons are named this way because they not only fire when the animal itself makes a movement, but they also fire when someone else makes the same movement (Rizzolatti et al., 1996; Gallese et al., 1996).

Neuroimaging and electrophysiology studies show the existence of the mirror neurons in the premotor and motor cortex of humans as well (Harrison & Critchley, 2007). Earlier, it was thought that mirror neurons were participating only in imitations and action recognition. But later studies indicate that these neurons also indulge in higher level roles such as intention, cognition and emotion. For example, while watching emotional facial expressions, the mirror neuron activity is observed to be weak in patients with social cognitive deficits such as autism, or in patients with developmental psychopathy. In humans, facial expressions, especially the interpretation of facial expression of others carry important roles in the establishment of empathy. For this, somatosensory, motor, and limbic systems are all at work. Carr et al. (2003) has shown that amygdala and insula participates in facial expression observation, as well as execution. In a study by Wicker et al. (2003), when a person observes someone with disgust expression, the same disgust expression develops on his face while at the same time, the anterior insula portion of his brain activates. In another study by Singer et al. (2004), when a person observes a beloved one to be subjected to a painful shock stimulus, a co-activation occurs in the anterior insula and rostral anterior cingulate cortex. As a result, we can say that while people generate their own emotional resposes, they are affected by the emotional responses they observe on others.

LATERALIZATION

The existence of cerebral asymmetry among the complex cognitive cortical functions makes us speculate that a similar asymmetry may be exhibited for the generation, expression and management of emotions as well. In addition, studies with right or left hemisphere lesion patients indicate that there are differences in the right and left hemispheres with respect to emotional responses. For example, patients with lesions in the right hemisphere exhibit much less illness-related negative emotional responses such as depression, uncontrollable crying compared to the patients with left hemisphere lesions (Fedoroff et al., 1992; House et al., 1990; Jorge & Robinson, 2002). Patients with left frontal lobe lesions are more inclined to have depression while patients with right frontal lobe lesions display symptoms related to mania (Robinson et al., 1984; Sackeim et al., 1982). In short, there exists a difference between the right versus left hemispheres of the brain with respect to positive versus negative affect. When one considers that right frontal systems are associated with negative (withdrawal-related) emotional states such as sadness, anger, fear, and disgust, but left frontal regions are associated with positive (approach-related) emotional states such as happiness, the lesions in the corresponding areas are better understood (Davidson, 2001; Davidson and Irwin, 1999: Ahern and Schwartz, 1985; Davidson et al., 1990).

Apart from this, it has also been shown that the right hemisphere of the brain is more effective in the perception and expression of emotions. The predominant speech production and processing/understanding areas are located in the left hemisphere, Broca's and Wernicke's areas, respectively. However, the counterpart of the Wernicke's area in the right temporal lobe is specially known to take part in the comprehension or discimination of emotional content in speech. By the help of the structures in this area, we are capable to sense the underlying emotions within the talks of people speaking in a language that is illegitimate to us. Similarly, the counterpart of Broca's area in the right temporal lobe is implicated in the processing of emotional intonations of speech. Patients with lesions in this area present with monotonic speech, making it almost impossible to identify whether they are angry or happy while talking. Similarly, although the left hemisphere is more active in face recognition, the right hemisphere is more active in the recognition of facial expressions (Haxby et al., 2000).

CONCLUSION

Although streotypical in many animals, emotional behaviour in humans is very different. Previous experiences, mood, expectations and social environment may alter the emotional response. For example, riding a roller coaster may induce fear in one person, but little or no reaction in others. In reality, exclusive mechanisms underlying individual emotional responses have not been understood well. Probably the main reason underlying this is the engagement of a multitude of structures in very different functional roles. Presumably the amygdala and its neocortical input-output connections play a significant role in the upstream processes of emotion. In addition, while the subjective experience of emotion requires intact cerebral cortex, the emotional expression does not require the cortical processes, because the neuronal circuitry between the amygdala, hypothalamus and brain stem are implicated in the emotional expression.

REFERENCES

Adolphs, R., Tranel, D., Damasio, H., & Damasio, A. (1994). Impaired recognition of emotion in facial expressions following bilateral damage to the human amygdala. *Nature, 372*(6507), 669–672. doi:10.1038/372669a0

Adolphs, R., Tranel, D., Hamann, S., Young, A. W., Calder, A. J., & Phelps, E. A. (1999). Recognition of facial emotion in nine individuals with bilateral amygdala damage. *Neuropsychologia, 37*, 1111–1117. doi:10.1016/S0028-3932(99)00039-1

Ahern, G. L., & Schwartz, G. E. (1985). Differential lateralization for positive and negative emotion in the human brain: EEG spectral analysis. *Neuropsychologia, 23*, 745–755. doi:10.1016/0028-3932(85)90081-8

Altemus, M., Deuster, P. A., Gallıven, E., Carter, C. S., & Gold, P. W. (1995). Suppression of hypothalmic-pituitary-adrenal axis responses to stress in lactating women. *The Journal of Clinical Endocrinology and Metabolism, 80*, 2954–2959. doi:10.1210/jc.80.10.2954

Amaral, D. G., Behniea, H., & Kelly, J. L. (2003). Topographic organization of projections from the amygdala to the visual cortex in the macaque monkey. *Neuroscience, 118*, 1099–1120. doi:10.1016/S0306-4522(02)01001-1

Argiolas, A. (1992). Oxytocin stimulation of penile erection. Pharmacology, site, and mechanism of action. *Annals of the New York Academy of Sciences, 652*, 194–203. doi:10.1111/j.1749-6632.1992.tb34355.x

Barbas, H. (2007). Flow of information for emotions through temporal and orbitofrontal pathways. *Journal of Anatomy, 211*, 237–249. doi:10.1111/j.1469-7580.2007.00777.x

Bechara, A., Damasio, H., & Damasio, A. R. (2000). Emotion, decision making and the orbitofrontal cortex. *Cerebral Cortex, 10*(3), 295–307. doi:10.1093/cercor/10.3.295

Berman, M. E., & Coccaro, E. F. (1998). Neurobiologic correlates of violence: relevance to criminal responsibility. *Behavioral Sciences & the Law, 16*(3), 303–318. doi:10.1002/(SICI)1099-0798(199822)16:3<303::AID-BSL309>3.0.CO;2-C

Berridge, K. C. (2003). Pleasures of the brain. *Brain and Cognition, 52*, 106–128. doi:10.1016/S0278-2626(03)00014-9

Blood, A. J., & Zatorre, R. J. (2001). Intensely pleasurable responses to music correlate with activity in brain regions implicated in reward and emotion. *Proceedings of the National Academy of Sciences of the United States of America, 98,* 11818–11823. doi:10.1073/pnas.191355898

Bownds, D. M. (1999). *Biology of Mind - origins and structures of mind, brain, and consciousness.* Maryland: Fitzgerald Science Press.

Breiter, H. C., Gollub, R. L., Weisskoff, R. M., Kennedy, D. N., Makris, N., & Berke, J. D. (1997). Acute effects of cocaine on human brain activity and emotion. *Neuron, 19*(3), 591–611. doi:10.1016/S0896-6273(00)80374-8

Bush, G., Luu, P., & Posner, M. I. (2000). Cognitive and emotional influences in anterior cingulate cortex. *Trends in Cognitive Sciences, 4,* 215–222. doi:10.1016/S1364-6613(00)01483-2

Bussey, T. J., Everitt, B. J., & Robbins, T. W. (1997). Dissociable effects of cingulate and medial frontal cortex lesions on stimulus reward learning using a novel Pavlovian autoshaping procedure for the rat: Implications for the neurobiology of emotion. *Behavioral Neuroscience, 111*(5), 908–919. doi:10.1037/0735-7044.111.5.908

Caldwell, J. D. (1992). Central oxytocin and female sexual behavior. *Annals of the New York Academy of Sciences, 652,* 166–179. doi:10.1111/j.1749-6632.1992.tb34353.x

Carmichael, M. S., Humbert, R., Dixen, J., Palmisano, G., Greenleaf, W., & Davidson, J. M. (1987). Plasma oxytocin increases in the human sexual response. *The Journal of Clinical Endocrinology and Metabolism, 64,* 27–31. doi:10.1210/jcem-64-1-27

Carr, L., Iacoboni, M., Dubeau, M. C., Mazziotta, J. C., & Lenzi, G. L. (2003). Neural mechanisms of empathy in humans: a relay from neural systems for imitation to limbic areas. *Proceedings of the National Academy of Sciences of the United States of America, 100,* 5497–5502. doi:10.1073/pnas.0935845100

Carter, C. S. (1992). Oxytocin and sexual behavior. *Neuroscience and Biobehavioral Reviews, 16,* 131–144. doi:10.1016/S0149-7634(05)80176-9

Chouchourelou, A., Matsuka, T., Harber, K., & Shiffrar, M., (2006). The visual analysis of emotional actions. *Social Neuroscience, 1*(1), 63-/74.

Damasio, A. R. (1994). *Descartes' error: emotion, reason, and the human brain.* New York: Grosset / Putnam.

Davidson, R. J. (2001). Towards a biology of personality and emotion. *Annals of the New York Academy of Sciences, 935,* 191–207. doi:10.1111/j.1749-6632.2001.tb03481.x

Davidson, R. J., Ekman, P., Saron, C. D., Senulis, J. A., & Friesen, W. V. (1990). Approach-withdrawal and cerebral asymmetry: emotional expression and brain physiology I. *Journal of Personality and Social Psychology, 58,* 330–341. doi:10.1037/0022-3514.58.2.330

Davidson, R. J., & Irwin, W. (1999). The functional neuronatomy of emotion and affective style. *Trends in Cognitive Sciences, 3,* 11–21. doi:10.1016/S1364-6613(98)01265-0

Davidson, R. J., Jackson, D. C., & Kalin, N. H. (2000). Emotion, plasticity, context, and regulation: perspectives from affective neuroscience. *Psychological Bulletin, 126*(6), 890–909. doi:10.1037/0033-2909.126.6.890

Di Chiara, G., & Imperato, A. (1988). Drugs abused by humans preferentially increase synaptic dopamine concentrations in the mesolimbic system of freely moving rats. *Proceedings of the National Academy of Sciences of the United States of America, 85,* 5274–5278. doi:10.1073/pnas.85.14.5274

Domes, G., Heinrichs, M., Michel, A., Berger, C., & Herpertz, S. C. (2007). Oxytocin improves "mind-reading" in humans. *Biological Psychiatry, 61,* 731–733. doi:10.1016/j.biopsych.2006.07.015

Downer, J. L., & De, C. (1961). Changes in visual gnostic functions and emotional behavior following unilateral temporal pole damage in the "split-brain" monkey. *Nature, 191,* 50–51. doi:10.1038/191050a0

Esslen, M., Pascual-Marqui, R. D., Hell, D., Kochi, K., & Lehmann, D. (2004). Brain areas and time course of emotional processing. *NeuroImage, 21,* 1189–1203. doi:10.1016/j.neuroimage.2003.10.001

Fedoroff, J. P., Starkstein, S. E., & Forrester, A. W. (1992). Depression in patients with acute traumatic injury. *The American Journal of Psychiatry, 149,* 918–923.

Ferguson, J. N., Aldag, J. M., Insel, T. R., & Young, L. J. (2001). Oxytocin in the medial amygdala is essential for social recognition in the mouse. *The Journal of Neuroscience, 21*(20), 8278–8285.

Ferguson, J. N., Young, L. J., & Insel, T. R. (2002). The neuroendocrine basis of social recognition. *Frontiers in Neuroendocrinology, 23,* 200–224. doi:10.1006/frne.2002.0229

Firestone, L. L., Gyulai, F., Mintun, M., Adler, L. J., Urso, K., & Winter, P. M. (1996). Human brain activity response to fentanyl imaged by positron emission tomography. *Anesthesia and Analgesia, 82*(6), 1247–1251. doi:10.1097/00000539-199606000-00025

Gallese, V., Fadiga, L., Fogassi, L., & Rizzolatti, G. (1996). Action recognition in the premotor cortex. *Brain, 119,* 593–609. doi:10.1093/brain/119.2.593

Guyton, A. C., & Hall, J. E. (2006). The Autonomic Nervous System and the Adrenal Medulla. In *Textbook of Medical Physiology* (11th ed., pp. 748–760). Philadelphia, Pennsylvania: Elsevier Inc.

Hagemann, D., Waldstein, S. R., & Thayera, J. F. (2003). Thayer Central and autonomic nervous system integration in emotion. *Brain and Cognition, 52,* 79–87. doi:10.1016/S0278-2626(03)00011-3

Harrison, N. A., & Critchley, H. D. (2007). Affective neuroscience and psychiatry. *The British Journal of Psychiatry, 191,* 192–194. doi:10.1192/bjp.bp.107.037077

Haxby, J. V., Hoffman, E. A., & Gobbini, M. I. (2000). The distributed human neural system for face perception. *Trends in Cognitive Sciences, 4,* 223–233. doi:10.1016/S1364-6613(00)01482-0

Heinrichs, M., Baumgartner, T., Kirschbaum, C., & Ehlert, U. (2003). Social support and oxytocin interact to suppress cortisol and subjective responses to psychosocial stress. *Biological Psychiatry, 54,* 1389–1398. doi:10.1016/S0006-3223(03)00465-7

Holland, P. C., & Gallagher, M. (2003). Double dissociation of the effects of lesions of basolateral and central amygdala on conditioned stimulus-potentiated feeding and Pavlovian-instrumental transfer. *The European Journal of Neuroscience, 17,* 1680–1694. doi:10.1046/j.1460-9568.2003.02585.x

Holstege, G., Georgiadis, J. R., Paans, A. M., Meiners, L. C., van der Graaf, F. H., & Reinders, A. A. (2003). Brain activation during human male ejaculation. *The Journal of Neuroscience, 23,* 9185–9193.

Horwitz, N. H. (1998). John F. Fulton (1899-1960). *Neurosurgery, 43*(1), 178–184. doi:10.1097/00006123-199807000-00129

House, A., Dennis, M., Warlow, C., Hawton, K., & Moltneux, A. (1990). Mood disorders after stroke and their relation to lesion location. *Brain, 113,* 1113–1129. doi:10.1093/brain/113.4.1113

Huber, D., Veinante, P., & Stop, R. (2005). Vasopressin and oxytocin excite distinct neuronal populations in the central amygdala. *Science, 308,* 245–248. doi:10.1126/science.1105636

Izard, C. E. (2009). Emotion theory and research. *Annual Review of Psychology, 60,* 1–25. doi:10.1146/annurev.psych.60.110707.163539

Jorge, R., & Robinson, R. G. (2002). Mood disorders following traumatic brain injury. *NeuroRehabilitation, 17*, 311–324.

Klein, D. F., Skrobola, A. M., & Garfinkel, R. S. (1995). Preliminary look at the effects of pregnancy on the course of panic disorder. *Anxiety, 1*, 227–232.

Klüver, H., & Bucy, P.C. (1939). Preliminary Analysis of Functions of the Temporal Lobes in Monkeys. *Archives of Neurology and Psychiatry, 42* (6), 979-1 000.

Knutson, B., Fong, G. W., Adams, C. M., Varner, J. L., & Hommer, D. (2001). Dissociation of reward anticipation and outcome with event-related fMRI. *Neuroreport, 12*, 3683–3687. doi:10.1097/00001756-200112040-00016

Knutson, B., Wolkowitz, O. M., Cole, S. W., Chan, T., Moore, E. A., & Johnson, R. C. (1998). Selective alteration of personality and social behavior by serotonergic intervention. *The American Journal of Psychiatry, 155*(3), 373–379.

Kosfeld, M., Heinrichs, M., Zak, P. J., Fischbacher, U., & Fehr, E. (2005). Oxytocin increases trust in humans. *Nature, 435*(7042), 673–676. doi:10.1038/nature03701

Kringelbach, M. L., O'Doherty, J., Rolls, E. T., & Andrews, C. (2003). Activation of the human orbitofrontal cortex to a liquid food stimulus is correlated with its subjective pleasantness. *Cerebral Cortex, 13*, 1064–1071. doi:10.1093/cercor/13.10.1064

Lane, R. D., & Nadel, L. (2006). Facial Expression, Emotion, and Hemispheric Organization. In Kolb, B., & Taylor, L. (Eds.), *Cognitive Neuroscience of Emotion* (pp. 62–83). Oxford University Press.

LeDoux, J. (1995). Emotion: Clues from the brain. *Annual Review of Psychology, 46*, 209–235. doi:10.1146/annurev.ps.46.020195.001233

LeDoux, J. (2000). Emotion circuits in the brain. *Annual Review of Neuroscience, 23*, 155–184. doi:10.1146/annurev.neuro.23.1.155

LeDoux, J. (2007). The amygdala. *Current Biology, 17*(20), R868–R874. doi:10.1016/j.cub.2007.08.005

Linnoila, V. M. I., & Virkkunen, M. (1992). Aggression, suicidality, and serotonin. *The Journal of Clinical Psychiatry, 53*(supp. 10), 46–51.

Lovallo, W. R., & Sollers, J. J. III. (2000). Autonomic nervous system. In Fink, G. (Ed.), *Encyclopedia of stress (Vol. 1*, pp. 275–284). San Diego: Academic Press.

Mathew, R. J., Wilson, W. H., Coleman, R. E., Turkington, T. G., & DeGrado, T. R. (1997). Marijuana intoxication and brain activation in marijuana smokers. *Life Sciences, 60*(23), 2075–2089. doi:10.1016/S0024-3205(97)00195-1

McCarthy, M. M., McDonald, C. H., Brooks, P. J., & Goldman, D. (1996). An anxiolytic action of oxytocin is enhanced by estrogen in the mouse. *Physiology & Behavior, 60*(5), 1209–1215. doi:10.1016/S0031-9384(96)00212-0

Morris, J.S., Frith, C.D., Perrett, D.I., Rowland, D., Young, A.W., Calder, A.J., & Dolan, R.J. (1996). A differential neural response in the human amygdala to fearful and happy facial expressions. *Nature, 31*, 383(6603), 812-815.

Murphy, M. R., Checkley, S. A., Seckl, J. R., & Lightman, S. L. (1990). Naloxone inhibits oxytocin release at orgasm in man. *The Journal of Clinical Endocrinology and Metabolism, 71*, 1056–1058. doi:10.1210/jcem-71-4-1056

Neumann, I. D., Kromer, S. A., Toschi, N., & Ebner, K. (2000). Brain oxytocin inhibits the (re) activity of the hypothalamo–pituitary–adrenal axis in male rats: Involvement of hypothalamic and limbic brain regions. *Regulatory Peptides, 96*, 31–38. doi:10.1016/S0167-0115(00)00197-X

Oatley, K., & Jenkins, J. M. (1996). *Understanding emotion*. Cambridge, MA: Blackwell.

Okun, M. S., Bowers, D., Springer, U., Shapira, N. A., Malone, D., & Rezai, A. R. (2004). What's in a 'smile?' Intra-operative observations of contralateral smiles induced by deep brain stimulation. *Neurocase, 10*, 271–279. doi:10.1080/13554790490507632

Öztürk, Ö., Eraslan, D., & Kayahan, B. (2005). Emosyon ve temel insan davranışlarının evrimsel gelişimi. *Yeni Symposium, 43* (1), 14-19.

Padoa-Schioppa, C., & Assad, J. A. (2006). Neurons in the orbitofrontal cortex encode economic value. *Nature, 441*(7090), 223–226. doi:10.1038/nature04676

Papez, J. W. (1937). A proposed mechanism of emotion. *Archives of Neurology and Psychiatry, 38*, 725–743.

Peciña, S., & Berridge, K. C. (2000). Opioid eating site in accumbens shell mediates food intake and hedonic 'liking': Map based on microinjection Fos plumes. *Brain Research, 863*, 71–86. doi:10.1016/S0006-8993(00)02102-8

Pedersen, C. A. (1997). Oxytocin control of maternal behavior. Regulation by sex steroids and offspring stimuli. *Annals of the New York Academy of Sciences, 807*, 126–145. doi:10.1111/j.1749-6632.1997.tb51916.x

Pedersen, C. A., Vadlamudi, S. V., Boccia, M. L., & Amico, J. A. (2006). Maternal behavior deficits in nulliparous oxytocin knockout mice. *Genes Brain & Behavior, 5*(3), 274–281. doi:10.1111/j.1601-183X.2005.00162.x

Pitkanen, A., Savander, V., & LeDoux, J. E. (1997). Organization of intra-amygdaloid circuitries in the rat: an emerging framework for understanding functions of amygdala. *Trends in Neurosciences, 20*, 517–523. doi:10.1016/S0166-2236(97)01125-9

Pollick, F. E., Paterson, H. M., Bruderlin, A., & Sanford, A. J. (2001). Perceiving affect from arm movement. *Cognition, 82*, B51–B61. doi:10.1016/S0010-0277(01)00147-0

Rizzolatti, G., Fadiga, L., Fogassi, L., & Gallese, V. (1996). Premotor cortex and the recognition of motor actions. *Brain Research. Cognitive Brain Research, 3*, 131–141. doi:10.1016/0926-6410(95)00038-0

Robinson, R. G., Kubos, K. L., Starr, L. B., Rao, K., & Price, T. R. (1984). Mood disorders in stroke patients. Importance of location of lesion. *Brain, 107*, 81–93. doi:10.1093/brain/107.1.81

Rolls, E. T. (2000). The orbitofrontal cortex and reward. *Cerebral Cortex, 10*(3), 284–294. doi:10.1093/cercor/10.3.284

Rolls, E. T., Kringelbach, M. L., & de Araujo, I. E. (2003a). Different representations of pleasant and unpleasant odours in the human brain. *The European Journal of Neuroscience, 18*, 695–703. doi:10.1046/j.1460-9568.2003.02779.x

Rolls, E. T., O'Doherty, J., Kringelbach, M. L., Francis, S., Bowtell, R., & McGlone, F. (2003b). Representations of pleasant and painful touch in the human orbitofrontal and cingulate cortices. *Cerebral Cortex, 13*, 308–317. doi:10.1093/cercor/13.3.308

Sackeim, H. A., Greenberg, M. S., Weiman, A. L., Gur, R. C., Hungerbuhler, J. P., & Geschwind, N. (1982). Hemispheric asymmetry in the expression of positive and negative emotions. Neurologic evidence. *Archives of Neurology, 39*, 210–218.

Sato, W., Yoshikawa, S., Kochiyama, T., & Matsumura, M. (2004). The amygdala processes the emotional significance of facial expressions: an fMRI investigation using the interaction between expression and face direction. *NeuroImage, 22*, 1006–1013. doi:10.1016/j.neuroimage.2004.02.030

Schmidt, L. A., & Fox, N. A. (1999). Conceptual, biological, and behavioral distinctions among different categories of shy children. In Schmidt, L. A., & Schulkin, J. (Eds.), *Extreme fear, shyness and social phobia* (pp. 47–66). Oxford: Oxford University Press.

Schultz, W. (2000). Multiple reward signals in the brain. *Nature Reviews. Neuroscience, 1*(3), 199–207. doi:10.1038/35044563

Singer, T., Seymour, B., O'Doherty, J., Kaube, H., Dolan, R. J., & Frith, C. D. (2004). Empathy for pain involves the affective but not sensory components of pain. *Science, 303*(5661), 1157–1162. doi:10.1126/science.1093535

Stern, K., & McClintock, M. K. (1998). Regulation of ovulation by human pheromones. *Nature, 392*(6672), 177–179. doi:10.1038/32408

Turner, R. A., Altemus, M., Enos, T., Cooper, B., & McGuinness, T. (1999). Preliminary research on plasma oxytocin in normal cycling women: investigating emotion and interpersonal distress. *Psychiatry, 62*(2), 97–113.

Wallis, J. D., & Miller, E. K. (2003). Neuronal activity in primate dorsolateral and orbital prefrontal cortex during performance of a reward preference task. *The European Journal of Neuroscience, 18*, 2069–2081. doi:10.1046/j.1460-9568.2003.02922.x

Wedekind, C., Seebeck, T., Bettens, F., & Paepke, A. J. (1995). MHC-dependent mate preferences in humans. *Proceedings. Biological Sciences, 260*(1359), 245–249. doi:10.1098/rspb.1995.0087

Whalen, P.J., Kagan, J., Cook, R.G., Davis, F.C., Kim, H., Polis, S., McLaren, D.G., Somerville, L.H., McLean, A.A., Maxwell, J.S., & Johnstone, T. (2004). Human amygdala responsivity to masked fearful eye whites. *Science, 17*, 306 (5704), 2061.

Wicker, B., Keysers, C., Plailly, J., Royet, J. P., Gallese, V., & Rizzolatti, G. (2003). Both of us disgusted in My insula: the common neural basis of seeing and feeling disgust. *Neuron, 40*, 655–664. doi:10.1016/S0896-6273(03)00679-2

Williams, J. R., Carter, C. S., & Insel, T. (1992). Partner preference development in female prairie voles is facilitated by mating or the central infusion of oxytocin. *Annals of the New York Academy of Sciences, 652*, 487–489. doi:10.1111/j.1749-6632.1992.tb34393.x

Williams, J. R., Insel, T. R., Harbaugh, C. R., & Carter, C. S. (1994). Oxytocin administered centrally facilitates formation of a partner preference in female prairie voles (Microtus ochrogaster). *Journal of Neuroendocrinology, 6*(3), 247–250. doi:10.1111/j.1365-2826.1994.tb00579.x

Young, A. W., Hellawell, D. J., Van De Wal, C., & Johnson, M. (1996). Facial expression processing after amygdalotomy. *Neuropsychologia, 34*(1), 31–39. doi:10.1016/0028-3932(95)00062-3

Zahm, D. S. (2000). An integrative neuroanatomical perspective on some subcortical substrates of adaptive responding with emphasis on the nucleus accumbens. *Neuroscience and Biobehavioral Reviews, 24*(1), 85–105. doi:10.1016/S0149-7634(99)00065-2

Zald, D. H. (2003). The human amygdala and the emotional evaluation of sensory stimuli. *Brain Research. Brain Research Reviews, 41*, 88–123. doi:10.1016/S0165-0173(02)00248-5

ADDITIONAL READING

Adolphs, R., & Heberlein, A. S. (2002). Emotion. In Ramachandran, V. S. (Ed.), *Encyclopedia of the Human Brain* (pp. 181–191). USA: Elsevier Science Publishing.

Bear, M. F., Connors, B. W., & Paradiso, M. A. (2007). Brain Mechanisms of Emotion. In *Exploring the brain* (pp. 563–584). Lippincott Williams & Wilkins.

Hari, R., & Kujala, M. V. (2009). Brain basis of human social interaction: from concepts to brain imaging. *Physiological Reviews*, *89*(2), 453–479. doi:10.1152/physrev.00041.2007

Kandel, E. R., Schwartz, J. H., & Jessell, T. M. (2004). Emotional States and Feelings. In Iversen, S., Kupfermann, I., & Kandel, E. R. (Eds.), *Principles of Neural Science* (pp. 982–997). New York: McGraw-Hill Companies, Inc.

Lewis, M., Haviland-Jones, J. M., & Barrett, L. F. (2008). Emotional Networks in the Brain. In LeDoux, J. E., & Phelps, E. A. (Eds.), *Handbook of Emotions* (pp. 159–179). The Guilford Press.

Oatley, K. Keltne,r D., & Jenkins, J.M. (2006). *Understanding Emotions*. Blackwell publishing Ltd. Madlen MA USA.

Picard, R. W. (2000). *Affective Computing*. Cambridge, MA: MIT press.

Power, M., & Dalgleish, T. (2008). *Cognition and Emotion: From order to disorder*. Psychology Press.

Purves, D. (2008). Emotions. In Purves, D., Augustine, G. J., Fitzpatrick, D., Hall, W. C., LaMantia, A. S., McNamara, J. O., & White, L. E. (Eds.), *Neuroscience* (pp. 733–759). Sinauer Associates, Inc.

Rubinson, K., & Lang, E. J. (2008). The Autonomic Nervous System and Its Central Control. In Koeppen, B. M., & Stanton, B. A. (Eds.), *Berne & Levy Physiology* (pp. 218–230). Mosby Elsevier.

KEY TERMS AND DEFINITIONS

Lateral: Away from the midline
Posterior: Backside of the body
Dorsal: The backside of the animal's body. In two-legged animals, the term posterior may be used interchangeable with the term dorsal, but four-legged animals dorsal is synonymous with superior (above)
Ventral: The belly side of animals.
Homeostasis: Maintenance of internal stability

ENDNOTES

[1] Long lasting brain seizure.
[2] This type of facial paralysis is also named as facial nerve's upper motor neuron syndrome

APPENDIX

NEUROCHEMICALS, PHEROMONES AND EMOTION

In nuclei of amygdala, the allocation of some neuromodulator and hormone receptors (including glu-cocorticoid and estrogen hormones) differs. Many peptide receptors (opioid peptides, oxytocin, vaso-pressin, corticotropin releasing factor and neuropeptide Y) are also located in amygdala. It is crucial to understand how these chemical systems interact in order to settle amygdala's response. Here, we will give examples of some eminent chemicals' effects.

In a dangerous/stressful situation the body can use all its potential with the intention of overcoming this situation. In case of danger, amygdala and other brain regions excite hypothalamic neurons and cause the release of corticotrophin releasing factor (CRF). Release of CRF excites the release of adrenocorticotropin (ACTH) from hypophisis, thus the cortisol release from adrenal glands increase. Cortisol spreads all over the body through blood stream and gets attached to the receptors located in the hippocampus in particular. When attached with adequate amount of cortisol, these receptors produce an effect of negative feedback on hypothalamus and so inhibit the CRF release. Keeping the cortisol level stable like this, hippocampus regulates the stress response which amygdala has triggered. If stress takes long, this prolonged stress may impair hippocampus' functions. In various researches it is confirmed that prolonged stress constricts the dendrites, which eventually causes cell deaths in hippocampus. Therefore, the functions depending on hippocampus, such as explicit memory, get seriously impaired. The constriction of dendrites is usually seen in CA3 region of hippocampus. The neurogenesis in dentate gyrus stops. These two conditions may illuminate the volume decrease in hippocampus in the other situations where stress and cortisol are increased. Stress does not only impair hippocampus functions, but it also impairs prefrontal cortex functions. The transmission in prefrontal cortex is mediated by glutamate which is an excitatory neurotransmitter. There are also inhibitory circuits in prefrontal region. Most of these inhibitory links are located in the output neurons situated in deeper layers. However, the most important neurotransmitter which provides the neuromodulation between excitatory and inhibitory circuits is dopamine. Animal experiments where dopamine effect is blocked with some dopamine antagonist chemicals resulted as if the prefrontal cortex was removed. In case of danger, the cells which release serotonin and norepinephrine are also activated and therefore serotonin and norepinephrine release is increased. These chemicals provide mostly the neuromodulation. In the instant of danger, since septum and hippocampus are active; enhancing the synaptic process, serotonin and norepinephrine cause vigilance, increased attention and anxiety. On the contrary, the decrease of serotonin level is correlated with enhanced aggression. For instance, in people who committed violent crime, serotonin level is found to be reduced (for reviews, see Linnoila & Virkkunen, 1992; Berman & Coccaro, 1998). In another study, Knutson et al. (1998) gave serotonin reuptake inhibitor to some of the volunteers, whereas they gave placebo to the other group. The volunteers were asked to fill some personal tests and then to play cooperative games in pairs. The group which took the serotonin reuptake inhibitor showed reduced hostility index and reduced negative effect on their personal tests. Moreover they showed fair amount of cooperation and affiliation.

One of the hormones which influence emotions and behaviors is oxytocin, which shows a neurotransmitter effect in the brain. Oxytocin actually means "quick birth" (*oxys*—quick and *tokos*—childbirth in Greek) because of its uterotonic activity. Oxytocin is released from supraoptic and paraventricular nuclei of hypothalamus into the posterior hypophisis (neurohypophysis) and interfuses into the blood stream from this point. This hormone has receptors on numerous brain regions such as limbic system, brain stem and olfactory system; and it is very influential on the autonomic nervous system, especially on parasymphatetic system. Oxytocin is mainly in charge of lactation, uterus contraction, maternal bonding and sexual interaction. Its effects on brain structures are also shown in various animal studies. For example, oxytocin enhances social memory in rodents (Ferguson et al., 2001; Ferguson et al., 2002), while it reduces anxiety in social interactions (Neumann et al., 2000). Moreover, it has a role on pair-bonding. In a study conducted on prairie voles, Williams et al. (1992; 1994) demonstrated that oxytocin injection into some specific brain regions enhanced single partner selection, whereas oxytocin antagonist injection caused a reduction. Similarly, oxytocin is very crucial for affiliation in maternal care. For instance, Pederson and colleagues showed that oxytocin activity blockage disrupted maternal care (Pedersen, 1997; Pedersen et al., 2006). Various studies emphasized oxytocin's role on sexual interaction. For example, for female rats, intracerebral infusion of oxytocin acts on hypothalamus and facilitates sexual behaviors (Caldwell, 1992). In another study conducted on rabbits and monkeys, oxytocin is showed to be the most important agent for the stimulation of penile erection (Argiolas, 1992). It can be said that oxytocin's central role is to mediate social behaviors depending on amygdala. For instance, oxytocin inhibits the excitatory current which goes to brainstem from amygdala, and hence reduces the fear (McCarthy et al., 1996; Huber et al., 2005).

Similarly in humans, oxytocin suppresses anxiety which causes stress (Heinrichs et al., 2003). In a study about stress, Altemus et al. (1995) demonstrated that lactating mothers showed reduced stress response to the given exercises compared to mothers who nourish their babies with bottle. Likewise, mothers, who have a panic disorder, showed relief of symptoms during lactation (Klein et al., 1995). Furthermore, in terms of interpersonal relations, oxytocin provides a raise of the feeling of trust in taking risk, in humans (Kosfeld et al., 2005). Domes et al. (2007) showed that oxytocin enhance the ability of understanding others' affective mental conditions from their facial expressions.

Apart from maternal oxytocin increase, oxytocin secretion can also be increased with touching (Turner et al., 1999). Interestingly, during both male and female sexual stimulation and orgasm, oxytocin secretion increases (Carmichael et al., 1987; Carter, 1992; Murphy et al., 1990). Moreover, oxytocin leads people to fidelity, monogamous sentiments, and that is why oxytocin is thought to be the biological substrate of love.

Pheromones

Odor has both visceral and behavioral effects on humans. To retch or to vomit because of a harmful odor or salivation and increased gastric activity because of a charming odor can be given as examples of visceral motor responses. Chemical signals that are transported through air are perceived by olfactory sensory neurons on the nasal cavity and are transferred to the olfactory bulb. The information coming from the olfactory bulb is transmitted directly and through thalamus to the neocortex. The afferent pathway which goes to orbitofrontal cortex through thalamus is responsible for the perception and discrimination of the odor; whereas the pathway which goes to amygdala and hippocampus regulates the emotional and motivational aspects of the odor.

It is assumed that the effects of odor on emotions can be via the mediation of the pheromones. Pheromones' etymologic origin stems from Greek words phrein (to carry) and horman (to excite). Although for numerous animals the functions of pheromones are understood very well, its importance for human beings is not yet clarified. There are various studies which illustrates the existence of pheromones in humans. In a study of Stern & McClintock (1998), a group of women who did not use any odor (donors) put a cotton pad on their armpit during 8 hours. When these odorless compounds are then smelled by another group of women (recipients), the menstrual cycle of the women from the recipient group extended or diminished in accordance with the menstrual cycle of the women from the donor group. Furthermore, with a similar experimental design, when the recipient women smelled men odors, the synchronization of the menstrual cycle is disrupted. Moreover relatives can recognize each other by their odors. Mother and infant can also differentiate their odors from others. While a similar structure can also be seen in siblings, this effect is not perceived among spouses. Therefore these studies demonstrate that body odors can determine kinship information on a deep genetic level. On this issue, Wedekind et al. (1995) has conducted a very interesting experiment. MHC (major histocompatibility complex) is a gene group which is coded for the human immune system and its differences are expressed via HLA types. Wedekind and colleagues made a group of women to smell t-shirts of men from different HLA groups. At the end, these women preferred the t-shirts of men who have the different HLA type than theirs.

Chapter 2

Functions of Unconscious and Conscious Emotion in the Regulation of Implicit and Explicit Motivated Behavior

Mark Ashton Smith
Girne American University, Turkey

ABSTRACT

In this chapter the objective is to taxonomize unconscious and conscious affective and emotional processes and provide an account of their functional role in cognition and behavior in the context of a review of the relevant literature. The position adopted is that human affect and emotion evolved to function in motivational-cognitive systems and that emotion, motivation and cognition should be understood within a single explanatory framework. A 'dual process' account that integrates emotion, motivation and cognition, is put forward in which emotion plays different functional roles in implicit motivations and explicit motivations.

INTRODUCTION TO THE BIOPSYCHOLOGY OF MOTIVATION

Biopsychological research on emotional and motivational processes has undergone an unprecedented growth spurt in the last couple of decades (Schultheiss & Wirth, 2008). Biopsy-

DOI: 10.4018/978-1-61692-892-6.ch002

chology is an insightful and fruitful discipline one for understanding the nature of human affect and motivation, and provides a theoretical foundation for understanding the functioning of not only emotional, motivational and cognitive processes that are shared with other higher mammals, but also those that may be uniquely human. A strategy of this chapter will be to develop a novel dual-process theoretical account of human motivation, emotion and cognition through the data and theoretical insights of biopsychology, and then assess this theory in the light of social and cognitive psychological research.

Biopsychology combines affect and motivation within a common explanatory framework, providing explanations of both in terms of specific functions of the brain in control of behavior. There is extensive use of mammalian animal models such as rats, mice and monkeys, with the assumption that brain functioning for basic motivational and affective processes is highly similar across species. This assumption is justified in as far as the functional architecture; neurotransmitter and endocrine systems implicated in motivated behaviors are highly similar across different mammalian species. Many mammalian motivations are readily explained in common evolutionary terms. They are *adaptive,* directing organisms towards or away from stimuli of obvious significance for survival and reproduction. This is true not only of basic motivations like hunger and thirst but also of motives such as paternal care, affiliation, dominance and sex. There is a clear evolutionary *continuity* of motivations. Either human motivations are close homologues of motives that exist in other mammals, or they are obviously derived from such motives. Humans' hunger for a wider and more culturally informed selection of foods than other apes, and human sexual motivations are independent of the biological need to reproduce. Human dominance motivations are more complex than the socially motivated dominance behaviors of our closest relatives the chimpanzees (Wrangham & Peterson, 1996). But there are obvious continuities that enable us to explain and predict human brain function and behavior, and theorize in evidence-based ways about how such motives have become more complex in the course of human evolution.

Approach and Avoidance Motivation

Central to biopsychological theories of motivation is the idea that motivated behavior comes in two modes: *approach* mode aimed at attaining incentives or rewards, and *avoidance* mode aimed at avoiding aversive disincentives or punishments. Rewards and punishments can be understood as the *unconditioned stimuli* towards which all Pavlovian and instrumental learning is ultimately directed. In the case of punishments or disincentives, these include poisons or rancid food, sources of disease, physical injury and pain, defeat in intra or inter-sex competition, or social rejection. In the case of rewards, these include nutrients for hunger motivation, water for thirst, orgasm for sexual motivation, social closeness for affiliation motivation, and being on top of a social hierarchy for dominance motivation.

These rewards and punishments are critical to an organism's genetic survival. Animals need to find food for energy, drink to quench thirst, and mate to pass on their genes to offspring. In order to do this they need to compete with and dominate other same-sex members of their species. These are recurrent adaptive goals in mammalian life over millions of years of evolutionary history. All mammals desire the rewards associated with fulfilling these functions, feel compelled to attain them repeatedly, and show invigorated responding where their behavior can be instrumental to attaining them. Evolution has equipped mammals with specialized neurobiological systems to coordinate and support the attainment of these classes of incentives. They have been described by biopsychologists in considerable detail for drinking, feeding, affiliation, dominance and sex (review, Schultheiss & Wirth, 2008).

Physiological Needs and Goal Object Incentives

Motivated behavior is complex and *dynamic* due to the interaction of several factors that determine it.

These include the interplay of competing motives, and the presence of cues in the environment that predict the availability or presence of rewards or punishments. Of particular interest for our current topic is a dissociation common to all specialized motivation systems: motivated behavior can be determined by both (1) the animal's physiological *need state* – for example how deficient in nutrients or water an animal is; and (2) the *incentive (or disincentive) value* of the goal object or state – that is, the 'goal status' of the reward governing instrumental performance which may exert an effect independently from need state. A need state is not necessary for the motivation to eat: rats will gorge themselves on hamburgers even when they are sated (Panksepp, 1998). Thus an animal may become motivated to eat either because of a state of nutrient depletion indicated by hunger, because it recognizes or experiences a food as tasty or desirable, or a combination of both. Moreover, the incentive value of a goal object is not fixed; it may change dynamically for an individual depending on the individual's need state.

Wanting and Liking

Biopsygical research has revealed two consecutive and functionally dissociable phases or aspects of motivational processes: 1. A *motivation phase* during which the organism works instrumentally to attain a reward or avoid a punishment. This motivated action could be as simple as taking steps to a water hole and starting to drink, or as complex as socially coordinated hunting of an elusive prey in a tree canopy. 2. A *consummation phase* in which there is an evaluation of the hedonic (pleasure-pain or 'affective') qualities that accompany the consumption of – or contact with – the incentive or disincentive (Berridge, 1996; Craig, 1918). Berridge (1996) has labeled these separable aspects of motivation *wanting* and *liking* respectively. While it seems intuitive that you want what you like and like what you want, research shows that both aspects of motivation

are dissociable. Drug addicts, for example, may feel compelled to obtain and take their drug even though they no longer take any pleasure from the act – a case of wanting without liking (Robinson & Berridge, 2000). And people respond both subjectively and objectively to eating tasty food with signs of liking and pleasure, irrespective of whether they are hungry and have been motivated to find the food in the first place or not – i.e. same liking with differences in wanting (Epstein et al., 2003).

Related to this distinction is the dissociation of a goal's *instrumental incentive value* from its *hedonic value*. For example, when a hungry rat is trained to respond for food by pressing a lever, and is then sated before being tested again in extinction (in the absence of food), it will lever press just as vigorously as a hungry rat (i.e. exhibit just as much *wanting*) even though it does have a physiological need for the food, *until* the point it experiences the reduced hedonic value of the food due to the fact it is sated (Balleine & Dickinson, 1991). After this direct hedonic ('liking' or 'disliking') experience, the incentive value will recalibrate appropriately with the motivational state of the animal, but without the direct hedonic experience, the two 'value' systems can operate independently.

Rats' hedonic reactions fluctuate in similar ways to human subjective pleasure in response to changing need states (Berridge, 2000). Just as food is more pleasurable to us when hungry, sweet tastes elicit more 'liking' reactions when rats are hungry than when full, as exhibited in oro-facial reactions (Steiner et al., 2001). Regular chow for a rat will have a higher hedonic value when it is starving than when it is sated – a phenomenon Cabanac (1971) has termed *alliesthesia*, i.e. the changing subjective evaluation of the same reward over time. In functional terms, *alliesthesia* can be seen as tracking the utility of a given reward depending on the changing need states of the animal.

These two aspects of motivation – 'wanting' and 'liking' – are subserved by different brain circuits. Evidence suggests that the motivation phase is mediated by the mesolimbic dopaminergic system, while the consummation phase is subserved by circuitry integrating 'liking' hotspots involve the orbitofrontal cortex for subjectively felt hedonic experience (Bozarth, 1994; Schultheiss & Wirth, 2008; Smith et al., 2009). Along with the amygdala in the temporal lobe that functions to form associations between affectively neutral stimuli that predict affectively charged events or stimuli, these systems constitute the core of the brain's *incentive motivation network* (Berridge, 1996)[1]. Figure 1 shows the location of the structures in this circuit in the human brain. For interested readers, a detailed look at the components of this network is presented in appendix. In their review of the field, Schultheiss & Wirth (2008) summarize the basic operation of this network as follows: "motivational processes rely on these three structures to act in concert so that cues that

predict (amygdala) stimuli that have been experienced as pleasant (orbitofrontal cortex) elicit behavioral invigoration (mesolimbic dopamine system) directed at reward attainment" (p. 28).

CATEGORIZATION OF MOTIVATION

Implicit vs. Explicit Motivation in Humans

Building on previous work by McClelland and colleagues (1980; 1989; Weinberger & McClelland, 1990) within a biopsychological framework, Schultheiss (2001, 2008), has presented an account of *implicit* and *explicit* human motives that draws on the widely applied distinction between implicit and explicit modes of cognition and affect (Gazzaniga, 1985; LeDoux, 2002; Nisbett & Wilson, 1977; Squire & Zola, 1996). On this account,

Figure 1. Sagittal cut of the human brain at the midline, with approximate locations of key structures of the incentive-motivation circuit of the IMS. (Dopamine: DA, ventral tegmental area: VTA, nucleus accumbens: NA, amygdala: A, orbitofrontal cortex: OFC, S: striatum) The mesolimbic dopamine system originates in the ventral tegmental area of the midbrain, and projects to the nucleus accumbens. The amygdala and orbitofrontal cortex send projections to the nucleus accumbens. The OFC is densely reciprocally connected to the amygdala

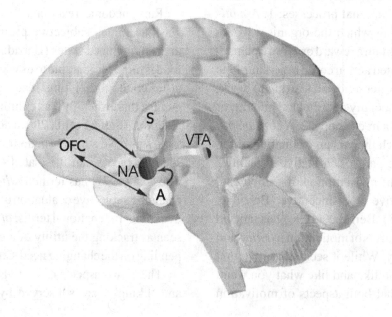

implicit motives respond to *nonverbal cues and incentives* and have an impact on behavior and processes that are not controlled by, or accessible to, the individual's verbally represented goals or self-concept. Implicit motives are revealed using *non-declarative* measures that include physiological autonomic responses (e.g., changes in blood pressure, hormone release, muscle tone), and acquisition of new stimulus-stimulus associations and goal-directed behaviors through Pavlovian and instrumental learning of the type reviewed above. Explicit motives, by contrast, are more recently evolved and respond to *verbal symbolic cues* and influence measures that tap into a person's verbally represented sense of self and the attitudes, judgments, decisions, and goals that are associated with it. Declarative measures for this include valence judgments, decision making behavior, assessments of self-regulatory control, and reports of personal goals. The biopsychological basis of this system will be reviewed below.

In humans there are measurable trait differences in implicit motivational needs. Individuals high in a need for *power* (closely related to 'dominance' needs of other mammals and sharing much of the same brain circuitry) obtain pleasure from being dominant over or having an impact on others physically, emotionally or socially and are averse to social defeat or submission. Individuals high in the need for *affiliation* (another mammal-wide motivational need with shared brain circuitry) value affectionate or intimate relationships with others and experience rejection or self-directed hostility as alarming and unpleasant (McClelland, 1987; Schultheiss, 2008; Winter, 1996).

Not surprisingly, implicit motives influence a lot of interpersonal behavior (review, McClelland, 1987). For example, there is evidence that implicit motives for affiliation or power/dominance influence non-verbal interactions in a way that emerges dynamically from the interaction of the affective signaling of these motives through facial expressions (Hess, Blairy & Kleck, 2000; Stanton, Hall, & Schultheiss, *in press*).

Brain structures mediating implicit motivations in all mammals include as a functional core the incentive-motivation system reviewed above. In addition, there are motivation-specific endocrine, peptide and neuromodulator systems, such as those differentially controlling the release of testosterone, epinephrine & norepinephrine in those high in dominance / power motivation, or those controlling the release of oxytocin in those high in affiliation motivation needs (review, Schultheiss & Wirth, 2008). These implicit motive systems influence (i) what types of incentives are experienced as rewarding or aversive, (ii) what and in what way incentives are energizing or invigorating in motivated action and physiological response and (iii) cognitively, what incentives and cues to incentives are oriented to and selectively attended to, with cascading effects for memory and learning (McClelland, 1987; Schultheiss, et al. *in press*).

Unconscious vs. Conscious Motivation

A key finding that emerges in the human implicit motive literature is that implicit motives operate to a large extent unconsciously – an assumption that has guided the field from the 1950s onwards. Rolls (1999) suggests that most cognitive processing serves the purposes of non-conscious implicit affective-motivational processes rooted in programs for genetic survival; conscious, goal directed, explicit motivation is the exception rather than the rule, serving largely to override implicit processes.

In this context, 'unconscious motivation' means that people do not have introspective access to the incentives that are particularly rewarding for them and that motivate their behavior in a way that they do to the goals that underlie their explicit motivations (Schultheiss & Brunstein, 2001). Nor do they have introspective access to, or control over, the means adopted to attain the incentives. Even for as basic a motivational system as feeding, people have little accurate understanding or awareness of what drives their appetites, or what makes them start or stop eating (Berridge, 1996). Self-reports of motivations contradict behavioral data and externally validated measures of individual differences in implicit motives (e.g. the Thematic Apperception Test (TAT), or the Picture Story Exercise (PSE)), do not correlate with scores from self report measures designed to measure the same motivational needs. It is striking that the variance shared between self-report and SE measures of implicit motives is *less than 1%* on average (Spangler, 1992).

Biopsychology of Implicit Motivation

Animal models of motivated behavior do not directly reveal the relationship between brain states and subjective affective or emotional states such as pleasure or pain that accompany aspects of motivation. The subjective impact of rewards as *felt* pleasure has been considered essential (Young, 1959) or irrelevant (Skinner, 1953) to their effect on behavior. Many contemporary biopsychologists accept the notion of subjective hedonic experience, at least at a *functional* level of description, just as cognitive representations and processes are conceived by cognitive scientists at a functional level of description that is distinct from what occurs in the neurocircuitry of the brain (Smith & Kossyln, 2006). This position has been implicit in my review of the field.

From a functional perspective it is clear that affect or emotion in biopsychological theory is a valid psychological construct. In the absence of any experience of affective reaction to an outcome in a particular motivational state, it can be argued that animals have no basis on which to assign an incentive or disincentive value (Balleine & Dickinson, 1998), and that motivated behavior is initiated through associations with the pleasure induced by a reward or the pain (physical or psychological) induced by a punishment (Schultheiss et al., *in press*). Recent accounts consider physiological and nonverbal expressions in the face,

voice or movement as independent indicators of affect. All higher mammals show 'liking' affective responses to sweet, tasty food (lip licking) and 'disliking' responses to unpalatable food (nose wrinkle, tongue protrusion) (Berridge, 2004), but it remains controversial whether these behavioral indicators imply that the emotions are consciously experienced in a way that resembles human felt emotion.

In the human case, while individuals are typically not aware of the implicit motives that control their behavior, the extent to which the motives are or are not satisfied does impact conscious experience of wellbeing, satisfaction or pleasure. For example, women high in intimacy motivation report lower levels of gratification when living alone than women low in intimacy motivation (McAdams & Bryant, 1987). In general, individuals experience more emotional well-being to the extent that their personal goals and life situation gives them opportunities to satisfy their implicit needs (review, Schultheiss et al, *in press*). But this response is not an instantiation of the 'liking' that accompanies the consummation of an incentive. There are methodological difficulties in measuring momentary conscious affective responses in situations where implicit motives are frustrated or satisfied, but EMG measures of facial expressions have been used to demonstrate the hedonic 'liking' or 'disliking' in human implicit motives. Individuals high in the power motive exhibit more pronounced negative affective responses in the form of frown muscle activity when confronted with a dominant person than people low in power motivation (Fodor, Wick, & Hartsen, 2006). And individuals with a strong affiliation motive react with more frequent smiles to positive social interactions than do people low in affiliation motivation (McAdams, Jackson & Kirshnit, 1984). Various studies have shown that emotional experience is affected by intentionally adopting different facial emotional expressions (Adelmann & Zajonc, 1989; Matsumoto, 1987) and according to the facial-feedback hypothesis, facial muscle activity is essential for the occurrence of emotional experience (Buck, 1980). It is parsimonious to assume that facial expressions accompany consciously felt emotional responses in implicit motivational contexts too. These emotions may also be detected by physiological (autonomic) responses such as blood pressure and electrodermal activity – both gauges of overall emotional arousal (Stern, Ray, & Quigley, 2001).

But critically these emotional experiences of pleasure or pain are not self-consciously labeled, declaratively encoded, and explicitly related to the actions resulting in them. This kind of emotional response I will propose is *phenomenally* conscious in the sense of subjectively experienced or 'felt', but not *reflectively* conscious and accessible to verbal report, reasoning and executive processes. This distinction parallels the philosopher Ned Block's influential distinction between *phenomenal consciousness* and *access consciousness* (Block, 1997). Phenomenal consciousness (P-consciousness) is experience, and the phenomenally conscious aspect of a state is what it is like to *be* in that state. Access consciousness (A-consciousness), by contrast, is availability for use in reasoning and rational guidance of speech and action (Block, 1995).

While orbitofrontal / limbic cortex mediated hedonic responses ('liking') may be subjectively experienced in this phenomenal sense, subcortical, mesolimbic DA system affective activation ('wanting') seems not to require conscious experience of any sort. Evidence for this is suggested by results from a study by Winkielman, Berridge & Willbarger (2005) in a widely cited and theoretically provocative paper on 'unconscious affect'. The implicit motive they looked at was thirst. In the first experiment, thirsty and non-thirsty participants were informed they were doing a gender discrimination task, in which a male or female face (with a neutral emotional expression) would appear on the monitor and the participant had to press a key as soon as they had identified the gender. But this task was a foil. Unknown to

the participants, happy, angry or neutral face *subliminal* primes - of which they had no conscious awareness - were presented for a brief 16 msecs just before being replaced by the neutral male or female faces. After 8 trials participants were offered a sweet beverage and were asked to rate their mood and arousal level. Thirsty participants poured more than twice the amount of the beverage after happy subliminal primes than angry primes, and after pouring, they drank 171% more of the beverage after happy primes than after angry primes. A follow up experiment showed that subliminal primes also strongly affected participants' willingness to pay for a drink and their ratings of how much they wanted to drink more. Despite the large impact of the happy vs. angry affective primes on thirsty participants' drinking behaviour, there was no impact of these primes on participants' 'deliciousness' or 'sweetness' ratings of the drink after tasting it. Moreover, there were no observed differences between happy vs. angry prime groups in mood or arousal ratings before and after priming: subjective experience did not change, despite marked behavioural-motivational changes.

The results of this study suggest that the subliminal primes did not affect the drink's *hedonic value* for thirsty participants – i.e. how much it was consciously 'liked'. If they did, the happy face primes would have caused higher ratings of 'deliciousness' than angry faces, but there was no such difference. The observed differences in 'willingness to pay' and 'wanting more beverage' are more obviously indices of the 'wanting' aspect of motivation than the 'liking' aspect. Thus we can conjecture that there was no OFC activation difference due to the subliminal primes; rather, the primes affected how much participants were invigorated in their motivation to consume the reward (how behaviourally 'turned on' they were) by the affective prime - a function mediated by the mesolimbic DA system. And this affective response was entirely *unconscious*.

In summary, the evidence suggests that emotion has a functional role in both the motivational 'wanting' phase, and the consummation 'liking' phase for implicit motives, and that these roles can be dissociated (Berridge, 1996). On the account proposed here, conscious emotion is confined to the cortically mediated 'liking' phase of the incentive-motivation system. It is not self-reflexive, introspectable, and accessible to control processes. This kind of emotion has a function in determining incentive values, and guiding behavior through hedonic anticipation. Unconscious emotion – as a low level 'valence' or 'affective' cue – exerts its effects by activating the mesolimbic DA system in the 'wanting' phase of the implicit motivation.

Biopsychology of Explicit Motivation

Unlike implicit motivation, explicit motivation – voluntary, goal directed action with self-attributed motivations – is conscious and accessible to introspection and executive control. If you are motivated to learn how to make wine or learn Chinese you know what goal is motivating you, what the satisfaction conditions are, what instrumental actions you may adopt to attain the goal, and whether or not you are progressing with respect to that goal. You can spontaneously and voluntarily pursue such goals, and know that you are doing so. Explicit motives respond to *verbal symbolic cues* and have an effect on measures that tap into a person's verbally represented sense of self and the attitudes, judgments, decisions, and goals that are associated with it. The lateral prefrontal cortex (LPFC) plays a central functional role in explicit motivation. The human LPFC supports a number of 'higher level' brain functions, including speech (Broca's area), working memory, prepotent response inhibition, memory encoding and retrieval and motor planning (Tanji & Hoshi, 2008). The LPFC subserves self-regulation through the formulation of explicit, verbally represented, goals and plans for their enaction. The human LPFC is a more recently evolved and differentiated part of

the prefrontal cortex – that is itself more elaborated in primates relative to other mammals. The LPFC guides behaviour through the formulation of verbally represented goals and plans for their enaction. Individuals with LPFC lesions find it difficult to initiate and execute voluntary behaviour, particularly if it is complex (Luria, 1973). In the influential 'goal maintenance model' of prefrontal working memory function (Braver, Cohen & Barch, 2002; Miller & Cohen, 2001), this brain region is proposed to serve both a representational / storage and control function: it maintains representations in the form of rules or goals, and has a 'top-down' influence that coordinates perception, attention and action to attain those goals. Feedback connections *bias* the associations activated in response to perceptual input, in a way that can override default automatic, implicit responses that may be in competition for control of thought and behaviour. This model is consistent with a wide range of both human and primate data (Miller & Cohen, 2001), and has been implemented in computational models that simulate human and primate performance in working memory tasks (O'Reilly et al., 2002).

The human LPFC represents and enacts verbally programmed goals that can regulate or override implicit motivations. Nonverbal stimuli with strong incentive properties, such as facial expressions, elicit activation of the amygdala in humans (Adolphs & Tranel, 2000), and activate the mesolimbic DA system (Critchley et al., 2000). However, as soon as the participant is able to verbally label the expression, the LPFC becomes activated and amygdala activation decreases (Ochsner et al., 2002). Engagement of the LPFC's verbal-symbolic functions in dealing with an emotionally arousing stimulus appears to dampen down activity in the implicit motivational responses driven by the amygdala and the mesolimbic DA system (Lieberman, 2003), shielding explicit goals from interference by incentive driven implicit motivational impulses. This 'damping down' of affective-motivational reactivity – particularly in the context of competitive dominance motives – is consistent with an evolutionary account developed by evolutionary anthropologist Brian Hare. On this account selective pressures in the course of human evolution have specifically targeted the amygdala and associated limbic motivational systems, exerting a 'self-domesticating' effect that has enabled the evolution of uniquely human cognitive flexibility and control (review, Hare, 2007).

DUAL PROCESS THEORIES

In the remainder of this chapter I will develop the thesis that the implicit versus explicit motivation distinction provides the basis of a comprehensive dual-process account of human behavior that integrates motivation, emotion and cognition. Dual processing accounts been developed to account for behavioral dissociation data in learning (e.g. Reber, 1993), attention (Schneider & Shiffrin, 1977), reasoning (Evans, 2003), decision making (Kahneman & Frederick, 2002) and social cognition (Chaiken & Trope, 1999). In these accounts a cognitive mode that is rapid, automatic, parallel and effortless is contrasted with one that is slow, sequential and controlled / voluntary. Both modes are understood as independent, and often conflicting, sources of control for behavioral response. Dual processes have been labeled in a number of ways: implicit-explicit (Evans & Over, 1996; Reber, 1993), experiential-rational (Epstein, 1994), emergence-control (Carver & Scheier, 1998), heuristic-systematic (Chen & Chaiken, 1999), and associative-rule-based (Sloman, 1996; Smith & Decoster, 2000). According to Smith & Decoster's dual process model, the fast versus slow distinction is reversed in the *learning* process: an 'associative processing mode' slowly learns general Pavlovian and operant regularities, while the 'rule based processing mode' engages in intentional retrieval of explicit / declarative, symbolically represented information to guide

processing and can quickly form representations as episodic or semantic representations of unique or novel events (e.g. Tulving, 2002). On this account, the rule based mode uses culturally transmitted knowledge as its 'program' (Smolensky, 1988), and since only one rule can guide behavior at a time, it is more effortful and time-consuming than associative processing. According to Stanovich's (1999) conceptualization, what he calls 'System 1 thinking' is heavily contextualized and not subject to logical-normative constraint, while 'System 2 thinking' is abstract, decontextualized and logically constrained. The automatic system is often described as evolutionarily old, shared with other mammals and independent of individual differences in intelligence, whereas the controlled system is evolutionarily recent, uniquely human and related to heritable differences in fluid intelligence and working memory capacity (review, Evans, 2006).

While there is broad agreement in the dual process literature of the existence of a rule based executive processing system subserved by the lateral prefrontal cortex and engaging a limited capacity working memory system, there is controversy surrounding labeling all forms of unconscious, automatic and rapid cognitive processes as belonging to the same alternative system (review, Evans, 2006). There are some processes (appraisals or skilled actions) that start off explicit under conscious control and later become automated – for example, in learning to drive a car. These processes have been investigated extensively in the *automaticity* literature on attention and skill acquisition (Bargh & Chartrand, 1999; Monsell & Driver, 2000; Schneider & Shiffrin, 1977). Explicit goals can also be primed unconsciously and automatically (review, Shah, 2005). But as reviewed above, other automatic and unconscious processes associated with implicit motives relating to, for example, affiliation or dominance interactions can continue to exert influence on behavior without engaging the rule-based, executive control system.

Dual Process Account of Motivational Systems

One way of circumventing these theoretical tensions, as well as providing an integrated motivation-emotion-cognition framework, is to reframe traditional dual process accounts with their information processing focus in terms of the duality of implicit and explicit *motivation*. On this reading, implicit vs explicit motivation systems may provide a more fruitful explanatory framework for taxonomizing the dual nature of cognition, rather than properties of the information processing such as automaticity and speed. The rationale for this taxonomy is that it is *behavior* that is targeted by selective forces, not the underlying information processing mechanisms, and for a complex behavior to be selected it must be *motivated*. The claim is that the explicit motivational system evolved in the context of relatively recent culturally-based, and normatively regulated, behaviors. This taxonomy also integrates motivation, emotion and cognition in a way that is not done in traditional dual process accounts that focus on cognition.

On this dual process account the 'Implicit Motivation System' (IMS) designates the set of implicit motives and their mediating information processing and affective neural-endocrine mechanisms. This system incorporates a diverse collection of specialized, biologically evolved, motivational-emotional systems, subserving a variety of recurrent adaptive problems in our ancestral environment, with diverse phylogenetic origins. Brain structures mediating implicit motivations include as a functional core the incentive-motivation system mentioned in the first part of this chapter. In addition to this there are motivation-specific endocrine, peptide and neuromodulator systems, such as those mediating oxytocin release in affiliation interactions.

Some human implicit motives relating to hunger, affiliation, dominance and sexual attraction are elaborations of motives found universally in all higher mammals. These have been studied extensively, both in mammals and humans (review, Schultheis & Wirth, 2008). Other implicit motives such as the 'achievement' motive (Thrash & Elliot, 2002) may be uniquely human, having evolved after the divergence with our common ancestor with modern day chimpanzees some 6–7 million years ago. Other contenders for uniquely human implicit motives which may be both universal and function implicitly without direct introspective access include conformity / group identification, ethnocentrism (review MacDonald, 2008), cooperation (Tomasello, 2007), or the need for coherence and meaning (Proulx & Heine, 2009). Importantly, many or all of these motives relate to the uniquely group-based nature of *Homo sapiens* socio-ecology.

IMS motives detect goal relevant cues, extract goal relevant instrumentally and classically conditioned contingencies in relevant environments, and produce biologically adaptive behaviors either through a combination of evolutionary hard-wiring and implicit learning. The cognition underlying this system is not introspectively accessible, nor under executive control. We may *infer* the operation of implicit motives, just as we may rationalize them, by observing our behavior and formulating plausible hypotheses. But the goals and motives we attribute are not encoded in a way that is accessible and controllable in the way that verbally mediated explicit motives are.

By contrast, the 'Explicit Motivational System' (what I shall call the 'Normative Motivational System' (NMS) for reasons described below) regulates behaviour via explicit, verbally encoded, motives – linguistically programmed rules or instructions, personal goals or standards, or culturally specified goals or norms. This uniquely human self-regulation system engages executive control processes, and depends on working memory and the capacity to reason through 'if-then' causal contingencies and counterfactuals. The goals and motivated behaviours in this system are introspectively accessible, self-attributed and subject to reflexive control. While contingencies and skills can be learned implicitly in the development of expertise in this mode, what distinguishes this kind of 'implicit' non-conscious and automatic cognition from implicitly-*motivated* cognition is that the latter is *gated* by executive, verbally explicit, processes involving self-attributed motivations, and is open to conscious 'reprogramming' in a self-reflexive, verbally reportable way.

On this account, the question of interest is not whether a cognitive process is conscious and slow or unconscious and fast, but how *normatively regulated, introspectively accessible* (open to conscious, verbal report) and subject to *intentional control* and *re-programming* it is.

Normativity is a critical concept on this account. Adopting a framework developed by the psychologist Charles Kalish (2006) who draws extensively from the philosopher John Searle's analysis of normativity (2001), I define the normativity that regulates behaviour as any culturally based norm or standard that regulates action via verbally encoded representations that denote or imply goodness, desirability, correctness or what ought to be (Kalish, 2006). The existence of a norm implies a *reason* for action (Searle, 2001), and embraces, on this account, not only moral norms (e.g. obligations or duties), and institutional norms (e.g. best practices for social roles, or standards of excellence for institutional performances), but also epistemic norms (e.g. the truth of an explanatory account), or any application of a rule, instruction or procedure involving correctness or appropriateness criteria (e.g. in learning how to drive). The extension of the term 'normativity' is thus very wide – and consequently controversial.

In broad terms the IMS-NMS distinction lies in how relatively 'biological' vs 'cultural' a motivated behaviour is – whether governed by innate and adaptive functions such as dominance or affiliation fitness promoting strategies, or by culturally mediated goals, norms and standards, such as 'performing competently and ethically at work'. Defining characteristics of the IMS and NMS are listed in Figure 2.

Figure 2. The Implicit Motivation System, IMS and Normative (Explicit) Motivation System, NMS: A dual process account

Implicit Motivation System (IMS)	Normative Motivation System (NMS)
Implicit motive driven	Explicit motive driven
Non-verbally encoded	Verbally encoded
Inaccessible to introspection & verbal report	Accessible to introspection & verbal report
Non executive processing	Executive processing
Emotion as reinforcer in incentive-motivational system	Emotion as information in executive self regulation
Incentive value regulated	Normatively regulated
Biological adaptation: Modular & domain specific	Cultural adaptation: General purpose, flexible & domain general

The IMS and NMS may be mutually support-ing, as when someone with strong affiliation motives works in a cooperative, caring profession. But often they may dissociate or be in conflict, such as when someone with a high affiliation needs adopts an explicit goal to lead an aggressive and competitive campaign in commerce. Indi-viduals experience more overall emotional well-being to the extent that their explicit goals and life situation gives them opportunities to satisfy their implicit motives (review, Schultheiss et al, *in press*).

THEORIES ON INFORMATIONAL ASPECTS OF EMOTION

In developing the proposed dual process account I will now interpret three influential theoretical 'emotion-as-information' accounts of the function of emotion in IMS-NMS terms: 1. Damasio's Somatic Marker Hypothesis for decision making, 2. Baumeister's Feedback Theory of emotion, 3. Carver and Scheier's Self-Regulation Theory of behavior. I will argue that two criteria for differ-entiating the NMS from the IMS are important in all of these accounts: 1. The principle of *emotion as information*. 2. The principle of *normative self-regulation*.

In 'emotion-as-information' theories the con-scious 'felt' character of emotional experience is used as information to guide decision making and strategic, goal directed actions. In some inferential accounts, a person forms a judgment about some-thing (an action, experience, object, or attribute) by asking 'How do I feel about it?' and uses the feeling as a short-cut to a judgment that guides sub-sequent behavior. In other inferential accounts, the role of emotion in decision making occurs because individuals perform actions to manage (maintain, change, remove) their emotional experience (for reviews, see Winkielman et al., 2007; Andrade, 2005; Erber & Markunas, 2006). In neither type of account does emotion act as a direct impulse

for behavior; rather, through feedback, emotion supplies information for cognitive processes that control behavior.

Damasio's Somatic Marker Hypothesis

Antonio Damasio and colleagues have proposed an influential theory for the functional role of emotion in decision making they have called the 'Somatic Marker Hypothesis' (Damasio, 1994; Damasio, 1996; Naqvi, Shiv & Bechara, 2006). On this account the amygdala triggers emotional and autonomic bodily states in response to rewards and punishments caused by deliberate, goal directed actions. These emotional states become linked to representations of the actions that brought them about in the ventromedial prefrontal cortex (VMPFC) – a part of the orbitofrontal cortex. Dur-ing decision making the DLPFC makes represen-tations of different action possibilities accessible in working memory. Via connections with the VMPFC, these action representations reenact the emotional/bodily states that have been associated with them in past experience. In the process of forming 'somatic markers' used for subsequent decision making, the bodily states associated with different actions are either mapped to the insula cortex subserving conscious desires or aversions for deciding for or against a particular action, or to the mesolimbic DA system where affective biases on decision making are unconscious. In support of this model, humans with VMPFC damage are impaired on a number of tests of emotional reac-tivity to stimuli, and are unable to use emotions to aid in decision making in 'personal, financial and moral arenas' (Damasio, 1994).

Interpreting the Somatic Marker Hypothesis in NMS Terms

According to the Somatic Marker Hypothesis, emotion plays a critical informational role in guid-ing decision making, contrary to the traditional idea that emotion impairs decision making and is in conflict with rationality. Somatic markers may guide decision making unconsciously and automatically, but this automaticity is apparently conditional on executive 'emotion-as-information' processing driven by explicit motives – such as strategically attempting to make money in the Iowa gambling task, or in real-world contexts to be financially solvent, hold down a job, maintain relationships and a reputation (Bechara et al., 1994).

Although not discussed explicitly, Damasio and colleagues stress the significance of the normative. They observe that damage to the VMPFC impacts long-range outcomes in 'interpersonal, financial and moral' spheres – all areas strongly regulated by social norms and normative standards of 'appropriate' or 'correct' behavior. This emphasis on cultural life and the role of emotion in navigating interpersonal and normative complexities is also apparent in Baumeister and colleagues' Feedback Theory which we will now review in some detail.

Baumeister and Colleagues' Feedback Theory

Damasio's Somatic Marker Theory finds a close parallel in Baumeister and colleagues' Feedback Theory of emotion. His focus is on subjectively felt emotion – i.e. 'full blown, conscious emotional experience' (Baumeister et al., 2007). According to this account subjectively felt emotions function to stimulate reflective cognitive processing after some event or experience to aid 'lesson learning' and the 'formation of associations between affect and various emotional responses'. While Baumeister and colleagues recognize the existence of unconscious, automatic affective processes that may directly impel behavior, full-blown, felt emotion, on their account, did not evolve to directly impel behavior. A review of the literature indicates that the evidence for a 'direct causation' function of emotional experience is weak (Schwarz & Clore, 1996). Emotion typically functions to

have an *indirect* impact on behavior by stimulating counterfactual reflection and evaluation, and enabling strategic anticipation of emotion. After a decision is enacted, emotional responses provide feedback for appraisal and cognition about the action that resulted in the emotion – or counterfactual actions and their emotional consequences (e.g. "if only I'd not done *this*, but done *that*, then I wouldn't have ended up feeling so guilty"). This reflective process promotes learning by helping to 'reprogram' weightings for decision making and what Baumeister and colleagues call 'if-then contingency rules' for behavior. Positive emotions reinforce some rules, and negative emotions promote counterfactual thinking and rule reprogramming. Representations of if-then actions are left with 'traces' or 'affective residues' (analogous to Damasio's 'somatic markers') of the positive or negative emotions that the actions caused. These function automatically and to a large extent unconsciously to guide subsequent decision making and planned action. This learning process, Baumeister points out, is similar to learning by reinforcement. But there is a crucial difference: the representational medium is symbolic and linguistic, allowing counterfactual thinking and means-ends reasoning.

According to the Feedback Theory, behavior is often determined by the flexible, strategic pursuit or avoidance of *anticipated* positive or negative emotional outcomes in an emotional self-regulatory way. For this reason anticipated emotions are typically more important than actual emotions in the 'on-line' regulation of behavior. As Baumeister and his colleagues formulate it: 'behavior pursues emotion' (Baumeister et al., 2007, p. 172). Pursuing anticipated positive emotions and avoiding negative ones is a useful heuristic for effective decision making and explicit goal pursuit. This kind of emotional self-regulation is strategic and mediated by executive processes, not automatic and impulsive; it is related to uniquely human autobiographical episodic memory systems and a domain general capacity for 'mental time travel' (Suddendorf & Corballis, 2007). It is a function of the NMS, on this dual-process account, not the IMS.

Evidence for the Feedback Theory of emotion is found in 'mood freeze' studies demonstrating that what appears to be direct effect of an emotion on behavior (such as sadness or anger) is, in fact, cognitively mediated and based on beliefs about what actions will result in mood repair. Manucia, Baumann & Cialdini (1984), for example, replicated the usual finding that people in sad moods help others more than those in neutral moods (Cunningham, Steinberg, & Grev, 1980). But they found that when participants were led to believe that a pill would immobilize their sad mood, and they did not expect to feel better by helping, they no longer helped. Subsequent studies have used the mood freeze procedure to examine a number of other emotion-behavior patterns and found a similar result (review, Baumeister et al., 2008).

The Feedback Theory predicts that emotions elicit counterfactual thinking and improve decision making. In her review of the literature, Roese (1997) concluded that negative emotional experience is the "chief determinant of the... activation of counterfactual processing" (p. 135). There is evidence for the impact of counterfactual thinking on 'learning lessons' (i.e. 'reprogramming' actions) to avoid repeating a misfortune in the future (Landman et al, 1995; Markman et al, 1993). Decision makers evaluate their outcomes relative to what *might* have been if they had chosen differently (Roese & Olson, 1995). In their review paper, Janis and Mann (1977) proposed that anticipated regret changes the decision making process towards greater vigilance and information gathering – leading to better decisions.

If emotion provides feedback to facilitate rule reprogramming then it should be most common when learning is taking place to facilitate memory. This prediction is supported by the evidence. Wood, Quinn & Kashy (2002) found that people reported more intense emotions when engaged in novel behaviors than when they performed

habitual ones. The heightened emotional intensity with novel behaviors is associated with a significant increase in thinking about what one is doing. And emotionally charged events are better remembered than neutral events (review, McGough, 2000). Memory is facilitated by both positive (Christianson, 1986) and negative (Christianson & Loftus, 1987) emotions.

Interpreting Baumeister's Feedback Theory in NMS Terms

Baumeister and colleagues distinguish between (i) simple positively and negatively valenced 'automatic affect' that is unreflective, fast-acting, and may be entirely unconscious, and (2) more complex 'full blown' conscious emotion that is slow to arise and is heavily saturated with cognitions and evaluations. They argue that the former may simply activate basic approach and avoidance systems, while the latter promotes reflection, learning and strategic self-regulation in the ways we have outlined above. Their Feedback Theory is an account of the latter, not the former. Since emotion on this account is an information source for working memory dependent *cognitive analysis* – with attributions, counterfactual thinking, and subsequent anticipation of behavioral options through mental stimulation, it can interpreted in terms of the explicit NMS. According to Baumeister and colleagues, while emotional states are not in themselves explicit goals, they act in the service of attaining explicit goals and their functional role depends on "cognitive appraisal to become translated into specific programs for what, exactly, should be done" (2007, p. 170).

A recurring emotion given considerable weight in the Feedback Theory is *guilt* – a uniquely human 'self conscious' emotion, tied to the idea of personal responsibility or accountability, and playing a social-regulatory role in the context of social norms and interpersonal obligations. I believe this emotion is prototypical in the Feedback Theory. The relationship between guilt and social regulation by normative standards is made explicit: "Guilt prompted the person to reflect on what he or she had done, to reevaluate the decision process in light of social norms and obligations, and possibly to extract lessons and conclusions about how a different course of action might have yielded better emotional outcomes" (Baumeister et al., 2008, p. 173). According to a sampling study by Baumeister, Reis and Delespaul (1995), people reported minor degrees ('twinges') of guilt on average about two hours per day, indicative of its critical regulatory function in human social-cultural life. People learn what will make them feel guilty and then change their behavior to avoid it; in this way behavior is brought in line with socially valued behaviors (Baumeister, Stillwell, & Heatherton, 1994).

Other emotions discussed in Baumeister and colleagues' account such as anger are explained in the same social-normative way. While the emotion of *pride* is not explored in this account, it is similar to Baumeister's prototype emotion guilt. It constitutes another uniquely human emotion that, like guilt, is understood relatively late in development. It is closely implicated in self-regulation by normative standards, and is associated with the notion of personal responsibility. Pride, as a pro-social, achievement-oriented emotion, is correlated with culturally advantageous traits such as agreeableness, conscientiousness and self esteem (Tracy & Robins, 2007).

Baumeister and colleagues' 2008 review paper concludes with the statement that conscious emotion evolved as "an advanced cognitive apparatus for figuring out how to negotiate…through the unique, remarkable opportunities and pitfalls of… intricate social and cultural systems" (p. 198). This framing of the topic is similar to Damasio and colleagues' account, and finds an obvious interpretation in terms of the proposed NMS.

Carver and Scheier's Self-Regulation Theory

In Carver and Scheier's (1990; 1998) Self-Regulation Theory of behavior as a goal-directed feedback control process, both the *emotion as information* and the *normative self-regulation* principles are critical: "Positive and negative affects are posited to convey information about whether the behavior being engaged in is going *well* or *poorly*" (Carver, 2001, p. 345). 'Well' or 'poorly' is defined relative to an internally represented 'reference value' – a standard, norm or goal. And as the authors observe, "Much of human behavior is a matter of isolating a point of reference, and then trying to conform to it" (1998, p. 47).

On this account, consciously experienced valenced emotion is information for the effectiveness of ongoing, goal directed voluntary action. Essentially, emotions provide feedback as to how fast one is moving towards a valued goal: positive emotions signal progress that is considered appropriate or better than appropriate, while negative emotions signal progress that is slower than expected or desired. In this way, as in Baumeister's Feedback Theory of emotion, pursuing emotional feedback can be a good heuristic for effective goal pursuit. Supporting evidence for this model is reviewed in Carver & Scheier, 1998, chapters 8 and 9, in experiments in which feedback of progress towards a goal is manipulated over an extended time while emotions are measured.

Goal pursuit on this account is conceived as coherent and hierarchical, with 'program level' goals (executed actions, such as 'eat low fat foods') at the lower levels of the hierarchy, and more abstract and motivating goals relating to an idealized, hoped-for, or 'ought' based, *sense of self* (such as 'be fit and healthy') at the highest level of the hierarchy. Thus on the Self-Regulation Theory, the principle of normative regulation is closely linked to the construct of the *self*. Self-serving goals can be both 'private' (personal values and standards, and private goals) and 'public' (communal, collective or interdependent goals, such as being socially accepted) (Carver & Scheier, 1998; Wylie, 1968).

The Self-Regulation Theory of goal directed behavior, like the Somatic Marker Theory of decision making and the Feedback Theory of emotion, finds a clear mapping onto the proposed NMS in the motivational dual process account. It presupposes explicit motivational processes, and hinges on the *emotion as information* and *normative self-regulation* principles underpinning the hypothesized NMS.

The Biopsychological Basis of the NMS

Recent evolutionary accounts of the basis of uniquely human cognition as depending on collective intentionality and normativity (Moll & Tomasello, 2007; Tomasello & Rakoczy, 2003) are consistent with the hypothesis that the DLPFC functions as a 'point of entry' for the social-cultural regulation of behaviour. Following DLPFC lesions there may be a relative sparing of the ability to respond motivationally to innate or learned nonverbal social cues such as facial expressions, emotional tone in speech, or gestures – important cues for *implicit* motivational processes. But normatively regulated explicit goal pursuit is severely impaired, with a loss of the "ability to coordinate … behavior with that of others flexibly through the pursuit of verbally shared goals or to adapt … behavior to changing demands and expectations of their sociocultural environment" (Schultheiss & Wirth, 2008).

Thus in addition to the known working memory / executive function of the DLPFC, it can be hypothesized to have a function that is inherently socio-cultural and normative. Conscious human emotion is highly sensitive to social-normative standards, and the ability to track normative standards is arguably uniquely human. It may depend on what Tomasello and his colleagues have called a capacity for 'shared intentionality' or 'collec-

tive intentionality' – the ability to understand and participate in cultural activities, with normatively regulating standards and practices (e.g. Tomasello & Carpenter, 2007; Tomasello & Rakoczy, 2003). It is this ability that Tomasello believes is at the core of what distinguishes human from non-human cognition. This notion of collective intentionality is understood on Tomasello's account to underlie not just the adoption of conventions of a moral or institutional sort, but also the ability to use artefacts and to the linguistic symbols that are the basis of human communication.

A well known class of experimental task that reveals DLPFC activation is the interference task in which a participant makes a forced choice to stimulus while simultaneously trying not to to be influenced by an irrelevant stimulus dimension. In the Stroop task, participants have to name the ink colour of a list of colour words such as 'red' or 'blue'. When the colour of the ink and the colour word are different ('incongruent') performance is slower and less accurate than when the colour and word match ('congruent'). This is because word reading is relatively more automatic than colour naming and the since the word is hard to ignore it activates the associated response. During incongruent trials, responses associated with the colour compete with those associated with the word, and DLPFC mediated attentional control is required to overcome the conflict, selectively maintaining representations of the task requirements and biasing downstream processing towards what is appropriate. On the IMS-NMS dual process account, this conflict resolution in favour of acting according to an explicit instruction reflects the functioning of the NMS system. Following a rule, and being concerned with 'correctness' in this goal, is a normative and explicit process.

In response to the question 'how is the DLPFC control itself regulated' van Veen & Carter (2002; 2006) and Bongers and Dijksterhuis (2008) have argued that the amount of conflict occurring plays a central role in how much executive attentional control is exerted or withdrawn, and the brain substrate for conflict monitoring is the anterior cingulate cortex (ACC). When conflict is detected the PFC is alerted to exert control and resolve the conflict in a 'conflict control loop'. On the Stroop task, neuroimaging studies have shown that the ACC is activated both during error trials of the Stroop task, and during correct, incongruent trials (Kerns et al., 2004; van Veen & Carter, 2002).

In support of the thesis that normativity plays a central role in this type of regulatory executive process, there is evidence that the conflict-control loop operates for a diverse range of 'conflicts', all of which involve some normative standard of what is 'appropriate' or 'valid' (review van Veen & Carter, 2007). Green and his colleagues provide evidence that during *moral dilemmas* a subcortical 'emotional' response competes with a utilitarian 'rational' response, the ACC detects the conflict and engages the lateral PFC to resolve the conflict in favour of the cognitive response (Green et al., 2004). A conflict-control loop has also been suggested to play a role in the phenonmenon of *cognitive dissonance*. The ACC detects conflicts between attitudes and behaviour (the dissonance) of the self and activates the PFC to reduce the dissonance to maintain a consistent self-image. Fugelsang & Dunbar (2005) have also suggested that in the domain of causal reasoning, when new data about causal relations conflicts with a model that is currently believed, this engages attention via an ACC-prefrontal cortex conflict-control loop.

Two inferences can be drawn from this conflict-control loop data: (1) The controlled conformity to explicit, verbally formulated rules (Stroop task), as well as causal reasoning, moral judgment and cognitive dissonance, are all *uniquely human* cognitive processes. (2) A common principle in all these cases of ACC-prefrontal conflict-control activation is that of a regulating evaluation based on some *rule* or *normative standard* – either what is *correct* in terms of following instructions in the Stroop task, what is *justified* with moral dilemmas, or what is *accountable* for the self concept in terms of cognitive dissonance, or what is *valid*

or *justified* in terms of causal mental models. We can predict that the same system will be activated in other normative domains – for instance when performance (measured by speed or quality) on a task does not match up to some benchmark standard – as described in Carver & Scheier's Self-regulation Theory. While this conception of normativity, embracing rule following and epistemic validity, is broad – it is in keeping with accounts developed by both philosophers and psychologists (e.g. Kalish, 2006; Searle, 2001).

By virtue of mechanisms similar to overlearning in the automaticity literature, explicit motives might in time operate unconsciously and automatically, with goals of explicit origin being activated and running to completion outside of awareness (review, Shah, 2005). But on this biopsychological account there is nonetheless a continuous ACC monitoring for 'error'. Evaluations of failures, mistakes, inappropriate actions or factual inconsistencies will render goal related information highly accessible, prompting conscious awarness of the goal, what has gone wrong, and how the situation might be corrected (for a related idea, see Bongers & Dijksterhuis, 2008).

How might emotion function in such 'conflict-control loops'? Normative failures result in negative emotions – concern, irritation, guilt, anxiety or anger – depending on the nature of the goal and how central it is to the sense of self, represented in the MPFC (Zhu et al., 2007). This could occur either during goal pursuit in a performance monitoring mode consistent with Carver and Scheier's Self-regulation Theory, or 'after the event' in a reflective feedback mode consistent with Baumeister and colleagues' Feedback Theory. Depending on the normative significance of the conflict between the action and the standard, these emotions may become more or less consciously salient, compelling and arousing, with the most intense negative emotions eliciting more sustained and elaborate goal-focused evaluation, problem solving and counterfactual thinking as described in detail by Baumeister and colleagues (2007). Emotions in this system motivate behavior, either via feedback for 'how *well* am I performing in pursuing this goal' or via the anticipation and avoidance of negative emotions in the way described by Baumeister and colleagues (2007). Felt emotions may become associated with representations of actions via the VMDLC, as proposed by Damasio and colleagues in their Somatic Marker Theory of decision making (Damasio, 1996). Although it has not been investigated in connection to anterior cingulate or limbic cortex functioning, when goal directed action results in an unexpected degree of accomplishment or normative success, it is likely that a monitoring process may result in feelings of satisfaction, elation, or pride, reinforcing the voluntary actions that led to those emotions. Studies investigating whether the anterior cingulate activates when normatively regulated performance is going *better than expected* are needed here.

Evolutionary Origins of the IMS and NMS

The dual process IMS vs NMS account proposed in this chapter can also be understood in terms of the contrast between domain general intelligence and domain specific mechanisms, or 'informationally encapsulated modules' (Fodor, 1983). While domain general systems are designed to attain evolutionary goals in uncertain, novel and changing environments, informationally encapsulated modules are specialized to handle specific inputs and generate particular solutions to recurrent adaptive problems, using highly stable patterns of evolutionarily significant information (Chiappe & McDonald, 2005). Implicit motive neuro-endocrine systems can be understood as predominantly domain specific mechanisms, having evolved over millions of years of mammalian competition for resources, inter and intra-sexual competion, pair-bonding and affiliation needs (Geary & Huffman, 2002). By contrast, the domain general, language based NMS has a primarily *cultural* function – enabling rapid assimilation,

innovation and transmission of cultural knowledge and skill, and the adoption of cultural norms (Tomasello, 1999). This co-evolution of this explicit mode of motivated cognition and behavior in conjunction with symbolic language may underpin the powerful bootstrapping process underlying human technical and institutional progress that has been called 'cummulative cultural evolution' (Tomasello, 1999; Moll & Tomasello, 2007). Explicit motives are inherently language mediated according to the biopsychologists Schultheiss and Wirth (2008). Language is well designed to encode and communicate normative evaluations and standards. In accordance with Tomasello's conception of language, linguistic symbols are themselves tool-like devices and normatively regulated (Tomasello, 1999). In factor analytic studies of the the underlying structure of word meaning, an *evaluative* (good vs bad) dimension comes out as the first factor, accounting for most of the variance (Osgood, Suci, & Tanenbaum, 1957).

We can further speculate that this normative affective and motivational system has its uniquely human origins in what Tomasello and colleagues call 'collective intentionality' – the ability to participate in a collective culture with shared meanings and goals – and the social approval and disapproval regulating behavior in a cultural context. Moreover, it may have been an adaptive advantage for the rapid, cumulative cultural evolution of knowledge and skill (Tomasello, 1999) that normative standards with a public, communal origin could become internalised' for self-regulation – for example, from public shame to private guilt or from external pride to internalized perfectionism.

Unconscious and Conscious Emotion

I will conclude this chapter with a closer look at how unconscious and conscious affect and emotion may be taxonomized in the context of the dual process IMS-NMS account that has been presented.

A distinction is often drawn in the emotion literature between (1) *affect*, that is an automatic, simple, rapid (sub second), and valenced (positive/negative; liked/disliked), and (2) 'full blown' emotion as conscious feeling, typically characterized by physiological changes such as bodily arousal, and differentiated into specific subjectively felt unitary states, which may nonetheless be experienced as complex, with a blend of emotions. Emotions in this highly processed sense are slower to arise and dissipate than affective responses, and are heavily saturated with cognitions, including attributions, inferences and especially evaluations. Dual process accounts of emotion based on this distinction have been proposed that parallel dual process theories of automatic vs controlled modes of cognition (review, Baumeister et al., 2007). On the motivational dual process account I have presented, affect and emotion in these senses are not mapped one-to-one onto the IMS and NMS respectively, as will now be explained.

A helpful way to taxonomize consciousness has been formulated by the philosopher Ned Block. He distinguishes between 'phenomenal consciousness' and 'access consciousness'. Phenomenal consciousness (P-consciousness) is experience, and the phenomenally conscious aspect of a state is what it is like to *be* in that state. Access consciousness (A-consciousness), by contrast, is defined as 'availability for use in reasoning and rationally guiding speech and action' (Block, 1995).

On our account, emotion in the 'full blown' sense is always both P-conscious in that it is experienced with a rich phenomenology, *and* A-conscious in that it functions as information for metacognition, domain general reasoning and executive control. This type of fully elaborated emotion is confined to the NMS, and – on this account – its ultimate origin is in the evolution of collective intentionality and culture. But not all emotion is conscious in this joint P-conscious and A-conscious sense in the NMS. In as far as emo-

tion guides decision making via 'somatic markers' (Damasio) or 'traces' or 'affective residues' (Baumeister) the emotion is affect-like. In this case it may not be P-conscious but it does, nonetheless, play an important role in A-consciousness to the extent that it helps constrain decision making and reasoning.

For the IMS, emotion as affect (automatic, rapid and valenced) encodes affectively significant perceptual cues to biologically based rewards or punishments that have been shown to play a critical role in subcortical, mesolimbic DA system activation – i.e. 'wanting'. These domain and stimulus-specific affective processes are unconscious and inaccessible to introspection or verbal report, as Winkielman and colleagues have demonstrated in their affective subliminal priming study (1995). Affect here is neither P-conscious (i.e. subjectively felt), nor A-conscious (i.e. accessible to reasoning, decision making and speech). Conscious emotion can, however, play a functional role in the IMS as the hedonic 'P-conscious' experience that accompanies goal consummation. The evidence suggests this kind of emotional experience is not A-conscious however: it is non-reflective and is not utilized by executive processes in reasoning and planning. This hedonic response – which varies as a function of need state – is essential for determining a goal's subsequent *incentive value* in instrumental behavior. This kind of emotion is likely to be mediated by the VMPFC, possibly in association with amygdala-hypothalamic-endocrine systems controlling autonomic arousal. It may be common to all mammals. Since VMPFC reward areas can become activated by conditioned as well as unconditioned incentives, stimuli *associated* with rewards during the 'homing in' process, can also elicit P-conscious, but non A-conscious, hedonic (pleasure or pain) feelings.

In summary, on this proposal human emotion is multifaceted in terms of its consciousness-related and executive processing properties. It plays a central role in both the IMS and the NMS, and can be unconscious and conscious in both systems.

CONCLUSION

In the first half of this chapter I reviewed the literature on the functional and neurobiological basis of implicit motives, indicating the ways in which they can exert control over behavior. Emotion in this context is better understood either as associative cues integral to *reinforcement-motivational* mechanisms that operate unconsciously, or as *non-reflective* hedonic experience of pleasure or pain. By contrast, emotion functions as *information* for cognitive inference and executive control in the NMS. Three theories I have reviewed above provide accounts of emotion in this 'explicit' mode of cognition and behavior, not the 'implicit' mode. The role of emotion in implicit motives is neglected in these accounts, in part because of the traditional distance between the disciplines of biopsychology and cognitive / social psychology.

While there is an obvious biological basis of implicit motives and emotions, and the brain mechanisms of these motivational systems are relatively well understood, the claim that explicit, normatively regulated motives have their own distinct evolutionary origins and neural mechanisms is more controversial. It may plausibly be assumed that implicit motives relating to survival, reproduction, affiliation and competition for resources, ultimately account for all motivated behavior; that more cultural, abstract and explicit goals such as 'getting qualified' or 'getting married' are linked by chains of reinforcement to implicit motives such as dominance or sexual desire. But the IMS-NMS dual process account is making a different claim. The three theories reviewed above suggest that there may be more recently evolved explicit motivation-emotion system – interpenetrated with explicit cognition – that is to an extent *autonomous* from the implicit motivation system. This system is hypothesized to motivate behavior through self-

reflectively, consciously experienced emotional feedback, and the anticipation of felt emotional states in explicit goal directed behavior. In terms of anatomical localization, this more recently evolved circuitry interconnects the dorsolateral prefrontal cortex (DLPFC) and anterior cingulate cortex (ACC) in an executive process circuit for working memory and 'conflict control'.

REFERENCES

Adelmann, P. K., & Zajonc, R. B. (1989). Facial efference and the experience of emotion. *Annual Review of Psychology, 40*, 249–280. doi:10.1146/annurev.ps.40.020189.001341

Adolphs, R., & Tranel, D. (2000). Emotion recognition and the human amygdala. In Aggleton, J. P. (Ed.), *The amygdala. A functional analysis* (pp. 587–630). New York: Oxford University Press.

Aharon, I., Etcoff, N., Ariely, D., Chabris, C. F., O'Connor, E., & Breiter, H. C. (2001). Beautiful faces have variable reward value: Fmri and behavioral evidence. *Neuron, 32*(3), 537–551. doi:10.1016/S0896-6273(01)00491-3

Balleine, B., & Dickinson, A. (1991). Instrumental performance following reinforcer devaluation depends upon incentive learning. *Quarterly Journal of Experimental Psychology, Section B. Comparative Physiological Psychology, 43*(3), 279–296.

Balleine, B., & Dickinson, A. (1998). Consciousness: The interface between affect and cognition. In Cornwell, J. (Ed.), *Consciousness and Human Identity* (pp. 57–85). Oxford: Oxford University Press.

Baumeister, R. F., Reis, H. T., & Delespaul, P. A. E. G. (1995). Subjective and experiential correlates of guilt in everyday life. *Personality and Social Psychology Bulletin, 21*, 1256–1268. doi:10.1177/01461672952112002

Baumeister, R. F., Stillwell, A. M., & Heatherton, T. F. (1994). Guilt: An interpersonal approach. *Psychological Bulletin, 115*, 243–267. doi:10.1037/0033-2909.115.2.243

Baumeister, R. F., Vohs, K. D., DeWall, C. N., & Zhang, L. (2007). How emotion shapes behavior: Feedback, anticipation, and reflection, rather than direct causation. *Personality and Social Psychology Review, 11*(2), 167–203. doi:10.1177/1088868307301033

Berridge, K. C. (1996). Food reward: Brain substrates of wanting and liking. *Neuroscience and Biobehavioral Reviews, 20*, 1–25. doi:10.1016/0149-7634(95)00033-B

Berridge, K. C. (2000). Measuring hedonic impact in animals and infants: microstructure of affective taste reactivity patterns. *Neuroscience and Biobehavioral Reviews, 24*, 173–198. doi:10.1016/S0149-7634(99)00072-X

Berridge, K. C. (2004). Motivation concepts in behavioral neuroscience. *Physiology & Behavior, 81*(2), 179–209. doi:10.1016/j.physbeh.2004.02.004

Blood, A. J., & Zatorre, R. J. (2001). Intensely pleasurable responses to music correlate with activity in brain regions implicated in reward and emotion. *Proceedings of the National Academy of Sciences of the United States of America, 98*(20), 11818–11823. doi:10.1073/pnas.191355898

Bongers, K., & Dijksterhuis, A. (2008). Consciousness as a trouble shooting device? The role of consciousness in goal-pursuit. In Morsella, J. B. E., & Gollwitzer, P. (Eds.), *The Oxford Handbook of Human Action* (pp. 589–604). New York: Oxford University Press.

Bozarth, M. A. (1994). Pleasure Systems in the Brain. In Warburton, D. M. (Ed.), *Pleasure: The politics and the reality* (pp. 5–14). New York: John Wiley & Sons.

Braver, T. S., Cohen, J. D., & Barch, D. M. (2002). The role of the prefrontal cortex in normal and disordered cognitive control: A cognitive neuroscience perspective. In Struss, D. T., & Knight, R. T. (Eds.), *Principles of frontal lobe function* (pp. 428–448). Oxford: Oxford University Press. doi:10.1093/acprof:oso/9780195134971.003.0027

Buck, R. (1980). Nonverbal behavior and the theory of emotion: The facial feedback hypothesis. *Journal of Personality and Social Psychology, 38*, 811–824. doi:10.1037/0022-3514.38.5.811

Cabanac, M. (1971). Physiological role of pleasure. *Science, 173*(2), 1103–1107. doi:10.1126/science.173.4002.1103

Cardinal, R. N., Parkinson, J. A., Hall, J., & Everitt, B. J. (2002). Emotion and motivation: The role of the amygdala, ventral striatum, and prefrontal cortex. *Neuroscience and Biobehavioral Reviews, 26*, 321–352. doi:10.1016/S0149-7634(02)00007-6

Carver, C. S., & Scheier, M. F. (1998). *On the self-regulation of behavior.* New York: Cambridge University Press.

Carver, S. C., & Scheier, M. F. (1990). Principles of self-regulation: Action and emotion. In Higgins, E. T., & Sorrentino, R. M. (Eds.), *Handbook of motivation and cognition: Foundations of social behavior* (*Vol. 2*, pp. 3–52). New York: Guilford Press.

Chaiken, S., & Trope, Y. (1999). *Dual-process theories in social psychology.* New York, NY: Guildford Press.

Chen, S., & Chaiken, S. (1999). The heuristic-systematic model in its broader context. In Chaiken, S., & Trope, Y. (Eds.), *Dual-process theories in social psychology.* New York: Guildford Press.

Chiappe, D., & MacDonald, K. (2005). The evolution of domain-general mechanisms in intelligence and learning. *132, 1*, 5-40.

Christianson, S.-A. (1986). Effects of positive emotional events on memory. *Scandinavian Journal of Psychology, 27,* 287–299. doi:10.1111/j.1467-9450.1986.tb01207.x

Christianson, S.-A., & Loftus, E. F. (1987). Memory for traumatic events. *Applied Cognitive Psychology, 1,* 225–239. doi:10.1002/acp.2350010402

Craig, W. (1918). Appetites and aversions as constituents of instincts. *Biological Bulletin of Woods Hole, 34,* 91–107. doi:10.2307/1536346

Critchley, H. D., Daly, E., Phillips, M., Brammer, M., Bullmore, E., & Williams, S. (2000). Explicit and implicit neural mechanisms for processing of social information from facial expressions: A functional magnetic resonance imaging study. *Human Brain Mapping, 9,* 93–105. doi:10.1002/(SICI)1097-0193(200002)9:2<93::AID-HBM4>3.0.CO;2-Z

Cunningham, M. R., Steinberg, J., & Grev, R. (1980). Wanting to and having to help: Separate motivations for positive mood and guiltinduced helping. *Journal of Personality and Social Psychology, 38,* 181–192. doi:10.1037/0022-3514.38.2.181

Damasio, A. (1994). *Descartes' error: Emotion, reason, and the human brain.* New York: Grosset/Putnam.

Damasio, A. R. (1996). The somatic marker hypothesis and the possible functions of the prefrontal cortex. *Philosophical Transactions of the Royal Society of London. Series B, Biological Sciences, 351*(1346), 1413–1420. doi:10.1098/rstb.1996.0125

de Araujo, I. E., Kringelbach, M. L., Rolls, E. T., & Hobden, P. (2003). Representation of Umami taste in the human brain. *Journal of Neurophysiology, 90*(1), 313–319. doi:10.1152/jn.00669.2002

Depue, R. A., & Collins, P. F. (1999). Neurobiology of the structure of personality: Dopamine, facilitation of incentive motivation, and extraversion. *The Behavioral and Brain Sciences, 22,* 491–569. doi:10.1017/S0140525X99002046

Epstein, L. H., Truesdale, R., Wojcik, A., Paluch, R. A., & Raynor, H. A. (2003). Effects of deprivation on hedonics and reinforcing value of food. *Physiology & Behavior, 78,* 221–227. doi:10.1016/S0031-9384(02)00978-2

Epstein, S. (1994). Integration of the cognitive and psychodynamic unconscious. *The American Psychologist, 49,* 709–724. doi:10.1037/0003-066X.49.8.709

Evans, J. St. B. T. (2003). In two minds: Dual process accounts of reasoning. *Trends in Cognitive Sciences, 7,* 454–459. doi:10.1016/j.tics.2003.08.012

Evans, J. St. B. T. (2006). Dual system theories of cognition: Some issues. In R. Sun (Ed.), *Proceedings of 28th annual meeting of the cognitive science society.* (pp. 202-7). Mahwah, N.J.: Erlbaum.

Evans, J. St. B. T., & Over, D. E. (1996). *Rationality & Reasoning.* Hove: Psychology Press.

Everitt, B. J. (1990). Sexual motivation: A neural and behavioural analysis of the mechanisms underlying appetitive and copulatory responses of male rats. *Neuroscience and Biobehavioral Reviews, 14*(2), 217–232. doi:10.1016/S0149-7634(05)80222-2

Fodor, E. M., Wick, D. P., & Hartsen, K. M. (2006). The power motive and affective response to assertiveness. *Journal of Research in Personality, 40,* 598–610. doi:10.1016/j.jrp.2005.06.001

Fodor, J. (1983). *The modularity of mind.* Cambridge, MA: MIT Press.

Francis, S., Rolls, E. T., Bowtell, R., Mc-Glone, F., O'Doherty, J., & Browning, A. (1999). The representation of pleasant touch in the brain and its relationship with taste and olfactory areas. *Neuroreport, 10,* 453–459. doi:10.1097/00001756-199902250-00003

Fugelsang, J. A., & Dunbar, K. N. (2005). Brain-based mechanisms underlying complex causal thinking. *Neuropsychologia, 43,* 1204–1213. doi:10.1016/j.neuropsychologia.2004.10.012

Gazzaniga, M. (1985). *The social brain.* New York, NY: Basic Books.

Geary, D. C., & Huffman, K. J. (2002). Brain and cognitive evolution: Forms of modularity and functions of mind. *Psychological Bulletin, 128,* 667–698. doi:10.1037/0033-2909.128.5.667

Greene, J. D., Nystrom, L. E., Engell, A. D., Darley, J. M., & Cohen, J. D. (2004). The neural bases of cognitive conflict and control in moral judgment. *Neuron, 44,* 389–400. doi:10.1016/j.neuron.2004.09.027

Hare, B. (2007). From nonhuman to human mind. What changed and why? *Current Directions in Psychological Science, 16*(2), 60–64. doi:10.1111/j.1467-8721.2007.00476.x

Hess, U., Blairy, S., & Kleck, R. E. (2000). The influence of facial emotion displays, gender, and ethnicity on judgments of dominance and affiliation. *Journal of Nonverbal Behavior, 24*(4), 265–283. doi:10.1023/A:1006623213355

Homer,. (1990). *The Iliad* (Fagles, R., Trans.). New York: Viking.

Ikemoto, S., & Panksepp, J. (1999). The role of nucleus accumbens dopamine in motivated behavior: A unifying interpretation with special reference to reward-seeking. *Brain Research. Brain Research Reviews, 31*(1), 6–41. doi:10.1016/S0165-0173(99)00023-5

Janis, I. L., & Mann, L. (1977). *Decision making: A psychological analysis of conflict, choice and commitment.* New York: Free Press.

Kahneman, D., & Frederick, S. (2002). Representativeness revisited: Attribute substitution in intuitive judgement. In Gilovich, T., Griffin, D., & Kahneman, D. (Eds.), *Heuristics and biases: The psychology of intuitive judgement* (pp. 49–81). Cambridge, UK: Cambridge University Press.

Kahneman, D., & Tversky, A. (1982). The simulation heuristic. In Kahneman, D., Slovic, P., & Tversky, A. (Eds.), *Judgment under uncertainty* (pp. 201–208). Cambridge, UK: Cambridge University Press.

Kerns, J. C., Cohen, J. D., MacDonald, A. W. III, Cho, R. Y., Stenger, V. A., & Carter, C. S. (2004). Anterior cingulate conflict monitoring and adjustments in control. *Science, 303,* 1023–1026. doi:10.1126/science.1089910

Killcross, S., Robbins, T. W., & Everitt, B. J. (1997). Different types of fear-conditioned behaviour mediated by separate nuclei within amygdala. *Nature, 388*(6640), 377–380. doi:10.1038/41097

Koepp, M. J., Gunn, R. N., Lawrence, A. D., Cunningham, V. J., Dagher, A., & Jones, T. (1998). Evidence for striatal dopamine release during a video game. *Nature, 393*(6682), 266–268. doi:10.1038/30498

Kringelbach, M. L. (2005). The orbitofrontal cortex: Linking reward to hedonic experience. *Nature Reviews. Neuroscience, 6,* 691–702. doi:10.1038/nrn1747

Landman, J., Vandewater, E. A., Stewart, A. J., & Malley, J. E. (1995). Missed opportunities: Psychological ramifications of counterfactual thought in midlife women. *Journal of Adult Development, 2,* 87–97. doi:10.1007/BF02251257

LeDoux, J. E. (1996). *The emotional brain.* New York: Simon & Schuster.

LeDoux, J. E. (2002). *The synaptic self.* New York, NY: Viking.

Lieberman, M. D. (2003). Reflective and reflexive judgment processes: A social cognitive neuroscience approach. In Forgas, J. P., Williams, K. R., & Hippel, W. v. (Eds.), *Social judgments: Implicit and explicit processes* (pp. 44–67). New York: Cambridge University Press.

Luria, A. R. (1973). *The working brain. And introduction to neuropsychology.* New York: Basic Books.

Manucia, G. K., Baumann, D. J., & Cialdini, R. B. (1984). Mood influences on helping: Direct effects or side effects? *Journal of Personality and Social Psychology, 46,* 357–364. doi:10.1037/0022-3514.46.2.357

Markman, K. D., Gavanski, I., Sherman, S. J., & McMullen, M. N. (1993). The mental simulation of better and worse possible worlds. *Journal of Experimental Social Psychology,* (29): 87–109. doi:10.1006/jesp.1993.1005

Matsumoto, D. (1987). The role of facial response in the experience of emotion: More methodological problems and a meta-analysis. *Journal of Personality and Social Psychology, 52,* 759–768. doi:10.1037/0022-3514.52.4.769

McAdams, D. P., & Bryant, F. B. (1987). Intimacy motivation and subjective mental health in a nationwide sample. *Journal of Personality, 55*(3), 395–413. doi:10.1111/j.1467-6494.1987.tb00444.x

McAdams, D. P., Jackson, J., & Kirshnit, C. (1984). Looking, laughing, and smiling in dyads as a function of intimacy motivation and reciprocity. *Journal of Personality, 52,* 261–273. doi:10.1111/j.1467-6494.1984.tb00881.x

McClelland, D. C. (1980). Motive dispositions. The merits of operant and respondent measures. In Wheeler, L. (Ed.), *Review of personality and social psychology* (*Vol. 1,* pp. 10–41). Beverly Hills, CA: Sage.

McClelland, D. C. (1987). *Human motivation.* New York: Cambridge University Press.

McClelland, D. C., Koestner, R., & Weinberger, J. (1989). How do self-attributed and implicit motives differ? *Psychological Review, 96,* 690–702. doi:10.1037/0033-295X.96.4.690

McGaugh, J. L. (2000). Memory—a century of consolidation. *Science, 287,* 248–251. doi:10.1126/science.287.5451.248

Medvec, V. H., Madey, S. F., & Gilovich, T. (1995). When less is more: Counterfactual thinking and satisfaction among Olympic medalists. *Journal of Personality and Social Psychology, 69,* 603–610. doi:10.1037/0022-3514.69.4.603

Miller, E. K., & Cohen, J. D. (2001). An integrative theory of prefrontal cortex function. *Annual Review of Neuroscience, 24,* 167–202. doi:10.1146/annurev.neuro.24.1.167

Mischel, W., Ebbesen, E. B., & Zeiss, A. R. (1973). Selective attention to the self: Situational and dispositional determinants. *Journal of Personality and Social Psychology, 27,* 129–142. doi:10.1037/h0034490

Mogenson, G. J., Jones, D. L., & Yim, C. Y. (1980). From motivation to action: Functional interface between the limbic system and the motor system. *Progress in Neurobiology, 14,* 69–97. doi:10.1016/0301-0082(80)90018-0

Moll, H., & Tomasello, M. (2007). Co-operation and human cognition: The Vygotskian intelligence hypothesis. *Philosophical Transactions of the Royal Society, 362,* 639–648. doi:10.1098/rstb.2006.2000

Monsell, S., & Driver, J. (2000). *Control of cognitive processes*. Cambridge, MA: MIT Press.

Naqvi, N., Shiv, B., & Bechara, A. (2006). The role of emotion in decision making. *Current Directions in Psychological Science, 15*(5), 260–264. doi:10.1111/j.1467-8721.2006.00448.x

Nisbett, R., & Wilson, T. (1977). Telling more than we can know: Verbal reports on mental processes. *Psychological Review, 84*(3), 231–259. doi:10.1037/0033-295X.84.3.231

O'Doherty, J. P. (2004). Reward representations and reward-related learning in the human brain: insights from neuroimaging. *Current Opinion in Neurobiology, 14*, 769–776. doi:10.1016/j.conb.2004.10.016

O'Reilly, R. C., David, C., Noelle, D., Braver, T. S., & Cohen, J. D. (2002). Prefrontal cortex in dynamic categorization tasks: Representational organization and neuromodulatory control. *Cerebral Cortex, 12*, 246–257. doi:10.1093/cercor/12.3.246

Ochsner, K. N., Bunge, S. A., Gross, J. J., & Gabrieli, J. D. (2002). Rethinking feelings: An fmri study of the cognitive regulation of emotion. *Journal of Cognitive Neuroscience, 14*(8), 1215–1229. doi:10.1162/089892902760807212

Olds, J., & Milner, P. (1954). Positive reinforcement produced by electrical stimulation of septal area and other regions of rat brain. *Journal of Comparative and Physiological Psychology, 47*, 418–427. doi:10.1037/h0058775

Panksepp, J. (1998). *Affective neuroscience: The foundations of human and animal emotions*. New York: Oxford University Press.

Panksepp, J. (2005). On the embodied neural nature of core emotional affects. *Journal of Consciousness Studies, 12*, 8–10, 158–184.

Pecina, S., Cagniard, B., Berridge, K. C., Aldridge, J. W., & Zhuang, X. (2003). *Hyperdopaminergic mutant mice have higher "wanting" but not "liking" for sweet rewards. Journal of Neuroscience, 23(28)*, 9395-9402. *Reber, A. S. (1993). Implicit learning and tacit knowledge*. Oxford: Oxford University Press.

Proulx, T., & Heine, S. J. (2009). Connections from Kafka: Exposure to schema threats improves implicit learning of an artificial grammar. *Psychological Science, 20*, 1125–1131. doi:10.1111/j.1467-9280.2009.02414.x

Robinson, T. E., & Berridge, K. C. (2000)... *Addiction (Abingdon, England), 95*(Supplement 2), S91–S117.

Roese, N. J. (1997). Counterfactual thinking. *Psychological Bulletin, 121*, 133–148. doi:10.1037/0033-2909.121.1.133

Roese, N. J., & Olson, J. M. (1995). *What might have been: The social psychology of counterfactual thinking*. Mahwah, NJ: Lawrence Erlbaum.

Rolls, E. T. (1999). *The brain and emotion*. Oxford: Oxford University Press.

Rolls, E. T. (2000). The orbitofrontal cortex and reward. *Cerebral Cortex, 10*(3), 284–294. doi:10.1093/cercor/10.3.284

Rolls, E. T. (2004). The functions of the orbitofrontal cortex. *Brain and Cognition, 55*(1), 11–29. doi:10.1016/S0278-2626(03)00277-X

Rolls, E. T., O'Doherty, J., Kringelbach, M. L., Francis, S., Bowtell, R., & McGlone, F. (2003). Representations of pleasant and painful touch in the human orbitofrontal and cingulate cortices. *Cerebral Cortex, 13*, 308–317. doi:10.1093/cercor/13.3.308

Salamone, J. D. (1994). The involvement of nucleus accumbens dopamine in appetitive and aversive motivation. *Behavioural Brain Research, 61*, 117–133. doi:10.1016/0166-4328(94)90153-8

Schneider, W., & Shiffrin, R. M. (1977). Controlled and automatic human information processing I: Detection, search and attention. *Psychological Review, 84*, 1–66. doi:10.1037/0033-295X.84.1.1

Schultheiss, O. C. (Ed.). (2001). *An information processing account of implicit motive arousal* (*Vol. 12*). Greenwich, CT: JAI Press.

Schultheiss, O. C. (2008). Implicit motives. In O. P. John, R. W. Robins & L. A. Pervin (Eds.), *Handbook of Personality: Theory and Research* (3 ed., pp. 603-33). New York: Guilford.

Schultheiss, O. C., & Brunstein, J. C. (2001). Assessing implicit motives with a research version of the TAT: Picture profiles, gender differences, and relations to other personality measures. *Journal of Personality Assessment, 77*(1), 71–86. doi:10.1207/S15327752JPA7701_05

Schultheiss, O. C., Rösch, A. G., Rawolle, M., Kordik, A., & Graham, S. (in press). *Implicit motives: Current research and future directions. To appear in Urdan, T* (Karabenick, S., & Pajares, F., Eds.). *Vol. 16*). Advances in Motivation and Achievement.

Schultheiss, O. C., & Wirth, M. M. (2008). Biopsychological aspects of motivation. In J. Heckhausen & H. Heckhausen (Eds.), *Moivation and Action* (2 ed., pp. 247-71). New York: Cambridge University Press.

Schultz, W., Dayan, P., & Montague, P. R. (1997). A neural substrate of prediction and reward. *Science, 275*, 1593–1599. doi:10.1126/science.275.5306.1593

Schwarz, N., & Clore, G. L. (1996). Feelings and phenomenal experiences. In Higgins, E. T., & Kruglanski, A. (Eds.), *Social psychology: Handbook of basic principles* (pp. 433–465). New York: Guilford.

Shah, J. Y. (2005). The automatic pursuit and management of goals. *Current Directions in Psychological Science, 14*(1), 10–13. doi:10.1111/j.0963-7214.2005.00325.x

Skinner, B. (1953). *Science and Human Behavior.* New York: Macmillan.

Sloman, S. A. (1996). The empirical case for two systems of reasoning. *Psychological Bulletin, 119*, 3–22. doi:10.1037/0033-2909.119.1.3

Smith, E. E., & Kossyln, S. M. (2006). *Cognitive psychology: Mind and Brain.* Upper Saddle River, NJ: Prentice Hall.

Smith, E. R., & DeCoster, J. (2000). Dual-process models in social and cognitive psychology: Conceptual integration and links to underlying memory systems. *Personality and Social Psychology Review, 4*(2), 108–131. doi:10.1207/S15327957PSPR0402_01

Smith, K. S., Mahler, S. V., Pecina, S., & Berridge, K. C. (2009). Hedonic Hotspots: Generating Sensory Pleasure in the Brain. (capital letters?). In Kringelbach, M. L., & Berridge, K. C. (Eds.), *Pleasures of the Brain* (pp. 1–35). New York: Oxford University Press.

Smolensky, P. (1988). On the proper treatment of connectionism. *The Behavioral and Brain Sciences, 11*, 1–74. doi:10.1017/S0140525X00052432

Spangler, W. D. (1992). Validity of questionnaire and TAT measures of need for achievement: Two meta-analyses. *Psychological Bulletin,* (112): 140–154. doi:10.1037/0033-2909.112.1.140

Squire, M., & Zola, S. M. (1996). Memory, memory impairment, and the medial temporal lobe. *Cold Spring Harbor Symposia on Quantitative Biology, 61*, 185–195.

Stanovich, K. E. (1999). *Who is Rational? Studies of Individual Differences in Reasoning.* Mahway, NJ: Lawrence Elrbaum Associates.

Stanton, S. J., Hall, J. L., & Schultheiss, O. C. (In press). Properties of motive-specific incentives. In Schultheiss, O. C., & Brunstein, J. C. (Eds.), *Implicit motives*. New York: Oxford University Press.

Steiner, J. E., Glaser, D., Hawilo, M. E., & Berridge, K. C. (2001). Comparative expression of hedonic impact: affective reactions to taste by human infants and other primates. *Neuroscience and Biobehavioral Reviews*, *25*, 53–74. doi:10.1016/S0149-7634(00)00051-8

Stern, R. M., Ray, W. J., & Quigley, K. S. (2001). *Psychophysiological recording* (2 ed.). New York: Oxford University Press.

Suddendorf, T., & Corballis, M. C. (2007). The evolution of foresight: What is mental time travel and is it unique to humans? *The Behavioral and Brain Sciences*, *30*, 299–313. doi:10.1017/S0140525X07001975

Tanji, J., & Hoshi, E. (2008). Role of the lateral prefrontal cortex in executive behavioral control. *Physiological Reviews*, *88*, 37–57. doi:10.1152/physrev.00014.2007

Thrash, T. M., & Elliot, A. J. (2002). Implicit and self-attributed achievement motives: concordance and predictive validity. *Journal of Personality*, *70*(5), 729–755. doi:10.1111/1467-6494.05022

Tice, D. M., Bratslavsky, E., & Baumeister, R. F. (2001). Emotional distress regulation takes precedence over impulse control: If you feel bad, do it! *Journal of Personality and Social Psychology*, *80*, 53–67. doi:10.1037/0022-3514.80.1.53

Tomasello, M. (1999). *The cultural origins of human cognition*. Cambridge, MA: Harvard University Press.

Tomasello, M., & Carpenter, M. (2007). Shared intentionality. *Developmental Science*, *10*(1), 121–125. doi:10.1111/j.1467-7687.2007.00573.x

Tomasello, M., & Rakoczy, H. (2003). What makes human cognition unique? From individual to shared to collective intentionality. *Mind & Language*, *18*(2), 121–147. doi:10.1111/1468-0017.00217

Tracy, J. L., & Robins, R. W. (2007). The psychological structure of pride: A tale of two facets. *Journal of Personality and Social Psychology*, *92*, 506–525. doi:10.1037/0022-3514.92.3.506

Tulving, E. (2002). Episodic memory: From mind to brain. *Annual Review of Psychology*, *53*, 11–25. doi:10.1146/annurev.psych.53.100901.135114

Underwood, B., Moore, B. S., & Rosenhan, D. L. (1973). Affect and self-gratification. *Developmental Psychology*, *8*, 209–214. doi:10.1037/h0034158

van Veen, V., & Carter, C. S. (2002). The timing of action-monitoring processing in the anterior cingulate cortex. *Journal of Cognitive Neuroscience*, *14*, 593–602. doi:10.1162/08989290260045837

van Veen, V., & Carter, C. S. (2006). Conflict and cognitive control in the brain. *Current Directions in Psychological Science*, *15*(5), 237–240. doi:10.1111/j.1467-8721.2006.00443.x

Vuilleumier, P., Richardson, M. P., Armony, J. L., Driver, J., & Dolan, R. J. (2004). Distant influences of amygdala lesion on visual cortical activation during emotional face processing. *Nature Neuroscience*, *7*(11), 1271–1278. doi:10.1038/nn1341

Weinberger, J., & McClelland, D. C. (1990). Cognitive versus traditional motivational models: Irreconcilable or complementary? In Higgins, E. T., & Sorrentino, R. M. (Eds.), *Implicit motives 45, Handbook of motivation and cognition: Foundations of social behavior* (*Vol. 2*, pp. 562–597). New York, NY: Guilford Press.

Whalen, P., Rauch, S. L., Etcoff, N. L., McInerney, S. C., Lee, M. B., & Jenike, M. A. (1998). Masked presentations of emotional facial expressions modulate amygdala activity without explicit knowledge. *The Journal of Neuroscience, 18,* 411–418.

Winkielman, P., Berridge, K. C., & Wilbarger, J. (2005). Unconscious affective reactions to masked happy versus angry faces influence consumption behavior and judgments of value. *Personality and Social Psychology Bulletin, 31,* 121–135. doi:10.1177/0146167204271309

Winter, D. G. (1996). *Personality: Analysis and interpretation of lives.* New York: McGraw-Hill.

Wood, W., Quinn, J., & Kashy, D. (2002). Habits in everyday life: Thought, emotion, and action. *Journal of Personality and Social Psychology, 83,* 1281–1297. doi:10.1037/0022-3514.83.6.1281

Wrangham, R., & Peterson, D. (1996). *Demonic Males: Apes and the Origins of Human Violence.* Boston, MA: Houghton Mifflin.

Young, P. (1959). The role of affective processes in learning and motivation. *Psychological Review, 66,* 104–125. doi:10.1037/h0045997

KEY TERMS AND DEFINITIONS

Priming: An effect in which exposure to a stimulus influences response to a subsequent stimulus. It can occur following perceptual, semantic, or conceptual stimulus repetition.

US: A stimulus evoking an unlearned, innate and often reflexive responseCS - is previously neutral stimulus that, after becoming associated with the unconditioned stimulus, eventually comes to trigger a conditioned response.

ACC: Anterior cingulate cortex, is the frontal part of the cingulate cortex, that resembles a "collar" around the corpus callosum.

OFC: Orbitofrontal cortex, is the broad area in the lower (ventral) central (medial) region of the prefrontal cortex. Also referred to as the ventromedial prefrontal cortex (VMPFC).

DLPFC: Dorsolateral prefrontal cortex, is a major division of the prefrontal cortex, including the lateral portions of the upper region of the prefrontal cortex.

ENDNOTE

[1] In a classical fear conditioning experiment, a conditioned stimulus (For ex: CS=neutral tone) precedes an unconditioned stimulus (For ex: US=electric shock). After several trials, the conditioned stimulus alone is adequate to trigger the response given to the unconditioned stimulus.

APPENDIX: INCENTIVE MOTIVATION NETWORK

The Mesolimbic Dopamine System

The mesolimbic dopamine system originates with neurons in the dopamine producing ventral tegmental area (VTA) on the floor of the midbrain. The axons of these cells terminate in the bottom of pallidum and the nucleus accumbens of the lower striatum, and the limbic prefrontal cortex. The nucleus accumbens also receives inputs from the amygdala and orbitofrontal cortex (OFC), both of which assess affect-related sensory properties of a stimulus. The nucleus accumbens has been characterized as a gateway through which sensory information influences motivational motor response preparation in the basal ganglia (Mogenson, Jones, & Yim, 1980). Conditioned and unconditioned *reward* stimuli induce a brief release of DA in the nucleus accumbens and prefrontal cortex but the dopamine is released in the presence of the actual reward only initially. Once the US-CS link has been learned, the DA is released only to the reward predictive CS, and this 'transference' mechanism is iterated for second order conditioning, and so on (Schultz, Dayan & Montague, 1997). In this way the DA release in the nucleus accumbens is involved in learning chains of (Pavlovian) stimulus associations that 'home in' on a reward.

The mesolimbic DA system associates these learned chains with instrumental actions that are directed at the rewards they predict. While the nucleus accumbens is not needed for knowledge of the contingency between instrumental actions and their outcomes, it influences instrumental behavior strongly by allowing Pavlovian CSs to affect the level or intensity of instrumental responding, known as Pavlovian–instrumental transfer (Cardinal et al., 2002). Studies on rats in which the mesolimbic DA system is lesioned or genetically engineered to have higher than normal dopamine levels, or DA agonists or antagonists are used to manipulate the action of the DA neurotransmitter in the accumbens, reveal that this system functions to (a) facilitate learning that an action results in a reward; (b) invigorate reward directed instrumental behaviors once they have been learned; and (c) reduce distractibility during these actions (Ikemoto & Panksepp, 1999; Pecina et al., 2003). Moreover, neither DA reducing (or blocking) nor DA increasing manipulations had an effect on the rats' affective 'liking' responses as measured by the amount of sucrose solution they consumed once they had reached the reward. Biopsychological research also shows that just as this system facilitates approach behaviors directed to rewards, it also facilitates avoidance behaviors – actions taken to avoid disincentives or punishments (Ikemoto & Panksepp, 1999; Salamone, 1994).

Synaptic activity in the accumbens has also been shown to be related to incentive seeking in humans. In brain imaging studies, increased brain activation in the nucleus accumbens has been observed in response to varied incentives including playing a computer game, beautiful opposite-sex faces, and listening to pleasurable music (Aharon et al, 2001; Blood & Zatorre, 2001; Koepp et al, 1998). According to Depue and Collins' (1999) influential theory of the personality trait 'extraversion', extraverts have a greater capacity for mesolimbic DA system activation, whether naturally stimulated by incentive signals or artificially induced through DA agonists – and are thus more 'turned on' and behaviorally invigorated by incentives. People high in extraversion respond with greater 'wanting' to incentives than introverts.

In summary the mesolimbic DA system functions to enhance goal directed instrumental learning and invigorate goal-directed behavior ('wanting' a reward). It facilitates behavior guided by incentives but it does not play a functional role in the hedonic response to the incentive itself ('liking' a reward).

The Orbitofrontal Cortex

The most likely candidate for the coding of the subjective 'liking' phase of motivation is the orbitofrontal cortex (OFC) (Kringelbach, 2005), although the causal circuitry involved is extensive, and other limbic forebrain areas such as the anterior cingulate and insula cortex may also play a role in subjective affect (Smith et al., 2009). Neurochemical signals in a number of 'hedonic hotspots' throughout the brain cause amplification of core 'liking' reactions to sweetness, including the nucleus accumbens, ventral pallidum, and brainstem. Hedonic circuits connect these 'hotspots' into integrated loops and relay them to limbic regions of prefrontal cortex, including the orbitofrontal cortex, and back again, for translation into feelings of pleasure and cognitive representations (Smith et al., 2009).

The OFC receives multimodal and highly processed sensory information and is densely reciprocally connected to the basolateral amygdala. Different types of reinforcers are coded by anatomically distinct areas of the OFC. Brain imaging studies on humans have shown that there are anatomically distinct reward areas for monetary gains (medial OFC) and monetary losses (lateral OFC) (reviewed in Rolls 2000; 2004). In humans the orbitofrontal cortex is activated by pleasant tastes and odors, pleasant touch sensations, and other pleasurable stimuli (de Araujo et al., 2003; Francis et al., 1999; O'Doherty, 2004; Rolls et al., 2003). Orbitofrontal cortex activity in rats, monkeys and humans also tracks changes in pleasure with constant food intake and the alliesthetic reductions in hedonic value caused by eating foods to satiety (Smith et al., 2009). For example, single neuron recording studies have shown that as a monkey becomes satiated on a given reinforcer (glucose syrup), neuronal firing rate in glucose specific cells in the OFC drops – a neural correlate of alliesthesia (Rolls, 2000; 2004). This evidence suggests that the OFC mediated hedonic response functions to reset the incentive values of goal objects, after an integration of information about the rewards' preexisting incentive value with the animal's need states.

OFC reward areas can become activated by conditioned as well as unconditioned incentives (e.g. sounds or sights that predict tasty food) indicating that stimuli associated with rewards can be just as liked as the actual goal of the instrumental action (Rolls, 2000; 2004). Stimuli that an animal learns are *predictive* of rewards (or punishments) – such as the sight of a food as well as the taste – can therefore have an incentive value as well as the rewards themselves. The OFC appears to be able to break or even reverse learned CS-reward associations very rapidly, as soon as the reward value of a conditioned incentive changes (Rolls, 2000; 2004). Lesions of the OFC destroys an individual's ability to track changing CS-reward contingencies and emotional responses may become dissociated from changing stimulus conditions, and persevere for long periods (Rolls, 1999).

Consistent with this *consummation phase* interpretation of OFC function are the brain-stimulation reward studies in which an electrode is implanted into a brain region and the animal can activate the flow of current at the electrode tip by pressing a lever. If a brain area is found where the animal is observed to continue pressing the lever compulsively as if the stimulation produces a pleasurable sensation it is taken as an indication that a brain reward area has been found. Laboratory animals will lever press at high rates (over 6,000 times per hour) to obtain brief stimulation pulses to certain brain regions (Olds and Milner, 1954). Brain stimulation reward effects have been documented for many OFC sites, suggesting pleasurable (as well as rewarding and reinforcing) emotions are experienced if these sites are activated. The amount of lever pressing an animal does to stimulate food related OFC reward sites, unlike reward sites in subcortical areas such as the nucleus accumbens, has been found to vary with the need state of the animal: if the animal is hungry it presses the lever vigorously, but when the animal has eaten, lever pressing ceases (Rolls, 1999). Thus the OFC integrates information about the reward's baseline incentive value with the animal's physiological need states, and this reflects the subjective experience of liking.

The Amygdala

The amygdala is the third major structure of the mammalian affective-motivational circuit, and it functions to form or strengthen associations between affectively neutral stimuli (CS) that reliably predict affectively charged events or stimuli (US). In the process the predictive stimuli take on affective significance themselves and via projections to the mesolimbic DA system can induce and invigorate motivated behaviors. According to Schultheiss & Wirth (2008), the amygdala can be characterized as a motivational 'homing-in' device allowing individuals to (a) learn rapidly about cues that signal proximity to a goal object, and (b) act in such a way that takes the individual from more distal to more proximal reward-predictive cues until the reward can be consumed – or conversely, to respond to punishment predictive warning signals either by freezing with increased vigilance or working actively at avoidance.

Loss of the amygdala leads to an inability to assess the motivational value of an object from a distance ('psychic blindness'). It is a key brain structure in Pavlovian conditioning, enabling Pavlovian associations to be formed between stimuli that do not initially carry any motivational meaning such as the sight of a juice drink (conditioned visual cue) with unconditioned rewards or punishers, if the former reliably predict the latter, such as the pleasant taste of the juice if it is drunk (UC reward) (LeDoux, 1996). It is also essential for second order reinforcement learning (Everitt, 1990). The amygdala receives input from almost all stages of sensory processing, and its response to lower level representations can guide motivated gaze – that is, enhanced focus on emotionally arousing features of the environment (Vuilleumier et al, 2004).

The amygdala is made up of a number of interconnected nuclei, two of which are key to emotional and motivated responses to CS and US. Through its central nucleus, the amygdala influences *emotional responses* mediated by hypothalamic and brainstem structures that can be characterized as physiological *arousal*. These responses include the release of stress hormones (e.g., cortisol) via the endocrine system, an increase in arousal and vigilance via activation of major neurotransmitter systems such as dopamine, and autonomic nervous system responses such as, pupil dilation, and increased blood pressure (LeDoux, 1996, 2002). Through its *basolateral nucleus* the amygdala influences the invigoration of *motivated action* to CS and UC through its projections to the nucleus accumbens. These two functions have been dissociated through lesion studies (Killross, Robbins & Everitt, 1997).

This concludes our review of what is known about the mammalian 'incentive motivation network'.

Chapter 3
Emotional Axes:
Psychology, Psychophysiology and Neuroanatomical Correlates

Didem Gökçay
Middle East Technical University, Turkey

ABSTRACT

For applications in affective computing, the quantitative representation provided by the dimensional view of emotions is very valuable. The dimensional account of emotions has gained impetus over the last decade, due to the consistent observation of two principal axes, valence and arousal, from several experiments on semantic maps. Interestingly, these two orthogonal components differentially modulate human physiology as measured by skin conductance, startle eyeblink and event related potentials. Furthermore, in the human brain there exists distinct localizations for valence/arousal-related emotion evaluation processes. Our current knowledge regarding these two basic components of emotion is presented in this chapter. The emotional palette varies widely through development and across populations. Two different models (Circumplex and PANA) have been coined to account for the vast distribution of data clustered across emotional categories. In this chapter, these models are also discussed comparatively.

INTRODUCTION

It has been slightly over a decade since the investigations regarding the role of emotions in cognitive functionality has gained popularity. Earlier, 'traditional approaches to the study of cognition emphasized an information-processing view that has generally excluded emotion' (Phelps, 2006). Then Damasio (1999) introduced the Somatic

Marker Hypothesis indicating that emotions interfere with the information processing streams of our brain through preserved somatic signals relating to the body-state structure and regulation either consciously or unconsciously. Nowadays the computer metaphor, which has inspired the human cognition studies is definitely augmented by a new player: affect. Although the main areas in the human brain that subserve emotional processing are already identified at the gross level (Pessoa, 2008), the nature of their interaction with

DOI: 10.4018/978-1-61692-892-6.ch003

each other, and the nature of their interference with cognitive processes remain elusive. This chapter is an attempt to clarify the dimensional approach to emotional processing, which can be briefly summarized as follows: The representation and expression of emotions is possible through a few orthogonal components. A data point along these components refer to the instantiation of a specific emotion, and emotion instances can be clustered creating emotional categories such as happiness, sadness, fear or anger. In the following sections, details about the main components of emotions will be introduced. However, it is important to mention that other than the dimensional account provided here, there is still ongoing research attempting to identify distinct physiological signatures that represent basic emotions. Most recent reviews in this regard can be found in Kreibig (2010) and Stephens et. al. (2010).

PRINCIPAL COMPONENTS OF AFFECT

The Layout of the Semantic Space

During the course of evolution, humans generated sophisticated responses for communicating the meaning of the situations they encounter. Many of these intentionally coded responses such as gestures, gross body movements and facial expressions are non-linguistic. Together with language, all of these expressions serve a single purpose: communicating the meaning of the complex environment that humans dwell. Through a series of experiments held during 1950's (Osgood, 1957), Osgood and his colleagues shed light on the nature of the redundancy embodied in the semantic space. According to Osgood, the semantic space consists of 2-5 principal components. Although there is some dependency between these components (as discussed later in the section on proposed models), after several decades and a plethora of experiments - not only involving verbal stimuli but

also involving sounds and pictures- two principal components prevail: valence (pleasantness) and arousal (activity).

The semantic space seems to be extremely wide, if we initiate voluntary free speech with a question such as: 'What does SOPHISTICATED mean?'

'It's being **clever** *and* **wise** *about people and things... It's sort of* **smooth** *and* **polished**, **graceful** *but not* **awkward**...**poised**, **savvy**' *(Osgood, 1957, p.18).*

On another front, associations indirectly bring out a somewhat similar response: 'What other things make you think of SOPHISTICATED?'

'Lady, cocktails, music, **educated**, **clever**, **smart**' *(Osgood, 1957, p.18-19)*

Although free expression is richer in terms of meaning, the overlap between free expression and associations point in the same direction: There exists a limited set of adjectives to be used to attribute meaning to a given verbal input. So Osgood and his colleagues started out to devise a methodology to generate a representative and standardized set of verbal responses across subjects. Needless to say, the ability for the human brain to generalize and think using metaphors helped this cause. 'Cotton' and 'stone' can be easily put on a scale of 'soft-hard' but so does 'mother' and 'bodyguard'. Similarly, 'loss' and 'win' can be directly defined on a scale of 'unfair-fair' but so does 'thunder' and 'breeze', albeit through metaphors. A representative layout of the entire semantic space can then be constructed through these semantic differences.

The 'semantic differential' technique is generated through the use of polar (i.e. opposite in meaning) adjective pairs each serving as an individual semantic dimension. For example in a semantic space of n dimensions, the adjective pairs might be: 1. 'good-bad', 2. 'soft-hard', 3. 'slow-fast',

Table 1. 4 principal factors extracted from the semantic space and some sample adjectives that contribute to these factors

Factor I (Evaluation)	Factor II (Potency)	Factor III (Activity)	Factor IV (Not named)
Good-bad	Hard-soft	Active-passive	Private-public
True-false	Strong-weak	Fast-slow	Small-large
Positive-negative	Opaque-transparent	Hot-cold	Constrained-free

…, n. 'bright-dark'. Each dimension is scaled the same way, for example on a 7 point Likert scale. Therefore, when we are asked to produce a response with respect to a given word (for ex. 'sun'), we will have to evaluate at what locations it would fit in each of these n scales. When several words representative of a vocabulary are evaluated in this manner, some of these n dimensions will group together and receive similar ratings almost all the time. By using factor analysis (or principal component analysis), we can determine which of these n different dimensions are correlated, and reduce the entire n-dimensional semantic space into m orthogonal dimensions such that m<<n. It is important to mention that each of the reduced m dimensions consists of a weighted (rotated) form of the original n dimensions. For example, the 'good-bad', 'bright-dark' dimensions specified above may receive high weightings in one of the emerging two principal components, pleasantness, whereas the 'slow-fast' dimension may receive a weighting close to zero for this component, because it is unrelated to this dimension.

The variance of the entire n dimensional data space may not be captured by the reduced m components. However, when eigenvalues corresponding to the rotated m dimensions are all greater than 1, we can safely assume that the reduced space is representative, although the new semantic space may now reflect approximately 50-80% of the variance of the original space. In one of their studies on 100 subjects, Osgood and his colleagues (Osgood, 1975, p.47-53), collected ratings from 20 new words (as well as those in a

previous study) along 76 dimensions. Four major dimensions are obtained which explained 41.1%, 20.5%, 16.0% and 11.5% of the variance respectively. Although these factors are not named, by studying the dimensions that contribute with high weightings to these factors, it becomes clear that the first three factors go along with the original naming of Osgood and his colleagues: Evaluation, Potency, and Activity. Table 1 (sampled from Osgood, 1957 p.53) illustrates a few adjective pairs contributing to these reduced four principal components.

As seen from this table, it is possible to obtain more than 2 principal components, however, among these components, Evaluation and Activity have been repeatedly emerging in follow-up studies whereas the variances represented by the other two components had not been replicated with the same consistency or turned out to be negligible in different samples/studies of the semantic space. There are some adjective pairs such as 'excitable-calm', which receive high weightings from multiple factors. Due to this, it is important to note that the data oriented along the new axes in the reduced space might have interactions. Nevertheless, the basic two components, named as Evaluation and Activity are consistently replicated for subject populations across different ages (Osgood, 1975, p. 58) and cultures (Osgood, 1975, chap. 4).

The semantic space studies at our times can be performed with more words and more dimensions, owing to the accessibility of high computing power. One of the most recent extensive vocabulary compilations done by Samsonovic and Ascoli (2010) yielded three axes: "good-bad" (valence), "calm-excited" (arousal), and "open-closed" (freedom). In this study, the dictionary of synonyms and antonyms extracted from the thesaurus of MS Office and Princeton WordNet are used. The word list is constructed by starting from an initial seed word, adding the corresponding synonyms and antonyms to the list in an iterative fashion. Synonyms and antonyms are assembled into bidirectional pairs and words with less than two synonym/antonym links are cleared, yielding with 15000-20000 core words for English. Then varying n from 10 to 100, the location of each word in the core list is computed automatically from a function which measures the word's distance from the given n dimensions through the number of its synonym/antonym links. After all the core words are mapped onto the n dimensional space, the principal components are extracted, once again returning valence and arousal as two prominent factors.

Among all semantic space studies of English, the most widely used one is inarguably ANEW (Bradley and Lang, 1999a). In this study, Bradley and Lang assumed that the three principal components of the semantic map are valence, arousal and dominance. With this assumption, on a 9 point scale, they collected evaluations from the subjects directly on these three principal components, rather than a higher dimensional adjective-pair scale space. A total of 1034 words are evaluated and the evaluation on the three scales are facilitated by the use of an icon named SAM, which contains a range of different expressions at different scale points (a smile … frown on SAM's face to represent the valence scale, a jittery … calm sketch on SAM's body to represent the arousal scale and a small … large SAM figure to represent the dominance scale). The data distribution emerging from this semantic map directly puts the words on the reduced semantic space consisting of three orthogonal axes, so there is no need for factor analysis. Affective word norms can be generated

in this fashion, by averaging the ratings of all subjects for each word and scale.

Another study is worth mentioning due to the different technique employed in generating the original n dimensional semantic space. As mentioned above, meaning is a construct derived from not only words but also from gestures and facial expressions. Fontaigne et. al. (2007) created a 144 dimensional affective space by using distinct verbal descriptions derived from the main characteristics of emotions such as: appraisals of events, psychophysiological changes, motor expressions, action tendencies, subjective experiences. Some sample verbal descriptions are as follows: 'treated unjustly', 'irrevocable loss' (appraisal of events), 'felt heartbeat slowing down', 'blushed' (psychophysiological change), 'frowned' (motor expression), 'produced abrupt body movements', 'spoke faster' (action tendency), 'felt nervous', 'felt tired' (subjective experience). On the other hand, 24 emotion words are chosen to be rated along these 144 dimensions on a 9 point Likert scale. These emotion words are: anger, anxiety, being hurt, compassion, contempt, contentment, despair, disappointment, disgust, fear, guilt, happiness, hate, interest, irritation, jealousy, joy, love, pleasure, pride, sadness, shame, stress, surprise. Subsets of emotion words are administered to 198 subjects and their ratings are collected on all 144 dimensions. After factor analysis, 4 principal components are extracted: Evaluation, Potency, Activity and Unpredictability. Altogether, these components explained for 75.4% of the variance of the distribution in the original affective space.

The semantic map studies in English are repeated over the years for other languages as well. BAWL-R (Vo et.al., 2009) contains imageability, valence and arousal ratings for approximately 2900 German words (2,107 nouns, 504 verbs, 291 adjectives). In another study on German words (Lahl et. al., 2009), Internet is utilized to collect concreteness, valence and arousal ratings for 2,654 German nouns from 3,907 subjects. Spanish version of ANEW is made available by Redondo et.

Figure 1. a) Mert icon for data collection along the affective axes, b) The distribution of TUDADEN data across valence and arousal axes

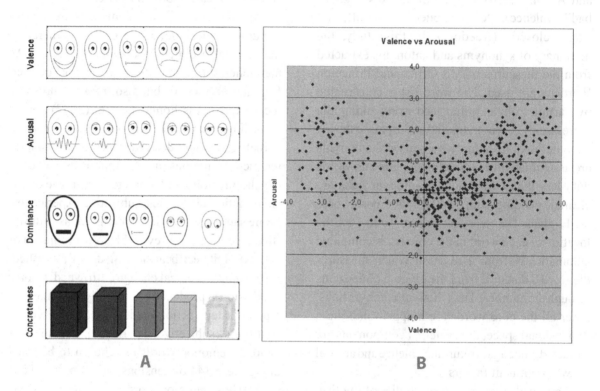

al (2007), providing mean affective ratings on the 3 major axes valence, arousal, dominance from 720 subjects. In our lab, through a joint study with M.A. Smith (Gokcay and Smith, 2007), we used a methodology similar to ANEW for generating mean evaluations for 1240 Turkish words from a subject pool of 170. Parallel sessions technique of MS Access is used to generate 200 word ratings from each subject for 4 dimensions valence, arousal, dominance and concreteness, and all of the ratings are merged into the same database called TUDADEN. Figure 1a illustrates the MERT icon we used for collecting online evaluations for each scale. Mean ratings of the words are plotted in the scatter-plot seen in figure 1b for the valence and arousal scales. In this graph, each point corresponds to a single word's valence and arousal ratings averaged across all subjects. It is important to note that not all the data quadrants are filled when ratings are collected from the

subjects directly in the reduced space of principal components. This is an important feature that is discussed below, in the section on models of the principal affective components.

When the adjective lists contributing to the principal affective components are considered, one might think that the principle components extracted from the semantic space are byproducts of verbal/cognitive processes rather than affective processes. This thought might have been agreeable if these principal components were obtained exclusively for the word lists but not for auditory or visual stimuli. However, as discussed in the section on ANS responses below, numerous studies conducted on visual and auditory stimuli reveal that words, pictures and sounds with similar valence and arousal ratings cause similar changes in the autonomic responses of subjects. Therefore the validity of the affective principal components has been verified across multiple stimulus modalities. IAPS (Lang et.al. 2008) and IADS (Bradley and Lang, 1999b, Redondo et.al, 2008), consisting of pictures and sounds respectively, provide two widely used stimulus sets with ratings along the three principal components, valence, arousal and dominance. A study conducted by Faith and Thayer (2001) supports very clearly that the principal components extracted from the semantic space relate to affect because in this study, subjects provided conscious, reflexive evaluations regarding their emotions in response to facial expressions, IAPS pictures, mental imagery and music. The evaluations are made for 15 emotion terms: afraid, agitated, amused, angry, aroused, disgusted, happy, interested, pleasant, relaxed, sad, serene, still, surprised, tired. Principal component analysis revealed 4 factors with eigenvalues above 1, explaining 35.8%, 15.4%, 10.2% and 7.2% of the variance. When emotional categories with high weightings for these factors are investigated, once again, the first two factors are found to be valence and arousal, while the other two factors turned out to be uninterpretable.

It still remains open whether verbal self-reports in response to emotionally loaded stimuli reflect the phenomenological feelings induced on the subjects or reflect just semantic understanding of the emotional words that are being rated. Barett (2004) investigated this aspect by conducting a series of experiments asking each subject to cross-rate emotion words as well as self-report their instantaneous feelings in response to: 1. A set of emotion-laden slides, 2. Pre-designed emotion inducing scenarios in their lab environment, 3. A beeper inquiring the subject's current emotional state for a 60 day period. To obtain a baseline, subjects rated the relationship between 16 emotion words on a 7 point Likert scale. In these semantic ratings, there was an overall bias for differentiation along the arousal axis. Subjects also rated their current emotional feelings in one of the above-mentioned three experimental setups for 88 emotion-related adjectives. For these

reflexive ratings, there was an overall bias for more differentiation along the valence axis. In sum, Barett (2004) showed that self-report ratings not only relate to phenomenological feelings, but also identify individual differences between the subjects.

Overall, collection of emotional evaluations over emotional verbal descriptions has proven to be a valid methodology to delineate the major components of our affective map.

Models for the Principal Affective Components

While the existence of two major emotional axes is inarguable, how to model the data distribution after reducing the original data distribution from n dimensions down to 2 dimensions has been problematic. The controversy created over modeling is centered on multiple issues:

1.   Why does the two dimensional data distribution sometimes fill all quarters, but at other times fill only two quarters?
2.   Is there a correlation between valence and arousal?
3.   How does the data in the two dimensions relate to the six basic emotions: happiness, sadness, fear, anger, surprise and disgust?
4.   What is the variability of the data distribution within and between subject populations?

Figure 2 is developed in an effort to answer these questions altogether. In this figure, our sample data distribution from TUDADEN (Gokcay and Smith, 2008) is merged with axes names taken from Russell (1980) and Watson et. al. (1999) along with 24 commonly used emotional categories (including the six basic emotions). Russell (1980) named the two principal emotional axes such that, the horizontal axis measures misery versus pleasure (valence) and the vertical axis measures sleepiness versus arousal (arousal). He also considered that there is another two di-

Figure 2. The axes and emotion categories of the Circumplex model, along with the axes and data distribution of the PANA model

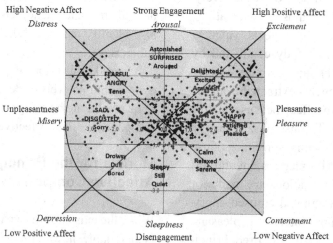

mensional orthogonal coordinate system rotated 45 degrees. In this system, one axis measures depression versus excitement and the other axis measures distress versus contentment. Russell always referred to the main axes as pleasure versus arousal, considering the other pair of axes as a means for explaining the data distribution within quarters. On the other hand, as seen in Figure 2, Watson et. al. (1999) posited that the main axes are the ones rotated 45° CCW. They named the first main axis as: PA (positive affect) which is used to measure low positive affect versus high positive affect. The second axis was named as: NA (negative affect) measuring low negative affect versus high negative affect. The other axes in Watson et.al.'s (1999) coordinate system were used as scales of pleasantness and engagement.

Issue 1: Models of data distribution

According to the **Circumplex model** (Russell 1980), when the original data in the n dimensional emotional space is projected into the two dimensional reduced space along the valence and arousal axes, the data distribution becomes similar to a doughnut shape. Although we are unable to show this in figure 2, we have shown how these data clusters would be distributed within point clouds of discrete emotions. For example, within the vicinity of the arousal axis, we expect a data distribution that reflects emotion terms similar to sleepy, still, quiet when arousal is low and astonished, surprised, aroused when arousal is high. All other point clouds anticipated within the circumplex distribution are observable from Figure 2. There exist several studies in support of this model (Barett, 2004; Terraciano et.al. 2003; Fontaine et.al. 2007, Faith and Thayer, 2001, Sauter, 2006).

According to the **PANA model** (Watson et. al., 1999), the main axes are the positive affect and negative affect axes, obtained by 45 degree rotation of the valence/arousal axes. The data distribution on these axes resemble a bumerang shape as seen from figure 1 b. In this approach, discrete emotional categories are not the main founding factors underlying behaviour, but approach and avoidance is. The points clustered within the vicinity of high positive affect are obtained from responses to stimuli that create approach behaviour. On the other hand, the avoidance behaviour is initiated as a result of the emotional evaluation represented by the points clustered around high negative affect. There are several studies supporting this type of data distribution (Bradley ANEW, Bradley IADS, Lang, 2008, Mikels, 2005; Libkuman, 2007; Rubin, 2009; Redondo2, 2008; Redondo1, 2007; Vo, 2009).

The study conducted by Rubin and Talarico (2009) point out the common methodologies between researches that support the Circumplex model versus PANA model. In studies which return data that comply with the Circumplex model, emotional ratings are done in a high dimensional space where n is varying between 15-140 and then the data distribution in two dimensions is obtained by principal component analysis. On the other hand, in studies which comply with the PANA model, the emotional ratings are collected directly on the two reduced dimensions. This observation indicates that there might be two different processes for evaluating the emotion scales: In the first process, the subjects go through extensive inquiries regarding the stimulus that is currently presented. In the second process, the subjects are presented a limited opportunity to weigh the emotional value of the stimulus (pleasantness versus intensity (arousal)). Therefore in the second process, the subjects have to filter-out all the other factors, deciding only about the importance of the stimulus in regards to a more goal-oriented framework. Needless to say, the evaluations performed weighing more attributes are richer, however the evaluations performed weighing only two attributes is faster and satisfy the crucial approach/avoidance need of humans.

Issue 2: Correlation between valence and arousal

When the Circumplex model is considered, the data does not comply with a specific valence/arousal pattern, so a correlation between the quantities measured by valence and arousal is not supported. However, when the PANA model

is considered, there is a clear pattern for the data distribution, indicating an interaction between these two axes. In Vo (2009), the nature of this interaction is revealed by curve-fitting. For this specific study, arousal is found to be related to valence with a quadratic function: $0.15x^2-0.25x+2.53$, $R^2=0.37$ (similar to the dashed line in figure 2). Conceptually, valence is distributed in a bi-polar fashion such that arousal increases when valence extends towards extremely positive or extremely negative values. But for low values of valence, regardless of the polarity, arousal is almost always low.

Issue 3: The relationship of the models with six basic emotions

Given emotional evaluations on either emotional words or valence/arousal axes, emotional categories are clustered into point clouds as illustrated in figure 2 (Among these emotional classes, six basic emotions are shown with capital letters). Unfortunately, the PANA model's ability in capturing emotional categories is limited. The scatter of the data is sparse in the lower quadrants (representing drowsy, dull, bored, sleepy, still, quiet, calm, relaxed, serene) as well as the left hand side of the valence axis (sad, sorry, disgusted). On the other hand, in the Circumplex model, although the data may not always be homogeneously distributed, almost all quadrants are represented. Hence this model supports the existence of six basic emotions, and a much larger emotional palette. As indicated before, the underlying concept behind the PANA model is goal-oriented behavior. If we approach from this direction, the emotional categories which does not reinforce goal-oriented behaviour (such as bored, calm, sad) become obsolete, whereas the emotional categories that support approach (such as excited, happy) and avoidance (such as fearful, angry) are essential. Interestingly, there have been several statistical attempts for predicting the distribution of valence/arousal from emotional categories or vice versa using words (Stevenson et. al., 2007), sounds (Stevenson and James, 2008) and pictures (Mikels et. al. 2005, Libkuman et. al. 2007) as stimuli. However, the predictive power between the principal components and distinct emotional categories is not found to be as high as expected. This might be partially due to the scarce representation of some emotional categories. Another factor prohibiting automatic emotion identification from the emotional axes is the variability involved in the data distribution between individual subjects, as well as populations.

Issue 4: Variability of the data distribution within and between subject populations

Variability of the emotional evaluation within the same individual occurs during the course of the day, or during larger time periods. It is also possible for some subjects to be more arousal oriented while others are more valence oriented. And finally among populations, some trends can be observed due to personality traits or other gross factors such as professional training. Watson et. al. (1999) studied variation of the arousal and valence ratings in their PANA model during the course of the day within 2 hour intervals. The ratings along the negative affect axis did not show much change throughout the day, but the ratings along the positive affect axis changed such that the ratings are low early in the morning and late at night, but higher during the day until the evening. Posner et. al. (2005) investigated the Circumplex distribution in school children, and found that in this population the data is collapsed along the valence axis. Unpleasantness extent of the valence axis coded fear, anger and sadness, while the Pleasantness extent coded excitement, happiness and contentment, without much difference along the arousal axis for these emotions. Terraciano et. al. (2003) studied personality traits based on the data distribution along the Circumplex. In the facet O3 (Openness to Feelings) of the Revised NEO Personality Inventory, individual differences in attentiveness to inner feelings and affective experi-

ences is assessed where high scorers experience deeper and more differentiated emotional states. Subjects with high scores on the O3 returned a wider range of emotions distributed along the Circumplex, while subjects with low O3 returned emotions distributed similar to the PANA model, occupying only the upper two quadrants.

Overall, depending on the population, we can say that when the n dimensional data collected from multiple subjects (or from the same subject over a period of time) is reduced to 2 dimensions by PCA, the scaling of the data distribution across the axes, as well as the location of the specific emotion clusters may differ. Some subjects may have a flatter emotion class distribution across the valence or arousal axis (Barett, 2004), whereas other subjects may have a distribution reflecting the Circumplex in a better way. In addition, the location of the emotional classes might be shifted across quadrants.

NERVOUS SYSTEM RESPONSES TO AFFECTIVE STIMULI

Autonomic Nervous System (ANS) Responses

A while ago, Lang et.al. (1993) showed that our body's autonomic response to emotionally evocative stimuli differs with respect to the valence or arousal content of the stimuli. While arousal modulates sweating as measured by skin conductance response (SCR), valence modulates startle as measured by eyeblink (startle eyeblink reflex). Table 2 summarizes the change of psychophysiology measurements with respect to the major affective components.

In an experimental paradigm which inspired psychophysiology research onwards, Lang et. al. (1993) measured psychophysiological signals in response to affective pictures chosen from IAPS. Pictures are shown for 6 sec, and then the screen goes dark for a variable period between 20-35 sec

Table 2. Psychophysiological measures related to the two principal components, valence and arousal

Emotional Axis	Contributing factor	Observed correlation
Valence	Startle eyeblink magnitude	Negatively correlated with increasing valence
	Startle eyeblink latency	Positively correlated with increasing valence
Arousal	Skin conductance magnitude	Positively correlated with increasing arousal
	Pupil dilation	Increase in dilation for high arousal stimuli with respect to neutral stimuli

while ratings are collected using the affective scales (valence, arousal) printed on the SAM icon. The skin conductance response is measured for the entire 6 sec as well as a baseline period of 2 sec beforehand. This response has a slowly rising and slowly falling pattern. The startle eyeblink response is not collected in this study, but a similar measure, facial muscle activity, (corrugator) is. Other measures such as heart rate, facial muscle response (zygomatic), viewing time are also collected. Recently, a replication of this study is done by Sanchez-Navarro (2008), in which startle eyeblink response is collected. The startle is induced by an acoustic white noise probe which comes on randomly either 3.5 or 4.5 sec after stimulus onset. This response builds up abruptly, hence must be sampled at a high frequency of 900-1000 Hz.

In both studies, factor analysis among all the pschophysiology data as well as the subjects' valence and arousal ratings revealed two principal components: valence and arousal. The valence axis was loaded positively by the valence ratings, and negatively by the corrugator/startle eyeblink magnitude. On the other hand, the arousal axis was loaded positively by the arousal ratings, skin conductance magnitude and viewing time. These findings implicate that even without looking at the individual emotional evaluations from the subjects, by inspecting the startle eyeblink and skin conductance responses, emotional appraisal of the subject can be predicted respectively in terms of valence and arousal.

- **Startle eyeblink response:** The magnitude of the eyeblink response is larger for unpleasant stimuli, and smaller for pleasant stimuli. Therefore there exists a negative correlation between the valence values and eyeblink magnitude (Lang. et. al, 1993). Another study (Sanchez-Navarro, et. al. 2008) which took the startle latency into account returned a high weighting for startle latency along the valence axis after factor analysis. Correlation of startle latency with valence resulted in a positive linear trend causing increased startle latencies for increasing values of valence. Interestingly, a different trend in eyeblink modulation is observed when static pictures are used versus the utilization of dynamic pictures. Lang and Bradley (2010) observed that in a predator prey simulation, when pictures of a closing gun are shown back to back, the startle eyeblink magnitude becomes increasingly inhibited, reversing the negative correlation between startle magnitude and valence.

- **Skin conductance response:** The magnitude of the skin conductance response is larger for intensely arousing stimuli, and smaller for stimuli with less arousal intensity. Therefore there exists a positive correlation between the arousal intensity and skin conductance response (Lang. et. al, 1993). In a recent study (Bradley. et. al., 2008) it is observed that pupil dilation is strongly correlated with arousal. After the presentation of a visual stimulus, a con-striction reflex of the pupil occurs due to the intensity change. Successively, as the stimulus is being viewed, the pupil starts to dilate. Pupil dilation is modulated by arousal intensity, as long as the valence values are high in a bipolar fashion: high in pleasantness or high in unpleasantness.

Before concluding this section, it is important to note that the interaction between valence and arousal is observed in psychophysiological data as well. When factor analysis is performed, the measures which load the valence axis with high weights do not receive completely negligible weights along the arousal axis and vice versa. It is commonly observed that valence-related measures load the arousal axes and vice versa with weights approximately in the range of 0.15. It is also worth to mention that, due to the limited space, only a few major autonomic responses are discussed here. Several different measures relating to respiration and cardiac pulsation are also found to be correlated with valence and arousal, as listed exhaustively in Kreibig (2010).

Brain Activation Patterns

Event Related Potentials (ERP) or functional Magnetic Resonance Imaging (fMRI) reveal the brain's physiological response to emotion-laden stimuli (Please see key terms and definitions for brief descriptions of the ERP signal and fMRI signal). Since in this chapter, we are exclusively interested in how emotional axes are manifested, we will concentrate on the manipulation and localization of brain activity with respect to plain evaluative processing of the principal axes, valence and arousal, leaving out how complex cognitive processes such as memory, decision-making are affected by emotions.

Prediction of Emotional Axes from the ERP Signals

In a most recent review (Oloffson et. al. 2008), ERP results obtained over decades for visual stimuli are compiled together. The literature based on event related potientials (ERP) indicates that the processing of affective stimuli distributed along the two principal components valence and arousal differ. Overall, the results show that the valence component modulates subtly the early part (100-150 msec) of the ERP signal whereas the arousal component modulates strongly the late part (300-1000 msec). In an effort to illustrate how the ERP signal changes, we have devised a sketch in figure 3. Since this type of processing pertains to both subliminally (duration 25-35 msec) and consciously (duration comparable to seconds) presented affective stimuli, affective processing can be considered as being an integral part of perception. (Oloffson et. al. 2008) interpret the early changes in the ERP signal as a reflection of selective attentional processes. However, they believe that the late modulation is due to a demand for attentional resource allocation –caused by appetitive and aversive action requirements as well as enhanced memory processing.

- **Changes in ERP due to valence:** In general, unpleasant stimuli is found to have stronger effects than pleasant or neutral ones, producing larger positive amplitudes around 100 msec (P1). This early modulation points to amygdala focused negativity processing. The ERP processing in this time range is also shown to be affected by stimulus complexity (Bradley et. al 2007), which is in line with the attentional processes in charge with saliency detection.
- **Changes in ERP due to arousal:** An arousal related positivity occurs in the ERP signal within the range of 200 msec (Please see discussion in Oloffson et. al., 2008). Usually 200-300 msec range of the

Figure 3. A sketch of the ERP signal in response to affective stimuli occurring at t=0 (Adapted from Rozenkrants and Polich (2008))

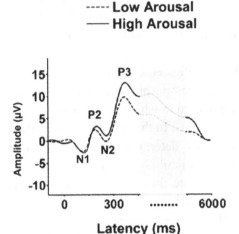

ERP signal is affected by stimulus discrimination and response selection processes, however, a negativity is reported for arousing stimuli in comparison to neutral stimuli in this time frame regardless of valence (for both pleasant or unpleasant pictures) and task (either passive viewing or target detection). Later, starting from 300 msec on, a strong arousal induced positive signal (P300) builds up, and remains potentiated for a long period in the range of seconds. Cutberth et. al (2000) asked subjects to view pleasant and unpleasant highly arousing stimuli, as well as neutral stimuli for about 6 sec and then evaluate the valence and arousal of these pictures. Pleasant stimuli consisted of erotic images and unpleasant stimuli consisted of violence. A negative build up in the ERP signal is observed for unpleasant images approximately 100 msec after picture onset, and a positive increase in the ERP signal is observed for all emotional pictures (regardless of valence) after 300 msec, which remained high for the entire 6 sec. In another study,

Rozenkrants and Polich (2008) constructed an emotional visual oddball paradigm. Subjects are asked to press a button when they detect a picture among continually presented images of patches. The patches occurred with a rate of 60% and pictures occurred with a rate of 40%. The pictures consisted of 4 categories: Pleasant and low arousal, unpleasant and low arousal, pleasant and high arousal, unpleasant and high arousal. The results were in alignment with those presented by Cutberth et. al (2000), such that the late positive potential was observed only for the high arousal categories, and was extended in the order of seconds. In an effort to summarize these findings, we have devised the generic transparent box in figure 3, showing that the distinction between the highly arousing versus neutral stimuli persists in the ERP signal for a duration of a few seconds.

In sum, the sustained late positive signal indicates the importance of the intensity of arousal. Interestingly the high ERP signal which extends for seconds persists mostly unhabituated even after 90 repetitions of the same stimulus (Lang and Bradley 2010). As pointed out by Oloffson et. al. (2008) as well as Lang and Bradley (2010), such a strong effect might be due to top-down processes in the production motivational responses.

Localization of Emotional Axes by fMRI

It is of great interest to find out whether the affective principal components are localized on dissociable brain systems. Current research indicates that valence and arousal are processed by distinct brain areas; however, the operation of these areas in the evaluation of emotions does not seem to be entirely separable. fMRI research on emotions center mostly on the localization of joint emotional and cognitive processes within decision making, memory, and attention, or perceptive processes modulated by emotion. Therefore, fMRI studies that focus exclusively on the evaluative processing of the principal axes, valence and arousal, are scarce. Here we will summarize only two studies in this regard.

In one study (Anders et.al., 2004), ANS outputs such as SCR, startle eyeblink are collected along with fMRI, as well as valence arousal ratings from the subjects while they viewed emotional and neutral pictures chosen from IAPS. The fMRI signal of each voxel in the brain is correlated with either ratings of the subjects or ANS responses. The ratings and ANS responses are used as separate regressors for the prediction of the observed fMRI signal (This procedure is called General Linear Model). High correlations of the fMRI signal with the valence ratings are observed within voxels around the Insula. On the other hand, voxels that correlated with the arousal ratings are observed around the Thalamus and Caudate. The startle eyeblink response was centered in the parietal region and Amygdala while the SCR response was centered in the orbitofrontal cortex (OFC).

In another study (Lewis et.al., 2007), fMRI is collected by using words from ANEW such that the words had either highly pleasant or highly unpleasant ratings with arousals ranging from neutral to high. The subjects are asked to perform a self-referential task and indicate with a button whether the presented word could be used to describe themselves. Regressors are defined using the ratings from ANEW. The fMRI signal in each voxel is attempted to be defined with these regressors. The voxels which can be defined with high values of both pleasant and unpleasant words (bipolar valence), are found to be located in the ventral and subgenual parts of the ACC. On the other hand, brain areas defined by the regressor constructed from the intensity of arousal are detected on Caudate, Ventral Striatum, Thalamus, Amygdala, Insula and brain stem (VT).

It is important to note that data acquisition through fMRI has a resolution on the order of seconds. The above reported brain areas respond-

ing to valence and arousal are observed to become active within ranges of 3-12 seconds.

A Neural Network Proposal Based on the Current Emotional Models and Neuroimaging Findings

Earlier, Phillips et.al. (2003, p.505), have suggested a processing pipeline for emotion appraisal and regulation in which stimulus processing occurs iteratively. In this model, initially, the emotional state is determined by appraisal. Then by excitatory or inhibitory modulation of the current emotional state, the next emotional state is determined, and also the appraisal step is reinitiated. This flow is repeated over and over defining successive emotional states through appraisal and regulation. Considering this pipeline, I have generated figure 4, to illustrate how key players in the brain may come together to generate the data distribution across the valence and arousal axes. Some of the key players as we know from the neuroscience and neuroimaging literatures (Posner et.al., 2005; Pessoa, 2008) are: Nucleus Accumbens (NA), Amygdala (Amg), Thalamus (Thal), Hypothalamus (Hypothal), Orbitofrontal Cortex (OFC), Lateral Prefrontal Cortex (LPFC), and Anterior Cingulate Cortex (ACC). Obviously for generality, we should add the Ventral Striatum -not just Accumbens- and Reticular Formation to the nodes, but for clarity of the figure, every component of the limbic system is not included.

According to figure 4, emotional evaluation proceeds as follows: Initially, the environmental input gets evaluated within our neural network consisting of the nodes inside the Appraisal box. Based on the ERP research, we know that this initial appraisal happens within the range of 300 msec. During initial appraisal, the Circumplex form of emotional state layout is produced in the 2 dimensional space of valence and arousal. However, as indicated by Norris et.al (2010), within our complex environment, valence can be activated bi-modally. For example, a thirsty animal may evaluate the sight of a pond as positive and arousing, but this animal may also realize that predators are nearby, adding a negative and arousing evaluation for the entire situation. Norris et. al (2010) postulates that valence is a bi-variate entity, which is modeled in our network as positive valence (+VAL) and negative valence (-VAL). I claim that the initial appraisal is fast, and captures all of the circumplex, providing detailed emotional differentiation. In this evaluation, NA, AMG, Thal might have higher weights than the other nodes of our network (as indicated by bold borders). At this point the second stage starts, which inputs all the current output from the brain nodes, as well as the emotional state indicated by the outputs of the arousal (ARO) and valence nodes (±VAL). The second stage of processing consists of goal-oriented/motivational or regulatory analysis. In this stage, the inputs to the network are processed to reach a target. This target might be a better emotional state (as in regulation) or the initiation of an approach/avoid response. Needless to say, prefrontal mechanisms as represented by LPFC and ACC have a higher weight at this stage. This is why these nodes are shown bold-weighted. This type of processing is

late, on the order of 3-6 seconds as we know from the ERP literature, and generates an emotional evaluation as represented by the PANA model. Going back to our example above, the ACC and LPFC interact to resolve the conflict between drinking from the pond to satisfy the animal's thirst versus escaping elsewhere to avoid the predators. Iterations between the appraisal and motivation phases occur through the recurrent connections of the outputs as indicated on the left part of figure 4. The role of the OFC might change over the iterations, becoming highly weighted in one phase versus the other. It is important to mention that, although not shown in this figure, the network nodes have lateral connections among themselves at every processing stage.

Obviously the model described herein is completely hypothetical, since such a model has not been implemented yet. However, in its current form, it supports the early (valence modulation) and late (arousal modulation) processes observed in the ERPs as well as the bi-modal activation of the valence component observed in both fMRI (Lewis et.al., 2007), and pupil dilation (Bradley et. al., 2008), along with both Circumplex and PANA data distributions. In order to test this

Figure 4. A neural network model of iterative evaluative processes in emotion

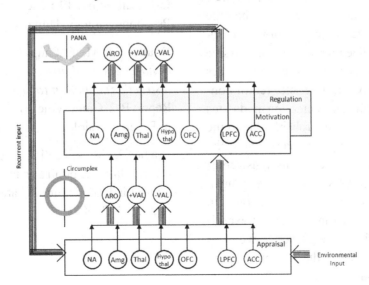

model, experiments should be designed to dissociate the appraisal and motivational processes. Needless to say, to identify which brain areas play what kind of a role, at what time, the data collection has to be made in a multi-modal fashion, preferably using simultaneous EEG and fMRI. Furthermore, in these experiments, complex stimuli rather than single words or pictures should be used, to reflect the situations in daily life representing all sorts of emotions around the circumplex. This model might also be extended by using replicas of the boxes to represent right and left hemispheres. As known in the emotion research, the right and left hemispheres assume differential roles in emotional processing and this can be incorporated into our model as well (see Harmon-Jones et. al (2010) for a recent review on emotional lateralization).

CONCLUSION

Over the last few decades, factor analyses of emotion words, as well as ANS/ERP/fMRI responses to affective stimuli, have consistently found two main factors that account for most of the emotional variance: valence and arousal. The data distributed along these axes reflect how emotions are evaluated: when the data occupies all quadrants, emotional differentiation is at is best, when the data occupies only the top two quadrants, a motivational tendency due to appetitive or aversive exposures is revealed. However, behavioral studies of attention, memory, priming, etc. return conflicting results regarding how emotion modulates cognitive processes. This is probably due to the lack of standardized attempts for manipulating the experiments across a matrix of conscious versus unconscious, appraisal versus motivation-related, and voluntary versus spontaneous behaviours. In addition, the stimuli used in the current experiments are too simplistic, using discrete events or happenings, despite the fact that humans operate in dynamically situated complex environments which reflect a larger emotional palette. Inarguably, these factors should be taken into account to deepen our knowledge regarding the effect of emotional processes in cognition. Our improved understanding in this regard will definitely enhance the applications within the newly emerging field of affective computing.

REFERENCES

Anders, S., Lotze, M., Erb, M., Grodd, W., & Birbaumer, N. (2004). Brain Activity Underlying Emotional Valence and Arousal: A Response-Related fMRI Study. *Human Brain Mapping*, *23*, 200–209.

Barrett, L. F. (2004). Feelings or Words? Understanding the Content in Self-Report Ratings of Experienced Emotion. *Journal of Personality and Social Psychology*, *87*(2), 266–281.

Bradley, M. M., Hamby, S., Low, A., & Lang, P. J. (2007). Brain potentials in perception: picture complexity and emotional arousal. *Psychophysiology*, *44*, 364–373.

Bradley, M. M., & Lang, P. J. (1999a). *Affective norms for English words (ANEW): Instruction manual and affective ratings*. Technical Report C-1. Gainesville, FL: The Center for Research in Psychophysiology, University of Florida.

Bradley, M. M., & Lang, P. J. (1999b). *International affective digitized sounds (IADS): Stimuli, instruction manual and affective ratings*. Technical Report B-2. Gainesville, FL: Center for Research in Psychophysiology, University of Florida.

Bradley, M. M., Miccoli, L., Escrig, M. A., & Lang, P. J. (2008). The pupil as a measure of emotional arousal and autonomic activation. *Psychophysiology*, *45*, 602–607.

Cuthbert, B. N., Schupp, H. T., Bradley, M. M., Birbaumer, N., & Lang, P. J. (2000). Brain potentials in affective picture processing: covariation with autonomic arousal and affective report. *Biological Psychology, 52,* 95–111.

Damasio, A. R. (1996). The Somatic Marker Hypothesis and the Possible Functions of the prefrontal cortex. *Philosophical Transactions of the Royal Society of London. Series B, Biological Sciences, 351,* 1413–1420.

Faith, M., & Thayer, J. F. (2001). A dynamical systems interpretation of a dimensional model of emotion. *Scandinavian Journal of Psychology, 42,* 121–133.

Fontaine, J., Scherer, K., Roesch, E., & Ellsworth, P. (2007). The world of emotions is not two-dimensional. *Psychological Science, 18*(12), 1050–1057.

Gökçay, D., & Smith, M. A. (2008). TÜDADEN:Türkçede Duygusal ve Anlamsal Değerlendirmeli Norm Veri Tabanı. *Proceedings of Brain-Computer Workshop,* 4.

Harmon-Jones, E., Gable, P. A., & Peterson, C. K. (2010). The role of asymmetric frontal cortical activity in emotion-related phenomena: A review and update. *Biological Psychology, 84,* 451–462.

Kreibig, S. D. (2010). Autonomic nervous system activity in emotion: A review. *Biological Psychology, 84,* 394–421.

Lahl, O., Göritz, A. S., Pietrowsky, R., & Rosenberg, J. (2009). Using the World-Wide Web to obtain large-scale word norms: 190,212 ratings on a set of 2,654 German nouns. *Behavior Research Methods, 41*(1), 13–19.

Lang, P. J., & Bradley, M. M. (2010). Emotion and the motivational brain. *Biological Psychology, 84*(3), 437–450.

Lang, P. J., Bradley, M. M., & Cuthbert, B. N. (2008). *International affective picture system (IAPS): Affective ratings of pictures and instruction manual.* Technical Report A-8. Gainesville, FL: University of Florida.

Lang, P. J., Reenwald, M. K. C., Bradley, M. M., & Hamm, A. O. (1993). Looking at pictures: Affective, facial, visceral, and behavioral reactions. *Psychophysiotogy, 30,* 261–273.

Lewis, P. A., Critchley, H. D., Rotshtein, P., & Dolan, R. J. (2007). Neural Correlates of Processing Valence and Arousal in Affective Words. *Cerebral Cortex, 17,* 742–748.

Libkuman, T. M., Otani, H., Kern, R., Viger, S. G., & Novak, N. (2007). Multidimensional normative ratings for the International Affective Picture System. *Behavior Research Methods, 39,* 326–334.

Mikels, J. A., Fredrickson, B. L., Larkin, G. R., Lindberg, C. M., & Reuter-Lorenz, P. A. (2005). Emotional category data on images from the International Affective Picture System. *Behavior Research Methods, 37*(4), 626–630.

Norris, C. J., Gollan, J., Berntson, G. G., & Cacioppo, J. T. (2010). The current status of research on the structure of evaluative space. *Biological Psychology, 84,* 422–436.

Olofsson, J. K., Nordin, S., Sequeira, H., & Polich, J. (2008). Affective picture processing: An integrative review of ERP findings. *Biological Psychology, 77,* 247–265.

Osgood, C. E., May, W. E., & Miron, M. S. (1975). *Cross cultural univrsals of affective meaning.* University of Illinois Press.

Osgood, C. E., Suci, G. J., & Tannenbaum, P. H. (1957). *The measurement of meaning.* University of Illinois Press.

Pessoa, L. (2008). On the relationship between emotion and cognition. *Nature Reviews. Neuroscience, 9,* 148–158.

Phelps, E. A. (2006). Emotion and Cognition: Insights from Studies of the Human Amygdala. *Annual Review of Psychology, 57,* 27–53.

Phillips, M. L., Drevets, W. C., Rauch, S. L., & Lane, R. (2003). Neurobiology of Emotion Perception I: The Neural Basis of Normal Emotion Perception. *Biological Psychiatry, 54,* 504–514.

Posner, J., Russell, J. A., & Peterson, B. (2005). The circumplex model of affect: An integrative approach to affective neuroscience, cognitive development, and psychopathology. *Development and Psychopathology, 17*(3), 715–734.

Redondo, J., Fraga, I., Padrón, I., & Comesaña, M. (2007). The Spanish adaptation of ANEW (Affective Norms for English Words). *Behavior Research Methods, 39*(3), 600–605.

Redondo, J., Fraga, I., Padrón, I., & Piñeiro, A. (2008). Affective ratings of sound stimuli. *Behavior Research Methods, 40*(3), 784–790.

Rozenkrants, B., & Polich, J. (2008). Affective ERP Processing in a Visual Oddball Task: Arousal, Valence, and Gender. *Clinical Neurophysiology, 119*(10), 2260–2265.

Rubin, D. C., & Talarico, J. M. (2009). A comparison of dimensional models of emotion: Evidence from emotions, prototypical events, autobiographical memories, and words. *Memory (Hove, England), 17*(8), 802–808.

Russell, J. A. (1980). A circumplex model of affect. *Journal of Personality and Social Psychology, 39*(6), 1161–1178.

Samsonovic, A. V., & Ascoli, G. A. (2010). Principal Semantic Components of Language and the Measurement of Meaning. *PLoS ONE, 5*(6), e10921.

Sánchez-Navarro, P. J., Martínez-Selva, J. M., Torrente, G., & Román, F. (2008). Psychophysiological, Behavioral, and Cognitive Indices of the Emotional Response: A Factor-Analytic Study. *The Spanish Journal of Psychology, 11*(1), 16–25.

Sauter, D. A., Eisner, F., Calder, A. J., & Scott, S. K. (2006). Perceptual cues in nonverbal vocal expressions of emotion. *Quarterly Journal of Experimental Psychology, 63,* 2251–2272.

Stephens, C. L., Christie, I. C., & Friedman, B. H. (2010). Autonomic specificity of basic emotions: Evidence from pattern classification and cluster analysis. *Biological Psychology, 84,* 463–473.

Stevenson, R. A., & James, T. W. (2008). Affective auditory stimuli: Characterization of the International Affective Digitized Sounds (IADS) by discrete emotional categories. *Behavior Research Methods, 40*(1), 315–321.

Terracciano, A., McCrae, R. R., Hagemann, D., & Costa, P. T. Jr. (2003). Individual Difference Variables, Affective Differentiation, and the Structures of Affect. *Journal of Personality, 71*(5), 669–703.

Võ, M. L.-H., Conrad, M., Kuchinke, L., Urton, K., Hofmann, M. J., & Jacobs, A. M. (2009). The Berlin Affective Word List Reloaded (BAWL-R). *Behavior Research Methods, 41,* 534–538.

Watson, D., Wiese, D., Vaidya, J., & Tellegen, A. (1999). The Two General Activation Systems of Affect: Structural Findings, Evolutionary Considerations, and Psychobiological Evidence. *Journal of Personality and Social Psychology, 76*(5), 820–838.

KEY TERMS AND DEFINITIONS

Valence: One of the principal affective axes, which is also referred as pleasentness or evaluation

Arousal: One of the principal affective axes, which is also referred as activity

Circumplex: A model of the distribution of emotion data along the valence and arousal axes which looks like a doughnut, and fills all quadrants

PANA: A model of the distribution of emotion data along the valence and arousal axes which looks like a bumerang having arms situated at a 45 degrees angle with respect to the main axes

SCR Response: A psychophysiological measure of the autonomic nervous system, derived from sweat

Startle Eyeblink Response: A psychophysiological measure of the autonomic nervous system, derived from eyeblink magnitude in response to a white noise burst

ERP Signal: A signal obtained from eeg, by averaging all data that applies to a certain category of stimuli. The independent measure is time that starts with stimulus onset. This signal has a msec resolution in time.

fMRI Signal: A signal obtained from MR, by applying a repetitive task condition and measuring the blood oxygenation level which somewhat predicts gross neural activity. This signal has mm resolution in space and is recorded for all the voxels in the brain. In time, the resolution is on the order of 2-3 sec.

Section 2
Emotional Frameworks and Models

Chapter 4
Evolution of Affect and Communication

Matthias Scheutz
Tufts University, USA

ABSTRACT

This chapter examines the utilization of affective control to support the survival of agents in competitive multi-agent environments. The author introduces simple affective control mechanisms for simple agents which result in high performance both in ordinary foraging tasks (e.g., searching for food) and in social encounters (e.g., competition for mates). In the proposed case, affective control via the transmission of simple signals can lead to social coordination. Therefore, this case prevents the need for more complex forms of communication like symbolic communication based on systematic representational schemata.

INTRODUCTION

Affect, or more precisely, *affective control*, is wide-spread in nature. From simple homeostatic control, to need-based control, to simple mood-based control, to basic and complex emotional control, and various other forms, affective control mechanisms of varying complexity underlie all behavior in animals. In humans, affective states are deeply intertwined with cognition and are an essential part of human mentality. And affective states often play a critical role in social behavior, from simple displays of prowess, to sexual attraction, to aggressive encounters, to social attachment, and many others. The challenge for cognitive science and its various defining disciplines including philosophy, psychology, artificial intelligence, and neuroscience is to explain what affective control is, what kinds of affective control occur in nature, how affective control can be implemented, and

DOI: 10.4018/978-1-61692-892-6.ch004

how it is implemented in biological organisms – we call this the "affect challenge".

The "affect challenge" comes on the heels of much conceptual disagreement in psychology alone (but also in philosophy and artificial intelligence) about what affect concepts are. For example, the difference between *moods* and *emotions* has been explained in various non-exclusive ways: Ekman (1994) only sees them as differing in terms of time-scale with moods being longer-lasting than emotions, while for Davidson (1994) emotions bias actions while moods bias cognition; yet another explanation is offered by Frijda (1994) who distinguishes moods and emotions based on their intentionality, i.e., emotions have an object towards which they are directed, while moods are non-intentional states. To appreciate the extent of the disagreement, one does not even have to compare classes of affective states such as emotions or moods; it suffices to look at any of the classes itself, e.g., the class of emotions. As succinctly put by Delancey (2002, p. 3), "there probably is no scientifically appropriate class of things referred to by our term emotion. Such disparate phenomena—fear, guilt, shame, melancholy, and so on—are grouped under this term that it is dubious that they share anything but a family resemblance." And, in fact, several authors have noted that there is not even agreement about what "basic emotions" are supposed to be (e.g., Ortony & Turner, 1990; Griffiths, 1997).

The "affect" challenge is, however, not limited to understanding affect concepts and the functional role of affective control processes instantiating these affect concepts in agent architectures. It also includes giving accounts of why affect is so pervasive in nature, and thus why certain forms of affective control might be better than other forms of control. In fact, we believe that understanding the dynamics of affective control processes and their utility for controlling and managing an agent's body (e.g., against the backdrop of survival and procreation) will help in answering many open questions about the nature of individual and social behavior. For example, understanding the nature of affective control will help elucidate the different ways in which affective and cognitive processes (such as reasoning, problem-solving, and decision-making) can interact. Moreover, a detailed account of affective control processes in individuals will also help to explain the dynamics and regulatory roles of emotion processes in social interactions (e.g., in aggressive exchanges). Most importantly, the utility and limits of affective control will allow us to determine, at least in part, possible evolutionary pressures leading to the evolution of higher-level cognition.

While we are currently a long way from being able to answer the above questions, we believe that it is possible to make headway on a smaller set of questions whose answers will contribute to making progress on the larger picture. For example, we can investigate whether the display of affective states will lead to better performance in cooperative tasks or better conflict resolution strategies in competitive tasks in multi-agent environments. We can also attempt to determine which affective control states will or are likely to evolve in cooperative and competitive multi-agent environments. And we can investigate the trade-offs between simple affective control and more complex deliberative control requiring representational mechanisms in the control architecture.

In this chapter, we focus on the utility of affective control states for ensuring an agent's survival in competitive multi-agent environments. We argue that for simple agents, simple affective control mechanisms can be defined that will result in high performance both in ordinary foraging tasks (e.g., searching for food) and in social encounters (e.g., competition for mates). As a result, we make the case that affective control via the transmission of simple signals can lead to social coordination that obviates the need for more complex forms of communication (i.e., symbolic communication based on systematic representational schemata). Methodologically, to avoid the conceptual difficulties associated with affect concepts, we will start by analyzing affect concepts in terms of *architectural capacities of agent architectures*, i.e., we explicate the architectural assumptions underlying a particular affect concept. Based on these architectural definitions, we can then define agent control architectures with mechanisms that can instantiate affect concepts, and we can implement these architectures in artificial agents in a simulated environment where agents have to perform survival tasks. Systematic experiments with these simulated agents and subsequent statistical analyzes of the results based on clearly defined performance measures then allow us to investigate the trade-offs between different architectures based on a variety of individual, social, and environmental factors (Scheutz, 2004c, 2004b).

The method of performing simulation experiments in order to investigate agent properties and be able to make claims about their likely evolution has been termed *synthetic ethology* (MacLennan, 1991) and was originally used to study the evolution of communication in a multi-agent artificial simulation environment. In a similar vein, the term "synthetic psychology" was coined (Braitenberg, 1984) to refer to the method of designing, building, and observing the behavior of artificial agents ("vehicles") in order to study psychological principles, in general, and the difference between observable behavior and mechanisms that bring about that behavior, in particular. In our study of the evolution of affect and communication, we will use a combination of both methodologies together with a third dimension that one could call "synthetic philosophy" – the method of attempting to understand and define mental concepts, in particular affect concepts, in terms of properties of agent architectures (and environmental processes, to the extent that they are part of the control loop).

We start by introducing a very general notion of affective control, followed by a description of how simple affective control states can be implemented in an agent control architecture for simple agents performing foraging and conflict resolution tasks in a competitive multi-agent environment.

We then summarize results from a large number of experiments we have performed over one decade that together provide strong evidence for the utility of simple affective control in simple organisms and thus the likely evolution of affective control systems. At the same time, we summarize results about the utility of communication showing that "representational" communication (i.e., communication that uses systematic symbolic representations to encode meanings) is unlikely to evolve for simple organisms.

BACKGROUND

Different forms of affective control have been been studied over the years. Pfeifer (1988) and Sloman and Croucher (1981) are among the early investigations in artificial intelligence that laid the foundations for what is now known as "affective computing" (Picard, 1997). Researchers have started to study "affective" user interfaces, "believable" synthetic characters and life-like animated agents with emotions, affective or affect-aware instructional and virtual agents, and others (e.g., see Trappl, Petta, & Payr, 2001 for a more recent overview). While the motivations for the various research directions and their specific aims are naturally quite different (e.g., making animated characters more believable by endowing them with emotional facial expressions vs. understanding the utility of affect processes for action selection), there is a tacit assumption common to all the different approaches that affective control, in one form or another, can be useful for and might have important applications in artificial agents. We have previously compiled a list of twelve potential roles of emotions for artificial agents (Scheutz, 2004e):

1. *alarm mechanisms* (e.g., fast reflex-like reactions in critical situations that interrupt other processes)

2. *action selection* (e.g., what to do next based on the current emotional state)

3. *adaptation* (e.g., short or long-term changes in behavior due to affective states)

4. *learning* (e.g., affective evaluations used for reinforcement learning)

5. *motivation* (e.g., creating motives as part of an emotional coping mechanism)

6. *social regulation* (e.g., using emotional signals to achieve social effects)

7. *goal management* (e.g., creation of new goals or reprioritization of existing ones)

8. *strategic processing* (e.g., selection of different search strategies based on overall affective state)

9. *memory control* (e.g., affective bias on memory access and retrieval as well as decay rate of memory items)

10. *information integration* (e.g., emotional filtering of data from various information channels or blocking of such integration)

11. *attentional focus* (e.g., selection of data to be processed based on affective evaluation)

12. *self model* (e.g., affect as representations of "what a situation is like for the agent")

This list, although not intended to be exhaustive, does point to the varied functional nature of affect mechanisms, from architectural roles to roles in social regulation. While surprisingly little work has focused on investigating roles 7 through 12 (although there are exceptions, e.g., (Gratch & Marsella, 2004)), work on interfaces, user interactions, human-robot interactions and other human-computer interaction fields has focused primarily on the sixth role, social regulation. In artificial intelligence, most work has been concerned with the first five roles, in particular, attention has been given to affective or emotional action selection, both in simulated agents (e.g. Gadanho, 2003) and robotic agents (Murphy, Lisetti, Tardif, Irish, & Gage, 2002). Similarly, quite a bit of work has investigated the utility of evaluations that are internally generated and

reflect some aspect of the internal environment (rather than the external environment) for reinforcement learning (although most reinforcement learning models in artificial intelligence do not call the evaluations "affective"). For example, Grossberg's general *CogEM* models (e.g., Grossberg & Schmajuk, 1987) of learning cognitive, emotional, and motor properties can account for several effects in Pavlovian fear conditioning (e.g., secondary conditioning or attentional blocking), but have not been directly applied to empirical data (e.g., data from fear conditioning studies with rats). Other more targeted models of the amygdala, which performs several functions in emotion processing, assume a dual pathway model of emotional processing and were tested in auditory fear conditioning and simulated lesion studies (LeDoux, 1996). There are also attempts to include simulated bodily processes in artificial agents, e.g., simulated hormones for emotional control (Cãnamero, 1997).

One difficulty with affect models is that it is often not clearly articulated why these are models of affect and what particular affective states they are models of (which sometimes leads to labels of implemented states that are familiar from human psychology such as "surprise" when, in fact, the implemented state in the model is nothing like what one would consider human surprise, e.g., Scheutz, 2002a). Rather than leaving it up to the interpretation of the reader (and risking misinterpretation), we have tried to be very specific about kinds of states we were concerned with in our work. Specifically, in Sloman, Chrisley, & Scheutz (2005) we introduced a critical high-level distinction between two very different kinds of control states in an agent architecture, those of *desire-like* and *belief-like* states, to be able to single out a general class of states that we took to be what we ordinarily intend by "affective", namely desire-like states:

A desire-like state D of a system S is one whose function it is to get S to do something to preserve or to change the state of the world—which could include part of S (in a particular way dependent on D). Examples include preferences, pleasures, pains, evaluations, attitudes, goals, intentions, and moods.

Contrast this to belief-like states:

A belief-like state B of a system S is one whose function is to provide information that could, in combination with one or more different sorts of desire-like states, enable the desire-like states to fulfill their functions. Examples include beliefs (particular and general), percepts, memories, and fact-sensor states.

Affective states, being desire-like states, are thus at the heart of what causes an organism to act, either to maintain a state or to change a state. Specifically, depending on whether the organism is trying to preserve a condition, as compared to changing it, allows us to distinguish two broad classes of affective states, namely *positive* and *negative* affective states. More specifically,

A state P of a system S is a positively affective state if being in P or moving towards being in P changes the dispositions of S so as to cause processes which increase the likelihood of P persisting, or which tend to produce or enhance processes that bring P into existence or maintain the existence of P.

Again, in contrast

A state N of a system S is a negatively affective state if being in N or moving towards being in N changes the dispositions of S so as to cause processes which reduce the likelihood of N persisting, or which tend to resist processes that bring N into existence.

Given this simple conceptual apparatus, we can now define different affect concepts in terms of

architectural mechanisms and investigate ways to implement them in agent architectures. By construing affect concepts as intrinsically architecture-based, it is possible to account for similarities and subtle differences of a great variety of affect concepts that are labeled the same in ordinary language and in large parts of the literature. A question like "Is system *S* capable of having *fear*? " now becomes "Is system *S* capable of having *fear*? ", where *fear* is a "fear concept" specified in terms of functional capacities of an agent architecture. Such a move will not only eliminate ambiguities in language usage ("your agent model does not implement fear, it implements anxiety"), but also allow us to say when affect concepts of a particular kind are implemented (and can be instantiated) in an agent, as we are able to check whether the architecture controlling the agent supports the affect concepts specified functionally in terms of architectural requirements.

In general, for us to be able to understand the nature of affective states as they occur in biological systems, we need to (1) what affective states are and what different kinds of affective states there are, (2) how and why affective mechanisms came about, and (3) what their function (if they have a function) is in information processing architectures. This questions can be widened from biological to artificial systems by adding the question (4) how affect mechanisms can be incorporated into agent architectures and implemented in artificial agents. Conceptual analyses of affective states are mostly targeted at answering questions (1) and (3), investigations in the empirical sciences mostly attempt to answer questions (2) and (3). Successful implementations of AI models, on the other hand, which employ typically simple affective states to control the behavior of simulated or real agents, provide partial answers to questions (3) and (4), but do not answer questions (1) or (2).

We believe that answers to these questions will likely not come forth from independent inquiries, but from the interplay of conceptual analyses, empirical findings and concrete experiments with agent architectures. The proposed research strategy, then, is to start with a notion of affective state that is applicable to natural systems, determine/define its function in a particular agent architecture, and subsequently try to explore the properties of this state for concrete agents in different environments with the goal of extending the notion to more complex cases. This includes investigating ways in which slight changes in environments can change the trade-offs between design options for the architecture and hence for the functional role of the affective state. Such explorations of "neighborhoods in design and niche space" (e.g., Sloman, 2000) will help us understand what the competitive advantage of a particular change in architecture or mechanism might be in a particular environment, and how the benefits change in slightly different environments.

We now start with a more detailed illustration of how one can define agent architectures that can instantiate affect concepts in terms of control components and then proceed to defining specific architectures for biologically plausible survival tasks that we can use to answer questions about the evolution of affect and communication.

SIMPLE AFFECTIVE CONTROL

First and foremost, we need *control elements*, for affect as construed above essentially deals with the control of agents. Secondly, the control elements need to be connected to other components in a way that allows them to influence the behavior and/or behavioral dispositions of the controlled agent. Finally, the *control loop* consisting of one or more control elements, the controlled components and the environment needs to be such that the functional description of the affect concepts matches the dispositional characteristics determined by the architectural layout as well as the interactions of the agent with its environment. In the following, we will focus on two rough classes of affective states, *motivational* and *emotional*

states, and construe their states in general control-theoretic terms.

"Motivations" (in their most general functional description) are *desire-like states* in that they influence and bias an agent's behavioral dispositions in such a way as to contribute to the realization of a state of the environment (including the agent) desired by the agent. They are caused by the disparity between an agent's desire state and the state of the environment, and are themselves causes for actions that are intended to change the state of the environment so as to make it agree with the agents' desires. Whether a state of an agent's control system (as determined by its architecture) is a motivational state, then, depends essentially on the state's causal connection to environmental states and its potential to influence the agent's actions.

By "simple motivational states" we intend to refer to motivational states that have little to no cognitive involvement and are primarily linked to "basic needs" of an agent (e.g., to maintain a certain charge level of the battery in a robot). For some of these states, the familiar term "drive" is appropriate, namely if the agent is driven in a mostly reactive way to act so as to eliminate the disparity between a desired and an actual state that was the cause for the motivational state (e.g., the adjustment of a homeostatic variable). For example, for a state of an agent's control system to qualify as a "hunger state" (i.e., an instance of a simple motivational state), roughly speaking the instantiation of this state needs to be caused by lack of energy, and needs to cause, in turn, food-seeking behavior (e.g., Lorenz & Leyhausen, 1973; McFarland, 1981). However, not all drives need to be linked to a "disparity" (e.g., play drives in dogs or cats may be triggered by boredom and thus may not be directly linked to any homeostatic imbalance), in which case they will not be (entirely) driven by motivations.

It is then possible to use outputs from gain controllers to influence motor control circuits to implement the kind of control system that will be able to instantiate such motivations. A "hunger state", for example, could be instantiated by a *proportional controller P* (e.g., Özbay, 2000) in the following way: input to P comes from an internal sensor S_e that measures the current energy level. P compares a set point e_{des} (i.e., the desired energy level), to the actual energy level e_{act} and scales the difference by a gain factor g_e:

$P = g_e \cdot (e_{des} - e_{act})$. The output then is a measure of the urgency with which the system requires energy. Hence, the intensity of the motivation is modeled by the magnitude of the output of the control circuit.

To be able to instantiate a hunger state, the controller P needs to be connected to components that control the agent's effectors in such a way that a positive output can influence and bias the agent's behavior towards food-seeking, where the intensity with which the agent searches for food depends on the magnitude of the output of P (reflecting the urgency with which food is needed).

Similar to motivational states, "emotions", in the most general functional description, are *desire-like states*. They, too, influence and bias an agent's behavioral dispositions. Yet, different from motivational states, which are linked to a disparity between a desired and an actual state, they do not have to be caused by any disparity (between an actual and a desired state). Furthermore, they themselves can be the states that the agent does or does not desire (whereas motivational states are directed towards or away from what the agent desires). A "fear state", for example, in and of itself is an undesirable state of an agent in that it indicates (potential) danger. As such, it causes the agent to behave in such a way as to prepare for or avoid the danger. Hence, while it can also be motivational in the sense that it may move the agent away from the cause of fear–this is the *desired state* with respect to the motivational state instantiated by a fear state–it is also emotional as it itself is not a desired state (i.e., it is a negatively valenced state). A fear state with no clearly discernible danger present, which

causes an agent to be more cautious and alert, may itself not instantiate a motivational state that is connected to a particular goal such as running away from a particular threat (i.e., a desired state of the world such as "run"). Furthermore, depending on the length of duration, such a state may be better construed as an instance of a mood state in that moods lack objects at which they are directed, contrary to emotional states (although the boundary between them is not clear-cut: it is not clear when exactly a fear state, i.e., something that is caused by a perception of a dangerous situation or object, turns into an anxiety-ridden mood-like state). Emotional and motivational states are, therefore, distinct, and emotional states may or may not instantiate motivational states.[1]

A simple fear state caused by the presence of dangerous objects in the environment, for example, could change the agent's behavioral dispositions in such as way as to make it keep a certain distance from these objects for a while. Note that, while the agent is changing its behavioral dispositions insofar as it is inclined to stay away from the cause of the fear, the dispositions are changed without making the agent achieve a particular goal (i.e., desired state), e.g., to get to an environment without these objects. In fact, it may be not be possible (or if possible, a bad move) to attempt to switch from a fear state to another (more pleasant or positively valenced) state in circumstances where the source of fear can either not be pinpointed or not be avoided altogether, and general caution over an extended period of time is a beneficial (if not the only) option.

Again, we can use outputs from gain controllers to implement a control system that can instantiate an emotional state such as the above-described simple form of fear. Specifically, the fear state can be instantiated by a controller C, which integrates over time the frequency of occurrence of fear triggering conditions: input to C comes from an internal sensor S_f that is activated (under normal circumstances) by a fear triggering condition (e.g., the sensor outputs a unit impulse, Özbay, 2000).

C integrates these inputs over time and outputs a signal that corresponds to the intensity of "fear", hence to the degree with which the system should change its behavioral dispositions to be more alert, action-ready, etc. The controller could, for example, have the response characteristic given by $g(t)=e^{-t}$ to a unit impulse generated by the sensor or the perceptual system detecting a dangerous stimulus.

An example of a controller for a simple fear mechanism is given by the following differential equation:

$$\frac{\partial Act}{\partial t} = S_f G_{sensor} Act + G_{decay} Act$$

where Act is the current activation level of the control system, G_{sensor} is the gain for the sensor input and G_{decay} is the discount value for past activations. Note that the decay here is important to allow the agent's behavioral dispositions return to normal when there have not been any triggers of fear in a while.

To be able to instantiate a fear state, the above controller C needs to be connected to components that control the agent's effectors in such a way that the positive output from C can influence and bias the agent's behavior towards avoiding or attempting to avoid dangerous objects, where the intensity with which the agent avoids or attempts to avoid these objects depends on the magnitude of the output of C (reflecting the agent's level of fear).

BIOLOGICALLY PLAUSIBLE AFFECTIVE AGENTS

The examples of motivational and emotional control mechanisms in the previous section were purposefully kept as simple as possible, for even though there is a large number of possible, much more complex affective control mechanisms that can be implemented in control circuits, we are here only interested in the simplest of control circuits that can instantiate affect concepts. For, as we will argue, these simplest of all control circuits are sufficient to allow simple agents to achieve their basic goals (of gathering food and surviving long enough to have offspring). Specifically, we now define a simple biologically inspired agent architecture that allows agents to achieve high levels of performance in foraging and conflict resolution tasks. The former task deals with the search for food, the latter with conflicts that arise when two or more agents contest a resource, given that resources are often scarce. Both tasks take place in the context of evolutionary survival tasks where agents have to collect resources in able to procreate and pass on their genes. This is because evolution discovered affective control mechanisms in the very same context of competition for survival. In fact, some neuroscientists believe that affects can be considered the major "emotional operating systems" that are defined by genetically coded neural circuits and the interactions among them (Panksepp, 1992, 1998).

We start with the basic perceptual system where a percept is viewed as generating "virtual forces" given by vector F. Force vectors point either in the direction of the percept or in the exact opposite direction depending on whether the agents perceives the object as *attractive* or *repulsive*. Moreover, the length $|F|$ determines the degree to which the agent is attracted to or repelled by the object. For example, if the perceived object is food, the agent will be generally attracted to it, but the strength of attraction might depend on how badly the agent needs food (i.e., how "hungry" the agent is). Similarly, if the object is another agent, a predator say, then the agent is repelled by it and the degree of repulsion will depend on the properties of the enemy (i.e., how strong, fast, etc., it is). Each perceptual force vector is then scaled by the distance (typically by using $1/d^n$ with d being the distance of the agent to the object and $n>1$ depending on the type of signal drop-off, typically $n=2$ for 3d-space or $n=3$ for the plane for most signals). Scaled perceptual force vectors for each kind of object are then summed and scaled again by a time-invariant or time-variant "gain value" to account for the interest the agent has in the particular modality. More formally, the overall summed force F_{tot} is given by

$$F_{tot} = \sum_{m} g_{m,\phi} \sum_{i_m=1}^{j_m} \frac{F_{i_m}}{d_{i_m}^{n_m}}$$

where $g_{m,\phi}$ is the (time-invariant or time-variant) gain value of the m-th modality possibly depending on ϕ, is the force vector to the i-th object in modality m, is the distance of the agent from the i-th object in modality m, and nm is the drop-off exponent for the m-th modality. If gm is a time-invariant, then the interest the agent has in modality m is the same regardless of the circumstances and ϕ is irrelevant. More often, however, g$m_{,\phi}$ will be time-variant and thus depend on other factors (e.g., time, energy levels, etc.) in which case ϕ stands for those parameters that vary over time to generate different gain values. For example, it might be that $\phi=c/le_w$ here le $_i$ s the energy level of the agent and the gain value indirectly depends on the energy stored in the agent. In that case, an agent will have higher g$m_{,\phi}$ values when its stored energy is low and thus have higher interest in food (relative to the other modalities). The vector sum over all summed modality force vectors will then reflect this change in interest in that it will overall bias the summed force vector Ftot_{in} the direction of the higher gain values, in that case the direction of food.

The total force vector is used by the agent to determine the direction in which it should go to satisfy its needs. Whether or not it will end up going in that direction, however, will depend on additional factors, e.g., on whether it has enough energy to move there, whether there is an obstacle in the way, etc. The agent's action system is the place where the final decision of what direction to move in is made. In the case of our simple agents, only available energy and physically possible motion are considered (although others are possible) to determine the speed and direction of an agent movement. Together, the perceptual and action system form the basic agent architecture for agents that can perform the foraging task. For one-resource foraging tasks, the foraging model then has two parameters: gm and nm for the gain and drop-off values of modality m, respectively. Each additional modality adds two more such parameters. And if there are time-variant gains, they might add more.

When resources are scarce (food, mates, territory, etc.) and multiple agents are interested in the same resource, conflicts naturally arise over those resources that need to be resolved. These contests typically involve various displays of aggression or prowess (e.g., Lorenz, 1977; Adamo & Hanlon, 1996; Hofmann & Schildberger, 2001). These expressions (e.g., facial expressions, gestures, etc.) can be construed as signals that *communicate the probability with which an animal will (continue to) fight,* where – roughly speaking – the strength of the displayed expression is directly related to the likelihood that the animal will keep fighting. Hence, for the conflict resolution task, we add another component that can determine what an agent should do if a resource is contested, i.e., when two or more agents want to eat the same food source. We also make agents display their *action tendency* and allow them to perceive the action tendency of other agents. The conflict model consists of one parameter to determine the agent's action tendency in a conflict situation: whether the agent wants to contest the resource and *fight* or whether the agent wants to move away from the resource and *flee*. We can express the agent's action tendency as the probability to fight P*(action=FIGHT)* and define a variety of different conflict policies. For agents who ignore the display action tendencies of other agents, we can define the following policies:

- *Timid agents* never fight: $P(action=FIGHT)=0$
- *Aggressive agents* always fight: $P(action=FIGHT)=1$
- *Asocial agents* play a mixed strategy: $P(action=FIGHT)=p$ with $0<p<1$

Note while agents might play a fixed policy over their life-time, they could also change it based on circumstance, e.g., depending on whether they were able to win previous contests or on how low their energy level is. For example, an agent could update its policy to become "more aggressive" (i.e., increase $P(action=FIGHT)$) to be able to increase the likelihood that it will get lucky in the future. We call such agents *adaptive* and add another parameter to the agent model that specifies how these agents change their policies over time. E.g., it might be possible for an agent to play the timid strategy until its energy level drops below a certain threshold, at which point it will start playing the aggressive strategy. Similarly, an agent might keep a tally of how many conflicts it has lost in the recent past and then increase or lower its aggression level based on how successful it was (e.g., mimicking what seems to happen in dominance relationships in social groups in nature).

Since agents will always display their action tendencies and since action tendencies are correlated with and thus predictive of the agent's actual choice and subsequent action (i.e., a high probability of fighting will often lead to "fight" decisions and outcomes), using perceived action tendencies to make decisions about one's own behavior can be beneficial. Hence, we can define several "social policies" that take both an agent's own and the perceived action tendencies into account:

- *Social agents* play a mixed strategy that depends on both their own and the perceived action tendency: $P(action=FIGHT)=f(p_s,p_o)$ where $f(p_s,p_o)$ is a policy depending on the agent's own (p_s) and the other agent's perceived (p_o) action tendencies with $0<p_s,p_o<1$[2]
- *Rational agents* play the limit-case social strategy with $P(action=fight)=1$ if $p_s>p_o$, $P(action=FIGHT)=0$ otherwise

We can also imagine that agents might play different strategies not only based on their own and their opponent's (perceived) action tendencies, but also on whether they perceive the other agent to be of their own versus another agent kind. We will call those agents "discriminating agents" and allow them to use two different strategies depending on whether the contesting agent is of their own or another kind. Finally, we have so far assumed that agents will display their action tendencies truthfully, but that does not have to be the case. Hence, we will also allow for agents to cheat and lie with their displays about their true action tendencies. Such "liar agents" will display one action tendency, but act on another. E.g., an agent might display that it is maximally aggressive $P(action=FIGHT)=1$, but really play a mixed strategy $P(action=FIGHT)=p_s$ with $0<p_s<1$.

The preceding foraging and conflict models combined allow agents to forage for food and resolve conflicts that arise in multi-agent environments when multiple agents contest the same resource. The final step is to add a procreation model which allows agents to have offspring. While models of various sophistication are possible, we only consider the simplest possible model here, where an agent will automatically produce an offspring asexually when its energy level is above a given *procreation threshold*. The energy for the new agent (which is less than the procreation threshold) will be subtracted from the parenting agent's energy store and a new agent will appear close proximity to the parent agent. The child agent will inherit all parent agent's traits, with the possibility of some of the traits being mutated (based on a predefined mutation rate on the trait). This way evolutionary processes can be defined that result from genetic adaptations over time in the context of the population dynamics of surviving agents.

EVIDENCE FOR THE UTILITY OF SIMPLE AFFECTIVE CONTROL

We are now in position to use results from simulation experiments with the affective agents defined above to make claims about the utility of affect control mechanisms and social signaling in the context of biologically plausible survival and procreation tasks that contain foraging and conflict subtasks. Specifically, we will base our claims on the success of different agent types, and consequently that of their architectures, as measured in terms of *the average number of surviving agents of a kind after a large number of agent generations* to establish that an agent kind is more likely to evolve – this is the standard evolutionary idea of *fitness*, i.e., that animals from a fitter species are more likely to procreate and pass on their genes than animals from a less fit species, which in turn might lead to the extinction of the less fit species when resources are scarce. In fact, we have been able to demonstrate that performance evaluations that measure foraging efficiency can be predictive of population dynamics and even evolutionary adaptations (Scheutz & Schermerhorn, 2005b).[3]

The general setup for all studies we will discuss below was a simulated unlimited 2D environment where agents have to forage for food in order to survive and procreate. Initially, specified numbers of agents and food sources are placed in the environment according to a given distribution (e.g., random, uniform, Gaussian, etc.) and then the simulation is run as a *discrete-time simulation* where, at the beginning of each simulation cycle, every agent gets to sense its environment and then decide on an action. All intended actions are then executed in parallel (with the possibility of an action failing if its enabling conditions are not given anymore). Since multiple agents are in

the same environment and food is often scarce, conflicts over food can arise, hence agents have to determine whether they want to engage in a conflict over a food item or leave the scene (conflicts can also happen about other agents, but we are not pursuing this direction here). Simulations are initialized with all initial parameters fixed and then run for a certain number of steps or until some termination criterion is reached (e.g., no more agent is alive). Then different variables in the simulation environment are used for measuring agent performance (e.g., the number of surviving agents, the overall energy stored in agents, etc.). Performance measures are averaged over a set of initial conditions that are taken to be samples from a large space of initial conditions. The averages can then be used to perform various statistical analyses (ANOVAs, ANCOVAs, MANOVAs, etc.) in order to determine the dependence of performance on a set of control, bodily, social, and environmental parameters (e.g., Schermerhorn & Scheutz, 2006, 2007b). Instead of reporting the details of the experimental setup together with the specific statistical results, we will for space reasons concentrate on higher-level summaries of our findings, referring the reader to the respective publications for details. This will allow us to generate a summary of a variety of related studies that together provide strong evidence for the claims we would like to advance.

In Scheutz & Sloman (2001), we demonstrated that simple motivational agents (with "hunger-like" and "thirst-like" control mechanisms) are likely to evolve from basic agents under many environmental variations such as the distribution and influx of energy and water sources in the environment as well as the number and distribution of other agents and obstacles. These "hunger-like" and "thirst-like" states were implemented by simple feedback control circuits connected to agent-internal energy-level and water-level sensors and mutation was allowed to operate on the output of these controllers to influence the way in which the control signal was used. In all evolutionary runs, the control output evolved to be used to implement positive time-variant gain values for force vectors pointing to food and water sources. Hence, the control circuit increased the agent's likelihood of moving towards food or water based on its needs, thus warranting the labels "hunger-like" and "thirst-like". Similarly, we demonstrated in Scheutz (2001) that simple "fear-like", but not "anger-like" states are likely to evolve, where the labels "fear-like" and "anger-like" were warranted because the agents evolved time-variant gain values for force vectors pointing to other agents and obstacles, thus causing them to move either away from or towards other agents and/or obstacles. We also showed that some of these connections can be learned during an agent's lifetime using simple associative learning mechanisms (Scheutz, 2000). These results were replicated and extended later in more systematic studies considering larger environmental variations (Scheutz, 2004e, 2004a).

We also investigated the trade-offs between simple reactive agents (with time-invariant gains), simple affective agents (with time-variant gains), and a third class of "deliberative" agents of varying complexity that were able to plan routes through the environment in order to acquire resources more efficiently. We showed that very simple deliberative mechanisms do not pay off in terms of overall performance, especially not if *relative performance* is considered, i.e., performance where the processing cost of using architectural mechanisms is taken into account – note that relative performance is ultimately what matters for evolutionary considerations because animals will need to spend energy for building, using, and maintaining any additional control circuits in their brains (Scheutz, Sloman, & Logan, 2000; Scheutz & Logan, 2001; Scheutz & Schermerhorn, 2002). These results were replicated in a variety of experiments investigating *foraging efficiency* in multi-agent territory exploration (MATE) tasks where a group of agents needed to collect as many resources either as quickly as possible

or until all resources were collected (Scheutz & Schermerhorn, 2003, 2004a, 2004b, 2005a, 2005b; Scheutz, 2004d). Specifically, we used MATE tasks to investigate the trade-offs among architectural mechanisms, sensory range, agent group size and environmental complexity. We found that complex control systems with (optimal or close-to-optimal) planning capabilities do not pay off in environments with low structure in the distribution of food sources when relative performance is considered. In fact, not even simple "predictive mechanisms" that attempt to anticipate which food item other agents are targeting lead to better relative performance in various tasks (e.g., Schermerhorn & Scheutz, 2007a), although they can sometimes lead to better absolute performance (Scheutz & Schermerhorn, 2005a). Collectively, these studies show that simple reactive agents that perform a "greedy" search are highly effective in foraging for food. Together with the previous results about the likely evolution of simple affective control states we can conclude that affective control states will likely evolve for foraging tasks given the low architectural cost of implementing them (e.g., often a simple neuron can implement time-variant gain control). The question, then, is whether affective social control using the simple signaling model we introduced in the previous section is sufficient for coordinating social groups, as compared to more sophisticated methods of communicating information.

In a first attempt to investigate the utility of signaling internal states to other agents, we showed that taking other agents' truthfully-displayed internal fear states into account can lead to significantly better performance in multi-agent foraging tasks where conflicts can arise over resources, as compared to groups that do not indicate their fear levels (Scheutz, 2002b). Later, we designed a general game-theoretic framework for conflict resolution in simple agents and showed that there are *fair* conflict resolution strategies (for a particular notion of *fairness*) that lead to Pareto-optimal behavior (Schermerhorn & Scheutz, 2003). Moreover, we showed that there were simple ways of implementing fair strategies based on keeping track of how often an agent won or lost a conflict in the past and making one-shot behavioral decisions about who should get a resource based on this tally, effectively playing an *adaptive rational* strategy. Such adaptive rational agents were superior to all other social and asocial agents in terms of the number of surviving agents after a certain number of generations in the conflict task (Scheutz, 2004d; Scheutz & Schermerhorn, 2004a). When agents are allowed to cheat, however, i.e., when they can wrongly indicate their action tendencies, then all truth-telling strategies will suffer (Scheutz & Schermerhorn, 2004b), which might be a reason why affective control in nature seems to be largely "hard-coded" to prevent organisms from cheating. We also analyzed the interactions between simple non-social affective control and social control through affective displays and conflict resolution strategies in order to determine the trade-offs between individual and social strategies and found that agents could make up for suboptimal strategies in the conflict task using specific gain values (behavioral propensities) in their foraging control that allowed them to avoid conflicts more frequently (Scheutz, 2006), thus providing evidence for the utility of simple (non-social) affective control (in the foraging task) in the light of conflicts, also possibly providing a way for agents to cope with cheaters in conflict tasks.

DISCUSSION

In sum, we found strong evidence that simple affective control mechanisms implemented in terms of feedback controllers based on internal and external sensors (e.g., energy-level sensors or action tendency sensors) whose outputs are used to modulate (time-variant) gain values of percept force vectors (e.g., food sources or other agents) lead to significantly superior performance compared to time-invariant gain values, and that

such control circuits are likely to evolve even in the context of competitive multi-agent environments with limited resources. Hence, the question arises whether there are circumstances in which either more complex deliberative mechanisms or more complex forms of communication are likely to evolve. We already mentioned evidence that more complex deliberative mechanisms (e.g., for planning trajectories through the environment to more efficiently collect food sources) do not have better relative performance than the considered affective mechanisms, and are thus not likely to evolve for simple agents in survival tasks (with foraging and conflict subtasks) in environments with low structure in the distribution of food sources. But this does not exclude the possibility of more complex control systems evolving in environments with more structure or in agents with more bodily limitations such as severely limited sensory ranges.

Given that more complex deliberative control systems evolved in nature, it seems clear that certain bodily, task, and/or environmental features must have provided enough evolutionary pressure for deliberative control mechanisms to evolve. For example, different from our simulations where food sources were stationary, it is likely that agents who need to deal with moving food sources (e.g., in a predator-prey scenario) will require more complex control systems for foraging and survival (e.g., to predict where prey is located/hiding, to anticipate the prey's evasive moves in a chase, etc.). While this is clearly an important direction to pursue, it is outside the scope of this chapter. Rather, we will examine the question whether more complex forms of communication would benefit the simple kinds of agents we have defined previously, given that we know that different forms of communication have evolved in nature for different purposes, in addition to signaling action tendencies in conflict situations as discussed above (e.g., signaling danger, indicating readiness for mating, reporting locations of food). Especially since we know that humans are capable of complex symbolic forms of communication, we believe that determining the evolutionary pressures for different forms of communication to evolve is particularly interesting in light of the results about affective control systems we have reviewed so far. In fact, given that signaling action tendencies alone can already achieve a very high level of coordination and performance in simple affective agents, it is not clear whether more complex forms of communication could significantly increase the performance of simple agents, especially if *relative performance* is considered.

For one, simple signals emitted from another agent such as "I see food here" or "I am likely going to fight" do not require much more in terms of processing on the receiving end (a simple perceptual system that can determine the signal's direction, quality and intensity is sufficient). Contrast such "deictic signals" (Perconti, 2002) with more complex messages of the form "Agent A sees food F at location X at time t", which require a much more complex architecture because agent names, food types, locations and times have to be explicit decoded from the message signals (typically assuming a systematic generative signal system). Clearly, such architectures come at an additional cost (for having, maintaining, and using the additional mechanisms). Moreover, the costs of communicating can also be substantive; an agent that needs to send signals at regular intervals over a given period of time might use up a significant portion of its energy reserves, possibly without any benefit if no other agent can hear the signals (for a longer version of this argument, see Scheutz & Schermerhorn, 2008). It should be clear, then, that claims about the evolvability of communication, in particular those about the *likelihood* of communication evolving, need to be very specific about the forms of communication they target – encoding direction and distance to food sources as well as food quality requires very different (sophisticated) mechanisms from simply

"annotating the environment" using pheromones like ants do.

We have investigated the utility of two major forms of communication: simple signaling, as described before, and more complex "representational messaging" where components of a communicated message require systematic representations of aspects of the environment (e.g., locations, food types, etc.). In various simulation studies, we compared simple agents with time-invariant gains with and without using signals for attracting (or repelling) other agents to (from) food sources in MATE tasks to agents that use more complex ways of communicating the location of food ("representational communication"). Overall, we found that representational communication is often not necessary to coordinate the behaviors of multiple agents in a social group (Schermerhorn & Scheutz, 2006) and that simple non-communicative predictive mechanisms can often significantly improve agent performance (Scheutz & Schermerhorn, 2005a), while adding representational communication to agents with and without this prediction mechanism does not improve the performance of the respective group. Moreover, we found that, in more structured environments where food occurs in clusters and communication does lead to better absolute performance, there is no performance difference between simple signaling and representational communication (Scheutz & Schermerhorn, 2008). And finally, even if the task complexity is increased so that multiple agents have to be at the same location in an environment at the same time, there are various simple non-communicative mechanisms that allow agents to coordinate and that lead to performance equal to, if not superior to, agents using representational communication (Schermerhorn & Scheutz, 2007a).

CONCLUSION

In this paper, we introduced a general notion of "affective states" that construed affect concepts as architecture-based concepts defined in terms of control mechanisms in agent architectures. We gave various examples of simple affective control states and defined several classes of simple affective agents for biologically plausible foraging and conflict resolution tasks in the context of a more general survival task. Based on the ideas of "synthetic ethology, psychology and philosophy", we reviewed the results of various previous studies with simulated agents and, based on this evidence, arrived at the conclusion that simple affective control mechanisms are very effective at guaranteeing agents a high absolute *and*, more importantly, relative performance in the survival task in competitive multi-agent environments with little structure. Consequently, we can claim that simple affective control states are very likely to evolve. In fact, simple affective control states turned out to be so efficient (in terms of the performance gains relative to the added cost of the control mechanisms compared to the performance of agents with time-invariant gains without additional costs) that the effectiveness of affective control is likely the cause for why evolution produced so many simple creatures that use only simple forms of signaling, if any (e.g., as measured in terms of the number of species or biomass). Comparatively, very few species were able to evolve more sophisticated control systems, including representational communication.

At present, it is not clear how and in what circumstances these more sophisticated control systems paid off relative to simpler affective control systems. One possibility is that constraints imposed on foraging tasks allowed agents to exploit them and evolve intermediate mechanisms that promised immediate performance gains. For example, we were able to show recently that the evolution of simple memories can lead to significant performance gains in foraging tasks where agents have to collect food and return it to a hive (Schermerhorn & Scheutz, 2009, 2005). Once such memories are in place, for whatever reason, agents will be able to use them in various ways. For example, they might be able to form associations between events and their affective evaluations of those events such that agents will be able to retrieve a memory item together with its affective value. This, in turn, might allow them to change gain values of force vectors in a more independent fashion compared to the fixed, determined way in which gain values are changed based on internal or external sensors. At present, this is all speculation, but it should be possible, at least in principle (if it turns out to be technologically infeasible due to an overly large number of parameters), to evaluate and ideally substantiate or refute such speculations in simulation studies with agents whose architectural parameters are systematic in the way we have done in the past. Such studies will not only contribute to a better understanding of the possible space of agent architectures and their performances, but also to a better understanding of our own mental concepts and their possible functions, including their evolutionary roles and, thus, the likelihood that instances of them would have evolved in nature.

REFERENCES

Adamo, S. A., & Hanlon, R. T. (1996). Do cuttlefish (cephalopoda) signal their intentions toconspecifics during agonistic encounters? *Animal Behaviour*, (52): 73–81. doi:10.1006/anbe.1996.0153

Braitenberg, V. (1984). *Vehicles: Experiments in synthetic psychology*. Cambridge, MA: The MIT Press.

Cãnamero, D. (1997). Modeling motivations and emotions as a basis for intelligent behavior. In L. Johnson (Ed.), *Proceedings of the first international symposium on autonomous agents (agents '97)* (pp. 148–155). New York: ACM Press.

Davidson, R. J. (1994). On emotion, mood, and related affective constructs. In (Ekman & Davidson, 1994) (pp. 56–58).

DeLancey, C. (2002). *Passionate engines: What emotions reveal about mind and artificial intelligence*. Oxford, UK: Oxford University Press.

Ekman, P. (1994). Moods, emotions, and traits. In (Ekman & Davidson, 1994) (pp. 56–58).

Ekman, P., & Davidson, R. J. (Eds.). (1994). *The nature of emotion: Fundamental questions*. New York: Oxford University Press.

Ferguson, E. (1982). *Motivation: An experimental approach*. Malabar, FL: Krueger Publishing Company.

Frijda, N. H. (1994). Varieties of affect: Emotions and episodes, moods, and sentiments. In (Ekman & Davidson, 1994) (pp. 56–58).

Gadanho, S. C. (2003). Learning behavior-selection by emotions and cognition in a multi-goal robot task. *Journal of Machine Learning Research, 4*(Jul), 385–412. doi:10.1162/jmlr.2003.4.3.385

Gratch, J., & Marsella, S. (2004). A domain-independent framework for modeling emotion. *Journal of Cognitive Systems Research, 5*(4), 269–306. doi:10.1016/j.cogsys.2004.02.002

Griffiths, P. (1997). *What emtions really are: The problem of psychological categories*. Chicago: Chicago University Press.

Grossberg, S., & Schmajuk, N. (1987). Neural dynamics of attentionally-modulated pavlovian conditioning: Conditioned reinforcement, inhibition, and opponent processing. *Psychobiology, 15*, 195–240.

Hofmann, H. A., & Schildberger, K. (2001). Assessment of strength and willingness to fight during aggressive encounters in crickets. *Animal Behaviour*, (62): 337–348. doi:10.1006/anbe.2001.1746

LeDoux, J. (1996). *The emotional brain*. New York: Simon & Schuster.

Lorenz, K. (1977). *Aggressivitt: arterhaltende eigenschaft oder pathologische erscheinung?* Aggression und Toleranz.

Lorenz, K., & Leyhausen, P. (1973). *Motivation and animal behavior: An ethological view*. New York: Van Nostrand Co.

MacLennan, B. (1991). Synthetic ethology: An approach to the study of communication. In C. G. Langton, C. Taylor, J. D. Farmer, & S. Rasmussen (Eds.), *Artificial life II: Proceedings of the second workshop on artificial life* (pp. 631–658). Redwood City, Calif.: Addison-Wesley.

McFarland, D. (1981). *The oxford companion to animal behavior*. Oxford: Oxford University Press.

Murphy, R. R., Lisetti, C., Tardif, R., Irish, L., & Gage, A. (2002). Emotion-based control of cooperating heterogeneous mobile robots. *IEEE Transactions on Robotics and Automation, 18*(5), 744–757. doi:10.1109/TRA.2002.804503

Ortony, A., & Turner, T. (1990). What's basic about basic emotions? *Psychological Review, 97*, 315–331. doi:10.1037/0033-295X.97.3.315

Özbay, H. (2000). *Introduction to feedback control theory*. London: CRC Press.

Panksepp, J. (1992). A critical role for 'affective neuroscience' in resolving what is basic about emotions. *Psychological Review*.

Panksepp, J. (1998). *Affective neuroscience-the foundations of human and animal emotions*. Oxford: Oxford University Press.

Perconti, P. (2002). Context-dependence in human and animal communication. *Foundations of Science, 7*, 341–362. doi:10.1023/A:1019613210814

Pfeifer, R. (1988). Artificial intelligence models of emotion. In V. Hamilton, G. H. Bower, & N. H. Frijda (Eds.), *Cognitive perspectives on emotion and motivation, volume 44 of series d: Behavioural and social sciences* (p. 287-320). Netherlands: Kluwer Academic Publishers.

Picard, R. (1997). *Affective computing.* Cambridge, Mass, London, England: MIT Press.

Schermerhorn, P., & Scheutz, M. (2003). Implicit cooperation in conflict resolution for simple agents. In *Agent 2003.* Chicago, IL: University of Chicago.

Schermerhorn, P., & Scheutz, M. (2005, June). The effect of environmental structure on the utility of communication in hive-based swarms. In *Ieee swarm intelligence symposium 2005* (pp. 440–443). IEEE Computer Society Press. doi:10.1109/SIS.2005.1501661

Schermerhorn, P., & Scheutz, M. (2006, May). Social coordination without communication in multi-agent territory exploration tasks. In *Proceedings of the fifth international joint conference on autonomous agents and multiagent systems (AAMAS-06)* (pp. 654–661). Hakodate, Japan.

Schermerhorn, P., & Scheutz, M. (2007a). Investigating the adaptiveness of communication in multi-agent behavior coordination. *Adaptive Behavior, 15*(4), 423–445. doi:10.1177/1059712307084690

Schermerhorn, P., & Scheutz, M. (2007b, April). Social, physical, and computational tradeoffs in collaborative multi-agent territory exploration tasks. In *Proceedings of the first ieee symposium on artificial life* (pp. 295–302).

Schermerhorn, P., & Scheutz, M. (2009, March/April). The impact of communication and memory in hive-based foraging agents. In *Proceedings of the 2009 IEEE symposium on artificial life* (pp. 29–36).

Scheutz, M. (2000). Surviving in a hostile multiagent environment: How simple affective states can aid in the competition for resources. In H. J. Hamilton (Ed.), *Advances in artificial intelligence, 13th biennial conference of the canadian society for computational studies of intelligence, ai 2000, montréal, quebec, canada, may 14-17, 2000, proceedings* (Vol. 1822, pp. 389–399). Springer.

Scheutz, M. (2001). The evolution of simple affective states in multi-agent environments. In D. Cañamero (Ed.), *Proceedings of AAAI fall symposium* (pp. 123–128). Falmouth, MA: AAAI Press.

Scheutz, M. (2002a). Agents with or without emotions? In R. Weber (Ed.), *Proceedings of the 15th international flairs conference* (pp. 89–94). AAAI Press.

Scheutz, M. (2002b). The evolution of affective states and social control. In Hemelrijk, C. K. (Ed.), *Proceedings of international workshop on self-organisation and evolution of social behaviour* (pp. 358–367). Monte Verità, Switzerland.

Scheutz, M. (2004a). An artificial life approach to the study of basic emotions. In *Proceedings of cognitive science 2004.*

Scheutz, M. (2004b). A framework for evaluating affective control. In *Proceedings of the ace 2004 symposium at the 17th european meeting on cybernetics and systems research* (p. 645-650).

Scheutz, M. (2004c). How to determine the utility of emotions. In *Proceedings of AAAI spring symposium 2004* (p. 122-127).

Scheutz, M. (2004d). On the utility of adaptation vs. signalling action tendencies in the competition for resources. In *Proceedings of aamas 2004* (pp. 1378–1379). New York: ACM Press.

Scheutz, M. (2004e). Useful roles of emotions in artificial agents: A case study from artificial life. In [New York: AAAI Press.]. *Proceedings of AAAI, 2004,* 31–40.

Scheutz, M. (2006, June). Cross-level interactions between conflict resolution and survival games. In *Proceedings of artificial life x* (pp. 459–465).

Scheutz, M., & Logan, B. (2001). Affective versus deliberative agent control. In S. Colton (Ed.), *Proceedings of the aisb'01 symposium on emotion, cognition and affective computing* (pp. 1–10). York: Society for the Study of Artificial Intelligence and the Simulation of Behaviour.

Scheutz, M., & Schermerhorn, P. (2002). Steps towards a theory of possible trajectories from reactive to deliberative control systems. In R. Standish (Ed.), *Proceedings of the 8th conference of artificial life* (pp. 283–292). Cambridge, MA: MIT Press.

Scheutz, M., & Schermerhorn, P. (2003, October). Many is more but not too many: Dimensions of cooperation of agents with and without predictive capabilities. In Proceedings of ieee/wic iat-2003 (pp. 378–384). Washington, DC: IEEE Computer Society Press. doi:10.1109/IAT.2003.1241105doi:10.1109/IAT.2003.1241105

Scheutz, M., & Schermerhorn, P. (2004a). The more radical, the better: Investigating the utility of aggression in the competition among different agent kinds. In *Proceedings of sab 2004* (pp. 445–454). Cambridge, MA: MIT Press.

Scheutz, M., & Schermerhorn, P. (2004b). The role of signaling action tendencies in conflict resolution. *Journal of Artificial Societies and Social Simulation*, *1*(7).

Scheutz, M., & Schermerhorn, P. (2005a). (in press). Many is more: The utility of simple reactive agents with predictive mechanisms in multiagent object collection tasks. *Web Intelligence and Agent Systems*, *3*(1), 97–116.

Scheutz, M., & Schermerhorn, P. (2005b, June). Predicting population dynamics and evolutionary trajectories based on performance evaluations in alife simulations. In *Proceedings of gecco 2005* (pp. 35–42). New York: ACM Press. doi:10.1145/1068009.1068015

Scheutz, M., & Schermerhorn, P. (2008, August). The limited utility of communication in simple organisms. In *Proceedings of artificial life xi* (pp. 521–528).

Scheutz, M., & Sloman, A. (2001). Affect and agent control: Experiments with simple affective states. In Zhong, N., Liu, J., Ohsuga, S., & Bradshaw, J. (Eds.), *Intelligent agent technology: Research and development* (pp. 200–209). New Jersey: World Scientific Publisher.

Scheutz, M., Sloman, A., & Logan, B. (2000). Emotional states and realistic agent behaviour. In Geril, P. (Ed.), *Proceedings of gameon 2000, imperial college london* (pp. 81–88). Delft: Society for Computer Simulation.

Sloman, A. (1992). Prolegomena to a theory of communication and affect. In Ortony, A., Slack, J., & Stock, O. (Eds.), *Communication from an artificial intelligence perspective: Theoretical and applied issues* (pp. 229–260). Heidelberg, Germany: Springer.

Sloman, A. (2000). Models of models of mind, in *Proceedings Symposium on How to Design a Functioning Mind* AISB'00, Birmingham, April 2000. In (pp. 1–9).

Sloman, A., Chrisley, R., & Scheutz, M. (2005). The architectural basis of affective states and processes. In Fellous, J., & Arbib, M. (Eds.), *Who needs emotions? the brain meets the machine*. New York: Oxford University Press.

Sloman, A., & Croucher, M. (1981). Why robots will have emotions. In *Proc 7th int. joint conference on AI* (pp. 197–202). Vancouver.

Trappl, R., Petta, P., & Payr, S. (Eds.). (2001). *Emotions in humans and artifacts*. Cambridge, MA: MIT Press.

ENDNOTES

[1] Note that we construe motivations to be directed towards a specific goal. In the case of an elevated "anxiety level", as present in anxiety disorders, this kind of goal appears to be absent. Given that the state of anxiety itself is not desired, the agent could be viewed as "motivated" to change this state. If motivation is construed in this wide sense, then many emotional states may also be a motivational states (see also Ferguson, 1982). This does not seem to apply to all emotional states, however, in particular not to the kinds of states Sloman calls "tertiary emotions" or "perturbances" (Sloman, 1992), which could result from a loss of control of higher-level resource management processes in the agent's control system.

[2] For a possible function f that has the rational agent strategy as a limit case, see (Scheutz & Schermerhorn, 2004b).

[3] There are, however, other measures that can be used for variants of the survival task (Scheutz & Schermerhorn, 2003).

Chapter 5
A Computational Basis for the Emotions

N Korsten
King's College London, UK

JG Taylor
King's College London, UK

ABSTRACT

In order to achieve 'affective computing' it is necessary to know what is being computed. That is, in order to compute with what would pass for human emotions, it is necessary to have a computational basis for the emotions themselves. What does it mean quantitatively if a human is sad or angry? How is this affective state computed in their brain? It is this question, on the very core of the computational nature of the human emotions, which is addressed in this chapter. A proposal will be made as to this computational basis based on the well established approach to emotions as arising from an appraisal of a given situation or event by a specific human being.

INTRODUCTION

Previous research in psychology and neuroscience has strived to reach the basis of the emotional process, but the resulting models and theories have often not been translated into a computational representation. In the literature, we can distinguish between those theories advocating a basic emotions approach, a dimensional approach and an appraisal based approach.

In the basic emotion theories (e.g. Plutchik (2001), Panksepp (1982)), it is assumed that different processes underlie a small set of basic emotions; more complex emotions would arise from subtle variations on these basic ones. If this were represented computationally, the dif-

DOI: 10.4018/978-1-61692-892-6.ch005

ferent basic emotions could have differring and separate underlying computational systems. In this vein, a computational model of fear has been proposed by Armony et al. (1995), based around the amygdala as a central structure in fear production, assuming that fear is caused specifically by a (potential) threat and different structures would be responsible for producing other emotions. This model is based on fear conditioning research by LeDoux (1992), in which it was shown that the amygdala is particularly active in this process. Although this model reproduces experimental results in detail, such specific neural modules have never been located for other emotions. It has later been proposed that the amygdala functions as a relevance detector (Sander et al., 2003) – where stimuli evoking fear tend to be highly relevant.

Dimensional theories state that an emotion is defined by its location in a multidimensional space, where the number and character of the dimensions varies, but tends to include some variation on valence (positive – negative) and arousal (high – low). Computationally, this would translate to a separation between different modules for the different dimensions, rather than a separation between the different emotions, where the output would not consist of categorised emotions but rather of gradual changes in emotional feelings and behaviour. Although it seems that neural responses to valence and arousal can indeed be dissociated (Grimm et al. (2006), Anders et al. (2004)), results are not so clear cut that it is possible to point to delineated neural substrates. Nevertheless, psychological research using a statistical technique to identify the principal contributors to a particular phenomenon (Principal Components Analysis) has pointed to the existence of precisely four dimensions (Fontaine et al., 2007).

A combination of these two approaches can be found in the work of Russell and Fieldman-Barrett (1999), where core affect is proposed as a two dimensional, permanently present emotional state that does not need to be directed at any particular object or event, whereas prototypical emotional episodes are event-driven and form categories. No explicit computational account is given of this theory, but it suggests some sort of sum or multiplication of the outputs of the dimensional and basic emotion systems as described above.

A more causal analysis of the emergence of emotions, appraisal theory, states that emotions are a function of the individual's interpretation of the situation in terms of (potential) harm or benefit to this individual. A recent, detailed account of appraisal theory is proposed in the Component Process Model (CPM) (Scherer (2001), Sander et al. (2005)), in which four different Stimulus Evaluation Checks (SEC) – each consisting of several more specific checks – produce different changes in the emotional state. In this account, the SEC's (Relevance, Implication, Coping potential and Normative Significance) are sequential, and each SEC can produce output to various neural systems. As such, a corresponding computational model would contain four modules that are connected in sequence, which each receive input from and produce output to several other neural systems. In such a system, there would not be any one specific emotional output; rather, the emotion would be dispersed across a range of neural systems, most of which would not be specifically 'emotional' in nature.

Ortony et al. (1988) have presented a more inherently computational model of the appraisal process, in which emotions are considered to be valenced reactions to either consequences of events, actions of agents or aspects of objects, whereby different other factors such as desirability and agency further discriminate emotions within these categories. A computational structure is clear from the outline of the model in Figure 1. However, there is no connection to potential neural correlates in this model. It should be noted that there is an assumption in this approach that the emotional outputs are categorised, whereas in the CPM this is explicitly not the case.

Thus, quantitative analyses of the emotional process are still scarce, despite the fact that many

Figure 1. Model by Ortony et al. (1988), where a classification of emotional outputs are based on (combined) valuations of consequences, expectations, present objects and events, both for the self and for the other

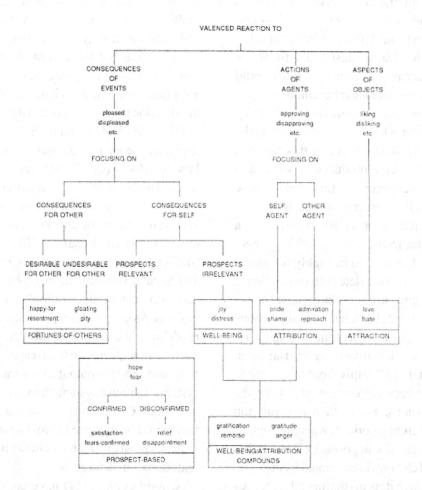

theories has been presented that would lend themselves to a quantitative interpretation. In the model we will present in the following sections, we have sought to fill this void in a manner interpretable from a neuroscience as well as a psychological background. The model we present incorporates aspects of the computational structures outlined above, and as such forms a blend of their associated theories. In it, we incorporate a set of concepts and contrasts similar to the model by Ortony et al. (1988) – such as action, consequence, valuation, other versus self, confirmation versus disconfirmation of expectations

– but these are combined differently in order to reach definitions for the different emotions.

Basis of Value Comparisons

Our proposal as to the computational origin of emotions is based on appraisal theory, as the emotional output relies on a set of continuous evaluations of the situation. We propose these evaluations to consist of value assessments – both current and predictive. The difference is that where appraisal theorists assume this to be, at its core, a complex cyclical process taking place across different neural systems, we propose a simple core computational basis of the emotional response. This proposal, first presented in Korsten (2009), is based on value as a core concept that has been related to emotion in psychology as well as neuroscience research.

In neuroscience, research related to value learning has been focused on the process of conditioning, in which an unconditioned stimulus (US) – a stimulus with an intrinsic positive or negative value to the subject – and a conditioned stimulus (CS) – a stimulus that is not intrinsically valuable to the subject – are associated through repeated concurrent or successive presentation, after which responses previously shown to the US only (such as freezing or approach behaviour) are also shown when the CS is presented. This is referred to as a conditioned response (CR). Thus, the CS adopts the value of the US by association. Although this is not an exclusively emotional process (it can occur automatically and subconsciously, and the UR can be non-emotional) the UR tends to consist of behaviours associated with emotion. Therefore, this provides a strong connection between emotion and value in the neuroscience literature, as the neural basis of this process has been investigated thoroughly, and outlined computationally (e.g. Suri et al. (1999), Armony et al. (1995)). The dopamine signal that has been found to function as a teaching signal in the storage of these associations in particular has been subject to much investigation, but some evidence has also been found also for the involvement of the orbitofrontal cortex (OFC) as the location of long term storage of these associations (Schoenbaum et al., 2005), and involvement of the amygdala in the process.

Appraisals - evaluations of the situation essential to appraisal theory - could be seen as values indicating ongoing or predicted beneficial or harmful effects of the stimulus in the process of being experienced. If we take fear, for example, this emotion could arise from the perception of a stimulus predictive of events that could be physically harmful to the individual. As such, the predicted value of events to come is, from this stimulus, negative; the individual has negative expectations in response to this stimulus. Thus, if we assign a numerical value to this expectation (the expected value) and compare it to whatever we consider a standard, normal value for our physical wellbeing (the normal value) we will find it to be lower. This discrepancy between the expected and normal values can be seen as computationally analogous to the emotion of fear. Similarly, other discrepancies can represent other emotions. Joy, for instance, represents a situation where the current state of events (actual value) is higher than normal, and disappointment represents the assessment that previous expectations (the second expected value) are not fulfilled. In these examples, four different value assessments have been involved:

- Actual value (act), representing the current state of affairs
- Expected value (exp1), representing a prediction based on the current stimulus
- Second expected value (exp2), representing a prediction based on previous stimuli
- Normal value (norm), representing a standard or norm for this value

In the following sections, we will show that discrepancies between these four values can differentiate between a large range of emotions and as such provide a quantitative framework for emotion production.

Individual Comparisons

One subset of emotions can arise from the physical state – and predictions as to the physical state – of the individual, and can be clearly identified in animals as well as humans. Beyond them are those more specifically recognisable as aroused in social situations, such as shyness or gratitude, or involved with the outcome of some action, as in guilt or regret. We will start by considering the emotions as arising from certain combinations of the four values mentioned at the end of the previous section reaching specific thresholds. We will then expand these processes to apply to the broader range of emotions by considering other aspects of valuations. We present in Table 1 putative threshold constraints for the arousal of the corresponding emotion.

This table illustrates how, through the assessment of different values, this framework could differentiate between an even larger range of emotions. We can justify the assignments in the table in more detail as follows:

Fear. This emotion can be thought of as a prediction of a future event that is negative when compared to normal circumstances. For example, a subject seeing a big, strong man holding a stick looking angrily in his direction may predict being beaten up and hurt, and therefore fearful. This is a prediction of the subject's physical comfort being lower than it would be in average normal circumstances. Barr-Zisowitz (2000) notes that: "For the most part, there is a consensus [in the literature] that sadness is distinguished from fear by being a response to an event that has already taken place, whereas fear anticipates an event to come." In terms of value comparisons, this equates for fear to the first expected value (expectation

Table 1. value comparisons for the reward / punishment value type

	reward / punishment
$exp1 < norm$	fear
$exp1 > norm$	hope
$act < norm$ & $exp1 > act$	anger
$act < norm$ & $exp1 =< act$	sadness
$exp2 < norm$ & $exp1 > exp2$	relief
$exp2 > norm$ & $exp1 < exp2$	disappointment
$act > norm$ & $exp2 < act$	surprise
$act > norm$	joy

for the future) being lower than the normal value: $exp1 < norm$.

Hope can be seen as the opposite of fear, so as a prediction that a future event is positive when compared to normal circumstances. This would occur when a subject is presented with a stimulus which would lead them to expect a reward in the near future, such as cooking smells and noises emanating from a kitchen. This equates to the first expected value (expectation for a future event) being higher than the normal value: $exp1 > norm$.

Joy, we can think of as the current situation being above average, regardless of past expectations for the current situation, or expectations for the future based on current stimuli. Therefore, $exp1$ and $exp2$ are not relevant here, and there is only the discrepancy of $act > norm$.

Anger may seem like a difficult emotion to classify in these terms, as it is generally regarded in relation to its associated response (attack) rather than to preceding events. However, it is still possible to imagine events that would typically lead to an angry response: being robbed, stubbing ones toe, being undeservedly humiliated. In all of these cases, a loss is involved that is perceived as unjustified and (should be) redeemable. In other words, the value of current events is perceived as below normal standards, but there is an expectation of improvement. In case of undeserved humiliation, the value level of self-esteem could be currently reduced, but expected to be increased again when a suitable response is made. On a purely functional level, an active, aggressive response is pointless if there is no potential for improvement. In this case, the actual value would be smaller than normal. However, the first expected value $exp1$ (the expectation for the event in the future) would be larger than the actual value: $act < norm$ and $exp1 > act$.

Sadness is, as quoted above, a "response to an event that has already taken place" (Barr-Zisowitz, 2000). This emotion is strongly associated with irretrievable loss of some kind, where irretrievable could be taken as low expectations for the future. Thus, it combines a low actual value with an equally low or lower expectation for the future (exp1). This low exp1 value contrasts it with anger: act < norm and exp1 <= act.

Relief can be thought of as fear not being fulfilled: if the angry man holding the stick coming towards the fearful subject turns out to only be carrying some firewood, the subject will feel relieved. In other words, the expected value was below the normal value (as is the case in fear) before, but now it has increased towards the normal value again. As for the example above, where the stimulus of the approaching angry man with the stick evokes fear, and at the event (arrival of the man with the stick) nothing happens, the value that was expected for this situation before (exp2) is lower than normal, but the currently expected value (exp1) is not reduced (or less so): exp2 < norm and exp1 > exp2.

Disappointment, in contrast to relief, can be thought of as hope not being fulfilled, so as a higher expectation than normal not coming true. This is analogous to relief as described above, which could be thought of as fear not coming true. In the example of the cooking smells emanating from the kitchen, disappointment would ensue if we then found out that the food was being prepared for someone else: the value we were expecting initially (exp2) is above the normal level, but the value we are currently expecting (exp1) is lower than that, leading to the following conditions: exp2 > norm and exp1 < exp2.

Surprise occurs when we are not expecting anything, and a positive event occurs, despite our lack of expectation. This means the actual value is higher than normal, and higher than we were expecting previously: act > norm and exp2 < act.

To extend the range of emotions being considered, we introduce two further aspects. Firstly, there is known to be a separation in the brain between the regions coding for the future reward value of stimuli (as in the OFC) and for that coding for aspects of the self. These latter areas have been suggested to reside in the mid-brain region

(Panksepp, 1999). Thus, we consider a new set of value maps (likely sited in mid-OFC) for predicted values associated with self-esteem and rewards/penalties for the self. Secondly, there are predictions of rewards or punishments for future actions as guided by internal motor models in the parietal-premotor system (sometimes called mirror neurons but more correctly part of the overall motor system) (Raos et al., 2004, 2007). We suggest that there is also a separate set of value maps related to (predicted) action outcomes in the OFC. Such predictions can also be applied to another person, as seen by direct observation by the subject. The resulting set of value maps and associated thresholds leads to the enlarged set of emotions as displayed in Table 2.

As above for reward and punishment, now follows a detailed description of how each emotion in the above table is connected to the comparisons in the first column (when different from those in the second column described above).

Self-esteem. Low or unstable self-esteem has been connected to anger and depression. As such, we hypothesise that positive changes in self-esteem have emotional consequences as well. In the literature, we can find a distinction between global self-esteem, self-evaluations and feelings of self-worth or state self-esteem. Global self-esteem is generally viewed as a personality trait determined in youth and adolescence (Brown et al., 2001), whereas self-evaluations refer to separate evaluations of the various abilities and characteristics of the self, and state self-esteem refers to temporary emotional states arising from positive or negative self-related stimuli. In this theory, we interpret global self-esteem as the normal value of self-esteem, and state self-esteem as the more variable actual and expected values of self-esteem, as these are responsive to incoming stimuli. As such, discrepancies between the innate global self-esteem value and the stimulus based state self-esteem values would give rise to emotions. Self-esteem is related not only to one's own judgment of the self, but also to that

Table 2. value comparisons and their associated emotions for different value types

	reward/ punishment	self-esteem	outcome of action	outcome of others action
exp1 < norm	fear	shyness	guilt	contempt
exp1 > norm	hope	confidence	hope	admiration
act < norm & exp1 > act	anger	anger	regret	empathy
act < norm & exp1 =< act	sadness	shame	regret	pity
exp2 < norm & exp1 > exp2	relief	gratitude	relief	
exp2 < norm & act <= exp2			guilt	schadenfreude
exp2 > norm & exp1 < exp2	disapp'tm't	disapp'tm't	frustration	pity
act > norm & exp2 < act	surprise	surprise	surprise	
act > norm	joy	pride, triumph	satisfaction	jealousy

of others; it is assumed here to be a highly social concept representing our own assessment of our status, our ranking in the pecking order.

Particular emotions are particularly related to the self, such as pride and shame. This has also been noted by other authors. They have termed this class of emotions 'self-conscious' (Lewis, 2000) or 'self-referential' (Zinck, 2008) emotions. Comparisons between different self-esteem value representations can lead to self-referential emotions in the following ways:

Pride could emerge from a stimulus giving rise to a high value of self-esteem, like a compliment or task well completed. This means the actual value of self-esteem is higher than the normal one: act > norm.

Shyness can be interpreted as a response to a threatening social situation in which we expect that our self-esteem could potentially be damaged. When giving a presentation, for example, one may feel shy and insecure if one has not prepared well and therefore expect to receive a dent in one's self-esteem if it turns out not to be appreciated by the audience: exp1 < norm.

Confidence could be taken as the opposite of shyness, in the sense that it is a response to a social situation in which we expect our self-esteem to be increased. One would feel confident when one has prepared well for a presentation one is giving, and

therefore expect the applause and compliments at the end: exp1 > norm.

Shame is strongly associated with public humiliation and a feeling of exposure. It could emerge in response to a reduced self-esteem when there is no expectation for this self-esteem to be redeemed: act < norm and exp1 =< act

Anger has been researched somewhat more thoroughly than other emotions as a consequence of changes in self-esteem values. Self-esteem has long been known to be involved in the development of feelings of anger. It has long been thought that it was low self-esteem per se that caused anger and aggression (Baumeister, Smart, & Boden, 1996) but more recently it has been suggested that an instability of (Franck & De Raedt, 2007) or/combined with threat to self-esteem (Kuppens & van Mechelen, 2007) creates violent responses. Baumeister et al. (1996) also point out that it is not low self-esteem per se, but a discrepancy between a global high self-esteem and a more temporary perception of a disagreement with this self-assessment somewhere in the outside world that gives rise to anger. As explained above, this could be equated to a discrepancy between the normal and actual value of self-esteem, where a lower actual that normal value would give rise to anger. However, as mentioned in the 'Anger' section above, it seems likely that feelings of anger also encompass an expectation of a higher value in the future: act < norm and exp1 > act.

Gratitude may be a counterintuitive item on this list, as it appears to be by definition a response to receiving a gift, which is not directly related to self-esteem. However, gratitude does not necessarily need to be focused on one particular person and /or gift, as we can feel grateful in general for e.g. our good health. We propose that gratitude is the response to a stimulus increasing the expected value of self-esteem (e.g. a compliment) when the subject is feeling shy or insecure (so has a low previous expectation of self-esteem). Let us add that receiving a gift does not always lead to an experience of gratitude, and can be interpreted as a stimulus that increases self-esteem: exp2 < norm and exp1 > exp2.

The reasoning behind the appearance of disappointment and surprise in this column in the table is similar to that applied previously for these emotions.

Outcome of Action

Some emotions, like guilt or regret, are immediately connected to our actions or choices and their associated goals and motivations. If we define a goal or motivation as the expected result of an action or choice, we can consider this action to be a stimulus evoking a particular expected value (the goal). After all, when a goal-directed action is performed, this implies that the expected result of this action has some motivational value. The following emotions can all be related to action/choice motivations and expectations in this manner:

Satisfaction is the emotion that arises when we know that our actions have had a positive result, or in other words, that we made the right choice: act > norm.

Guilt can be related to a negative consequence of an action, but depends strongly on the intent of the individual when performing the action. As an example, let us take an action that most people would feel guilty about: throwing an egg

at an innocent old lady. Regardless of whether or not the egg actually hits the old lady, it is the intent of doing something malicious that should already make us feel bad before the outcome of this action is known. What could reduce our guilty feelings is if the action was intended to have a positive effect (e.g. we were trying to hit the pickpocket that was trying to steal her bag at the time). In this case, our expectation was positive rather than negative. So we see that it is the expectation we have at the time of performing the action that makes us feel guilty (or not). In other words, if our expected value (as a consequence of an action) is lower than normal, we feel guilty: exp1 < norm. It should be noted that, contrary to fear, feelings of guilt continue if the outcome is indeed as negative as we expected: exp2 < norm and act <= exp2.

Frustration has an element of thwarted goal achievement: our actions do not have the expected result or we believe that our actions will not have the result that we expected. In other words, our expectations have been reduced. This is similar to disappointment. For example, when we perform an action from which we expect a reward, such as putting money in a candy machine, and we do not receive the reward (if the candy machine turns out to be broken) we feel frustrated. exp2 > norm and exp1 < exp2.

Regret, the feeling associated with wishing that we had not made a particular choice in the past, is related to an action or choice that has had a negative result. Contrary to guilt, where the past action is the focus of the emotion and the outcome is irrelevant, in regret it is the outcome that matters, and the expectations of the time of the action are ignored. It is possible to regret an action without feeling guilty about it, and vice versa. Let us suppose that in the earlier example where the egg is thrown at the old lady's bag thief, the egg accidentally hits the old lady instead of the bag thief. In this instance, the subject (the egg thrower) would probably regret his/her actions, but not feel guilty, as he/she was only trying to help the old lady. So regret is felt in cases where the actual value (the outcome of the action) is lower than normal, where our previous expectation (at the time of the action) is irrelevant: act < norm.

Actions of Others

Our evaluations of the actions of other people also play a role in the emergence of some emotions, like pity and jealousy.

Jealousy arises when another persons actions result in a disproportionate reward, or when he/she receives reward without having deserved it, in other words when his/her actions should not lead to a reward. The value of his/her possessions or wellbeing as a consequence of his/her action is higher than normal: act > norm.

Pity is created by the opposite situation: another person possesses less than he/she should, when his/her actions should have resulted in a higher reward or less punishment than he/she actually has. The value of his/her possessions or wellbeing, as a consequence of his/her actions, is lower than normal: act < norm. This is also the case when the expectation of reward is decreased relative to the previous expectation: exp2 > norm and exp1 < exp2.

Contempt is related to the likelihood that a person behaves in a way that is stupid, cowardly or otherwise not beneficial to themselves or others. When someone performs an action that we deem unwise or wrong, because we expect this action to result in a loss, we may feel contempt for this person: exp1 < norm.

Admiration, as the opposite of contempt, is related to the likelihood that a person behaves in a way that is clever, brave or otherwise beneficial to themselves or others. When someone performs an action that we deem wise or right, because we expect it to result in a reward or increase in wellbeing for themselves or others, we may admire this person: exp1 > norm.

Empathy is similar to pity, with the difference that in empathy we expect the subject to be able to cope on his/her own, and sympathise with his/her struggle, whereas pity suggests a victim that needs help: act < norm and exp1 > act.

Schadenfreude is an emotion that can follow contempt, if a persons unwise actions result in the expected punishment: exp2 < norm and act <= exp2.

Other Emotions

Some emotions have a prominent place in the emotion literature, but are missing from table 2. Perhaps the most notable one is disgust, which has often been named as one of the basic emotions. It could be argued that disgust is a drive rather than an emotion, as it is strongly related to body state, similarly to other drives like pain and hunger. Disgust may constitute a direct physical response to food or body related stimuli that are best avoided. The more abstract meaning of disgust whereby one can indicate to be disgusted with for example a person behaving immorally could be taken as a linguistic analogy rather than indicating a particular emotion. In this case, the actual emotion may be contempt.

Other notable omissions from the above list of emotions are love and hate. Although it is impossible to deny that these are actually true emotions, they do differ from the emotions listed above. Love and hate are not so much produced by one particular episode, but tend to be longer lasting states, attached to one particular individual; it is hardly possible to feel love or hate for a little while in response to a single stimulus. These emotions encompass not only a feeling, but also imply a commitment. Without this commitment, love is reduced to mere liking and hate is reduced to dislike, neither of which can be classed as fully fledged emotions, merely as evaluations.

A final emotion missing from the list above is embarrassment. Although it has been proposed that embarrassment is merely a milder version of shame, empirical study shows otherwise (Tangney et al., 1996): differences in ratings of subjects'

Figure 2. Representation of the structure of the simulink model. In the 'COMPARE normal' module, act, exp1 and exp2 are compared to the normal value, whereas in the 'COMPARE exp1-exp2-act' they are compared to one another. Both signals are passed on to the 'OUTPUT' module, in which they are combined to represent the different emotions as per table 2. Output from the 'COMPARE normal' module disinhibits the 'ctxt' module via the 'SI' module, maintaining a representation of stimuli that may no longer be present

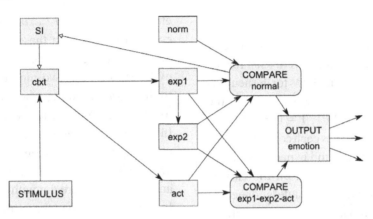

embarrassing and shameful experiences cannot be explained by intensity of affect alone, although exactly how embarrassment differs from shame is still not clear.

A question that arises is how, in a computational framework like this, the intensity of the emotion could be determined. The cases of fear, hope and joy, where only one value comparison is involved, seem relatively straightforward: it would be the size of this discrepancy that determines the intensity of the emotion. For the other emotions, it seems likely that both relevant comparisons contribute in some way to their intensity. Let us, for example, look at sadness, which we feel when confronted with an irretrievable loss. The amount of sadness we feel would both depend on the current reduction in our actual value (the perceived loss) and our expectation for the future: if we expect things to get worse, we will be more sad than if we expect things to stay the way they currently are.

Architecture & Simulations

The comparisons as described in the previous sections and summarised in table 2 can be calculated through the neurally inspired computational architecture outlined in Figure 2 (Korsten, 2009).

This architecture was implemented in Matlab Simulink, with a fixed step size of 0.01 and applying the Euler method of integration. Each neuron in the model is a simple graded-response neuron with a membrane equation of:

$$\tau \frac{\delta V}{\delta t} = -V - \rho I$$

where V is the neuron membrane potential, τ is the neuron time constant, I is the injected current from the neuron's various connections and ρ is a constant that regulates the voltage to current ratio. The output of each neuron is the positive part of a saturating sigmoidal non-linearity:

$$\text{output} = f(V(t))$$

$$f(\mathrm{x}) = \left[\left\{ \frac{1}{1 - e^{-\frac{x-\delta}{T}}} \right\} - \frac{1}{2} \right]$$

where θ is the threshold and T is the noise temperature. The following values were used for the parameters of the neuron equations for the neurons in the model, unless otherwise indicated in the next sections: ρ = 5; θ = 0.01; T = 1; τ = 20 ms.

The act and exp1 modules each contain a single node indicating the actual and expected value of one particular value type based on the current context. Each node in the ctxt module is connected to the act and exp1 modules. These connections are differentially weighted, so different contexts cause different activations of act and exp1. The exp2 module also contains a single node, receiving input from the exp1 module and containing a decaying representation of exp1. This is achieved through an increased τ value in this node, of 1000 ms, whereas this is 200 ms in the other nodes in the simulation. The *norm* module contains two

constants, indicating the higher and lower limit of the range of normal values.

These normal values are compared to the other three values in the *compare normal* module. This module contains six nodes, one for each comparison (act > norm, act < norm, exp1 > norm etc.). In the *compare exp1-exp2-act* module, a comparison between these three values occurs, also in six nodes (act > exp1, act < exp1, exp1 < exp2, etc.). These two modules produce output to the *output* module, where they are combined to form the assessments as presented in table 1. In this module, each of the nodes represents an emotion. Finally, the spontaneous inhibition (*SI*) module inhibits the *ctxt* module unless the actual and exp1 values are not within the normal range. In other words, once an emotional stimulus is present, the *SI* module will keep the *ctxt* module activated, through disinhibition, until the actual and exp1 values have returned to within a normal range. Please refer to Korsten (2009) for more details on exact weights and connectivity between the modules.

We will now present two simulated scenarios representative of a large range of value related

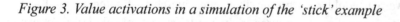

Figure 3. Value activations in a simulation of the 'stick' example

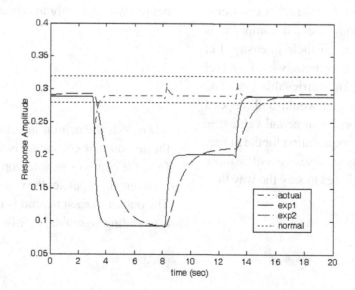

situations, including those containing a series of incremental increases and slow as well as fast changes in value, in- or decreases of act and exp1 resting on or crossing the normal value, and producing multiple emotional responses at once as well as in unison, weakly as well as strongly.

The first scenario concerns the example of the man and the stick presented earlier in this chapter, in which we define the point in time where the man with the stick appears as t1, the moment when the subject realises that the stick could be firewood as t2, and the point in time where the man with the stick reaches the subject as t3. Three different contexts exist in this example: the context where no danger has been noticed (before t1 and after t3), the one where an angry man with a weapon is walking towards us (t1 to t2), and the one where an angry man with firewood is walking towards us (t2 to t3). This situation was implemented in the model through different *ctxt – exp1* weights

Figure 4. Emotion activations in the simulation of the 'stick' example

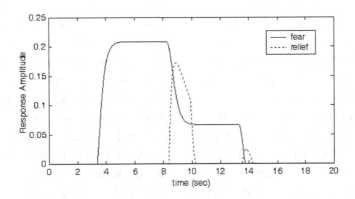

Figure 5. Value levels for the 'sprinter' example

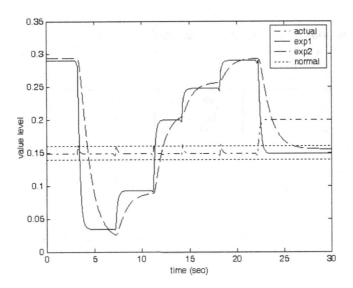

Table 3. Simulation weights for the 'sprinter' example.

Ctxt - exp1 weights	Ctxt – act weights	Activation time
0.3	0.15	0 - 3 18 - 22
0.05	0.15	3 - 7
0.1	0.15	7 - 11
0.2	0.15	11 - 14
0.25	0.15	14 - 18
0.15	0.2	22 - 30

(0.3, 0.1 and 0.2, respectively) combined with sequential activation of the different contexts, where time t1 occurs at t = 3 seconds after onset of the simulation, t2 = 8 sec, t3 = 13 sec. In this simulation, the lower normal value was 0.28 and the higher was 0.32. Figures 3 and 4 show activations of the value modules and emotion nodes in the output module, respectively.

Let us consider a second example of an emotion evoking situation as per the example of the man and the stick above: a professional sprinter running an important race. This is a highly emotionally charged situation, where the emotional experience would depend at least for a large part on the expectation of the reward of winning the race, as a consequence of the sprinter's action of running it. Before starting, the sprinter would psych herself up to be absolutely convinced that she can win the race (or, if there are opponents that she is sure are much stronger, that she can achieve a different goal like beating her more direct opponents). This would create a high expected reward value of the outcome of her action of running as fast as she can, where her normal value (average result in the past) may be to become fourth. Where she to get into the last position after a bad start, her expectations would be lower than normal, but as she overtakes each of her opponents in turn, her expectation would rise back to the level of winning the race. Were she to be overtaken at the last minute and end in second place, her exp1 and actual values would both reflect this second position, whereas exp2 would remain slightly higher.

Figure 6. Emotion activations for the 'sprinter' scenario

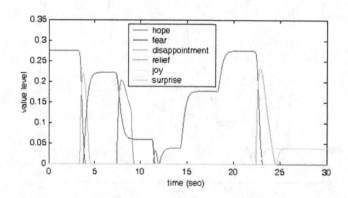

In this example of the sprinter, there is a whole range of different contexts, one for each position she holds in the race plus one before the start and after the finish. Simulation results for this scenario are presented in Figure 5, according to weights as presented in Table 3. Emotional outputs of this scenario are presented in Figure 6.

These results show quantitative criteria for the emergence and classification of emotions and as such could form a basis for 'affective computation'. Please note that a small discrepancy exists in the value of exp2, which sometimes rises slightly above previous values of exp1. This is due to the complex parameters of the neurally inspired simulation.

DISCUSSION

Predictions of this model go beyond the few examples mentioned in this chapter, and can in principle apply to any situation, predicting the particular emotion that will ensue in response to that particular situation, based on the value discrepancies implied by the context and stimuli perceived by the subject. Apart from these situation specific predictions, this model also contains implications as to which emotions may be considered basic; those emotions most generally included in the basic emotions (anger, fear, joy, sadness) all concern reward / punishment without involvement of the exp2 value. Furthermore, it is possible to predict which emotions can and cannot occur simultaneously for the same value type.

This theory has a strong interdisciplinary character; it can be expressed computationally, related to various psychological theories on emotion and is neurally inspired. Moreover, neural correlates for the model have tentatively been identified (Korsten, 2009). Also, it accounts for a range of emotional processes, encompassing short prototypical emotional episodes as well as longer lasting states. Nevertheless, this model does not account for attentional or perceptual influences on emotion and vice versa, or for any subtleties in the emotional response based on response inhibition, for instance. It is also unspecific as to how the emotional feeling – the perception of the emotion – arises. As such, it needs to be considered as a proposal for a core process rather than a complete theory encompassing all aspects of emotional functioning. It is our hope that future avenues of empirical research will focus on assessing the neuroscientific and psychological reality of this model, as well as mapping out the processes impacting on both the initial value assessments and the eventual emotional response.

REFERENCES

Anders, S., Lotze, M., Erb, M., Grodd, W., & Birbaumer, N. (2004). Brain activity underlying emotional valence and arousal: a response-related fMRI study. *Human Brain Mapping*, *23*, 200–209. doi:10.1002/hbm.20048

Armony, J. L., Servan-Schreiber, D., Cohen, J. D., & Ledoux, J. E. (1995). An anatomically constrained neural network model of fear conditioning. *Behavioral Neuroscience*, *109*, 246–257. doi:10.1037/0735-7044.109.2.246

Barr-Zisowitz, C. (2000). "Sadness" - Is There Such a Thing? In Lewis, M., & Haviland-Jones, J. (Eds.), *Handbook of emotions* (pp. 607–622). New York: Guilford Press.

Baumeister, R. F., Smart, L., & Boden, J. M. (1996). Relation of Threatened Egotism to Violence and Aggression: The Dark Side of High Self-Esteem. *Psychological Review*, *103*, 5–33. doi:10.1037/0033-295X.103.1.5

Brown, J. D., Dutton, K. A., & Cook, K. E. (2001). From the top down: Self-esteem and self-evaluation. *Cognition and Emotion*, *15*, 615–631.

Fontaine, J. R., Scherer, K. R., Roesch, E. B., & Ellsworth, P. C. (2007). The world of emotions is not two-dimensional. *Psychological Science, 18,* 1050–1057. doi:10.1111/j.1467-9280.2007.02024.x

Franck, E., & De Raedt, R. (2007). (in press). Self-esteem reconsidered: Unstable self-esteem outperforms level of self-esteem as vulnerability marker for depression. [Corrected Proof.]. *Behaviour Research and Therapy.* doi:10.1016/j.brat.2007.01.003

Grimm, S., Schmidt, C. F., Bermpohl, F., Heinzel, A., Dahlem, Y., & Wyss, M. (2006). Segregated neural representation of distinct emotion dimensions in the prefrontal cortex-an fMRI study. *NeuroImage, 30,* 325–340. doi:10.1016/j.neuroimage.2005.09.006

Korsten, N. (2009). *Neural Architectures for an Appraisal Basis of Emotion.* PhD thesis, London:King's College.

Kuppens, P., & van Mechelen, I. (2007). Interactional appraisal models for the anger appraisals of threatened self-esteem, other-blame and frustration. *Cognition and Emotion, 21,* 56–77. doi:10.1080/02699930600562193

Ledoux, J. E. (1992). Brain mechanisms of emotion and emotional learning. *Current Opinion in Neurobiology, 2,* 191–197. doi:10.1016/0959-4388(92)90011-9

Lewis, M. (2000). Self-Conscious Emotions: Embarrassment, Pride, Shame, and Guilt. In Lewis, M., & Haviland-Jones, J. (Eds.), *Handbook of emotions* (pp. 623–636). New York: Guilford Press, New York.

Ortony, A., Clore, G. L., & Collins, A. (1988). *The Cognitive Structure of Emotions.* Cambridge, UK: Cambridge University Press.

Panksepp, J. (1982). Toward a General Psychobiological Theory of Emotions. *The Behavioral and Brain Sciences, 5,* 407–467. doi:10.1017/S0140525X00012759

Panksepp, J. (1999). The Preconscious Substrates of Consciousness: Affective States and the Evolutionary Origins of the Self. In Gallagher, S., & Shear, J. (Eds.), *Models of the Self* (pp. 113–130). Exeter, UK: Imprint Academic.

Plutchik, R. (2001). The Nature of Emotions. *American Scientist, 89,* 344.

Raos, V., Evangeliou, M. N., & Savaki, H. E. (2004). Observation of action: grasping with the mind's hand. *NeuroImage, 23,* 193–201. doi:10.1016/j.neuroimage.2004.04.024

Raos, V., Evangeliou, M. N., & Savaki, H. E. (2007). Mental simulation of action in the service of action perception. *The Journal of Neuroscience, 27,* 12675–12683. doi:10.1523/JNEUROSCI.2988-07.2007

Russell, J. A., & Barrett, L. F. (1999). Core affect, prototypical emotional episodes, and other things called emotion: dissecting the elephant. *Journal of Personality and Social Psychology, 76,* 805–819. doi:10.1037/0022-3514.76.5.805

Sander, D., Grafman, J., & Zalla, T. (2003). The human amygdala: an evolved system for relevance detection. *Reviews in the Neurosciences, 14,* 303–316.

Sander, D., Grandjean, D., & Scherer, K. R. (2005). A systems approach to appraisal mechanisms in emotion. *Neural Networks, 18,* 317–352. doi:10.1016/j.neunet.2005.03.001

Scherer, K. R., Schorr, A., & Johnstone, T. (2001). *Appraisal Processes in Emotion: Theory, Methods, Research.* New York: Oxford University Press.

Schoenbaum, G., & Roesch, M. (2005). Orbitofrontal cortex, associative learning, and expectancies. *Neuron, 47,* 633–636. doi:10.1016/j.neuron.2005.07.018

Suri, R. E., & Schultz, W. (1999). A neural network model with dopamine-like reinforcement signal that learns a spatial delayed response task. *Neuroscience, 91,* 871–890. doi:10.1016/S0306-4522(98)00697-6

Tangney, J. P., Miller, R. S., Flicker, L., & Barlow, D. H. (1996). Are shame, guilt, and embarrassment distinct emotions? *Journal of Personality and Social Psychology, 70,* 1256–1269. doi:10.1037/0022-3514.70.6.1256

Zinck, A. (2008). Self-referential emotions. *Consciousness and Cognition, 17,* 496–505. doi:10.1016/j.concog.2008.03.014

Chapter 6
For a 'Cognitive Anatomy' of Human Emotions and a Mind–Reading Based Affective Interaction

Cristiano Castelfranchi
CNR, Italy

ABSTRACT

Human emotions are based on typical configurations of beliefs, goals, expectations etc. In order to understand the complexity of affective processing in humans, reactions to stimuli, perception of our bodily reaction to events or just the feeling related to something should be considered but this is not adequate. Besides, our body does not respond just to external stimuli (events); it reacts to our interpretation of the stimulus, to the meaning of the event as well. In order to build affective architectures we also have to model the body, and its perception. In this chapter, with the help of these facts, the author will analyze the cognitive anatomies of simple anticipation-based emotions in addition to some complex social emotions.

INTRODUCTION

In this chapter, we present, in a rather synthetic way and without the possibility of extensively discussing the literature:

a.   An explicit and analytical cognitive modeling of human emotions (cognitive 'anatomies' in terms of beliefs, goals, etc.);

b.   The limits of this fundamental approach, and the need for its embodiment: modeling and integrating the bodily motions and signals, and what we feel;

c.   Its application to computational models, artificial intelligence (AI), and human-computer interaction (HCI).

DOI: 10.4018/978-1-61692-892-6.ch006

The effects of complex emotions processed by humans go beyond reacting to stimuli, perceiving our bodily reaction to events, or feeling something. Especially complex human emotions are based on specific mental states; they are typical configurations of beliefs, goals, motives, expectations etc. In this chapter, we will analyze some typical mental configurations needed for (i) rather simple anticipation-based emotions ('hope', 'fear', 'disappointment', 'relief', 'joy') and (ii) complex social emotions like 'shame', 'envy', 'guilt', 'pity': their ingredients and their coherent structure. In particular, we will analyze shame and guilt in a very synthetic way.

We are in favor of a componential analysis of emotions (and in general, mental states and processes like 'expectation', 'need', 'trust', 'argument', etc.). This allows a systematic explicit model of the relationships within and among the substances to be modeled. However, one should also care about accounting for the unitary character of the mental-behavioral phenomena. On one side, being atomically decomposable, the complex mental states have their own emergent, specific, non-reducible properties and functions on the other side.

Our body does not respond to external stimuli or events based on pattern matching; it also reacts to our interpretation of the stimulus, to the meaning of the event; that is to a mental representation. In addition, the body reacts to merely endogenous representations, to mental events (like a counterfactual imagination). For example, it is always a thought that makes us blush. Of course for a complete real emotion, bodily activation and perception is necessary: at least in terms of the activation of the central memory trace of the bodily reaction (somatic marker), the evocation of some sensation. We feel our bodily response, but we ascribe it to that event or idea; this combination gives an emotional nature to both sides.

EXPECTATIONS AND RELATED EMOTIONS

Expectations vs. Predictions

'Expectations' are not just 'Predictions'; they are not fully synonyms. Therefore, we do not want to use expectations (like in the literature) just to mean predictions, that is, epistemic representations about the future. We consider, in particular, a 'forecast' as a mere belief about a future state of the world and we distinguish it from a simple hypothesis. The difference is in terms of degree of certainty: a hypothesis may involve the belief that future p is possible while a forecast has the belief that future p is probable. A forecast implies that the chance threshold has been exceeded.

Putting aside the degree of confidence (a general term for covering weak and strong predictions), for us expectations have a more restricted meaning (and this is why a computer can produce predictions or forecasts but do not have expectations). In 'expectations':

i.   the prediction is relevant for the predictor; he is concerned, interested, and that is why

ii.   he is expecting, that is the prediction is aimed at being verified; he is waiting in order to know whether the prediction is true or not.

Expectation is a suspended state after the formulation of a prediction[1]. If there is an expectation then there is a prediction, but not the other way around.

Epistemic Goals and Activity

In the prediction-expectation chain, first of all, the agent X, has the Goal of knowing whether the predicted event or state really happens (epistemic goal). She is waiting for this; at least for curiosity. This concept of 'waiting for' and 'looking for' is necessarily related to the notion of expecting and expectation, but not to the notion of prediction.

During the expectation process, either X is actively monitoring what is happening and comparing the incoming information (for example perception) to the internal mental representation; or X is doing this cyclically and regularly; or X will compare what happens with her prediction (epistemic actions) in any case at the moment of the future event or state. Because in any case she has the Goal to know whether the world actually is as anticipated and if the prediction was correct. Therefore, in order to represent 'expecting' and the true 'expectation' schematically, we can write:

Expectation(x,p) $\Rightarrow$ *Bel(x,p'')$^{t'}$ & Goal(x,p)*

where *Bel(x,p'')$^{t'}$* is the belief of x at t' that the predicted event p occurs at t'' (where $t'' > t'$) and *Goal(x,p)* denotes the goal of x from t' to t''' ($t''' > t''$) for *Know(x,p'')$\vee$Know(x,~p'')*.

Content Goals

This Epistemic/Monitoring Goal is combined with Goal that p: the agent's need, desire, or 'intention that' the world should realize. The Goal that p is true (or the Goal that Not p). This is really why and in which sense X is concerned and not indifferent, and also why she is monitoring the world. She is an agent with interests, desires, needs, objectives, on the world, not just a predictor. This is also why computers, that already make predictions, do not have expectations.

Expectations can be classified according to the relation between the goals and predictions. When the agent has a goal opposite to her prediction, she has a negative expectation. On the other hand, when the agent has a goal equal to her prediction she has a positive expectation.

In sum, expectations are axiological anticipatory mental representations, endowed with Valence: they are positive or negative or ambivalent or neutral. But in any case they are evaluated against some concern, drive, motive, goal of the agent. In expectations, we have to distinguish two components:

- On one side, there is a mental anticipatory representation, the belief about a future state or event, the mental anticipation of the fact, what we might also call pre-vision (to foresee).

  The format of this belief or pre-vision can be either propositional or imagery (or mental model of). At this point the function is pertinent rather than the format of the belief.

- On the other side, as we have just argued, there is a co-referent Goal (wish, desire, intention, or any other motivational explicit representation).

Given the resulting amalgam these representations of the future are charged of value. Their intention or content has a (positive or negative) 'valence'[2]. More precisely, expectations can be:

positive (goal conformable):

$$Bel(x, p^{t'})^{t<t'} \& Goal(x, p^{t'}) \quad \left[or\ Bel(x, \sim p^{t'})^{t<t'} \& Goal(x, \sim p^{t'}) \right]$$

negative (goal opposite):

$$Bel(x, p^{t'})^{t<t'} \& Goal(x, \sim p^{t'}) \quad \left[or\ Bel(x, \sim p^{t'})^{t<t'} \& Goal(x, p^{t'}) \right]$$

neutral:

$$Bel(x, p^{t'})^{t<t'} \& \sim Goal(x, p^{t'}) \& \sim Goal(x, \sim p^{t'}) \quad \left[or\ Bel(x, \sim p^{t'})^{t<t'} \& \sim Goal(x, p^{t'}) \& \sim Goal(x, \sim p^{t'}) \right]$$

ambivalent:

$$Bel(x, p^{t'})^{t<t'} \& Goal(x, p^{t'}) \& Goal(x, \sim p^{t'}) \quad \left[or\ Bel(x, \sim p^{t'})^{t<t'} \& Goal(x, p^{t'}) \& Goal(x, \sim p^{t'}) \right]$$

THE QUANTITATIVE ASPECTS OF MENTAL ATTITUDES

Decomposition of emotions in terms of beliefs and goals is not enough. We need quantitative' parameters. Frustration and pain have an intensity which can be more or less severe; the same holds for surprise, disappointment, relief, hope, joy etc. Since they are clearly related with what the agent believes, expects, likes, pursues, can we account for those dimensions on the basis of our (de)composition of those mental states, and of the basic epistemic and motivational representations? We claim so.

Given the two basic ingredients of any expectations (defined as different from simple forecast or prediction) Beliefs and Goals, we postulate that:

P1: Beliefs & Goals have specific quantitative dimensions; which are basically independent from each other.

Beliefs have strength, a degree of subjective certainty; the subject is more or less sure and committed about their content. Goals have a value, a subjective importance for the agent.

To simplify, we may have very important goals combined with uncertain predictions or pretty sure forecasts for not very relevant objectives etc. Thus, in our schematic notation, we should explicitly represent these dimensions of Goals and Beliefs:

$$Bel^{\%}(x,p^t)$$

$$Goal^{\%}(x,p^t)$$

where % represents the subjective importance or the value of the Goals and the subjective credibility and the certainty of the Beliefs.

Putting aside the Epistemic Goal, an expectation will be like this:

$$Bel^{\%}(x,p^t)\&Goal^{\%}(x,\sim p^t)$$

The subjective quality of those "configurations" or macro-attitudes will be very different precisely depending on those parameters. Also the effects of the invalidation of an expectation are very different depending on: (i) the positive or negative character of the expectation and (ii) the strengths of the components. Therefore, we postulate that:

P2: The dynamics and the degree of the emergent configuration or the macro-attitude are strictly a function of the dynamics and strength of its micro-components.

For example, when compared to the case of mere goal and high certainty, anxiety (Miceli and Castelfranchi, 2005) will probably be greater when the goal is very important and the uncertainty high and it is characterized by the need to know to reduce the uncertainty. In the following sections, we will characterize some of these emergent macro-attitudes.

Hope and Fear

In our account, 'hope' is a peculiar kind of positive expectation where the goal is rather relevant for the subject while the expectation (more precisely the prediction) is not sure at all but rather weak and uncertain[3]:

$$Bel^{low}(x,p^t)\&Goal^{high}(x,p^t)$$

Correspondingly one might characterize 'fear', as an expectation of something bad, i.e. against our wishes:

$$Bel^{\%}(x,p^t)\&Goal^{\%}(x,\sim p^t)$$

But it seems that there can be 'fear' at any degree of certainty and of importance.[4]

Of course, these representations are seriously incomplete. We are ignoring their affective and felt component, which is definitely crucial. We do not represent here the body, its states and signals to the control system; we are just providing their cognitive skeleton.

THE IMPLICIT COUNTERPART OF EXPECTATIONS

Since we introduce a quantification of the degree of subjective certainty and reliability of Belief about the future (the forecast) we get a hidden, strange but nice consequence. There are other implicit opposite beliefs and thus implicit expectation. For implicit belief we mean here a belief that is not written or contained in any database (short term, working, or long term memory) but is only potentially known by the subject since it can be simply derived from actual beliefs. For example, my knowledge that Buenos Aires is the capital of Argentina is an explicit belief that I have in some memory and I just have to retrieve it. On the contrary, my knowledge that Buenos Aires is not the capital of Greece is not in any memory, but can just be derived (when needed) from what I explicitly know. Until it remains implicit, merely potential, and until it is not derived, it has no effect in my mind. For instance, I cannot perceive possible contradictions: my mind is only potentially contradictory if I believe that p, I believe that q, and p implies Not q, but I didn't derive that Not q.

Now, a belief that "70% it is the case that p", implies a belief that "30% it is the case that Not p"[5]. This has interesting consequences on expectations and related emotions. The Positive Expectation that p, entails an implicit (but sometime even explicit and compatible) Negative Expectation, and vice versa:

$$Bel^{\%}(x, p^t) \& Goal^{\%}(x, p^t) \Rightarrow Bel^{\%}(x, \sim p^t) \& Goal^{\%}(x, p^t)$$

This means that any hope implicitly contains some fear, and that any worry implicitly preserves some hope. But also means that when one gets a relief because a serious threat which was strongly expected has not happened and the world is conforming to her desires, she also gets (or can get) some exultance. It depends on her focus of attention and framing: is she focused on her worry and evanished threat, or on the unexpected achievement? Inversely, when one is satisfied for the actual expected realization of an important goal, she also can get some measure of relief while focusing on the previous implicit worry. It is not necessary to feel both the given emotion (i.e. fear) and the complementary one (i.e. hope) in a sort of oscillation or ambivalence and affective mixture. Only when the belief is explicitly represented and the attention is focused on it at least for a moment the corresponding emotion can be generated.

Emotional Response to Expectation: The Strength of Disappointment

As we said, the effects of the invalidation of an expectation differ depending on: a) the positive or negative character of the expectation; b) the strengths of the components. Given the fact that X has previous expectations, how does this fact change her evaluation of and reaction to a given event?

Invalidated Expectations

We call invalidated expectation an expectation that results to be wrong. For instance, X now (t") believes that NOT p at time t' while she expects that p at time t':

Invalidating: $Bel(x, p^t)^{t<t} \Longleftrightarrow Bel(x, \sim p^t)^{t''>t}$

This crucial belief is the 'invalidating' belief. Relative to the goal component it represents a "frustration", "goal-failure". It is the frustrating belief: I desire, wish, want that p but I know that not p:

Frustration: $Goal(x, p^t) \& Bel(x, \sim p^t)$

Relative to the prediction belief, it represents the 'falsification', 'prediction-failure':

Invalidation: $Bel(x,p')^{t<t'} \& Bel(x,\sim p')^{t''>t'}$

$Bel(x,p')^{t<t'}$ represents the former illusion or delusion (X illusorily believed at time t that at t' p would be true).

This configuration provides also the cognitive basis and the components of "surprise": the more certain the prediction the more intense the surprise (Lorini and Castelfranchi, 2006; Machedo et alli, 2009). Given positive and negative expectations and the answer of the world, that is the frustrating or gratifying belief, we have either confirmation of the expectation or disappointment or relief.

Disappointment

Relative to the whole mental state of positively expecting that p, the invalidating & frustrating belief produces 'disappointment' that is based on this basic configuration (plus the affective and cognitive reaction to it):

Disappointment:
$$Goal^{\%}(x,p^{t'})^{t\&t'} \& Bel^{\%}(x,p^{t'})^t \& Bel^{\%}(x,\sim p^{t'})^t$$

At time t, X believes that at t' (later, t' > t) p will be true; but now – at t' – she knows that Not p, while she continues to want that p. Disappointment contains goal-frustration and forecast failure, surprise. It entails a greater suffering than simple frustration (Miceli and Castelfranchi, 1997) for several reasons:

i.   for the additional failure;
ii.   for the fact that this impact also on the self-esteem as epistemic agent (Badura's (1990) predictability and related controllability) and is disorienting;
iii.   for the fact that losses of a pre-existing fortune are worst than missed gains, and long expected and surely expected desired situation are so familiar and sure that we feel a sense of loss.

When the belief is stronger and well-grounded, the surprise gets more disorienting and restructuring and the consequences becomes stronger on our sense of predictability. When the goal becomes more important, the subject gets more frustrated.

In Disappointment these effects are combined:

The surer the subject is about the outcome & the more important the outcome is for her, the more disappointed the subject will be.

The degree of disappointment seems to be a function of both dimensions and components[6]. It seems to be felt as a unitary effect. Let's examine 4 situations in this regard, as and answer to the following question:

- *"How much are you disappointed?"*
  - *"I'm very disappointed: I was <u>sure</u> to succeed"*
  - *"I'm very disappointed: it was very <u>important</u> for me"*
  - *"Not at all: it was not <u>important</u> for me"*
  - *"Not at all: I have just tried; I was <u>expecting</u> a failure".*

Obviously, worst disappointments are those with great value of the goal and high degree of certainty. However, the surprise component and the frustration component remain perceivable and a function of their specific variables.

Relief

Relief is based on a negative expectation that results to be wrong. The prediction is invalidated but the goal is realized. There is no frustration but surprise. In a sense relief is the opposite of disappointment: the subject was down while expecting something bad, and now feel much better because this expectation is invalidated.

Relief:

$$Goal(x, \sim p^{t'}) \;\&\; Bel(x, p^{t'}) \;\&\; Bel(x, \sim p^{t'})\,^7$$

The harder the expected harm and the more sure the expectation (i.e. the more serious the subjective threat) the more intense the relief. More precisely, the higher the worry, the threat, and the stronger the relief. The worry is already a function of the value of the harm and its certainty.

Analogously, joy seems to be more intense depending on the value of the goal, but also on how unexpected it is. More specifically, for us 'joy' is not simply some form of happiness or some satisfaction for a goal achievement. It implies some excitation, in other words some significant arousal, which is precisely due to the fact that either the reward is higher than expected or the trust, the estimated probability, was not so high. In both cases, there is not only an achievement but also a positive surprise: something unexpected. For example, 'Exultance' seems a kind of joy, but due to a 'victory' against some perceived opposition, resistance, difficulty.

A more systematic analysis should distinguish between different kinds of surprise (based on different monitoring activities and on explicit vs. implicit beliefs), and different kinds of disappointment and relief due to the distinction between 'maintenance' situations and 'change/achievement' situations (Lorini and Castelfranchi, 2006).

More precisely (making constant the value of the Goal) the case of loss is usually worse than simple non-achievement. This is coherent with the theory of psychic suffering (Miceli and Castelfranchi, 1997) that claims that pain is greater when there is not only frustration but disappointment (that is a previous expectation), and when there is loss, not just missed gains, that is when the frustrated goal is a maintenance goal not an achievement goal. However, the presence of expectation makes this even more complicated.

APPRAISAL AND THE COGNITIVE STRUCTURE OF COMPLEX EMOTIONS

People's appraisal of the meaning of a given state of affairs for their well-being is concordantly assumed to be a condition for their experiencing an emotion (Frijda and Swagerman, 1987; Ortony, 1987). Each emotion would involve a particular kind of appraisal, as well as a specific set of action tendencies and (perceived) physiological changes.

Cognitive models of emotion should then try

- to identify the specific cognitive processes implied by different emotions,
- by analyzing the structure of beliefs and goals typical of each of them.

Our analysis addresses such cognitive components, both directly and, so to say, indirectly, through the cognitive devices or strategies people can employ to elicit or to cope with that feeling (Miceli and Castelfranchi, 1998).

The general anatomy (sub-components) of a complex emotion is as follows:

EMOTION *of x[before/towards y]for/about O*
BELIEFS
1. Bel about O
2. Bel about y
3. Bel (-/+ Evaluation O), ...,. Bel (-/+ Evaluation O),
4. Bel (-/+ Expectations O), ..., Bel (-/+ Expectations O)
MONITORED GOALS
5. Goal related to O or y → result: FRUSTRATION or REALIZATION
ACTIVATED GOALS (Action tendencies or *'impulses'*)
6. Goal in response to...
BODILY SENSATIONS
PLEASANT/UNPLEASANT FEELINGS
EMOTIONAL DISPLAY

Shame

Let's provide an instantiation of a complex emotion using the above framework. Shame is a quite relevant social (but not necessarily moral) emotion that is due to the worry for the failure and frustration of our goal of having a good face (image), of being well evaluated by the others that observe and judge us (Castelfranchi and Poggi, 1990).

We feel ashamed about something (O) and before somebody (Y) whose opinion about us we care of.

SHAME x before y for/about O
BELIEFS
1. Bel x O where O = (Predicate of x) *"I did act" / "I have feature f"*
2. Bel x (Knows y O) *"they know/might know O"*
3. Bel x (negativeEvaluation y O) *"for them O is a fault, is bad, is negative"*
4. Bel x (negativeEvaluation y x) *"my image is defective; they do not like me"*
5. Bel x (negativeEvaluation x O) *"O is a bad thing"* SHARED VALUE
6. Bel x (negativeEvaluation x x) *"I'm defective"*

MONITORED GOALS
7. Goal x (positiveEvaluation y x) *being well evaluated; esteem, good image* → FRUSTRATION

ACTIVATED GOALS
8. Goal x (reducing exposure)

As for the first belief, notice that it is not strictly necessary. In other words while shared interiorized values are absolutely necessary, there can be disagreement about the evaluated fact. Although blushing, X might be innocent; she didn't do anything wrong. It is possible to blush and feel ashamed for the mere suspect. This is why blushing is not a confession at all.

As for the goal of shame (the goal of having positive evaluations, from Y), we have to notice that how the more X cares of Y's judgment and the worst Y's evaluation is, the greater X's suffering and shame intensity.

The 5th ingredient is very important, which is the personal negative evaluation of O by X herself, in other words; value sharing. Therefore, this statement implies that both self- and social esteem is harmed.

One cannot be ashamed of O in front of Y if:

- he does not (at least unconsciously) sincerely share some NegativeEvaluation of O (Shared/ Interiorized Values).
- he does not care at all of Y's opinion (Goal of PositiveEvaluation from Y; face/image; esteem).

What mainly matters in SHAME is:

FRUSTRATION → 5. Goal x (positiveEvaluation y x)
being well evaluated; esteem, good figure/face.

Emotional Display of Shame

The Emotional display (posture, eyes, front, blushing) is very coherent with this complex mental state. The meaning of its non-verbal discourse (posture, eyes, front, blushing) is:

- *I care for your judgment; I care of being accepted in the group*
- *I recognize my fault, imperfection, flaw; I sincerely agree about its negativity;*
- *I sincerely share your values; I'm not an alien or a provocative; (consider that blushing cannot be simulated or inhibited);*
- *I do not oppose to you; I do submit to you;*
- *I'm suffering for my defect and your judgment; I'm sorry (I'm already paying for this)*
- *Be clement.* (Castelfranchi and Poggi, 1990)

In a similar manner, we present the complex anatomy of 'guilt' in the appendix.

The "Intersubjectivity" of Social Emotions

Apart from possible mirroring, empathy, identification, etc., that imply some shared sensation and feeling, it is important to underline the shared and mutual mental ground of social emotions, also in their 'cognitive anatomies'. A shared mind is also crucial but left out from the discussion here.

Notice for example how Shame – in our anatomy – presupposes shared mental representations:

- The belief about O is 'shared', following X (and X believes so) (1 & 2);
- The negative evaluation of O is necessarily shared (and X believes so);
- Also the goal of X being well evaluated (that is, for Y the goal that: X be good, correspond to the cultural standards) is shared.

Moreover, beliefs and goals are not only shared, but they are meta-represented (Y's mind in X's mind, and X's mind in Y's mind (following X)) and mutual. We do not fully represent this, for sake of simplicity.

- X believes that Y believes that she shares the value (and this is actually true, especially after X's blushing signal);
- X believes that Y believes/knows that X believes (1) (2); etc.

They have (and know/feel to have) the same values, the same beliefs, the same goals.

And this is not based on complex reasoning and inferences about the other's mind, but mainly is due to their sharing a given culture, with its scripts, norms, values, conventions and behavioral rules, and to the emotional/behavioral signals and their automatic understanding.

THE GESTALT NATURE OF COMPLEX MENTAL STATES

We are in favor of a componential analysis of emotions (and in general of mental states and processes, like 'expectation', or 'need', or 'trust', or 'argument', etc.) and this is what we refer as the cognitive anatomy. It allows a systematic explicit model of the relationships within that object and among objects. However, one should always also care about accounting for the 'unitary' character of those mental-behavioral phenomena. Although atomically decomposable, those complex mental states have their own emergent, specific, non-reducible properties and functions.

For example, a prediction is not *per se* an expectation, because it must be considered within a possible frame. It is a matter of the Gestalt nature of complex mental states. The side of a square is a linear segment; but: is any segment the side of a square? Not *per se*, only if considered, imagined, within that figure, as a component of a larger configuration that changes it meaning/role. Analogously: a belief about a future event is just part of an expectation, but it acquires a special color and function within the expectation Gestalt. Expectation is not simply the sum of a belief and a goal.

The fact that emotions are analyzable in parts and components (shared by other phenomena) does not necessarily deny their possible uniqueness and unitary/global nature. In our vocabulary they are Gestalts; there is an emergent, self-organizing form, which is not reducible to its parts and to their specific properties and functions. Decomposing a Gestalt is not reducing it to its components.

The new mental entity constitutes a Gestalt both phenomenally speaking, and functionally speaking: the whole has psychological and behavioral effects, properties, and functions that are new and specific; not just the results of the effects of its isolated parts. Moreover, within this whole the constituents change their nature, acquire a new color (or a role): they are - for example - no longer just segments but have the function of sides of the emerging form of square. In this sense, even the elements that precede and cause the formation of such new complex object, remain there as its parts; since they are no longer exactly the same object.

There is a synergy among the constituents which is bi-directional: from micro to macro (the global form and effects), and from macro to micro: the role/function within the whole, and the new perception of/perspective on the part. Not necessarily all the components are there; but this gives rise to different related emotions, or to variations of the same emotion from more simple and primitive forms to richer ones (Miceli and Castelfranchi, 2009).

For example, in which sense an expectation - that compound configuration of beliefs and goals - is a new mental object, a unitary object? Because it, as a whole, acquires new properties, effects, and functions that are not properties of its parts. Like a molecule has properties that are not properties of its component atoms. For example, the expectation as such (not simply the prediction, or the goal) is involved in decision making. Expectations as such are needed for formulating an intention. Expectations as such produce 'hope' or 'fear', 'disappointment' or 'relief'.

The same holds for more complex mental states like 'shame' or 'guilt': they have a lot of common components, or components shared with other emotions, but they have their own specific subjective experience, and specific and global functions and reactions.

RI-EMBODYING EMOTIONS

We believe that cognitive models have put aside for too long the problem of subjective experience, of feeling something. In our view quite obviously, to feel something is necessarily somatic; it presupposes having a body (including a brain), and receiving some perceptual signal from it. You cannot experience or feel anything without a body.

However, current approaches claiming the role of the body, and feelings, emotions, drives, (and several biological mechanisms) tend to put this as a radical alternative to cognition, as incompatible with the traditional apparatus of cognitive science (beliefs, intentions, plans, decision, and so on).

To fully characterize several important mental states (kinds of belief or kinds of goal, like needs and desires (Castelfranchi, 2007)) it is necessary to model the bodily information; but on the other side – as we try to argue in this contribution - also traditional mental representations are necessary.

'Felt' Mental States

Notice, for example, that we cannot feel goal, intention, objective, plan, aim! Why? And why on the contrary can we feel needs and desires? (and a bit extensively hopes, expectations, trust).

Our trivial answer is: because they involve some perceptual component, while not all mental representations (goals, beliefs, etc.) involve significant perceptually active components, but are more abstract, or more disembodied representations. What we mean is that we cannot feel a goal per se but we can feel some perceptual component related to having a goal (like some uneasiness, or some perceptual representation of the expected results). While notions like needs or desires focus precisely on these aspects/components (Castelfranchi, 2007), other goal-notions are more abstract and do not explicitly concern these perceptual aspects.

Desires imply some pleasure, but not only the pleasure experienced at the moment of the achievement of the goal and satisfaction of the desire. Desires imply a pleasure at the very moment of desiring something as a mental activity. It is a virtual reality pleasure. A true desire implies the anticipatory representation of the goal state in a sensory-motor format (let's say an image) and the simulation of the desired situation. This implies some (partial) imagined sensation (for example the taste of a food; the joy of a sexual encounter).

What you feel is this sensation: an anticipated part of the sensation you will experience; an illusory gratification. To desire is this, and this is why you can feel a desire while you cannot feel an intention. The term intention does not focus on the perceptual anticipatory representation of the result and of its perceptual components.

So our claim would be: always when we can use the word[8] 'to feel' some somatic marker[9] or some self-perception is involved. Probably this is too strong, since the language extends the use of words and introduces metaphors; but it should be basically true.

It is important to understand that the problem is not only to go beyond a cognitive/functionalist analysis of emotions to integrate other aspects, but the problem is that any functional explanation is incomplete if ignores the subjective or felt facet of emotions. The real problem is precisely the function of the internal perception, of the feeling of the bodily peripheral reactions and of the central response. Since a reactive system can do the job of an emotional system, why do we need emotions? Why do we need a system that perceives its own reactions? What is the role of this self-perception in the adaptive process?

The classical AI position about emotions enounced by Simon (1967) explains their function in terms of operating system interrupts prompting one processing activity to be replaced by another of higher priority, i.e. in terms of a reactive goal-directed system in an unpredictable environment. As Sloman and Croucher (1981) observe, the need to cope with a changing and partly unpredictable world makes it very likely that any intelligent system with multiple motives and limited powers will have emotions. We believe that this view is basically correct but seriously incomplete. This function is necessary to explain emotions but is not sufficient at all. In fact, to deal with this kind of functionality a good reactive system able to focus attention or memory and to activate or inhibit goals and actions would be enough. Current models of affective computing simply model the emotional behavior and the cognitive-reactivity function. Consider for ex. Picard's nice description of fear in a robot:

In its usual, nonemotional state, the robot peruses the planet, gathering data, analyzing it, and communicating its results back to earth. At one point, however, the robot senses that it has been physically damaged and changes to a new internal state, perhaps named 'fear'. In this new state it behaves differently, quickly reallocating its resources to drive its perceptual sensors and provide extra power to its motor system to let it move rapidly away from the source of danger. However, as long as the robot remains in a state of fear, it has insufficient resources to perform its data analysis (like human beings who can't concentrate on a task when they are in danger). The robot communication priorities, ceasing to be scientific, put out a call for help. (Picard, 1997).

What is lacking in this characterization of fear? Just the most typical emotional aspect: feeling. Feeling is a broader notion: we can feel a lot of things that are not emotions (for example needs). However, feeling is a kernel component of emotion: if we cannot feel x, we should/could even doubt that x is an emotion (Ortony, 1987). This puts out a serious question: since we can account for emotional functioning without modeling feeling, since a reactive change of the internal state, cognitive processing, and behavior is enough, why is feeling such a crucial component of human (and animal) emotions? Is it a mere epiphenomenon lacking any causal function in the process? Or which is its function and its reason?

We believe that computational models of emotions should answer precisely this theoretical question. Let us simply mention what we believe to be the main functions of the feeling component in emotion, i.e. of the fact the robot should sense those changes of its internal state and of its behavior. We believe that the main functions of feeling in emotions are the following ones:

- felt emotional internal states work as drives (Canamero, 1997) to be satisfied, i.e. to go back to the equilibrium (homeostasis) through action; Mower (1960) postulates that in learning, the animal learns precisely what behavior serves to alleviate the emotion associated to a given stimulus;
- felt emotional internal states work as positive or negative internal reinforcements for learning (they will be associated to the episode and change the probability of the reproduction of the same behavior); [10]
- felt emotional internal states associated to and aroused by a given scenario constitute its immediate, unreasoned, non-declarative appraisal (to be distinguished from a cognitive evaluation - Castelfranchi, 2000; Miceli and Castelfranchi, 2000)

In sum, the cognitivist dominant paradigm cannot any longer neglect the necessity for modeling subjective experience and feeling. The relation with the body seems to be crucial: beliefs, goals, and other mental (declarative) ingredients are necessary but not sufficient. For example, one cannot account for the intentional aspect of feeling the need for something without beliefs about what is needed and about the origin of some sensation of pain or uneasiness. Also a better and convincing functionalist analysis of emotions requires precisely explaining the functional role of feeling. Cognitive appraisal, modification of attention and cognitive processes, reactive changes of goals priorities, are not adequate.

Ri-Embodying 'Hope' and 'Fear'

In this paragraph we want to give some hints about the possible ri-embodiment of these mental states, claiming that their 'cognitive anatomy' is correct but insufficient. We will try to explain how the feeling aspect should be integrated with the epistemic and motivational ones.

Our claim is that

i.   those mental configurations may produce a reaction of the body (a 'motion' **M**): a bodily response to that mental/representational content or interpretation of the events[11];

ii. this bodily response is entero-perceived by the agent, there is a signal **S** from the body: subjective 'sensations' about what is happening into the body or internal environment;

iii. these **S** and **M** are recognized (or attributed) as due to that event (or rather, interpreted event).

Only this provides the full experience and state of having 'worries about', or 'being afraid of', or 'feeling fear for' the eventuality that p will happen.

The molecule $Bel^\%(x, p^t)$ & $Goal^\%(x, \sim p^t)$ is not enough for fear: Where are the quiver, the tremble or the stress? Or the tremor that can characterize joy, the trepidation of hope?

Let's call **S** the sensation arriving from our body reacting to the prospected idea of a serious threat. Suppose that the reaction of the body, **M**, is a tremble, quivering, and that x perceives back this signal of the status of his body, **S**; and that he interprets this reaction as related and due to that (bad) mental prospect or better to its content (the negative event p).

The complete picture is as follows:

Only at this point x really feels fear:

- on the one side, the simple negative expectation is affectively colored as 'fear', and
- on the other side, his tremor is a 'tremor of fear'.

Only the (causal) co-occurrence and association of the specific mental representation to the felt current bodily reaction (and possibly its cognitive attribution (**Bel**$_2$)) accounts for what does it mean to worry about/for something, or to be afraid of something. Only the felt bodily reaction (feeling

Figure 1. Beliefs - Body motion interaction

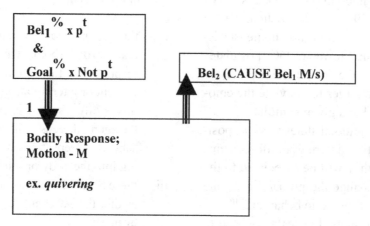

and motion) makes this mental state emotion; but only the beliefs and goals provide the emotion with its origin.

The prediction is that: The greater the perceived threat- that is the more important the goal and the stronger the expectation- (moreover, the closer the check of the expectation, the verification, the expected moment **t**) the stronger the bodily reaction, the tremor or the tension.

Real 'Hope'

Analogously, for having 'Hope' as a feeling, $Bel^{\%}(x, p^t) \& Goal^{\%}(x, p^t)$ is not enough. There is a reaction of the body (trepidation) to this prospect. And this trepidation is felt by X and related to that expectation. At that very moment X experiences hope (not just predicts a possible positive outcome). And only at that point (with this kind of body-mental-representation association) we have X's trepidation for hope.

The prediction is that: The more important the goal (and the closer the check of the expectation, the verification, the expected moment **t**) the stronger the trepidation.

The Impact of the Felt Motion on Beliefs and Goals

But there are also other strange effects of the bodily feedback. The signal from the body can be used as an evidence, as a perceptual information source for the Belief. The intensity of the bodily sensation can affect the certainty of the forecast: *'Since I feel fear, there should be danger'*. Hence: The stronger the motion that x feels, the stronger the Belief.

However, this is an 'anomalous' and not very rational source. In fact its credibility has collapsed on its intensity. The degree of worries becomes, more broadly, a measure of the threat. A measure about not only the probability of the event (in our terms: degree of the prediction), but that is also the belief about the seriousness of the harm (i.e. the amount of the goal to be jeopardized).

The feeling might also affect the value of the goal: perhaps, the stronger the fear the greater the perceived value of the threatened Goal.

In general, as we saw, we claim that feeling provides an anomalous (nonrational) basis for both the strength of the Beliefs and values of the Goals. For example in felt 'needs for O' (Castelfranchi, 1998) we claim that: The stronger the disturbing or painful sensation that x feels when he feels 'the need for O', the stronger and more cogent and

Figure 2. Bottom-up emotions

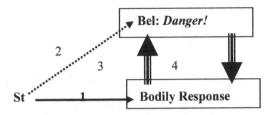

Figure 3. Top-down emotions

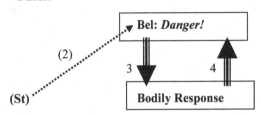

compulsory the Goal of 'having/obtaining O', that is not the usual way we calculate the importance of our Goals and their preference-order.

Different Paths for Different Kinds of 'Fear'

We do not claim that this path (evaluation and mental interpretation of an event or a mental prospect m => bodily response **M** to m => sensorial feedback of the bodily response **S** => attribution of M & S to m) is the only path conducing to an emotional experience. There are more basic or primitive emotions that are more stimulus driven, not based on a match or mismatch between a Belief and a Goal (Reisenzein, 2009) like in shame which is presented before. A simple low level pattern matching is enough for eliciting an emotional reaction, for example a reactive fright to an unexpected noise (such as explosion) or to a non identified object suddenly moving/jumping under my feet. We claim that in this case there is no real evaluation and prediction of a possible danger. There is just an automatic (and sometimes conditioned) fear-reaction to the stimulus.

However, at least in humans, this motion of the body (and its sensations like being chilled with fear, or automatic retraction, horripilation, etc.) is a signal S that is interpreted and can generate a Belief of threat, and this Belief used as a feedback may confirm the bodily reaction. But the path is rather different. We have here some sort of Bottom-up (and back) emotions which is given in Figure 2

with the path 1 + 3 + 4 (In parallel, the cognitive processing of St proceeds on path 2).

While the previous flow was rather Top-down (and back), as shown in Figure 3.

Stimulus can even be absent; some fear can be just the result of a mere idea.

EMOTIONS IN HUMAN MACHINE INTERACTION

Emotional Cognition and Affective Interactions

We have provided earlier a quite brief anatomy of complex social emotions in order to give the reader the flavor of such specificity and complexity. However, actually even the anatomy of more simple affective attitudes like hope, fear, disappointment, relief, was rather cognitively rich.

In fact, we claim that the ascription of such a background mental state to the other is a necessary requisite for emotion recognition and understanding. In this section we will argue on this necessity of a Theory of Mind (ToM) for an appropriate affective response and interaction.

Appropriate emotional interactions are based on the recognition of the mental stuff of the other agent: of her beliefs, suppositions, motives, expectations. We react to this, not just to an expressive face, posture, or intonation. Expressive and physiological cues should mainly be the signs for a diagnosis of mind. Without this Theory of Mind map we are rather powerless.

Suppose that the other party is surprised; in order to appropriately react to this, I have to understand Why ? What for ? Moreover, is the other party just surprised or disappointed or relieved? What was her expectation, desire or worry? Is she ascribing to me the responsibility of such disappointment? I have to relate my response to this mental background. Should I express solidarity, excuse, or irony towards the other's expectation and reaction?

As we said, for an appropriate affective interaction, the mere detection and recognition of an emotional expression and a reaction to it is not enough. We do not react just to the emotion, but to the emotion as well as its 'aboutness'.

In other words, the affective reaction to an affective state depends on the recognition of the cognitive content (intension) of the affective state, not only on its expression (and the cultural and pragmatic context), which is summarized in Figure 4.

Human Machine Interaction (HMI)

In sum, also for HMI: the detection and recognition of the symptom of an emotional state or reaction (speech prosody, heartbeat, facial expression) is not enough for an appropriate response. In fact, human and especially social emotions are based on a very rich and characteristic mental frame; on peculiar thoughts (the appraisal of current or possible events), on specific goals (frustrated or achieved), on action tendencies and activated impulses: what we call the "cognitive anatomy" of each emotion.

As for the HMI (and in particular H-Agent I) our claim is that:

- in HMI we are moving - also thanks to the Autonomous Agent (Ag) paradigm - from mere Interactivity to Collaboration;
- this more and more requires Ags able to have a some form of mind reading at least about the human user;
- thus, also the affective interaction cannot be merely behavioral and needs some level of mind-reading (if not felt empathy, shared sensations).

To model emotions, believable and appropriate faces and expressions are not enough. We have to build formal or computational models of the cognitive appraisal on which human emotions are based. The ability for Ags of building and reasoning upon explicit representations of the user's mind in terms of beliefs, expectations, desires, goals, needs, plans, values, etc.; in terms of social attitudes: like trust, diffidence, benevolence, hostility, etc.; and also in terms of the mental counterparts of speech acts, conventions, norms, roles, commitments, etc. is necessary for:

a.   modeling credible emotional states as internal states;

Figure 4. Reacting to the mental state not to the expressive signal

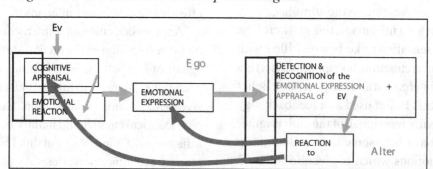

b. modeling the sophisticated interaction between the cognitive components of the emotions (basically, beliefs and goals) and their bodily component: the felt 'motion' from the body; going beyond the quite schematic dual system models;

c. modeling a more credible affective interaction, where the detection and recognition of the symptoms of an emotional state or reaction (voice, heart, face,…) is not enough for an appropriate response to it, and the Ag must be able to understand the mental and subjective ground of the expressive reaction: what the emotion is about, that is what the user has in mind while feeling that emotion, what she believes, what she was desiring and expecting, what she would like or is pushed to do, etc.

Emotional interaction (Ag-Ag; H-Ag; H-robot; HC; etc.) cannot be based only on the recognition of the expressive or physiological signals.

Ideally we should have embodied the artificial minds; that is, modeling artificial agents with a real body, endowed with interoception and proprioception, bodily felt reactions, and an internal dynamic environment; and able to perceive and recognize the body response of the other and to react to it with a body felt response. Or even better: agents able to perceive the body response of the other through their own corresponding body activation. However, this would not be enough at all both for having emotional machines and for an affective HCI.

To make this idea concrete, let us give just an example that might be directly applied to interaction with anthropomorphic Agent: the appropriateness of an empathic response.

Even an emphatic response is not always the right, appropriate response. This strongly depends on the interpretation of the intention of the other's expressed emotion. For example, if X expresses irritation and rage against Z (a third part), then an empathic and sympathetic response of Y, sharing

X's emotion, can be appropriate. This expresses support, solidarity, sympathy. But if the object of X's disappointment is precisely Y, Y's solidarity can be very inappropriate and irritating. The problem is: 'about what' and 'against who' X is furious? Is it about something that I personally did or provoked? Or is against X herself or a third agent?

If Y is the cause and the target of X's disappointment, a feeling of guilt, regret, and excuses could be much more appropriate than empathy in strict sense.

More precisely: suppose that X is disappointed and irritated against Y, this means that

Bel1 x (Done y act)
Bel2 x (Cause act_y ev1)
Bel3 x (Harm ev1 x)
With a consequent negative evaluation of Y
Bel4 (negEVALUATION x y)

If Y shares those beliefs, if he agrees about Bel1, Bel2, Bel3 he can react by expressing guilt, sorrow (*"I'm sorry"*) and excuses. But if Y disagrees about some of these Cognitive Appraisal ingredients, a different affective response is needed. For example, Y might be offended by X 'accusation': *"It is not my fault! How can you think this of me!"* (disagreement about at least Bel1 or Bel2, and thus Bel4). If Y *disagrees* about Bel3, the response can be completely different, not only verbally (*"But it is not bad! You didn't realize what really happened"*) but also as affective disposition: surprise and contrast. Suppose that X is disappointed and irritated against herself, the affective reaction of Y should again be quite different: *"It is not your fault" "it happens!"*… (friendly solidarity, consolation; or irony) And so on.

How can an Agent appropriately react to a perceived emotional state of the user without understanding what the user has in mind?

In sum: the affective reaction to an affective state depends on the recognition of the cognitive content (intention) of that affective state, not only on its expression. We do not react to the emotion, but to the emotion and its 'aboutness', which presupposes some mind reading ability.

Moreover, we claim the emotional signals and expressions communicate also about this: about the mental content (beliefs, goals) not only about the affective feeling and disposition of the subject. Inferences from behaviors (implicit behavioral communication; Tummolini et al, 2004) cooperate with the specialized expressive signals to make us understand the emotional state of the subject, its reasons, and what it is about. For example, from your face I recognize that you are furious, but perhaps only from your behavior I realize that you are furious against me.

CONCLUDING REMARKS (FOR HUMAN-AGENT INTERACTION)

The general conclusion is that we need a synthetic model of mental activity (and of emotion), able to assemble in a principled way both abstract and embodied representations, cognitive and dynamic dimensions. This is also necessary for the theory of emotions and for the theory of motivation that cannot be reduced to their bodily components, arousal, impulses, etc. but require specific beliefs, goals, expectations, explicit evaluations, and so on.

This strongly impacts the affective interaction too, which cannot be reduced to (and just modeled as) a felt empathic reaction: disgust elicits disgust, suffering elicits suffering, and so on; but requires some explicit mind reading and some appropriated reaction to the other's mental assumptions: beliefs, expectations, goals .

Do we really want a social interaction with our artificial creatures? Do we really want to support and mediate human interaction by the computer technology? There is no alternative: we have to explicitly and computationally model the mental proximate mechanisms generating the behaviors (both, the affective and the more reasoned and deliberated ones), and we have to address our response or our support-mediation to them, not just to the exterior behaviors and signals. No emotions without cognition and motivation, no interaction without understanding.

ACKNOWLEDGMENT

I would like to thanks Maria Miceli, Isabella Poggi, Rino Falcone, Emiliano Lorini, Luca Tummolini, Giovanni Pezzulo for their invaluable contribution to many of the ideas presented here.

REFERENCES

Bandura, A. (1990). Self-efficacy mechanism in human agency. *The American Psychologist, 37,* 122–147. doi:10.1037/0003-066X.37.2.122

Canamero, D. (1997) Modeling Motivations and Emotions as a Basis for Intelligent Behavior. *Autonomous Agents'98,* ACM Press, 148-55, 1997.

Castelfranchi, C. (1998). To believe and to feel: The case of "needs". In Canamero, D. (Ed.), *Emotional and Intelligent: The Tangled Knot of Cognition* (pp. 55–60). Menlo Park, CA: AAAI Press.

Castelfranchi, C. (2000). Affective Appraisal vs. Cognitive Evaluation in Social Emotions and Interactions. In A. Paiva (ed.) *Affective Interactions. Towards a New Generation of Computer Interfaces.* Heidelbergh, Springer, LNAI 1814, 76-106.

Castelfranchi, C. (2005). Mind as an Anticipatory Device: For a Theory of Expectations. BVAI 2005 Brain, vision, and artificial intelligence (First international symposium, BVAI 2005, Naples, Italy, October 19-21, 2005) (proceedings). *Lecture Notes in Computer Science, 3704,* 258–276. doi:10.1007/11565123_26

Castelfranchi, C., & Miceli, M. (2009). The Cognitive-Motivational Compound of Emotional Experience. *Emotion Review*, *1*(3), 221–228. doi:10.1177/1754073909103590

Castelfranchi, C., & Poggi, I. (1990). Blushing as a discourse: was Darwin wrong? In Crozier, R. (Ed.), *Shyness and Embarassement: Perspective from Social Psychology*. N.Y: Cambridge University Press. doi:10.1017/CBO9780511571183.009

Damasio, A.R. (1994) *Descartes' Error*. N.Y., Putnam's Sons, Frijda N. H. & Swagerman J. (1987) Can Computers Feel? Theory and Design of an Emotional System. *Cognition and Emotion, 1* (3) 235-57, 1987.

Lorini, E., & Castelfranchi, C. (2006). The Unexpected Aspects of Surprise. *IJPRAI*, *20*(6), 817–834.

Macedo, L., Cardoso, A., Reisenzein, R., Lorini, E., & Castelfranchi, C. (2009). Artificial Surprise. In Vallverdú, J., & Casacuberta, D. (Eds.), *Handbook of Research on Synthetic Emotions and Sociable Robotics: New Applications in Affective Computing and Artificial Intelligence.*

Miceli, M., & Castelfranchi, C. (1997). Basic principles of psychic suffering: A preliminary account. *Theory & Psychology*, *7*, 769–798. doi:10.1177/0959354397076003

Miceli, M., & Castelfranchi, C. (1998). How to Silence One's Conscience: Cognitive Defences Against the Feeling of Guilt. *Journal for the Theory of Social Behaviour*, *28*(3), 287–318. doi:10.1111/1468-5914.00076

Miceli, M., & Castelfranchi, C. (2000). The role of evaluation in cognition and social interaction. In Dautenhahn, K. (Ed.), *Human cognition and agent technology* (pp. 225–261). Amsterdam: Benjamins.

Miceli, M. e Castelfranchi, C. (2002). The mind and the future: The (negative) power of expectations. *Theory & Psychology,* 12 (3), 335-.366

Miceli, M., Castelfranchi, C. (2005) Anxiety as an epistemic emotion: An uncertainty theory of anxiety, *Anxiety Stress and Coping* (09957J0), 18,291-319.

Mower, O. (1960). *Learning Theory and Behavior*. New York: J. Wiley and Sons. doi:10.1037/10802-000

Ortony, A. (1987) Is Guilt an Emotion? *Cognition and Emotion*, I, 1, 283-98, 1987.

Pezzulo, G., Butz, M. V., Castelfranchi, C., & Falcone, R. (2008). Anticipation in Natural and Artificial Cognition. In Pezzulo, G., Butz, M.V., Castelfranchi, C. & Falcone, R. (Eds.), *The Challenge of Anticipation: A Unifying Framework for the Analysis and Design of Artificial Cognitive Systems* (LNAI 5225, pp. 3-22). New York: Springer.

Picard, R. (1997). *Does HAL cry digital tears? Emotion and computers;* HAL's Legacy: 2001's Computer as Dream and Reality, Cambridge, 279-303.

Reisenzein, R. (2009). Emotional Experience in the Computational Belief–Desire Theory of Emotion. *Emotion Review*, *1*(3), 214–222. doi:10.1177/1754073909103589

Simon, H. (1967). Motivational and emotional controls of cognition. *Psychological Review, 74*, 29–39. doi:10.1037/h0024127

Sloman, A., & Croucher, M. (1981) Why robots will have emotions. In Proceedings of *IJCAI'81*, Vancouver, Canada, 1981, p. 197

Staats, A. (1990). The Paradigmatic Behaviorism Theory of Emotions: Basis for Unification. *Clinical Psychology Review, 10*, 539–566. doi:10.1016/0272-7358(90)90096-S

Tummolini, L., Castelfranchi, C., Ricci, A., Viroli, M., & Omicini, A. (2004) What I See is What You Say: Coordination in a Shared Environment with Behavioral Implicit Communication. In G. Vouros (Ed.) *ECAI 04 Proceedings of the Workshop on Coordination in Emergent Societies* (CEAS 2004).

ENDNOTES

[1]   'Prediction' is the result of the action of predicting; but 'expectation' is not the result of the action of expecting; it is that action or the outcome of a prediction relevant to goals, it is the basis of such an action.

[2]   Actually the expectation entails a cognitive evaluation. In fact, since the realization of p is coinciding with a goal, it is 'good'. If belief is the opposite of the goal, it implies a belief that the outcome of the world will be 'bad'. Or the expectation produces an implicit, intuitive appraisal, simply by activating associated affective responses or somatic markers (Damasio, 1994). Or the expected result will produce a reward for the agent, and – although not strictly driving its behavior- it is positive since it will satisfy a drive and reinforce the behavior.

[3]   We may also have 'strong hope' but we explicitly call it strong precisely because usually hope implies low confidence and some anxiety and worry. In any case, 'hope' (like explicit 'trust') can never really be subjectively certain and absolutely confident. Hope implies uncertainty. More precisely, hope should be based on a belief of possibility rather than on an estimated probability of the event.

[4]   To characterize *fear* another component would be very relevant: the goal of avoiding the foreseen danger; that is, the goal of *doing* something such that Not p. This is a goal activated while feeling fear. But it is also a component of a complete fear mental state, not just a follower or a consequence of fear. This goal can be a quite specified action (motor reaction) (a cry; the impulse to escape; etc.); or a generic goal 'doing something' ("my God!! What can I do?!"). The more intense the felt fear, the more important the activate goal of avoidance.

[5]   In fact it is possible that there is an interval of ignorance, some lack of evidences; that is that I estimate with a probability of 45% that p and with a probability of 30% Not p, while having a gap of 25% neither in favor of p nor of Not p.

[6]   As a first approximation of the degree of Disappointment one might assume some sort of multiplication of the two factors: Goal-value * Belief-certainty. Similarly to 'Subjective Expected Utility': the greater the SEU the more intense the Disappointment.

[7]   Or – obviously - (Goal x pt') & (Bel x ¬pt') & (Bel x pt').

[8]   This is especially true in Italian (the semantic difference between "sentire" and "provare"); perhaps less true in English where really to "feel" seems quite close to "believe".

[9]   In Damasio's terminology (Damasion, 1994) a somatic marker is a positive or negative emotional reaction in the brain that is associated to and elicited by a given mental representation or scenario, making it attractive or repulsive, and pre-orienting choice. It may just be the central trace of an original peripheral, physiological reaction.

[10]   I assume, following along tradition on emotional learning, that in general positive and negative emotions are reinforcers; but notice that this does neither imply that we act in order to feel the emotion, which is not necessarily motivating us (it can be expected without being intended); nor that

only pleasure and pain, or emotions, are rewarding (Staats, 1990).

[11]   As we said, *also this* makes them like 'molecules' with their own global properties and effects, since the 'response' is to the whole pattern not to its components, and it is not just the sum of the specific reactions to the components.

APPENDIX

Anatomy of Guilt

The prototypical kind of Guilt is an unpleasant feeling, a sufferance for having been responsible of some harm to a victim. One feels guilt about something (O) and for somebody (Z) who is suffering or might suffer for that harm (Miceli and Castelfranchi, 1998).

GUILT x for/about O harming z [before y/z]
BELIEFS

1. Bel x O were O = (Did x act) *"I did act1"*
2. Bel x (Cause O (Fate of z)) *"act1 affected y's fate/condition"*
3. Bel x (Harm for z) *"it is a bad fate, a harm for z"*
4. Bel x (will/could Suffer z) *"z is suffering; will suffer; might suffer"*
5. Bel x (not deserved by z) *"z is a victim, did not deserve this harm"*
6. Bel x (Could have avoided x act) *"I could have avoided this"* (counterfactual)
7. Bel x (-Evaluation y O) *"for them O is a wrong, is bad, is negative"*
8. Bel x (-Evaluation y x) *"I'm a bad guy for him/them"*

MONITORED GOALS

9. Goal x: (Not being cause of an unfair harms)
10. Goal x (+Evaluation y x) *being well evaluated; moral estime, moral image*
11. -Evaluation x O *"O is a bad thing"* SHARED VALUE
12. -Evaluation x x *"I'm not good; I'm a bad guy"*

ACTIVATED GOALS (Action tendencies or *'impulses'*)

13. Goal (help x y) *"compensating; worrying about; to care of y"* →ANXIETY
14. Goal x (Expiate x) *"to atone; pay for..."* → ANXIETY
15. Goal x (Not Did x act) *counterfactual desire*; REGRET (IMPOSSIBLE Goal!)
16. Goal x (Not Does X act in the future): virtuous intention

Let's remark that guilt feeling presupposes the capacity for empathy: belief (4.) and (5.) activate an empathic attitude; X imagines and feels Y's sufferance, and this is one of the basis of Guilt intensity (the other are the degree of responsibility, the perceived gravity of the harm, the degree of unfairness).

Very crucial is also the counterfactual belief (6.); it is the core of the sense of responsibility. Moreover: since I could have avoided my act or the harm, I should have avoided it! (This is the internal reproach, the remorse, and also the basis for the good intention for the future).

To be more precise (6.) is a group of related beliefs: like *"I could/should have understood the consequences"*; *"I had some freedom; I was not forced to do so"* .

Also guilt feeling implies a negative evaluation of the action and of X (and thus a wound to self-esteem and – if somebody can know and judge (but it is not necessary for Guilt) – also shared values and a wound to social image. However, this is not the goal guilt feelings monitor and are about.

Guilt mainly is about causal links between our own action or fate with the other's bad fate, and focuses on our bad power (the power to harm, to be noxious); while shame focuses on our lack of power, inferiority, inadequacy, and defectiveness; and on face problems. Shame elicits a passive and depressive attitude; while Guilt an active and reparative attitude (M. Lewis, 1992). In guilt the preeminent role is played by the assumed responsibility.

One generally does not feel responsible for one's lack of power and inadequacy, which are often perceived as beyond one's control. Hence, the passive and depressive attitude. By contrast, one's injurious behavior, negative power and dispositions are seen as controllable and modifiable.

People can feel ashamed because of their ugliness or handicaps, but they don't feel guilty (unless they attribute themselves some responsibility for not trying enough to improve themselves or avoid bad consequences). Conversely, people tend to feel guilty, rather than ashamed, for their bad behavior or dispositions.

What mainly matters in GUILT is:

FRUSTRATION → 7. Goal: (Not being cause of an unfair harm)
moral self-esteem and reproach

Section 3
Affect in Non−Verbal Communication

Chapter 7
Towards a Technology of Nonverbal Communication:
Vocal Behavior in Social and Affective Phenomena

Alessandro Vinciarelli
University of Glasgow, UK

Gelareh Mohammadi
Idiap Research Institute, Switzerland

ABSTRACT

Nonverbal communication is the main channel through which we experience inner life of others, including their emotions, feelings, moods, social attitudes, etc. This attracts the interest of the computing community because nonverbal communication is based on cues like facial expressions, vocalizations, gestures, postures, etc. that we can perceive with our senses and can be (and often are) detected, analyzed and synthesized with automatic approaches. In other words, nonverbal communication can be used as a viable interface between computers and some of the most important aspects of human psychology such as emotions and social attitudes. As a result, a new computing domain seems to emerge that we can define "technology of nonverbal communication". This chapter outlines some of the most salient aspects of such a potentially new domain and outlines some of its most important perspectives for the future.

INTRODUCTION

Nonverbal communication is one of the most pervasive phenomena of our everyday life. On one hand, just because we have a body and we are alive, we constantly display a large number of nonverbal behavioral cues like facial expressions,

vocalizations, postures, gestures, appearance, etc. (Knapp & Hall, 1972; Richmond & McCroskey, 1995). On the other hand, just because we sense and perceive the cues others display, we cannot avoid interpreting and understanding them (often outside conscious awareness) in terms of feelings, emotions, attitudes, intentions, etc. (Kunda, 1999; Poggi, 2007). Thus, *"We cannot not communicate"*

DOI: 10.4018/978-1-61692-892-6.ch007

(Watzlawick et al., 1967) even when we sleep and still display our feelings (of which we are unaware) through movements, facial expressions, etc., or when we make it clear that we do not want to communicate:

If two humans come together it is virtually inevitable that they will communicate something to each other [...] even if they do not speak, messages will pass between them. By their looks, expressions and body movement each will tell the other something, even if it is only, "I don't wish to know you: keep your distance"; "I assure you the feeling is mutual. I'll keep clear if you do". (Argyle, 1979).

As nonverbal communication is such a salient and ubiquitous aspect of our life, it is not surprising to observe that computing technology, expected to integrate our daily life seamlessly and naturally like no one else, identifies automatic understanding and synthesis of nonverbal communication as a key step towards *human-centered* computers, i.e. computers adept to our natural modes of operating and communicating (Pantic et al., 2007; Pantic et al., 2008). This is the case of *Affective Computing*, where the aim is automatic understanding and synthesis of emotional states (Picard, 2000), of certain trends in *Human-Computer Interaction*, where the goal is to interface machines with the psychology of users (Reeves & Nass, 1996; Nass & Brave, 2005), of research in *Embodied Conversational Agents*, where the goal is to simulate credible human behavior with synthetic characters or robots (Bickmore & Cassell, 2005), and of the emerging field of *Social Signal Processing*, where the target is to understand mutual relational attitudes (*social signals*) of people involved in social interactions (Vinciarelli et al., 2008; Vinciarelli et al., 2009).

This list of domains is by no means complete, but it is sufficient to show how a *nonverbal communication technology* is actually developing in the computing community. Its main strength is an intense cross-fertilization between machine

intelligence (e.g., speech processing, computer vision and machine learning) and human sciences (e.g., psychology, anthropology and sociology) and its main targets are artificial forms of social, emotional and affective intelligence (Albrecht, 2005; Goleman, 2005). Furthermore, social and psychological research increasingly relies on technologies related to nonverbal communication to develop insights about human-human interactions, like in the case of large scale social networks (Lazer et al., 2009), organizational behavior (Olguin et al., 2009), and communication in mobile spaces (Raento et al., 2009).

This chapter aims at highlighting the most important aspects of this research trend and includes two main parts. The first introduces the main aspects of nonverbal communication technology and the second shows how this last is applied to the analysis of social and affective phenomena. The first part introduces a general model of human-human communication, proposes a taxonomy of nonverbal behavioral cues that can be used as perceivable stimuli in communication, and outlines the general process that nonverbal communication technology implements. The second part illustrates the most important phenomena taking place during social interactions, provides a survey of works showing how technology deals with them, and proposes the recognition of emotions in speech as a methodological example of the inference of social and affective phenomena from vocal (nonverbal) behavior. The chapter ends with a description of the emerging domain of Social Signal Processing (the most recent research avenue centered on nonverbal communication) and a list of application domains likely to benefit from the technologies described in this chapter.

PSYCHOLOGY AND TECHNOLOGY OF NONVERBAL COMMUNICATION

Nonverbal communication is a particular case of human-human communication where the means used to exchange information consists of nonverbal behavioral cues (Knapp & Hall, 1972; Richmond & McCroskey, 1995). This is appealing from a technological point of view because nonverbal cues must necessarily be accessible to our senses (in particular sight and hearing) and this makes them detectable through microphones, cameras or other suitable sensors, a *conditio sine qua non* for computing technology. Furthermore, many nonverbal behavioral cues are displayed outside conscious awareness and this makes them *honest*, i.e. sincere and reliable indices of different facets of affect (Pentland, 2008). In other words, nonverbal behavioral cues are the physical, machine detectable evidence of affective phenomena not otherwise accessible to experience, an ideal point for technology and human sciences to meet.

The rest of this section outlines the most important aspects of nonverbal communication from both psychological and technological points of view.

Psychology of Nonverbal Communication

In very general terms (Poggi, 2007), communication takes place whenever an *Emitter E* produces a *signal* under the form of a *Perceivable Stimulus PS* and this reaches a *Receiver R* who interprets the signal and extracts an *Information I* from it, not necessarily the one that *E* actually wanted to convey. The emitter, and the same applies to the receiver, is not necessarily an individual person, it can be a group of individuals, a machine, an animal or any other entity capable of generating perceivable stimuli. These include whatever can be perceived by a receiver like sounds, signs, words, chemical traces, handwritten messages, images, etc.

Signals can be classed as either *communicative* or *informative* on one hand, and as either *direct* or *indirect* on the other hand. A signal is said to be communicative when it is produced by an emitter with the intention of conveying a specific mean-

ing, e.g. the "thumb up" to mean "OK", while it is informative when it is emitted unconsciously or without the intention of conveying a specific meaning, e.g. crossing arms during a conversation. In parallel, a signal is said to be direct when its meaning is context independent, e.g. the "thumb up" that means "OK" in any interaction context, and indirect in the opposite case, e.g. crossing arms when used by workers in strike to mean that they refuse to work.

In this framework, the communication is said to be *nonverbal* whenever the perceivable stimuli used as signals are *nonverbal behavioral cues*, i.e. the myriad of observable behaviors that accompany any human-human (and human-machine) interaction and do not involve language and words: facial expressions, blinks, laughter, speech pauses, gestures (conscious and unconscious), postures, body movements, head nods, etc. (Knapp & Hall, 1972; Richmond & McCroskey, 1995). In general, nonverbal communication is particularly interesting when it involves informative behavioral cues. The reason is that these are typically produced outside conscious awareness and can be considered *honest signals* (Pentland, 2008), i.e. signals that leak reliable information about the actual inner state and feelings of people, whether these correspond to emotional states like anger, fear and surprise, general conditions like arousal, calm, and tiredness, or attitudes towards others like empathy, interest, dominance and disappointment (Ambady et al., 2000; Ambady & Rosenthal, 1992).

Social psychology proposes to group all nonverbal behavioral cues into five classes called *codes* (Hecht et al., 1999): *physical appearance, gestures and postures, face and eyes behavior, vocal behavior*, and *space and environment*. Table 1 reports some of the most common nonverbal behavioral cues of each code and shows the social and affective phenomena most closely related to them. By "related" it is meant that the cue accounts for the phenomenon taking place and/or influences the perception of the same phenomenon. The cues listed in this section are the most important, but

Table 1. This table shows the most common nonverbal behavioral cues for each code and the affective aspects most commonly related to them. The table has been published in Vinciarelli et al. 2009 and it is courtesy of A.Vinciarelli, M.Pantic and H.Bourlard

Nonverbal cues	Affective Behaviors							Tech.		
	emotion	Personality	status	dominance	persuasion	regulation	rapport	Speech analysis	Computer vision	biometry
Physical appearance										
Height			✓	✓					✓	✓
Attractiveness		✓	✓	✓	✓		✓		✓	✓
Body shape		✓		✓					✓	✓
Gesture and posture										
Hand gestures	✓	✓			✓	✓	✓		✓	✓
Posture	✓	✓	✓	✓	✓	✓	✓			
Walking		✓	✓	✓						
Face and eye behavior										
Facial expressions	✓	✓	✓	✓	✓	✓	✓		✓	✓
Gaze behavior	✓	✓	✓	✓	✓	✓	✓		✓	
Focus of attention	✓	✓	✓	✓	✓	✓	✓		✓	
Vocal behavior										
Prosody	✓	✓		✓	✓		✓	✓		
Turn taking	✓	✓	✓	✓		✓	✓	✓		
Vocal outbursts	✓	✓		✓	✓	✓	✓	✓		
Silence	✓		✓				✓	✓		
Space and environment										
Distance	✓	✓	✓		✓		✓		✓	
Seating arrangement				✓	✓		✓		✓	

the list is by no means exhaustive. The interested reader can refer to specialized monographs (Knapp & Hall, 1972; Richmond & McCroskey, 1995) for an extensive survey. In the following, codes and some of their most important cues are described in more detail.

Physical appearance: Aspect, and in particular attractiveness, is a signal that cannot be hidden and has a major impact on the perception of others. After the first pioneering investigations (Dion et al., 1972), a large body of empirical evidence supports the "*Halo effect*", also known as "*What is beautiful is good*", i.e. tendency to attribute socially desirable characteristics to physically attractive people. This has been measured through the higher success rate of politicians judged attractive by their electors (Surawski & Osso, 2006), through the higher percentage of individuals significantly taller than the average among CEOs of large companies (Gladwell, 2005), or through the higher likelihood of starting new relationships that attractive people have (Richmond & McCroskey, 1995). Furthermore, there is a clear influence of people somatotype (the overall body shape) on personality traits attribution, e.g., thin people tend to be considered lower in emotional stability, while round persons tend to be considered higher in openness (Cortes & Gatti, 1965).

Gestures and Postures: Gestures are often performed consciously to convey some specific meaning (e.g., the thumb up gesture that means "OK") or to perform a specific action (e.g., to point at something with the index finger), but in many cases they are the result of some affective process and they are displayed outside conscious awareness (Poggi, 2007). This is the case of *adaptors* (self-touching, manipulation of small objects, rhythmic movements of legs, etc.) that typically account for boredom, uncomfort, and other negative feelings, and self-protection gestures like folding arms and crossing legs (Knapp & Hall, 1972; Richmond & McCroskey, 1995). Furthermore, recent studies have shown that gestures express emotions (Coulson, 2004; Stock et al., 2007) and accompany social affective states like shame and embarrassment (Costa et al., 2001; Ekman & Rosenberg, 2005).

Postures are considered among the most reliable and honest nonverbal cues as they are typically assumed unconsciously (Richmond & McCroskey, 1995). Following the seminal work in (Scheflen, 1964), postures convey three main kinds of social messages: *inclusion and exclusion* (we exclude others by orienting our body in the opposite direction with respect to them), *engagement* (we are more involved in an interaction when we are in front of others), and *rapport* (we tend to imitate others posture when they dominate us or when we like them).

Face and gaze behavior: Not all nonverbal behavioral cues have the same impact on our perception of other's affect and, depending on the context; different cues have different impact (Richmond & McCroskey, 1995). However, facial expressions and, in more general terms, face behaviors are typically the cues that influence most our perception (Grahe & Bernieri, 1999). Nonverbal facial cues account for cognitive states

like interest (Cunningham et al., 2004), emotions (Cohn, 2006), psychological states like suicidal depression (Ekman & Rosenberg, 2005) or pain (Williams, 2003), social behaviors like accord and rapport (Ambady & Rosenthal, 1992; Cunningham et al., 2004), personality traits like extraversion and temperament (Ekman & Rosenberg, 2005), and social signals like status, trustworthiness (Ambady & Rosenthal, 1992). Gaze behavior (*who looks at whom and how much*) plays a major role in exchanging the floor during conversations, and in displaying dominance, power and status.

Vocal Behavior: Vocal behavior accounts for all those phenomena that do not include language or verbal content in speech. The vocal nonverbal behavior includes five major components: *prosody, linguistic* and *non-linguistic vocalizations, silences,* and *turn-taking patterns* (Richmond & McCroskey, 1995). Prosody accounts for *how* something is said and it influences the perception of several personality traits, like competence and persuasiveness (Scherer, 1979). Linguistic vocalizations correspond to sounds like "ehm", "ah-ah", etc. that are used as words even if they are something different. They typically communicate hesitation (Glass et al., 1982) or support towards others speaking. Non-linguistic vocalizations include cry, laughter, shouts, yawns, sobbing, etc. and are typically related to strong emotional states (we cry when we are very happy or particularly sad) or tight social bonds (we laugh to show pleasure of being with someone). Silences and pauses typically express hesitation, cognitive effort (we think about what we are going to say), or the choice of not talking even when asked to do so. Last, but not list, turn-taking, the mechanism through which people exchange the floor in conversations, has been shown to account for roles, preference structures, dominance and status, etc.

Space and Environment: Social and physical space are tightly intertwined and, typically, the distance between two individuals corresponds to the kind of relationship they have, e.g. *intimate* (less than 0.5 meters in western cultures),

Figure 1. This picture draws a parallel between the communication processes as it takes place between humans and as it is typically implemented in a machine. The correspondence does not mean that the process implemented in the machine actually explains and or described a human-human communication process, but simply helps to understand how technology deals with nonverbal communication

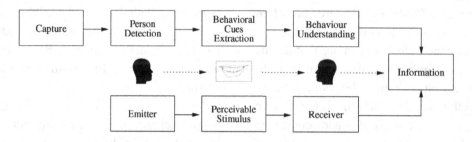

casual-personal (between 0.5 and 1.2 meters) or *socio-formal* (between 1 and 2 meters) following the terminology in (Hall, 1959). Furthermore, the kind of relationship between people sitting around a table influences the seating positions, e.g. people collaborating tend to sit close to one another, while people discussing tend to sit in front of one another (Lott & Sommer, 1967).

Technology of Nonverbal Communication

Is it possible to make technological value out of social psychology findings about nonverbal communication? This is a core question for domains like affective computing (Picard, 2000) and Social Signal Processing (Vinciarell et al., 2009; Vinciarelli, 2009), where nonverbal behavioral cues are used as a physical, *machine detectable* evidence of emotions and social relational attitudes, respectively. Both domains start from the simple consideration that we sense nonverbal behavioral cues (most of the times unconsciously) through our eyes and ears. Thus, it must be possible to sense the same nonverbal cues with cameras, microphones and any other suitable sensor. Furthermore, both domains consider that there is an inference process (in general unconscious) between the behavior we observe and the perceptions we develop in terms of emotional and social phenomena. Thus, automatic inference approaches, mostly based on

machine learning, could be used to automatically understand emotional and social phenomena.

Figure 1 shows the main technological components involved in approaches for automatic understanding of nonverbal communication. The scheme does not correspond to any approach in particular, but any work in the literature matches, at least partially, the process depicted in the picture. Furthermore, the scheme illustrated in Figure 1 is not supposed to describe how humans work, but only how machines can understand social and affective phenomena. Overall, the process includes four major steps described in more detail in the rest of this section.

Capture: Human behavior can be sensed with a large variety of devices, including cheap webcams installed on a laptop, fully equipped smart meeting rooms where several tens of microphones and cameras record everything happens (McCowan et al., 2003; Waibel et al., 2003), mobile devices equipped with haptic and proximity sensors (Raento et al., 2009; Murray-Smith, 2009), pressure captors that detect posture and movements (Kapoor et al., 2004), eyefish cameras capturing spontaneous interactions, etc. Capture is a fundamental step because, depending on the sensors, certain kinds of analysis will be possible and others not. However, what is common to all possible sensing devices is that they give as output *signals* and these must be analyzed automatically to complete the whole process.

Person detection: In general, signals obtained through capture devices portray more than one person. This is the case, for example, of audio recordings where more than one person talks, of video recordings where different persons interact with one another, etc. This requires a person detection step aimed at identifying what parts of the data correspond to which person. The reason is that nonverbal behavioral cues can be extracted reliably only when it is clear what individual corresponds to a signal under analysis. Person detection includes technologies like speaker diarization, detecting who talks when in audio data (Tranter & Reynolds, 2006), face detection, detecting what part of an image corresponds to the face of one person (Yang et al., 2002), tracking, following one or more persons moving in a video (Forsyth et al., 2006), etc. The application of one person detection technology rather than another one depends on the capture device, but the result is always the same: the signals to be analyzed are segmented into parts corresponding to single individuals.

Behavioral cues detection: The technological components described so far can be considered as a preprocessing phase that gives the raw data a form suitable for actual analysis and understanding of nonverbal communication. Behavioral cues are the perceivable stimuli that, in the communication process, are used by the emitter to convey information and by the receiver to draw information, possibly the same that the emitter wants to communicate. Detection of nonverbal behavioral cues is the first step of the process that actually deals with nonverbal behavior and it includes well developed domains like facial expression recognition (Zeng et al., 2009), prosody extraction (Crystal, 1969), gesture and posture recognition (Mitra & Acharya, 2007), head pose estimation (Murphy-Chutorian & Trivedi, 2009), laughter detection (Truong & Van Leeuwen, 2007), etc. (see Vinciarelli et al., 2009) for an extensive survey on techniques applied at all processing steps). These are the perceivable stimuli that we both

produce and sense in our everyday interactions to communicate with others.

Nonverbal behavior understanding: In the communication process, receivers draw information from perceivable stimuli. The information corresponds, in general, to what the emitter actually wants to convey, but this is not necessarily the case. Nonverbal behavior understanding corresponds to this step of the communication process and aims at inferring information like the emotional state or the relational attitude of the receiver from the nonverbal behavioral cues detected at the previous stage of the process. This step of the process relies in general on machine learning and pattern recognition approaches and it is the point where human sciences findings are integrated in technological approaches. Most of the efforts have been dedicated at the recognition of emotions (Picard, 2000) and social signals, i.e. relational attitudes exchanged by people in social interactions (Vinciarelli et al., 2009).

PSYCHOLOGY AND TECHNOLOGY OF FACE-TO-FACE INTERACTIONS

The most natural setting for nonverbal communication is face-to-face interaction, in particular conversations that are considered the "*primordial site of social interaction*" (Schegloff, 1987). As such, conversations are the natural context for a wide spectrum of social phenomena that have a high impact on our life as well as on the life of the groups we belong to (Levine & Moreland, 1998), whether these are work teams expected to accomplish some complex collaborative tasks, circles of friends trying to organize an entertaining Saturday evening, or families aimed at supporting the well being of their members.

This section focuses in particular on those social phenomena that have been not only investigated from a psychological point of view, but that have been the subject of technological research as well (Vinciarelli et al., 2008, 2009).

Psychology of Face-to-Face Interactions

Three main social phenomena recognized as fundamental by psychologists have been addressed by computer scientists as well, namely *roles*, *dominance* and *conflict* (or *disagreement*). This section provides a description of each one of them.

Roles are a universal aspect of human-human interaction (Tischler, 1990), whenever people convene to interact, they play roles with the (unconscious) goal of fulfilling others expectations (if you are the head of a group you are expected to provide guidance towards the fulfillment of group goals), give meaning to their behaviors (helping a patient as a doctor is a professional duty while helping the same patient as a family member is a form of love and attachment), and provide predictability to other interactants (when teachers enter their classroom it is likely they will give a lecture and this helps students to behave accordingly). Some roles correspond to explicit functions (like the examples given above) and can be easily identified and formalized, while others are more implicit and embody deeper aspects of human-human interaction like the *attacker*, the *defender* or the *gate-keeper* in theories of human interactions (Bales, 1950). From a behavioral point of view, roles corresponding to explicit functions tend to induce more regular and detectable behavioral patterns than others and are thus easier to be analyzed automatically (Salamin et al., 2009).

Conflict and disagreement are among the most investigated social phenomena because their impact on the life of a group is significant and potentially disruptive. In some cases, conflicts foster innovation and enhance group performance, but in most cases they have a contrary effect and can lead to the dissolution of the group (Levine & Moreland, 1998). From a social point of view, the most salient aspects of conflicts and disagreement are activities of some of the members that have negative effects on others, attempts of increasing power shares at the expense of others, bargaining

between members and formation of coalitions (Levine & Moreland, 1990). In terms of nonverbal behavior, conflicts are typically associated with interruptions, higher fidgeting and voice loudness typical of anger, pragmatic preference structures such that people tend to react to those they disagree with rather than to those they agree with (Bilmes, 1988; Vinciarelli, 2009), longer periods of overlapping speech, etc.

Dominance accounts for ability to influence others, control available resources, and have higher impact on the life of a group, whatever its goal is. Dominance can be interpreted as a personality trait (the predisposition to dominate others), or as a description of relationships between group members (Rienks & Heylen, 2006). While being a hypothetical construct (it cannot be observed directly), dominance gives rise to a number of nonverbal behavioral cues that allow observers to agree on who is (or are) the dominant individuals in a given group. These include seating in positions allowing direct observation of others like the shortest side of a rectangular table (Lott & Sommer, 1967), being looked at by others more than looking at others (Dovidio & Ellyson, 1982), talking longer than others (Mast, 2002), etc.

Technology of Face-to-Face Interactions

Given the centrality of small group interactions in psychology research, it is not surprising to observe that computing technology efforts aimed at the analysis of social and affective phenomena have focused on face-to-face interaction scenarios like meetings, talk-shows, job interviews, etc. (Vinciarelli et al., 2008, 2009). This section proposes a brief survey of the most important approaches dedicated to this problem in the literature, with particular attention to those dealing with role recognition, conflict and disagreement analysis, and dominance detection, i.e. those dealing with the social phenomena identified above as among the most important ones from a social psychology

Table 2. This table presents the main works where nonverbal behavioral cues have been used, in different contexts, to interpret automatically social interactions. Whenever possible, the table reports the amount of data used in the experiments and a performance measure

Article	Data	Performance
Role Recognition		
Salamin et al. (2009)	Broadcast+AMI (90h)	80% frame accuracy
Laskowski et al. (2008)	AMI (45h)	53% frame accuracy
Garg et al.(2008)	AMI (45h)	67.9% frame accuracy
Dong et al. (2007)	MSC (4h.30m)	75% role assignment accuracy
Liu (2006)	Broadcast (17h)	77.0% story accuracy
Banerjee & Rudnicky (2004)	Meetings (45m)	53.0% analysis segments accuracy
Barzilay et al. (2000)	Broadcast (17h)	80.0% story accuracy
Dominance Detection		
Jayagopi et al. (2009)	AMI subset (5h)	80% dominant person recognition rate
Rienks & Heylen (2006)	AMI and M4 subset (95m)	75% dominance level recognition rate
Rienks et al. (2006)	AMI-40	70% dominance level recognition rate
Otsuka et al. (2005)	Broadcast (17h)	N/A
Analysis of (Dis-) Agreement		
Vinciarelli (2009)	Canal9 (43h)	66% (dis-)agreement recognition rate
Hillard et al. (2003)	ICSI subset (8094 talk spurts)	78% (dis-)agreement recognition rate
Galley et al. (2004)	ICSI subset	86.9% (dis-)agreement recognition rate

point of view. Table 2 reports results and some of the experimental characteristics of the works surveyed in this section.

Role recognition is typically based on automatic analysis of speaking activity, the physical, machine detectable aspect of behavior that seems to be more correlated with the roles people play in a conversation. By speaking activity is meant here the simple act of speaking or remaining silent, the use of certain words rather than others, the tendency to speak while others are speaking, the number and length of turns during a conversation, etc. Temporal proximity of different speakers interventions is used in (Vinciarelli, 2007; Salamin et al., 2009) to build social networks and represent each person with a feature vector. This is then fed to Bayesian classifiers mapping individuals into roles belonging to a predefined set. A similar approach is used in several other works (Barzilay et al., 2000; Liu, 2006; Garg et al., 2008; Favre

et al., 2009) in combination with approaches for the modeling of lexical choices like the BoosT-exter (Barzilay et al., 2000) or the Support Vector Machines (Garg et al., 2008). Probabilistic sequential approaches are applied to sequences of feature vectors extracted from individual conversation turns in (Liu, 2006; Favre et al., 2009), namely Maximum Entropy Classifiers and Hidden Markov Models, respectively. An approach based on C4.5 decision trees and empirical features (number of speaker changes, number of speakers talking in a given time interval, number of overlapping speech intervals, etc.) is proposed in (Banerjee & Rudnicky, 2004). A similar approach is proposed in (Laskowski et al., 2008), where the features are probability of starting speaking when everybody is silent or when someone else is speaking, and role recognition is performed with a Bayesian classifier based on Gaussian distributions. The only approaches including features non-related to speaking activity are presented in (Zancanaro et al., 2006; Dong et al., 2007), where fidgeting is used as an evidence of role. However, the results seem to confirm that speaking activity features are more effective.

Conflict and disagreement analysis is a domain attracting increasingly significant interest in the last years (Bousmalis et al., 2009). Like in the case of roles, behavior evidences based on speaking activity seem to account reliably for conflict, agreement and disagreement, though psychology insists on the importance of facial expressions, head nods and bodily movements (Poggi, 2007). The coalitions forming during television debates are reconstructed in (Vinciarelli, 2009) through a Markov model keeping into account that people tend to react to someone they disagree with more than to someone they agree with. Similarly, pairs of talk spurts (short turns) are first modeled in terms of lexical (which words are uttered), durational (length, overlapping, etc.), and structural (spurts per speaker, spurts between two speakers, etc.) features and then classified as expressions of agreement or disagreement with a Maximum Entropy Model in (Hillard et al., 2003; Galley et al., 2004).

Dominance detection is one of the most extensively investigated problems in machine analysis of human behavior (Vinciarelli et al., 2009). In contrast with the other two problems considered above, speaking activity features are here accompanied by other nonverbal behavioral cues as well. This happens in (Otsuka et al., 2005), where Dynamic Bayesian Networks are used to model speaking based features (see description of role recognition) and gaze behavior (who looks at whom). Another multimodal approach (Jayagopi et al., 2009) combines speaking activity features with movement based cues (e.g., time during which a person moves, number of time intervals during which a person moves, etc.). In both approaches, movement and gaze help, but speaking features still seem to be the most effective. This seems to be confirmed by other works that achieve god

results by using only speaking activity features (Rienks et al., 2006; Rienks & Heylen, 2006).

A METHODOLOGICAL EXAMPLE: EMOTION RECOGNITION IN SPEECH

The above survey has shown that, from an automatic behavior analysis point of view, cues extracted from speech tend to be more effective than cues extracted from other communication modalities (gestures, movement, facial expressions, etc.). This is in contrast with the results of psychology experiments showing that vocal cues, while having a major impact on the perception of social and emotional phenomena, still have less influence than other behavioral cues, in particular facial expressions and gaze. The most likely reason is that speech analysis techniques are more robust than other technologies (e.g. facial expression analysis and gesture recognition) with respect to conditions in naturalistic interaction settings (e.g., people assuming unconstrained positions, moving, occluding one another, etc.). In other words, machines represent a bottleneck through which some cues, effective when perceived by humans, become difficult to detect and interpret.

For this reason, this section proposes the recognition of emotions in speech as a methodological example of technology of nonverbal communication. The domain has been investigated for long time in both psychology and computing science and the results, if not conclusive, still have a high degree of maturity.

Emotion and Vocal Behavior

Generally, the term "emotion" describes subjective feelings lasting for short periods of time, as well as mental and physiological states associated with a wide variety of feelings. No definitive taxonomy of emotions exists, though numerous taxonomies have been proposed; the two commonly used models are called *discrete* and *dimensional*. Most studies in the field of vocal effects of emotion have used the discrete model that groups all emotional states into few discrete categories: happiness, sadness, anger, fear, disgust and surprise. In the dimensional model, different emotional states are mapped in a two-or three-dimensional space. The two main dimensions are *valence* and *activity*; the third dimension is often power or control.

Darwin believed that the voice is the primary channel for expressing emotion in both humans and animals (Knapp & Hall, 1997). Studies of content free speech have shown that emotion perception depends on changes in pitch, speaking rate, volume and other paralinguistic characteristics of voice (Scherer, 2003). Davitn, as cited in (Knapp & Hall, 1997), said in 1964 that "Regardless of the technique used, all studies of adults thus far reported in the literature agree that emotional meanings can be communicated accurately by vocal expression". Significant efforts have been made to identify the vocal cues actually carrying emotional information (Scherer, 2003) and the result is that there is no "dictionary" of emotions in terms of paralinguistic cues, i.e. there is no one-to-one correspondence between observed cues and emotions being expressed. Furthermore, there are several factors interfering with vocal cues including verbal aspects of communication, culture dependency and the rest of nonverbal behavior; however, it has been possible to show which vocal features tend to be associated with which emotions (Knapp & Hall, 1997; Polzin & Waibel, 2000; Scherer, 2003). This is evident in Table 3, where the cues most commonly used in automatic emotion recognition are reported with the respective emotions they tend to be associated with.

Emotion Recognition in Speech

There is a long list of paralinguistic features employed for the recognition of emotions in speech (Knapp & Hall, 1997; Morrison et al., 2007;

Scherer, 2003; Ververidis & Kotropoulos, 2006) and they can be categorized into four main groups:

1. **Prosodic Features:** these are features which are reflecting rhythm, stress and intonation of speech. In acoustic terms, the three main classes of prosodic features are pitch, energy, and rhythm (Morrison et al., 2007). Rhythm is represented by various features like, number of pauses, ZCR (Zero-cross ratio which represents the number of times that the speech signal touches the level zero), speech rate (SR), voiced-segment length and unvoiced-segment length.

2. **Spectral-based features:** These are features accounting for the speech signal behavior in the frequency domain. MFCC (Mel-frequency Cepsteral Coefficients), LPC (Linear Prediction Coefficients), LPCC (Linear Prediction Cepstral Coefficients), PLP (Perceptual Linear Prediction), LFPC (Log Frequency Power Coefficients) and Energy in spectral bands are the most commonly applied spectral-based features, typicallly used in speech and emotion recognition (Oudeyer, 2003; Nwe et al., 2001; Nwe et al., 2003; Ververidis & Kotropoulos, 2006; Womack & Hansen, 1996).

3. **Articulatory-based features:** these are features measuring the changes in shape and structure of vocal tract during articulation, e.g., formants, which are a representation of the vocal tract resonance, and cross-section areas when the vocal tract is modeled as a series of concatenated lossless tubes (Ververidis & Kotropoulos, 2006; Womack & Hansen, 1996).

4. **Voice quality features:** Voice quality is the outcome of the human voice excitation; voice quality is the result of glottal pulse shape, its rate and time variations. In particular, voice quality features describe the properties of the glottal source. Jitter, shimmer (Li et al., 2007) and VQP (voice quality parameters)

Table 3. Paralinguistic features, used in recognition of different emotional states

	Joy	Boredom	Neutral	Sadness	Anger	Fear	Surprise	Stress	Depression	Happiness	Disgust	Annoyance	Frustration	Anxiety	Dislike
Pitch	✓	✓	✓	✓	✓	✓	✓	✓	✓	✓	✓	✓	✓	✓	✓
Intensity	✓	✓	✓	✓	✓	✓	✓	✓	✓	✓	✓	✓	✓	✓	✓
Rhythm	✓	✓	✓	✓	✓	✓	✓	✓		✓	✓	✓	✓	✓	✓
Formants		✓	✓	✓	✓	✓	✓	✓	✓	✓				✓	✓
Cross sectional Areas								✓							
MFCC		✓	✓	✓	✓	✓	✓	✓		✓					✓
LFPC			✓	✓	✓	✓				✓					✓
LPC	✓		✓	✓	✓	✓	✓				✓				
Spectral-band Intensity		✓	✓	✓	✓			✓	✓	✓	✓				
Cepstral Coefficients												✓	✓		
Voice Quality Parameters		✓	✓	✓	✓					✓				✓	

(Lugger & Yang, 2006) are used in emotion recognition as a representation of voice quality.

The features in these four main groups are called "*primary*", they are estimated on a frame basis and they reflect short-term characteristics of vocal behavior. Other features, called "*secondary*", are obtained from primary features by, e.g., estimating their average, median, minimum, maximum, range, variance, mean, contour, and, in more general terms, by extracting statistical information about the variation of primary features over a time interval.

Identifying exactly what features account for what emotion is not evident; however, Table 3 shows the paralinguistic features most commonly used for recognizing each emotion. Furthermore, Table 4 provides the most important results in terms of emotion recognition obtained so far in the literature.

Pitch, intensity and rhythm appear to be the most effective paralinguistic features in emotion recognition (Morrison et al., 2007). Pitch is the

Figure 2. Feature groups

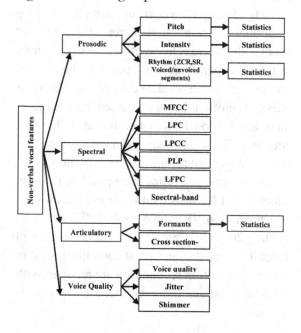

perceived fundamental frequency of voice and it is the rate of vibration of vocal folds (see Figure 3).

The pitch contour has been shown to vary depending on emotional state (Ang et al., 2002;

Table 4. Previous studies in emotional speech recognition

Study Groups	Emotional States	Feature Groups	Recognition Method	Accuracy (%)
Womack, & Hansen (1996)	Different stress conditions	Pitch, Rhythm, Cross Sectional Areas, Mel-based	Back-propagation Neural Network	91
Nicholson et al. (1999)	Joy, Neutral, Sadness, Anger, Fear, Surprise, Disgust, Teasing	Pitch, Intensity, LPC, Delta-LPC	OCO Neural Network ACO Neural Network Learning Vector Quantization	50 55 33
Amir et al., (2000)	Joy, Sadness, Anger, Fear, Disgust	Pitch, Intensity, Rhythm	Fuzzy Classifier	43.4
France et al. (2000)	Control, Depression, Suicidal Risk	Pitch, Intensity, Formants, spectral-band Intensity	Quadratic Classifier	70 (F), 77(M)
Polzin, & Waibel (2000)	Neutral, Sadness, Anger	Pitch, Intensity, Jitter, MFCC, + Verbal features	GMM Classifier	62
McGilloway et al. (2000)	Happiness, Neutral, Sadness, Anger, Fear	Pitch, Intensity, Spectral-band Intensity	Gaussian SVM Linear Discriminant	52 55
Lee et al. (2001)	Negative from Non-negative Emotions	Pitch, Intensity	KNN	80 (F), 76 (M)
Zhou et al. (2001)	Different stress conditions	Spectral-ban Intensity	HMM Classifier	91
New et al. (2001)	Happiness, Sadness, Anger, Fear, Surprise, Dislike	LFPC, Mel-based	HMM Classifier	78
Park et al. (2002)	Neutral, Anger, Surprise, Laugh	Pitch	Recurrent Neural Network	Not Reported
Ang et al. (2002)	Annoyance+Frustration vs. Else	Pitch, Intensity, Rhythm, Cepstral Coef.	Decision Tree	83
Oudeyer (2003)	Calm, Sadness, Anger	Pitch, Intensity, Spectral-band Intensity, MFCC	KNN Classifier Decision Tree (C4.5) Decision Rules/PART Kernel Density Kstar Linear Regression LWR Voted Perceptrons SVM VFI M5Prime Naive Bayes AdaBoost	90 93 94 90 86 85 89 75 94 84 92 91 95
Kwon et al. (2003)	Stress, Neutral / Happiness, Boredom, Neutral, Sadness, Anger	Pitch, Intensity, Rhythm, Formants, MFCC, Spectral-band Energy	Gaussian SVM	42.3
Ververidis (2004)	Happiness, Neutral, Sadness, Anger, Surprise	Pitch, Intensity, Formants	Bayes Classifier	51.6
Bhatti et al., (2004)	Happiness, Sadness, Anger, Fear, Dislike, Surprise	Pitch, Intensity, Rhythm	A standard Neural Network KNN Classifier Modular Neural Network	80.69 79.31 83.31
Schuller et al. (2005)	Joy, Neutral, Sadness, Anger, Fear, Disgust, Surprise	Pitch, Intensity, Rhythm, Spectral-band Intensity	StackingC	71.6
Hyun et al. (2005)	Joy, Neutral, Sadness, Anger	Pitch, Intensity, Rhythm	Bayes Classifier	71.1
Shami, & Kamel (2005)	Approval, Attention, Prohibition Weak, Soothing, Neutral	Pitch, Intensity, Rhythm, MFCC	KNN SVM	87 83
Morrison et al. (2007)	Happiness, Sadness, Anger, Fear, Dislike, Surprise	Pitch, Intensity, Rhythm, Formants	StackingC Unweighted Vote	72.18 70.54
Lugger & Yang (2008)	Happiness, Boredom, Neutral, Sadness, Anger, Anxiety	Pitch, Intensity, Rhythm, Formants, MFCC, VQ Parameters	Bayes Classifier	88.6

Table 4. continued

Study Groups	Emotional States	Feature Groups	Recognition Method	Accuracy (%)
Yang, & Lugger (2009)	Happiness, Boredom, Neutral, Sadness, Anger, Anxiety	Pitch, Intensity, Rhythm, Formants, Length, Harmony(derived from pitch), Voice Quality	Bayes Classifier	73.5
Rong et al. (2009)	Happiness, Sadness, Anger, Fear	Pitch, Intensity, Rhythm, MFCC	Decision Tree + Random Forest	72.25
Busso et al. (2009)	Neutral, Emotional	Pitch	Distance from Neutral speech model (GMM)	70

Lee et al., 2001; Mozziconacci & Hermes, 1995; Park et al., 2002; Polzin & Waibel, 2000). For example, neutral speech has narrower pitch range than emotional speech, i.e. people tend to change more their pitch while emotionally affected. This is particularly evident in angry speech that shows higher pitch range (Scherer, 1996), as well as increased mean pitch and intensity with respect to neutral speech (Scherer, 2003). The same can be observed for happiness while fear was discovered to have a high pitch median, wide pitch range, medium inflection range, and a moderate rate variation. Emotions characterized by lower arousal levels like sadness and disgust typically have lower physiological activation levels and this is evident in speech as well, e.g., sadness results into lower pitch mean and narrower pitch range. Disgust generally has a low pitch median, wide pitch range, lower inflectional range, and lower rate of pitch change during inflection (Mor-

rison et al., 2007; Rong et al., 2009; Scherer, 2003; Ververidis & Kotropoulos, 2006). Table 5 shows a summary of how different emotions affect pitch.

Voice intensity is another important paralinguistic feature that can be used as an emotional marker (McGilloway et al., 2000; Polzin & Waibel, 2000; Scherer, 2003). Voice intensity contour provides useful information to discriminate sets of emotions; For instance angry speech is shown to have a significant increase in energy envelope in contrast to sadness and disgust that typically lead to a decrease in intensity. Happiness is shown to have on intensity roughly the same affects as anger. Scherer (2003) notes that anger, fear and joy determine an increase in high frequency intensity while sadness determines, over the same parameter, a decrease. In summary, emotions with high excitation levels such as happiness, anger and surprise have typically higher intensity whereas sadness, fear and disgust have lower

Figure 3. Pitch Estimation

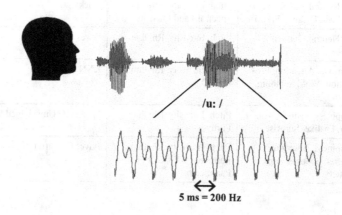

Table 5. Emotional states and pitch. The symbols show whether the pitch increases (> and >>), decreases (< and <<) or remain unchanged for a given emotion (=). The same symbols are used in the following tables 6 and 7

	Pitch		
	Mean	**Range**	**Variance**
Anger	>>	>	>>
Boredom		<	<
Disgust	<	$>_M,<_F$	
Fear	>>	>	>
Joy	>	>	>
Sadness	<	<	<
Stress	>		
Surprise	>=	>	

intensity (Rong et al., 2009; Ververidis & Kotropoulos, 2006). Table 6 is an abstract of intensity changes affected by different emotional states.

Rhythm-based characteristics of speech can be used as another index in motion recognition (Ang et al., 2002; Kwon et al., 2003; Schuller et al., 2005; Shami & Verhelst, 2007; Womack & Hansen, 1996; Yang & Lugger, 2009). Rhythm-based characteristics include length of voice/unvoiced segments, pauses between them, Zero Cross Ratio and speech rate.

In several studies it has been shown that speaking rate is higher in anger while on the other side it is lower in sadness; it is also noted that in sadness speech contains "irregular pauses" (Morrison et al., 2007). Table 7 reviews speech rate variation for different emotions.

Formants are among effective features in emotion recognition (France et al., 2000; Morrison et al., 2007; Kwon et al., 2003; Yang & Lugger, 2009). Formants are resonances of the human vocal tract. The frequency of resonance depends upon the shape and physical dimensions of vocal tract. Under different emotional states the length and width of vocal tract changes. It has been shown in previous studies that during anger, vowels are produced "with a more open vocal tract" and from that they concluded that the first formant frequency is higher in mean than natural speech. Neutral speech usually has a "uniform formant structure and glottal vibration pattern" which is in contrast with formant contours of sadness, fear and anger. Scherer (2003) found that in happiness first formant (F1) mean is decreased

Table 6. Emotional states and Intensity (see caption of Table 5 for an explanation of symbols)

	Intensity		
	Mean	**Range**	**High-freq. mean**
Anger	$>>_M,>_F$	>	>
Disgust	<		
Fear	>=		>
Joy	>	>	>=
Sadness	<	<	<
Stress	>		

Table 7. Emotional states and changes in speech rate (see caption of Table 5 for an explanation of symbols)

	Rhythm
	Speech Rate
Anger	><
Boredom	<
Disgust	>
Fear	><
Joy	>
Sadness	<
Surprise	=

but the bandwidth of F1 is increased while in sadness, fear and anger it is opposite (Scherer, 2003), Table 8.

CONCLUSIONS AND FUTURE PERSPECTIVES

The main reason why computing science is interested in Nonverbal Communication is that this represents an ideal interface between machines and some of the most important aspects of human psychology, in particular emotions and social attitudes. In this respect, automatic analysis, synthesis and modeling of nonverbal behavior concur towards human-computer confluence and have the potential for bridging the emotional

and social intelligence gap between humans and machines. As a result, there are at least two major computer communities working towards technology of nonverbal communication, i.e. affective computing (Picard 2000), dealing with emotions, and Social Signal Processing (Vinciarelli et al., 2008, 2009), dealing with social relational attitudes. Affective Computing is a well established domain and it has been extensively investigated for at least one decade. In contrast, Social Signal Processing is an emerging domain that aims at automatically understanding and synthesizing the social relational attitudes that people exchange during social interactions.

At its core, Social Signal Processing aims at answering three main questions:

- Is it possible to detect nonverbal behavioral cues in recordings of social interactions captured with microphones, cameras and other kinds of sensors?
- Is it possible to infer social signals from nonverbal behavioral cues as detected from data captured with different kinds of sensors?
- Is it possible to synthesize nonverbal behavioral cues eliciting desired social perceptions?

The first two questions pertain to the problem of analyzing social behavior and the involved technological components are those depicted in Figure

Table 8. Emotional states and Formants (see caption of Table 5 for an explanation of symbols)

	Formants			
	F1		**F2**	
	Mean	**Bandwidth**	**Mean**	**Bandwidth**
Anger	>		><	
Disgust	>	<	<	
Fear	>	<	<	
Joy	<	>		
Sadness	>	<	<	

1 and described in the section about psychology and technology of nonverbal behavior. The third question concerns the problem of embodiment of social behavior in Artificial Agents, Robots, Avatars, Artificial Characters and any other manufact supposed to simulate human behavior in human-machine interactions. While being in its early stages, Social Signal Processing has attracted significant attention in the business community for its potential impact on organizational sciences (Buchanan, 2007). Furthermore, major efforts are being made towards the creation of a publicly available web-based repository hosting the most important resources necessary to work on SSP, i.e. publications, benchmarks and tools (www.sspnet.eu).

Some issues still remain open and should be addressed in the next years. The first is the effect of context. It has been observed in a previous section that signals can be context dependent (or indirect). In current technology, the context is typically never modeled and the meaning of a given nonverbal cue can be misunderstood. On the other hand, the context is difficult to define and it is unclear how to address its modeling. Furthermore, social and affective aspects of behavior tend to be considered separately (SSP and Affective Computing are typically presented as separate domains) while they overlap to a certain extent and common aspects could be used to reinforce domain technologies.

Several application domains are likely to take significant profit from the development of technology of nonverbal communication (the list is not exhaustive): *multimedia content analysis* can rely on techniques for automatic understanding of social and affective phenomena to enrich the description of multimedia data content. This is particularly important because people and their interactions are among the most important cues we use to access reality and indexing the data in terms of social and affective phenomena is expected to bring retrieval systems closer to human needs (Dumais et al., 2003). *Computer mediated communication* (e.g., videoconferencing) will benefit

significantly from the transmission of nonverbal cues (which includes both automatic understanding and synthesis of nonverbal behavior) as their lack seems to be one of the main sources of unnaturalness in mediated communication like, e.g., the lack of gaze contact in videoconferences (Crowley, 2006). In a similar vein, *communication in mobile spaces* can benefit from the use of devices like gyroscopes and haptic sensors capable of stimulating natural nonverbal phenomena like mimicry and coordination (Murray-Smith, 2009). Early detection of cognitive and mental problems can be performed by identifying problems in nonverbal communication (e.g., lack of gestures accompanying speech or unnatural delays in reacting to others in conversation), thus automated systems for analysis of nonverbal communication can help in *healthcare*, particularly for aging related diseases like Alzheimer and Parkinson. *Videogames* have significantly increased their degree of interactivity in the last years and a better understanding of users via their nonverbal behaviors, as well as characters more convincing in the naturalness of their behaviors is likely to further improve gaming experience. *Marketing* is likely to benefit from the automatic analysis of customers behavior in retail spaces as well as from the identification of nonverbal cues capable of establishing a trust relationships between customers and sellers (Ambady et al., 2006). Furthermore, new application domains are likely to emerge like the development of tools for supporting and enhancing human-human communication, the creation of technologies for helping workers using communication (e.g., teachers) in their job. Last, but not least, the use of automatic approaches is likely to help psychologists to make their observations way more extensive and objective with respect to current standards mostly based on observation in the laboratory. These are just few examples, but many more can be identified by looking at how pervasive and ubiquitous computers are becoming in our everyday life.

ACKNOWLEDGMENT

This work is supported by the European Community's Seventh Framework Programme (FP7/2007-2013), under grant agreement no. 231287 (SSPNet). Furthermore, it is supported by the Swiss National Science Foundation through the Indo-Swiss Joint Research Project ``Cross-Cultural Personality Perception'' (Grant 122936), and through the National Centre of Competence in Research on Interactive Multimodal Information Management (IM2).

REFERENCES

Albrecht, K. (2005). *Social intelligence: The new science of success*. New York: John Wiley & Sons Ltd.

Ambady, N., Bernieri, F., & Richeson, J. (2000). Towards a histology of social behavior: judgmental accuracy from thin slices of behavior. In Zanna, M. (Ed.), *Advances in experimental social psychology* (pp. 201–272).

Ambady, N., Krabbenhoft, M., & Hogan, D. (2006). The 30-sec sale: Using thin-slice judgments to evaluate sales effectiveness. *Journal of Consumer Psychology*, *16*(1), 4–13. doi:10.1207/s15327663jcp1601_2

Ambady, N., & Rosenthal, R. (1992). Thin slices of expressive behavior as predictors of interpersonal consequences: a meta-analysis. *Psychological Bulletin*, *111*(2), 256–274. doi:10.1037/0033-2909.111.2.256

Amir, N., Ron, S., & Laor, N. (2000). Analysis of an emotional speech corpus in Hebrew based on objective criteria. In *Proceedings of the ISCA Workshop on Speech & Emotion* (pp. 29-33).

Ang, J., Dhillon, R., Krupski, A., Shriberg, E., & Stolcke, A. (2002). Prosody-based automatic detection of annoyance and frustration in human-computer dialog. In. *Proceedings of ICSLP*, *02*, 2037–2040.

Argyle, M., & Trower, P. (1979). *Person to person: ways of communicating*. HarperCollins Publishers.

Bales, R. (1950). *Interaction process analysis: A method for the study of small groups*. Addison-Wesley.

Banerjee, S., & Rudnicky, A. (2004). Using simple speech based features to detect the state of a meeting and the roles of the meeting participants. In *Proceedings of international conference on spoken language processing* (pp. 221-231).

Barzilay, R., Collins, M., Hirschberg, J., & Whittaker, S. (2000). The rules behind the roles: identifying speaker roles in radio broadcasts. In *Proceedings of the 17th national conference on artificial intelligence* (pp. 679-684).

Bhatti, M. W., Wang, Y., & Guan, L. (2004). A neural network approach for human emotion recognition in speech. In *Proceedings of the International Symposium on Circuits & Systems, ISCAS'04*, (Vol. 2, pp. II-181-4).

Bickmore, T., & Cassell, J. (2005). Social dialogue with embodied conversational agents. In van Kuppevelt, J., Dybkjaer, L., & Bernsen, N. (Eds.), *Advances in natural, multimodal, dialogue systems* (pp. 23–54). New York: Kluwer. doi:10.1007/1-4020-3933-6_2

Bilmes, J. (1988). The concept of preference in conversation analysis. *Language in Society*, *17*(2), 161–181. doi:10.1017/S0047404500012744

Bousmalis, K., Mehu, M., & Pantic, M. (2009). Spotting agreement and disagreement: A survey of nonverbal audiovisual cues and tools. In *Proceedings of the international conference on affective computing and intelligent interaction* (Vol. II, pp. 121-129).

Buchanan, M. (2007). The science of subtle signals. Strategy+Business, 48, 68–77.

Busso, C., Lee, S., & Narayanan, S. (2009). Analysis of emotionally salient aspects of fundamental frequency for emotion detection. *IEEE Transaction on Audio. Speech and Language Processing, 17*(4), 582–596. doi:10.1109/TASL.2008.2009578

Cohn, J. (2006). Foundations of human computing: facial expression and emotion. In *Proceedings of the ACM international conference on multimodal interfaces* (pp. 233-238).

Cortes, J., & Gatti, F. (1965). Physique and self-description of temperament. *Journal of Consulting Psychology, 29*(5), 432–439. doi:10.1037/h0022504

Costa, M., Dinsbach, W., Manstead, A., & Bitti, P. (2001). Social presence, embarrassment, and nonverbal behavior. *Journal of Nonverbal Behavior, 25*(4), 225–240. doi:10.1023/A:1012544204986

Coulson, M. (2004). Attributing emotion to static body postures: Recognition accuracy, confusions, and viewpoint dependence. *Journal of Nonverbal Behavior, 28*(2), 117–139. doi:10.1023/B:JONB.0000023655.25550.be

Crowley, J. L. (2006). Social Perception. *ACM Queue; Tomorrow's Computing Today, 4*(6), 43–48. doi:10.1145/1147518.1147531

Crystal, D. (1969). *Prosodic systems and intonation in English.* Cambridge: Cambridge University Press.

Cunningham, D., Kleiner, M., Bültho, H., & Wallraven, C. (2004). The components of conversational facial expressions. *Proceedings of the Symposium on Applied Perception in Graphics and Visualization* (pp. 143-150).

Dion, K., Berscheid, E., & Walster, E. (1972). What is beautiful is good. *Journal of Personality and Social Psychology, 24*(3), 285–290. doi:10.1037/h0033731

Dong, W., Lepri, B., Cappelletti, A., Pentland, A., Pianesi, F., & Zancanaro, M. (2007). Using the influence model to recognize functional roles in meetings. In *Proceedings of the 9th international conference on multimodal interfaces* (pp. 271-278).

Dovidio, J., & Ellyson, S. (1982). Decoding visual dominance: Attributions of power based on relative percentages of looking while speaking and looking while listening. *Social Psychology Quarterly, 45*(2), 106–113. doi:10.2307/3033933

Dumais, S., Cutrell, E., Cadiz, J. J., Jancke, G., Sarin, R., & Robbins, D. C. (2003). *Stuff I've seen: a system for personal information retrieval and re-use.* Proceedings of the 26th Annual International ACM SIGIR Conference on Research and Development in Information Retrieval (pp. 72-79).

Ekman, P., & Rosenberg, E. (2005). *What the face reveals: Basic and applied studies of spontaneous expression using the facial action coding system (facs).* New York: Oxford University Press.

Favre, S., Dielmann, A., & Vinciarelli, A. (2009). Automatic role recognition in multiparty recordings using social networks and probabilistic sequential models. In *Proceedings of ACM international conference on multimedia.*

Forsyth, D., Arikan, O., Ikemoto, L., O'Brien, J., & Ramanan, D. (2006). Computational studies of human motion part 1: Tracking and motion synthesis. *Foundations and Trends in Computer Graphics and Vision, 1*(2), 77–254. doi:10.1561/0600000005

France, D. J., Shiavi, R. G., Silverman, S., Silverman, M., & Wilkes, D. M. (2000). Acoustical Properties of speech as indicators of depression and suicidal risk. *IEEE Transactions on Bio-Medical Engineering, 47*(7), 829–837. doi:10.1109/10.846676

Galley, M., McKeown, K., Hirschberg, J., & Shriberg, E. (2004). Identifying agreement and disagreement in conversational speech: use of Bayesian Networks to model pragmatic dependencies. In *Proceedings of meeting of the association for computational linguistics* (pp. 669-676).

Garg, N., Favre, S., Salamin, H., Hakkani-Tur, D., & Vinciarelli, A. (2008). Role recognition for meeting participants: an approach based on lexical information and Social Network Analysis. In *Proceedings of the acm international conference on multimedia* (pp. 693-696).

Gladwell, M. (2005). *Blink: The power of thinking without thinking*. New York: Little Brown & Company.

Glass, C., Merluzzi, T., Biever, J., & Larsen, K. (1982). Cognitive assessment of social anxiety: Development and validation of a self-statement questionnaire. *Cognitive Therapy and Research*, *6*(1), 37–55. doi:10.1007/BF01185725

Goleman, D. (2005). *Emotional intelligence*. New York: Random House Publishing Group.

Grahe, J., & Bernieri, F. (1999). The importance of nonverbal cues in judging rapport. *Journal of Nonverbal Behavior*, *23*(4), 253–269. doi:10.1023/A:1021698725361

Hall, E. (1959). *The silent language*. New York: Doubleday.

Hecht, M., De Vito, J., & Guerrero, L. (1999). Perspectives on nonverbal communication-codes, functions, and contexts. In L. Guerrero, J. De Vito, & M. Hecht (Eds.), *The nonverbal communication reader - classic and contemporary readings* (p. 3-18). Waveland Press.

Hillard, D., Ostendorf, M., & Shriberg, E. (2003). Detection of agreement vs. disagreement in meetings: Training with unlabeled data. In *Proceedings of the north American chapter of the association for computational linguistics - human language technologies conference*.

Hyun, H. K., Kim, E. H., & Kwak, Y. K. (2005). Improvement of emotion recognition by Bayesian classifier using non-zero-pitch concept. *IEEE International Workshop on Robots and Human Interactive Communication*, ROMAN 2005, (pp. 312-316).

Jayagopi, D., Hung, H., Yeo, C., & Gatica-Perez, D. (2009). Modeling dominance in group conversations from non-verbal activity cues. *IEEE Transactions on Audio. Speech and Language Processing*, *17*(3), 501–513. doi:10.1109/TASL.2008.2008238

Kapoor, A., Picard, R., & Ivanov, Y. (2004). Probabilistic combination of multiple modalities to detect interest. In *Proceedings of the international conference on pattern recognition* (pp. 969-972).

Knapp, M., & Hall, J. (1972). *Nonverbal communication in human interaction*. Harcourt Brace College Publishers.

Kunda, Z. (1999). *Social cognition*. Boston: MIT Press.

Kwon, O. W., Chan, K., Hao, J., & Lee, T. W. (2003). Emotion Recognition by Speech Signals. In *Proceedings of International Conference EUROSPEECH* (pp. 125-128).

Laskowski, K., Ostendorf, M., & Schultz, T. (2008). Modeling vocal interaction for text independent participant characterization in multi-party conversation. In *Proceedings of the 9th isca/acl sigdial workshop on discourse and dialogue* (pp. 148-155).

Lazer, D., Pentland, A., Adamic, L., Aral, S., Barabasi, A., & Brewer, D. (2009). Computational social science. *Science*, *323*, 721–723. doi:10.1126/science.1167742

Lee, C. M., Narayanan, S., & Pieraccini, R. (2001). Recognition of negative emotions from the speech signals. In *Proceedings of IEEE Workshop on Automatic Speech Recognition and Understanding* (pp. 240-243).

Levine, J., & Moreland, R. (1990). Progress in small roup research. *Annual Review of Psychology*, *41*, 585–634. doi:10.1146/annurev.ps.41.020190.003101

Levine, J., & Moreland, R. (1998). Small groups. In Gilbert, D., & Lindzey, G. (Eds.), *The handbook of social psychology* (*Vol. 2*, pp. 415–469). New York: Oxford University Press.

Li, X., Tao, J., Johanson, M. T., Soltis, J., Savage, A., Leong, K. M., & Newman, J. D. (2007). Stress and emotion classification using jitter and shimmer features. In *Proceedings of IEEE International Conference on Acoustics, Speech & Signal Processing, ICASSP 2007* (Vol. 4, pp. IV-1081-4).

Liu, Y. (2006). Initial study on automatic identication of speaker role in broadcast news speech. In *Proceedings of the human language technology conference of the naacl, companion volume: Short papers* (pp. 81-84).

Lott, D., & Sommer, R. (1967). Seating arrangements and status. *Journal of Personality and Social Psychology*, *7*(1), 90–95. doi:10.1037/h0024925

Lugger, M., & Yang, B. (2006). *Classification of different speaking groups by means of voice quality parameters*. ITG-Sprach-Kommunikation.

Lugger, M., & Yang, B. (2008). Cascaded emotion classification via psychological emotions using a large set of voice quality parameters. In *Proceedings of IEEE International Conference on Acoustics, Speech & Signal Processing, ICASSP 2008* (pp. 4945-4948).

Mast, M. (2002). Dominance as expressed and inferred through speaking time: A metaanalysis. *Human Communication Research*, *28*(3), 420–450.

McCowan, I., Bengio, S., Gatica-Perez, D., Lathoud, G., Monay, F., Moore, D., et al. (2003). Modeling human interaction in meetings. In *Proceedings of IEEE international conference on acoustics, speech and signal processing* (pp. 748-751).

McGilloway, S., Cowie, R., & Douglas-Cowie, E. (2000). Approaching automatic recognition of emotion from voice: a rough benchmark. In *Proceedings of the ISCA Workshop on Speech and Emotion* (pp. 207-212).

Mitra, S., & Acharya, T. (2007). Gesture recognition: A survey. *IEEE Transactions on Systems, Man and Cybernetics. Part C, Applications and Reviews*, *37*(3), 311–324. doi:10.1109/TSMCC.2007.893280

Morrison, D., Wang, R., & De Silva, L. C. (2007). Ensemble methods for spoken emotion recognition in call-centres. *Speech Communication*, *49*, 98–112. doi:10.1016/j.specom.2006.11.004

Mozziconacci, S. J. L., & Hermes, D. J. (1995). A study of intonation patterns in speech expressing emotion or attitude: production and perception. In *Proceedings of 13th International Congress of Phonetic Sciences (ICPh'95)* (Vol. 3, pp. 178-181).

Murphy-Chutorian, E., & Trivedi, M. (2009). Head pose estimation in computer vision: A survey. *IEEE Transactions on Pattern Analysis and Machine Intelligence*, *31*(4), 607–626. doi:10.1109/TPAMI.2008.106

Murray-Smith, R. (2009). (to appear). Empowering people rather than connecting them. *International Journal of Mobile HCI*.

Nass, C., & Brave, S. (2005). *Wired for speech: How voice activates and advances the Human-Computer relationship*. Boston: The MIT Press.

Nicholson, J., Takahashi, K., & Nakatsu, R. (1999). Emotion recognition in speech using neural networks. In *Proceedings of ICONIP'99, 6th International Conference on Neural Information Processing* (Vol. 2, pp. 495-501).

Nwe, T. L., Foo, S. W., & De Silva, L. C. (2003). Speech emotion recognition using hidden Markov models. *Speech Communication*, *41*, 603–623. doi:10.1016/S0167-6393(03)00099-2

Nwe, T. L., Wei, F. S., & De Silva, L. C. (2001). Speech based emotion classification. In *Proceedings of IEEE Region 10 International Conference on Electrical &. Electron Technology, 1,* 291–301.

Olguin Olguin, D., Waber, B., Kim, T., Mohan, A., Koji, A., & Pentland, A. (2009). Sensible organizations: technology and methodology for automatically measuring organizational behavior. *IEEE Transactions on Systems, Man abd Cybernetics – Part B, 39* (1), 43-55.

Otsuka, K., Takemae, Y., & Yamato, J. (2005). A probabilistic inference of multiparty conversation structure based on Markov-switching models of gaze patterns, head directions, and utterances. In *Proceedings of ACM international conference on multimodal interfaces* (pp. 191-198).

Oudeyer, P. Y. (2003). The production and recognition of emotions in speech: features and algorithms. *International Journal of Human-Computer Studies, 59,* 157–183. doi:10.1016/S1071-5819(02)00141-6

Pantic, M., Nijholt, A., Pentland, A., & Huang, T. (2008). Human-Centred Intelligent Human-Computer Interaction (HCI2): how far are we from attaining it? *International Journal of Autonomous and Adaptive Communications Systems, 1*(2), 168–187. doi:10.1504/IJAACS.2008.019799

Pantic, M., Pentland, A., Nijholt, A., & Huang, T. (2007). Human computing and machine understanding of human behavior: A survey. In *Lecture notes in articial intelligence* (*Vol. 4451,* pp. 47–71). New York: Springer Verlag.

Park, C. H., Lee, D. W., & Sim, K. B. (2002). Emotion recognition of speech based on RNN. In *Proceedings of International Conference on Machine Learning & Cybernetics(ICMLC'02)* (Vol. 4, pp.2210-2213).

Pentland, A. (2008). *Honest signals: how they shape our world.* Cambridge, MA: MIT Press.

Picard, R. (2000). *Affective computing.* Cambridge, MA: The MIT Press.

Poggi, I. (2007). *Mind, hands, face and body: A goal and belief view of multimodal communication.* Weidler Buchverlag Berlin.

Polzin, T. S., & Waibel, A. (2000). Emotion-sensetive human-computer interfaces. In *Proceedings of the ISCA Workshop on Speech and Emotion* (pp. 201-206).

Raento, M., Oulasvirta, A., & Eagle, N. (2009). Smartphones: an emerging tool for social scientists. *Sociological Methods & Research, 37*(3), 426. doi:10.1177/0049124108330005

Reeves, B., & Nass, C. (1996). *The media equation: How people treat computers, television, and new media like real people and places. New York (USA).* NY, USA: Cambridge University Press New York.

Richmond, V., & McCroskey, J. (1995). *Nonverbal behaviors in interpersonal relations.* Allyn and Bacon.

Rienks, R., & Heylen, D. (2006). Dominance Detection in Meetings Using Easily Obtainable Features. [). New York: Springer.]. *Lecture Notes in Computer Science, 3869,* 76–86. doi:10.1007/11677482_7

Rienks, R., Zhang, D., & Gatica-Perez, D. (2006). Detection and application of in fluence rankings in small group meetings. In *Proceedings of the international conference on multimodal interfaces* (pp. 257-264).

Rong, J., Li, G., & Chen, Y. P. (2009). Acoustic feature selection for automatic emotion recognition from speech. *Information Processing & Management, 45,* 315–328. doi:10.1016/j.ipm.2008.09.003

Salamin, H., Favre, S., & Vinciarelli, A. (2009). Automatic role recognition in multiparty recordings: Using social aliation networks for feature extraction. *IEEE Transactions on Multimedia, 11*(7), 1373–1380. doi:10.1109/TMM.2009.2030740

Scheflen, A. (1964). The significance of posture in communication systems. *Psychiatry, 27,* 316–331.

Schegloff, E. (1987). Single episodes of interaction: an exercise in conversation analysis. *Social Psychology Quarterly, 50*(2), 101–114. doi:10.2307/2786745

Scherer, K. (1979). *Personality markers in speech.* Cambridge, MA: Cambridge University Press.

Scherer, K. (2003). Vocal communication of emotion: a review of research paradigms. *Speech Communication, 40,* 227–256. doi:10.1016/S0167-6393(02)00084-5

Schuller, B., Reiter, S., Muller, R., Al-Hames, M., Lang, M., & Rigoll, G. (2005). Speaker independent speech emotion recognition by ensemble classification. In *Proceedings of IEEE International Conference on Multimedia & Expo (ICME'05).*

Shami, M. T., & Kamel, M. S. (2005). Segment-based approach to the recognition of emotions in speech. *IEEE International Conference on Multimedia & Expo (ICME'05),* Amsterdam, The Netherlands.

Shami, M. T., & Verhelst, W. (2007). An evaluation of the robustness of existing supervised machine learning approaches to the classification of emotions in speech. *Speech Communication, 49,* 201–212. doi:10.1016/j.specom.2007.01.006

Surawski, M., & Osso, E. (2006). The eects of physical and vocal attractiveness on impression formation of politicians. *Current Psychology (New Brunswick, N.J.), 25*(1), 15–27. doi:10.1007/s12144-006-1013-5

Tischler, H. (1990). *Introduction to sociology.* Harcourt Brace College Publishers.

Tranter, S., & Reynolds, D. (2006). An overview of automatic speaker diarization systems. *IEEE Transactions on Audio, Speech, and Language Processing, 14*(5), 1557–1565. doi:10.1109/TASL.2006.878256

Truong, K., & Van Leeuwen, D. (2007). Automatic discrimination between laughter and speech. *Speech Communication, 49*(2), 144–158. doi:10.1016/j.specom.2007.01.001

Van den Stock, J., Righart, R., & de Gelder, B. (2007). Body expressions influence recognition of emotions in the face and voice. *Emotion (Washington, D.C.), 7*(3), 487–494. doi:10.1037/1528-3542.7.3.487

Ververidis, D., & Kotropoulos, C. (2006). Emotional speech recognition: resources, features, and methods. *Speech Communication, 48,* 1162–1181. doi:10.1016/j.specom.2006.04.003

Ververidis, D., Kotropoulos, C., & Pitas, I. (2004). Automatic emotional speech classification. In *proceedings of IEEE International Conference on Acoustics, Speech &. Signal Processing, 1,* I-593–I-596.

Vinciarelli, A. (2007). Speakers role recognition in multiparty audio recordings using social network analysis and duration distribution modeling. *IEEE Transactions on Multimedia, 9*(9), 1215–1226. doi:10.1109/TMM.2007.902882

Vinciarelli, A. (2009). Capturing order in social interactions. *IEEE Signal Processing Magazine, 26*(5), 133–137. doi:10.1109/MSP.2009.933382

Vinciarelli, A., Pantic, M., & Bourlard, H. (2009). Social Signal Processing: Survey of an emerging domain. *Image and Vision Computing Journal, 27*(12), 1743–1759. doi:10.1016/j.imavis.2008.11.007

Vinciarelli, A., Pantic, M., Bourlard, H., & Pentland, A. (2008). Social Signal Processing: State-of-the-art and future perspectives of an emerging domain. In *Proceedings of the ACM international conference on multimedia* (pp. 1061-1070).

Waibel, A., Schultz, T., Bett, M., Denecke, M., Malkin, R., Rogina, I., & Stiefelhagen, R. (2003). SMaRT: the Smart Meeting Room task at ISL. In *Proceedings of IEEE international conference on acoustics, speech, and signal processing* (pp. 752-755).

Watzlawick, P., Beavin, J., & Jackson, D. (1967). *The pragmatics of human communication*. New York: Norton.

Williams, A. (2003). Facial expression of pain: An evolutionary account. *The Behavioral and Brain Sciences, 25*(4), 439–455.

Womack, B., & Hansen, J. L. H. (1996). Classification of speech under stress using target driven features. *Speech Communication, 20,* 131–150. doi:10.1016/S0167-6393(96)00049-0

Yang, B., & Lugger, M. (2009). Emotion recognition from speech signals using new harmony features. Article in Press. *Signal Processing,* 1–9.

Yang, M., Kriegman, D., & Ahuja, N. (2002). Detecting faces in images: a survey. *IEEE Transactions on Pattern Analysis and Machine Intelligence, 24*(1), 34–58. doi:10.1109/34.982883

Zancanaro, M., Lepri, B., & Pianesi, F. (2006). Automatic detection of group functional roles in face to face interactions. In *Proceedings of international conference on multimodal interfaces* (pp. 47-54).

Zeng, Z., Pantic, M., Roisman, G., & Huang, T. (2009). A survey of affect recognition methods: audio, visual and spontaneous expressions. *IEEE Transactions on Pattern Analysis and Machine Intelligence, 31*(1), 39–58. doi:10.1109/TPA-MI.2008.52

Zhou, G., Hansen, J. H. L., & Kaiser, J. F. (2001). Nonlinear feature based classification of speech under stress. *IEEE Transactions on Speech and Audio Processing, 9*(3), 201–216. doi:10.1109/89.905995

KEY TERMS AND DEFINITIONS

Affective Computing: Domain aimed at modeling, analysis and synthesis of human emotions.

Emotion: Subjective feeling lasting for short periods of time, as well as mental and physiological state associated with a wide variety of feelings.

Nonverbal Communication: Form of communication based on nonverbal behavioral cues (facial expressions, vocalizations, gestures, postures, etc.)

Paralinguistic Features: Features extracted from speech data that account for nonverbal vocal behavior.

Social Interactions: Every form of interaction including at least two persons modifying their behavior accordingly to others.

Social Signal Processing- Domain aimed at modeling: analysis and synthesis of nonverbal behavior in social interactions.

Vocal Behavior: Ensemble of speech phenomena that do not include words or language (pauses, laughter, fillers, prosody, rhythm, intensity, etc.).

Chapter 8

Communication and Automatic Interpretation of Affect from Facial Expressions

Albert Ali Salah
University of Amsterdam, The Netherlands

Nicu Sebe
University of Trento, Italy

Theo Gevers
University of Amsterdam, The Netherlands

ABSTRACT

The objective of this chapter is to introduce the reader to the recent advances in computer processing of facial expressions and communicated affect. Human facial expressions have evolved in tandem with human face recognition abilities, and show remarkable consistency across cultures. Consequently, it is rewarding to review the main traits of face recognition in humans, as well as consolidated research on the categorization of facial expressions. The bulk of the chapter focuses on the main trends in computer analysis of facial expressions, sketching out the main algorithms and exposing computational considerations for different settings. The authors then look at some recent applications and promising new projects to give the reader a realistic view of what to expect from this technology now and in near future.

INTRODUCTION

In June 2009, Microsoft released a trailer of its latest project for Xbox 360 gaming console, called Project Natal. The video, an instant Facebook epidemic and a YouTube favourite, featured Peter Molyneux, the creative director of Microsoft Game Studios Europe, demonstrating a virtual agent called Milo. Using the sensing and processing capabilities of its hardware, the virtual agent communicated with the user as if the boundary of the screen is just a window, recognizing identity

DOI: 10.4018/978-1-61692-892-6.ch008

and speech, but also emotions, which enabled it to respond to the user with an impressive range of realistic behaviours. The innovation of the project was in its ambitious scope: creating a virtual agent that truly communicates with the user. The key to life–like communication was recognizing emotions of the user, and in return, generating states that carry affect information for the agent in human–readable form, i.e. in the body posture, vocal intonation, and most importantly, facial expression.

The recently flourishing field of social signal processing (Vinciarelli et al., 2009) targets a greater contextual awareness for computer systems and human–machine interaction, and drawing on cognitive psychology, places great emphasis on automatically understanding facial expressions. The human face is a window that allows peeking into diverse patterns of emotions that manifest themselves voluntarily and involuntarily, communicating affect or projected displays of personality. Even dissociated from gesture and voice (as in still face pictures), facial expressions convey complex, layered, and vital information. Consequently, it is a great challenge to create computer systems that can automatically analyse images to reveal the sometimes obvious and sometimes subtle messages engraved in faces. In this chapter we aim to provide the reader with a broad overview of how computer scientists have risen to this challenge, starting from relevant taxonomies and guidelines, briefly touching upon the cognitive aspects of affect and face recognition, summarizing recent advances in algorithmic aspects of the problem, giving pointers and tools for the initiate, and finally, discussing applications and the future of facial expression recognition.

CATEGORIZATION OF FACIAL EXPRESSIONS

The human face is a complicated visual object; it contains a lot of information with regards to

identity, communicative intent and affect, and humans can "read" these cues, even under difficult visibility conditions. We can for instance understand the emotions of a person we see for the first time. In this section we look at taxonomies of facial expressions, and point out to several important factors that need to be taken into account in evaluating facial expressions.

A facial expression can be the result of an emotional response (spontaneous), or a construct with communicative intent (volitional) (Russell & Fernandez–Dols, 1997). It can occur naturally, or it can be posed. In both cases, it can have different intensities, and it can be a mixture of pure expressions. These factors make the task of sorting out a facial expression difficult. Additionally, the categorization of expressions can be achieved in ever-finer levels. It is one thing to label the category of an expression as "happy", quite another to distinguish between a real smile (also called a Duchenne smile), a miserable smile, an angry smile, an embarrassed smile, and a dimpler. Finally, cultural differences in facial expressions also need to be taken into account.

Categorization of emotions predate computers by hundreds of years, but the roles of particular emotions in society are different for each culture; in India, for instance, it was believed that the basic emotions are sexual passion, anger, disgust, perseverance, amusement, sorrow, wonder, fear, and serenity. Facial expressions of these emotions are culture-dependent, but also the semantic counterparts of these emotions do not completely overlap with the current understanding of these words, adding to the difficulty of systematically categorizing emotions. Furthermore, the experimental settings under which any study is conducted and the ensuing databases on which we measure the success of a given method are not independent of cultural influences. For instance it is known that in some cultures the expression of emotion is more restricted for social reasons. Finally, as facial morphology also changes according to the anthropological group of a subject, it is natural to expect some principled variation across races and gender.

Adolphs (2002) cautions that the emotion categories used in everyday life may not result in the most appropriate categorization of emotion for scientific purposes. Yet, as opposed to language, automatic perceptual grouping of emotional cues is apt to produce meaningful structural relationships, as the semantic proximity of emotions is reflected in the structural proximity of their expressions. Presently, most emotion researchers use discrete categories to indicate the presence of one emotion in any given instance. This method requires singular labelling of the ground truth, as well as mostly exaggerated expressions in the evaluation data. Paul Ekman argued that **six basic emotional facial expression categories** are persistent across cultures (Ekman, 1993): happiness, sadness, anger, fear, surprise and disgust. While other taxonomies extend these basic emotions with contempt, shame, distress, interest, guilt, and many others, this six–emotion classification is the most commonly used taxonomy in the computer science literature pertaining to facial expression analysis.

We note here that the presence of emotion, even when measured in continuous scales, is usually seen as a momentary evaluation of the percept, instead of a spatio–temporal event unfolding in time. A more granular analysis must be able to

label subordinate components of a complex emotion, and the research is headed in this direction. One challenge is to create complex ground truth to measure methods that will attempt to gauge the accuracy of such an analysis.

The range of facial expressions is assumed to reflect the range of emotional displays in general, which is the primary reason we base facial expression categorization on taxonomies of emotional display. One important taxonomy is due to Russell (1980), and it dissects emotions that give rise to expressions along *arousal* and *valence* dimensions. Arousal controls the intensity of the emotion, whereas valence relates to its positive and negative connotations. This model enables a two-dimensional projection of emotional displays (See Figure 1). However, given a face image, it is difficult to precisely situate it in this projection. Note that of the six basic categories proposed by Ekman, only happiness has a positive valence. Another relevant approach is the OCC model (Ortony, Clore, & Collins, 1988), which proposes valenced reactions to consequences of events, actions of agents, and aspects of objects, based on relevant attributes thereof. Complex emotional theories usually take action semantics into account, which stresses the dynamic nature of emotions. For computer analysis, the incorporation of semantics is usually much more difficult due

Figure 1. Arousal- and valence-based categorization of emotions agrees with self-report studies. Here are 28 affect words distributed according to valence/arousal (left) and the same words distributed by a principal components analysis of self-reports (right). © 1980, Russell. Used with permission

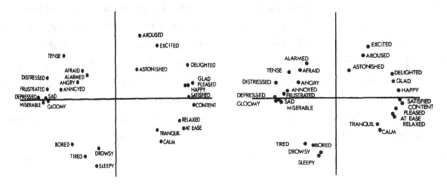

Table 1 Action Units (AU) in the Facial Action Coding System

AU	Descriptor	AU	Descriptor	AU	Descriptor
1	Inner Brow Raiser	2	Outer Brow Raiser	4	Brow Lowerer
5	Upper Lid Raiser	6	Cheek Raiser	7	Lid Tightener
8	Lips Towards Each Other	9	Nose Wrinkler	10	Upper Lip Raiser
11	Nasolabial Deepener	12	Lip Corner Puller	13	Cheek Puffer
14	Dimpler	15	Lip Corner Depressor	16	Lower Lip Depressor
17	Chin Raiser	18	Lip Puckerer	19	Tongue Out
20	Lip Stretcher	21	Neck Tightener	22	Lip Funneler
23	Lip Tightener	24	Lip Pressor	25	Lips Part
26	Jaw Drop	27	Mouth Stretch	28	Lip Suck
29	Jaw Thrust	30	Jaw Sideways	31	Jaw Clencher
32	Lip Bite	33	Cheek Blow	34	Cheek Puff
35	Cheek Suck	36	Tongue Bulge	37	Lip Wipe
38	Nostril Dilator	39	Nostril Compressor	43	Eyes Closure
44	Squint	45	Blink	46	Wink
(40)	Eyes Normally Open	(41)	Lid Droop	(42)	Slit

knowledge acquisition and representation issues. Consequently, computer scientists prefer to work with quantifiable schemes.

The **facial action coding system** (FACS) developed by Ekman and Friesen (1978) is the basis of much work on facial expression recognition today. According to this system, facial muscle movements are grouped into different action units (AU), and expressions are described in terms of these action units. Each action is attributed with an intensity value (on a 5–point scale). There are procedures for describing the timing of facial actions, as well as for describing expressions as events. Table 1 gives a revised list of AUs. Historically, AU 40 is indicated as optional, and AUs 41 and 42 are merged into 43 ("Eyes Closure", previously "Eyes Closed") in later versions. References to FACS recognizing 44 action units refer to the old version, which omits AUs 3 and 8. AU 3 is the "Brow Knit", which is later dropped from the classification, and AU 8 was re-inserted. One of the reasons of the popularity of FACS is that facial muscle movements are completely objective physiological

measures, and thus provide a solid basis for the formulation of emotion categories. Also, they are not restricted to displays of emotion, which increases their usability.

For other observational coding schemes and their comparison with FACS, the reader is referred to (Ekman & Rosenberg, 2005). We note here only that the FACS model only describes changes in facial configuration, and leaves temporal dynamics of these changes out of the picture. For relating facial expressions to emotions, Ekman and Friesen have later developed the EMFACS system, which specifies which facial actions are common for particular emotion displays. Obviously, the projection of emotional display to a low-dimensional space (as in the arousal/valence system) is an oversimplification, just like its classification by a few discrete categories (like Ekman's basic categories). Yet, as the state-of-the-art in autonomous categorization progresses, finer grained representations will become possible for use in computer systems.

There are several other concerns in categorizing expressions. The manifestation of affective states depends on a particular **context**. The specification of the context serves the dual purpose of disambiguation of the expressive display, and constraining the search space for the expression. For instance, the AmI project (Carletta, 2006) focuses on a particular meeting scenario, and the corpus that is collected within this application framework is annotated using the following categories: neutral, curious, amused, distracted, bored, confused, uncertain, surprised, frustrated, decisive, disbelief, dominant, defensive, supportive. These categories are not recognized as universal expressions, yet they are identifiable and consistently labelled within the particular meeting scenario context.

Expressions also have **temporal dimensions**. We do not feel surprise for a second, followed by a short burst of happiness, and immediately switch to disgust. A system that continuously evaluates affect needs to take into account the temporal unfolding of the expressions. An additional benefit of this approach would be to account for the "baseline effect", which stresses the relevance of the difference from the neutral state as opposed to the absolute feature locations for identifying emotions, especially when they are subtle. The differences and changes in the facial configuration can be used to describe emotional displays at a much higher granularity, allowing realistic contextual modelling. Going to contextual level is promising for two reasons: The actual switch from one expression to another can be more accurately recognized in the presence of other contextual cues. Conversely, reliable detection of an expression change can point to an external event of importance, thus leading to improved event categorization.

Most of the earlier research focuses on **posed** (or simulated) expressions. For better discrimination, the expressions under study are created by persons imitating a certain expression in an exaggerated way. There is however subtle differences between faked expressions and expressions caused by true emotions. Some recent research is tailored towards making this distinction explicit, for instance to understand whether an expressed emotion is honest or not. The temporal nature of emotional expressions also allows one to test for the authenticity of an emotional display. The so-called micro-expressions are involuntary cues that are persistently found in genuine expressions, yet are usually absent from faked ones. However, the spatio-temporal resolution of these cues is very fine, and it is very difficult to separate them from measurement noise, as their magnitudes are comparable under currently used experimental settings. On the other hand, a fake expression involves more conscious control, and thus is not prone to correlate highly with naturally occurring bodily gesture cues. Subsequently, multimodal analysis becomes a promising alternative to detect genuine emotion expressions.

An important point here is that people are equally successful in recognizing the category of genuine and posed emotional expressions. This suggests that posed expressions, while not exactly overlapping with their genuine counterparts, have their own semiotic function that works within the appropriate social context. It follows that an all-encompassing emotion recognition software needs to model both genuine and posed expressions, and to recognize both.

INTERPRETATION OF AFFECT FROM FACIAL CUES IN HUMANS

In this section we look at some biological and cognitive aspects of facial expression recognition in humans. We should at this point stress that the subjective feeling of an emotion and its expression on the face are two different things, where the latter is one manifestation of the former among many bodily signals like gestures, postures, and changes on the skin response. Thus, what we perceive from a face is either an involuntary manifestation of an emotional state, or the result of a deliberate effort at communicating an emotional signal. The urge

Figure 2. A human face is rarely perceived as completely neutral; even a two-weeks–old infant's face is full of "emotions"

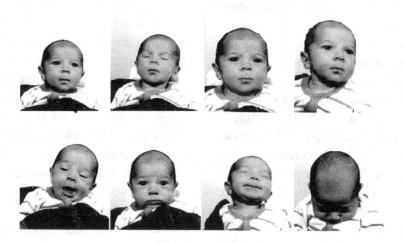

to associate affect with faces is so great that we 'recognize' expressions even on infant's faces, even though they are not yet associated with the emotions they represent in adults (See Figure 2). This association partly relies on innate biases implicit in the human visual system, and partly on the efficient way humans represent facial information. In humans, the subjective experience of an emotion, the production of its somatic expressions, and its recognition in other subjects are all tightly coupled, and influence each other. This allows for a degree of feedback that is beyond current computer systems, and enables differentiation of very subtle affective cues.

The goal of facial affect recognition systems is to mimic humans in their evaluations of facial expression. If a computer can learn to distinguish expressions automatically, it becomes possible to create interfaces that interpolate affective states from these expressions and use this information for better interfaces. We open a little parenthesis here. When we talk about 'learning' in the context of a computer, we usually mean a machine learning procedure, which is different from human learning. Here, what usually happens is that the computer is provided with a number of samples from a category to be learned (be it images of

faces with a particular expression or any other numeric representation), as well as a method of categorization. The learning algorithm tunes the parameters of the method to ensure a good categorization on these samples. The ensuing system, however, depends crucially on the quality of provided samples, in addition to the data representation, the generalization power of the learning method and its robustness to noise and incorrect labels in the provided samples. These points are shared by all computer systems working on face images, be it for the recognition of identity or expressions. We bear these in mind when investigating what the brain does with faces, and how it can be simulated with computers.

Recognition of relevant processes that partake in human recognition of faces and facial affect guides the designers of computer algorithms for automatic recognition of emotions from faces. For instance, it is known that humans have selective attention for the eyes and mouth areas, which can be explained by recognizing the importance of these areas for communicating affect and identity. Computer simulations by Lyons et al. (1999) have shown that feature saliency for automatic algorithms that evaluate facial affect parallels feature saliency for the human visual system.

How humans determine identity from faces is a widely researched area. One reason for this is that both low-level neurological studies and high-level behavioural studies point out to faces as having special status among other object recognition tasks. Kanwisher et al., (1997) have argued that there is an innate mechanism to recognize faces, and they have isolated the lateral fusiform gyrus (also termed the fusiform face area) to be the seat of this process. The proponents of the expertise hypothesis, on the other hand, argued that humans process a lot of faces, and this is the sole reason that we end up with such a highly specialized system (Gauthier et al., 1999).

The expertise hypothesis banks on a fundamental property of the human brain: the key to learning is efficient representation, and while we learn to recognize faces, the neural representation of faces gradually changes, becoming tailored to the use of this information. In other words, we become (rather than born as) face experts. But this also means that we are sensitive to cultural particularities we are exposed to, an example of which is the famous other-race effect. This is also true for affect recognition from facial expressions, which incorporate cultural elements. While the geometric and structural properties of a face might allow the viewer to distinguish the basic emotional content, cross–cultural studies have established that the cultural background of the viewer plays a large role in labelling the emotion in a face. Furthermore, perception of emotion-specific information cued by facial images are also coloured by previous social experience. In a recent study (Pollak et al., 2009), a number of children who have experienced a high-level of parental anger expression were shown sequences of facial expressions. They were able to identify the anger expression in the sequence earlier than their peers, using a smaller amount of physiological cues.

The traditional problems faced by face recognition researchers are illumination differences, pose differences, scale and resolution differences, and expressions (See Figure 3). These variables

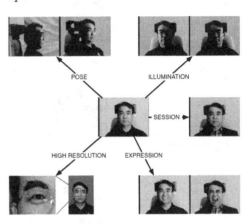

change the appearance of the face, and make the task of comparing faces non-trivial for the computer. While there is a consensus among brain researchers that recognizing facial identity and facial affect involve different brain structures (e.g. lateral fusiform gyrus for identity as opposed to superior temporal sulcus for emotional content, (Hasselmo, Rolls & Baylis, 1989)), these are not entirely independent (Bruce & Young, 1986). Many aspects of facial identity recognition and affect recognition overlap. This is also the case for computer algorithms that are created for recognition of identity or affect from face images. Hence, it should be no surprise that computational studies also recognize the need for different, but overlapping representations for these two tasks. For instance Calder and colleagues (Calder et al., 2001) have investigated a popular projection based method for classifying facial expressions, and determined that the projection base selected to discriminate identity is very different than the base selected to discriminate expressions. Also, while facial identity concerns mostly static and structural properties of faces, dynamic aspects are found to be more relevant for emotion analysis. In particular, the exact timing of various parts of an emotional display is shown to be an important cue in distinguishing real and imitation

Figure 4. Overview of computer analysis of facial expressions. Face images taken from the Jaffe database

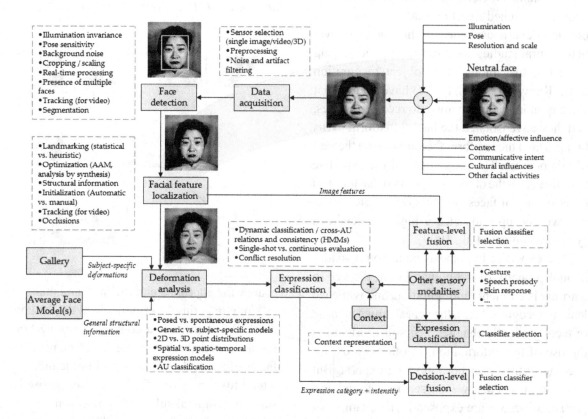

expressions (Cohn & Schmidt, 2004). Similarly, the dichotomy of feature–based processing (i.e. processing selected facial areas) versus holistic processing (i.e. considering the face in its entirety) is of importance. Features seem to be more important for expressions, and while in some case it can be shown that some expressions can be reliably determined by looking at a part of the face only (Nusseck et al., 2008), the dynamics of features and their relative coding (i.e. the holistic aspect) cannot be neglected.

Before moving to tools and techniques for computer analysis of facial expressions, we note here that all emotions were not created equal. Brain studies suggest different coding mechanisms for particular emotions. According to the valence hypothesis there is a disparity between the processing of positive and negative emotions, as well as the amount of processing involved for these

types in the left and right hemisphere of the brain (Borod et al., 1998). This is an evolutionarily plausible scenario, as rapid motor response following particular emotions (e.g. fear, anger) is important for survival. Blair et al. (1999) have found that the prefrontal cortex is more active for processing 'anger', as opposed to 'sadness'. Different cortical structures show differential activation for different emotion types under lesion and functional imaging studies. On the other hand, specific emotions do share common neural circuitry, as disproportionate impairment in recognizing a particular emotion is very rare, as shown by lesion studies (the reader is referred to (Adolphs, 2002) for examples and references).

This inequality is also reflected in displays of emotion. The configural distances from a neutral face are disproportionate for each emotion, with 'sadness' and 'disgust' being represented by more

Figure 5. The original frame and three synthesized representations. © 2009, Afzal et al. Used with permission

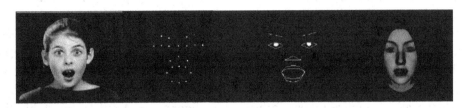

subtle changes (as opposed to for instance 'happiness' and 'fear'). In addition to this disparity, it is unlikely that emotions are encountered with the same background probability in everyday life. Thus, from a probabilistic point of view, it makes sense not to treat all six basic emotions on the same ground. The valence hypothesis suggests that 'happiness' (as a positive emotion) is a superordinate category, and should be pitted against negative emotions (fear, anger, disgust, sadness and contempt). Surprise can be divided into 'fearful surprise' and 'pleasant surprise'; it has been noted that 'surprise' and 'fear' are often confused in the absence of such distinction. Also, 'disgust' encompasses responses to a large range of socially undesirable stimuli. When it expresses disapproval for other people, for instance, it approaches 'anger'. These issues require careful attention in the design and evaluation of computer systems for facial expression analysis.

A STARTER'S KIT FOR COMPUTER ANALYSIS OF FACIAL EXPRESSIONS

In this section we give pointers to relevant methods for facial expression analysis in the literature and summarize the most important techniques, as well as challenges. Evaluation of facial expression relies on accurate face detection, face registration, localization of fiducial points in faces, and classification of shape and appearance information into expressions. As such, recognizing emotional

expressions from faces can be treated as a pattern recognition problem.

For a very extensive list of different approaches (including visual, as well as audio-based and multimodal approaches) to affect recognition, the reader is referred to (Zeng et al., 2009). For a more focused and very readable survey of facial expression analysis, see (Fasel & Luettin, 2003). Figure 5 summarizes the information flow of a facial expression analysis system, where each stage is annotated with design decisions and difficulties from this perspective (dashed boxes). The expressive face image contains variations due affective state, as well as variations due pose, illumination, scale and resolution. The data acquisition itself adds some noise, which can be significant in natural settings. Face detection is generally the first step in the processing pipeline, followed by determination of the pose, either via localization of facial landmarks, or via iterative fitting of a face model to the appearance. The analysis of the face image needs to dissociate subject-specific variation from expression-induced changes. Analysis of features (static or dynamic) can be supplemented with context, and via information fusion with other modalities.

Face Detection

Face detection is a crucial first step in facial expression analysis (Yang et al., 2002). The state-of-the-art in face detection is the Viola-Jones algorithm (Viola & Jones, 2004) that is freely available in the OpenCV library (see Databases and Tools section). The key idea behind this algorithm is to use a hierarchical Adaboost cascade classifier, which eliminates locations that obviously do not contain face images quickly, and to focus on likely candidates. A multi-resolution Haar wavelet basis is used, which is simple and fast to compute. The training is accomplished on a very large number of positive and negative samples (about forty thousand images for the OpenCV cascade).

The Viola-Jones algorithm has its limitations; since it is essentially a 2D face detector, it can only generalize within the pose limits of its training set. Also, large occlusions will impair its accuracy. It is however possible to train other cascades for faces with different pose variations with this method, as well as cascades for individual facial features. The one big advantage of this algorithm is in its speed, which is essential for real-time expression analysis. Additional cascades and more accurate detectors will come at a computational cost. (Bartlett et al., 2005) presents some improvements to this algorithm, for which the code is also freely available.

Facial Feature Localization

Analysis of detected faces often proceeds by locating several fiducial points on them. These features are called anchor points, or landmarks. Typically, eye and eyebrow corners, centre of iris, nose tip, mouth corners, and tip of the chin are located for face alignment. For expression analysis, a greater number of landmarks are usually required (typically between 20-60). Collectively, the landmark locations define the *shape* of the face, whereas the texture of the face is called its *appearance*. The configurations of facial landmarks are indicative of deformations caused by expressions. Subsequently, deformation analysis can reveal expression categories, provided that facial landmarks are accurately detected and they contain sufficient information for the recognition of a particular facial expression.

Finding facial landmarks automatically is a difficult problem, which faces all hurdles of face

recognition in a smaller scale, like illumination and occlusion problems (Salah et al., 2007). Constellation of facial landmarks is different for each face image. Part of the difference is due to the subjective morphology of the face, as different persons have different face shapes. Even for the same person, different images will have different configurations. Another part of this difference is due to camera angle and pose differences. There are also expression-based changes (of which some part may be attributable to emotion) and measurement noise, which is omnipresent. Commercial facial landmarking applications rely on tens of thousands of manually annotated images for training robust and fast classifiers.

The appearance of each landmark and the structural relationships between landmark points (i.e. configuration) are both taken into account in locating landmarks automatically. However, both appearance and structure is changed under expression variations, and in different ways. For this reason, most methods solve the simpler problem of landmarking the neutral face, and then track each landmark while the face is deformed under the influence of an expression. The deformation sequence then allows one to classify the expression category.

While landmark-based approach is the mainstream in 2D facial expression analysis, a recent study has shown that facial landmark distributions are not always sufficient to distinguish emotional expressions (Afzal et al., 2009). In this study, the authors asked their subjects to label faces according to five emotional expressions (interested, bored, confused, happy, and surprised). The contrasted representations were 1) face videos, 2) a point-light representation of the facial landmarks, 3) a stick-figure of these landmarks (appropriately connected), and 4) the mapped expression display with an Xface virtual agent (See Figure 5). Their findings show that 1) natural expressions are harder than posed expressions to identify, 2) expressions are best identified in the original videos, followed by stick-figure, point-

Figure 6. (a) Landmarks and corresponding triangular mesh model for AAM (Stegmann, 2002). (b) The wireframe model used in (Cohen et al., 2003)

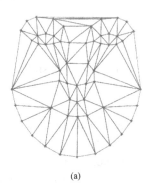

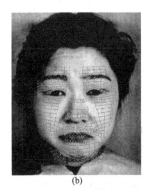

(a)   (b)

light and finally virtual agent representations, 3) subjective labels of expression categories are moderate for the original videos, but quite poor for other representations, 4) the accuracies vary greatly across different expressions.

Expression Classification from Images and Video

A large number of detection and classification approaches are developed for categorization of facial expressions from images. Typically, the first steps are face detection, landmark localization, and pre-processing for scale and illumination normalization. For image-based methods, if the neutral configuration of the face is not known, the appearance of the face (either global appearance, or features extracted from the landmark points), as well as configuration of the shape relative to an average shape are informative cues to classify expression. Different parts of the face contain different amounts of information, making segmentation into different regions a reasonable choice. For instance Figure 6 (b) shows a possible segmentation of the face based on relevance to expression recognition, as well as to facial motion.

A popular approach for face analysis that relates shape and appearance is the active appearance model (AAM) (Cootes et al., 2001). In this approach, the 'shape' (represented by a set of con-

nected landmarks, see Figure 6 (a)) and the 'appearance' of a face are jointly modelled. AAM is essentially an analysis-by-synthesis method; the correct parameterisation that represents a novel face is obtained by synthesizing face images from a generative model until these images look sufficiently close to the analysed image.

The method requires the initial generation of a shape and an appearance model. For this purpose, a set of training images are used, on which several landmarks are annotated. These images are rigidly aligned to an averaged shape, which is just a set of landmark locations. Then, each training image is warped to this shape. The 'appearance' model is obtained separately from the texture. In this method, a novel face can be represented by a mean shape and a mean appearance, plus linear combinations of shape and appearances present in the training set.

In practice, when a new face image is analysed with the AAM, the search for the best parametric representation is initialized with an average face. Then, the residual error is minimized by adjusting the parameters of the generative model iteratively, in a coarse-to-fine fashion, each time synthesizing a new face with modified shape and appearance parameters. When the best parameter configuration is obtained, the shape parameters indicate the landmark locations. These can then be used in classifying the expression of the face. Since AAM is not a full-blown 3D model, its accuracy starts to diminish rapidly for faces with pose differences beyond ±20° from the frontal pose. A detailed study of appearance models and subsequent modifications can be found in (Lee et al., 2009). Recently, Milborrow and Nicolls (2008) extended the AAM to create a very successful system for automatic facial landmark localization on frontal faces. This system requires over 60 annotated landmarks for each face during training, but once trained, shows remarkable generalization for frontal and neutral faces acquired in different conditions (see Table 3).

A related methodology is the analysis-by-synthesis approach, which tries to synthesise a face image that matches a query image as closely as possible, and optimizes the pose, illumination and expression parameters of a generative model for this purpose (Volker & Blanz, 1999). These unknown parameters are estimated iteratively, and a fully 3D model is maintained, which make this approach computationally expensive. There is a vast literature in face and facial expression synthesis, which are excluded from the present survey.

While earlier approaches favoured holistic analysis of the face images, AAM and other model-based approaches eventually received more attention. Another trend that exhibits itself is the extensive use of neural network classifiers in earlier work, as opposed to support vector machines (SVM), AdaBoost and dynamic Bayesian network (DBN) classifiers in more recent approaches. For instance (Bartlett et al., 2005) compares AdaBoost, SVM and linear discriminant analysis (LDA) classifiers on a range of features. The best results are obtained by initially deriving a very large number of features combined with clever feature selection methods. In their study, the authors use a bank of Gabor wavelet filters at 8 orientations and 9 spatial frequencies on face images scaled to 48x48 pixels. This processing results in about 160,000 features per face. Then the AdaBoost algorithm is used as a feature selection method to choose 900 features, which are fed

to an SVM classifier. A number of AU-detectors implemented with this approach are combined in a second stage to detect driver drowsiness (Vural et al., 2007) and to distinguish between real and faked pain (Littlewort et al., 2009). In (Whitehill et al., 2009), a similar setup is used for a smile detection application, but Haar wavelet filters (also called Box filters) are contrasted with Gabor filters. The authors remark that an AU-detector needs to be trained with 1,000-10,000 training samples for robust operation.

The dynamic nature of expressions results in improved detection from video, where the spatio–temporal dynamics of facial structures can be evaluated. The Cohn Kanade database of FACS annotated video sequences of emotions has been a major facilitator of facial expression research from dynamic cues (Kanade et al., 2000). Major tools for implementing such systems include algorithms for motion flow field computation and tracking and Bayesian approaches, for instance Markov models for characterizing dynamics of emotional states. In optical flow methods, the spatio-temporal motion-energy templates are taken as characteristic for expression classes, and used for recognition (Essa & Pentland, 1997). Kalman filters and realistic muscle models can be used to increase the stability of the optical flow model. (Fasel & Luettin, 2003), as well as (Cohen et al., 2003) include good surveys of earlier dynamic approaches to facial expression recognition. Here we describe a few relevant methods.

In (Zhang & Ji, 2005), facial features are tracked with the help of infrared cameras, and a number of muscle-movement-based heuristics. Following (Tian et al., 2001), a Canny edge detector is used to enhance the furrows of the face. A number of rules are employed to infer AUs from the tracked feature points. The AU detection results are combined with a DBN. The inference performed by the DBN takes into account the dynamic nature of AU transitions, and improves the final detection rate. In a subsequent work, (Tong et al., 2007) combine the Gabor-AdaBoost

Figure 7. Action units and basic expressions from the Bosphorus 3D face dataset. © 2008, Alyüz et al. Used with permission

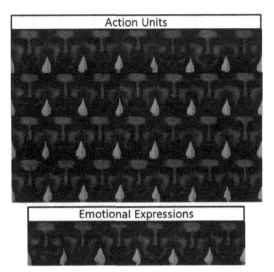

feature selection with DBNs. They select 200 Gabor wavelet coefficients from the processed face images via AdaBoost, but then discretize the continuous output of the AdaBoost classifiers into binary values. If the value of a particular classifier is 0, it means that particular AU is not present, where a value of 1 indicates the presence of the AU. These binary values are used as evidence in the DBN learned from the training set.

In (Valstar & Pantic, 2006), the Gabor-AdaBoost scheme is supplemented with a particle filter based tracker. This method robustly tracks the feature points over subsequent frames, albeit at a higher computational cost. In (Koelstra & Pantic, 2008) features are detected in the first frame, and tracked over the subsequent frames, where classification is performed with Gentleboost (a variant of AdaBoost) and HMMs in succession.

In (Cohen et al., 2003), a model-based face tracking approach is taken, where a wireframe model of the face is constructed (see Figure 6 (b)). In the first frame of the image sequence, facial features such as the eye corners and mouth corners are selected by the user. Assuming a neutral, frontal pose, this part of the model can also be automatically performed. The generic face model is then warped to fit the located facial features. Once the model is constructed and fitted, head motion and local deformations of the facial features such as the eyebrows, eyelids, and mouth can be tracked. The motion direction and intensity of the tracked points are used as observation vectors of a hidden Markov model (HMM). Each expression type has its own Markov model, and the model that produces the highest posterior probability for a given observed sequence is selected as the expression class. The authors also propose a second level HMM to model transitions between emotions, and use this model for automatic segmentation of the video sequences.

Expression Classification from 3D Faces

With the advances in 3D sensor technology 3D has become an attractive modality for face recognition. State–or–the–art databases created for 3D face recognition pay attention to expressions and facial movement. Figure 7 shows samples from the Bosphorus 3D face database, which is publicly available (see Databases and Tools section).

It is possible to process 3D faces in a way similar to 2D faces. A depth map representation can be obtained by mapping the depth of each 3D facial surface point to an intensity value, depending on the distance from the camera. This is called a 2.5D representation, and most 2D analysis techniques can be adapted for this representation. In order to harness the full power of the 3D representation, however, the points that represent the facial surface are aligned to a prototypical shape. While 3D information allows the computation of features like curvatures and shape indices, accurate landmark localization and deformation analysis remain to be challenging.

There are relatively few purely 3D approaches for expression analysis in the literature. (Soyel & Demirel, 2007) use a neural network classifier that receives six indicative feature distances as an input (i.e. distances between eye and mouth corners, mouth and eyebrow height, and the face span) and categorizes the facial expression into a basic emotion category or as neutral. Subject-specific information is not used, and accurate landmarks (84 points) are assumed. Under these conditions, they achieve more than 90% classification accuracy. In (Mpiperis et al., 2008) 3D point clouds are aligned to a base mesh, but the mouth boundaries are detected separately for expressions with open mouth, as this causes a great change in the appearance. The classification is obtained by probabilistically modelling each expression class as a generative model. (Tang & Huang, 2008) use multi-class AdaBoost schemes with different weak classifiers, and obtain 95% average accuracy on the BU-3DFE database (Yin et al., 2006). This approach also relies on manually located landmarks.

It is obvious that there is room for improvement in 3D facial expression analysis. New scanner technologies also allow the analysis of 3D information with temporal dynamics (so–called 4D approaches) by enabling recording of 3D scans at rates approaching video acquisition (Yin et al., 2008). Recent work shows that processing dynamic information is also useful in the 3D modality (Sun & Yin, 2009). Consequently, it becomes possible to evaluate spontaneous expressions, which was not possible (or very difficult) for static 3D snapshots, acquired from highly controlled 3D scanner setups.

Databases and Tools

Extensive research into face recognition has resulted in the collection of large numbers of datasets. Although most of these focus on the biometrics aspects, and are more suitable for identification experiments, some include facial expressions, and some are specifically tailored towards expression research. In Table 2 we summarize 12 databases that are open for research purposes. The primary modalities are single-shot images and videos depicting emotions. The Bosphorus database is obtained with a 3D scanner, and it is the most comprehensive 3D face database for expression research. The Canal 9 database is a collection of political debates, and provides for analysis in natural, as opposed to posed data collection settings.

Table 3 lists a number of open source (or freely distributed) software tools that are useful for facial expression research. Among these, we list tools for face detection and tracking (OpenCV, MPT), automatic facial feature point localization (Gabor-ffpd, STASM), active appearance models (AAM-API), expression annotation and labelling (SCORE, FEELTRACE), machine learning and pattern recognition (MPT, PRTools, WEKA, Torch, MSBNx). There are also links to embodied conversational agents (GRETA and XFace), and two repositories of tools and data from European framework projects (HUMAINE, SIMILAR/eNTERFACE).

Table 2 Databases for facial expression related research

Database	Type	Details	Location
Cohn-Kanade (CMU-Pitt)	video, annot.	100 subj., neutral+ six basic emotions, 500 sequences, FACS action units	http://vasc.ri.cmu.edu/idb/html/face/facial_expression/index.html
Green persuasive	video	eight discussions, 25-48 min. each, persuasiveness annotations	http://green-persuasive-db.sspnet.eu/
RU-FACS-1	video	100 subj., 2,5 min. recordings, FACS codes for 20% subjects, lie detection	http://mplab.ucsd.edu/?page_id=80
MPLab GENKI-4K	image	4000 images, annotated as smiling/non-smiling	http://mplab.ucsd.edu/?page_id=398
CMU PIE	image	68 subj., 41,368 images, 4 expressions, 43 illuminations, 13 poses	http://www.ri.cmu.edu/projects/project_418.html
Multi-PIE	image	337 subj., 750,000+ images, 6 expressions, 15 poses	http://multipie.org
Stegmann	image, annot.	37 subj. frontal neutral faces, 58 landmarks + shape model ground truth	http://www.imm.dtu.dk/~aam/datasets/face_data.zip
CAS-PEAL (R1)	image	1040 subj., 30.900 images, 5 expressions, accessories, 15 lighting directions	http://www.jdl.ac.cn/peal/
JAFFE	image	10 female Japanese models, 213 images of 7 expressions, intensity ratings	http://www.kasrl.org/jaffe.html
MPI	video	246 sequences of face actions taken simultaneously from 6 cameras	http://vdb.kyb.tuebingen.mpg.de/
Bosphorus	3d scans, image	105 subj., 4666 scans, 24 landmarks, action units and basic expressions	http://bosphorus.ee.boun.edu.tr/
BU-3DFE/ BU-4DFE	3d scans/ 3d video	100 subj., 2500 scans, basic expressions in four intensities, no landmarks 101 subj., 606 sequences of 100 frames each, basic expressions	http://www.cs.binghamton.edu/~lijun/Research/3DFE/3DFE_Analysis.html
MMI face	image, video	86 subj., 2894 sequences, posed and spontaneous expressions, audio incl.	http://www.mmifacedb.com/
Canal 9	video	72 political debates, total of 48 hours. speaker segmentation and group indication	http://canal9-db.sspnet.eu/

APPLICATIONS AND FUTURE TRENDS

Widespread use of face detection and recognition technology has enabled a range of applications, some foreseeable in near future, and some desired applications with long–term research aspects. There are practical applications for recognizing each emotion separately; for instance recognition of fear and happiness has different implications.

In this section we shortly look at applications of facial expression analysis in several interrelated domains, including social analysis, robotics, ambient intelligence, and gaming. The boundaries of these applications are fuzzy; there are games for ambient intelligence settings, and robots for social analysis. Our aim here is to make the reader aware of some of the possibilities where this technology can take us in the near future. A comprehensive survey is beyond our scope.

Applications in Social Analysis

For social sciences that analyse human behaviours, affect is a relevant dimension that needs to be accounted for. While computers are not as accurate as humans in assessing affect, automatic recognition of emotion lightens the burden of

Table 3 Some software tools usable for facial expression related research

Tool Name	Details	Location
OpenCV	C/C++ & Python library for real time computer vision (face detection)	http://sourceforge.net/projects/opencv/
MPT	C & MATLAB toolbox for machine perception tools (inc. eye detection and face tracking in video)	http://mplab.ucsd.edu/grants/project1/free-software/MPTWebSite/introduction.html
STASM	C++ library for finding features in frontal & neutral faces	http://www.milbo.users.sonic.net/stasm/index.html
Gabor-ffpd	MATLAB Gabor wavelet based facial feature point detector	http://www.doc.ic.ac.uk/~mvalstar/programs/sliwiga_ffpd.zip
AAM-API	C++ API for Active Appearance Models, related MATLAB tools	http://www2.imm.dtu.dk/~aam/
SCORE	Digital video coding and annotation tool inc. FACS annotations	http://mpscore.sourceforge.net/facs.php
FEELTRACE	Two dimensional (activation/evaluation) emotion labeling tool	http://emotion-research.net/download/Feeltrace%20Package.zip
Greta	Expressive embodied conversational agent, with face expression synthesis	http://perso.telecom-paristech.fr/~pelachau/Greta/
XFace	Expressive conversational agent, without a body	http://xface.itc.it/index.htm
PRtools	MATLAB toolbox for pattern recognition	http://www.prtools.org/
WEKA	Java toolbox of machine learning algorithms	http://www.cs.waikato.ac.nz/ml/weka/
Torch	C++ toolbox of machine learning algorithms	http://www.torch.ch/
MSBNx	Microsoft Bayesian Network editor and toolkit	http://research.microsoft.com/en-us/um/redmond/groups/adapt/msbnx/
HUMAINE	Source codes and data from HUMAINE network	http://emotion-research.net/toolbox/
eNTERFACE	Source codes and data from eNTERFACE Workshop series	http://www.enterface.net/results/

costly and error–prone data annotation process, it enables analysis of datasets composed of long multimodal observations, and also stands to provide quantitative, objective measurements. With advances in automatic classification of FACS action units from videos, there have already been cases of computers outperforming humans. For example, in a recent study on pain (Littlewort et al., 2009), 170 naïve human subjects were shown videos of real and faked pain, and could differentiate between these classes only 49% of the time (with standard deviation 13.7%). The automatic system based on AU analysis on the other hand had 88% correct discrimination rate for the same task. Since pain is very subjective, it is not difficult to see that automatic tools to analyse pain from facial expressions would be very useful for diagnostic purposes. A similar application is assisting human training in distinguishing between real and faked expressions, which is not only a useful social skill, but a job requirement in some cases.

Imagine yourself being equipped with a device that can 'read' other's facial expressions. Imagine further that you suffer from autism, and have trouble understanding expressions and interaction patterns of people around you. People with autism spectrum conditions (ASC) stand to gain much from such "empathy enhancing" technologies, especially if an unobtrusive and transparent interface can provide them with helping cues (El Kaliouby et al., 2006).

Clinical and psychological applications of facial expression analysis are not limited to autism research. (Ekman & Rosenberg, 2005) contains several studies relating to the analysis of depression, schizophrenia, psychosomatic disorders, suicidal tendencies, guilt expressions for psychotherapeutic interaction, and personality assessment. In these studies, facial expression is interpreted as a dependent variable of affect-related changes in the body, and automated tools are used in assisting diagnosis and therapy monitoring.

Affect assessment from facial cues can go beyond facial actions, as computers have access to sensors humans do not possess. For instance it has been shown that bio-heat modelling of facial imagery can reveal increased blood flow around the eyes (see Figure 8), which is a good indicator of stress, as well as cardiac pulse and heart rate

Figure 8. Thermal imaging of the face can reveal stress. © 2007, Pavlidis et al., adapted with permission

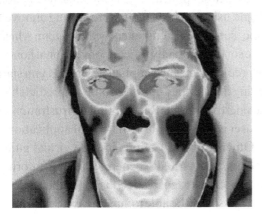

(Pavlidis et al., 2007). These indicators can be used in clinical studies, in games that can adapt to the user's stress levels, or even in criminal investigations.

Recent research directions in social signal processing employ facial expression analysis in assessment of group interaction dynamics. Relevant applications include automatic analysis of mood, coordinated patterns of interaction, mimicry, engagement, focus of attention, and dominance relations. Such indicators help for instance in automatic assessment of political discussions and campaign footages to predict the outcome of political debates, or for determining cognitive styles and personality aspects of individuals.

A related application is the automated analysis of impact for commercials. The cost of screening a commercial in a valuable slot (for instance during Super Bowl, the main sports event in US) can cost millions of dollars. Emotion–sensing technology has been harnessed for gauging the immediate impact of such expensive advertisements. It is also possible to measure affect directly in relation to the product. In one such application, Unilever has used video footages of people tasting different kind of food, and used the eMotion face expression analysis system developed at the University of Amsterdam (http://www.visual-recognition.nl/index.html) for obtaining objective and reproducible results.

A final application we would like to mention under this category is affect-based multimedia retrieval. Multimedia content analysis (MCA) tools enhanced with expression analysis can provide the means for qualitative search of material (querying for 'happy' episodes), highlight extraction, automatic life-logging and summarization (storing and retrieval of emotionally loaded content), and surveillance (retrieval of frames that contain people with angry or stressed expressions from a surveillance footage). The exponential growth of multimedia material accumulating on the Internet makes this type of affect-based indexing a very promising application (Hanjalic & Xu, 2005).

Applications in Robotics

One of the goals of robotics is to create robots that interact naturally with humans. Understanding affect is a very important requirement for these applications. To give one example, consider robots designed to help autistic children, as partners of interaction or as educational tools to teach children basic visual concepts (Dautenhahn & Werry, 2004). (Salter, 2009) reports a case of robot–child interaction where the child is distressed by the music played by the robot, and signals this emotion through facial and bodily gestures. Unless the robot understands this signal, and acts upon it by terminating the activity that is causing the stress, the interaction will have undesired consequences.

Affect is an integral part of human communication, and sensitivity to affect allows for more natural interaction. For this reason, robotics researchers seek to endow robots with the ability to respond to human psychological states like fear, panic, stress, or to allow the robot build a more accurate representation of the interacting human by taking into account focus of attention, gaze direction, engagement, boredom and such properties. A more responsive robot presents a richer experience for the interacting party.

The dyadic nature of affective communication requires the evaluation of emotion, as well as an internal emotion model. A good example is MIT's Kismet robot, which has mechanisms for recognizing precipitating events, appraising it for affective content, displaying a certain expression through its face, voice and posture, and finally a set of action tendencies that motivate its behavioural response (Breazeal, 2001). Modulation of action selection mechanisms is particularly important, because an emotional display by the human needs to be acknowledged by the robot for seamless interaction. This will be done by modulating the behaviour of the robot appropriately.

Applications in Ambient Intelligence

Ambient intelligence (AmI) represents a vision where people are surrounded by smart appliances and devices that respond to overt and covert signals of the user in intelligent ways. It deals with both understanding of a user's emotions, and with synthesizing emotions on virtual agents to create the impression of affect for a more natural communication interface. As such, there are many AmI applications that can benefit from facial expression analysis. In ambient environments like smart homes, the recognition of affect improves categorization of action context. By correlating affect and intentions, it becomes possible to constrain the search for the correct interpretation of signals.

Detection of anger, fatigue or boredom of the driver in a smart car is desirable for increasing safety (Ji et al., 2006). A simple camera positioned behind the wheel allows tracking of the driver's face and analysing the expression for such signals. An assumption that gained much experimental evidence is that human errors are correlated with negative affective states. Consequently, detecting these states is a path to minimizing such errors.

Improving user's performance is a goal for many ambient intelligence technologies, including personal wellness and assistive technologies. Ambient intelligence settings are also adequate for cognitive enhancement applications, providing their users with useful information. One problem AmI needs to deal with, which was apparent even in its earliest applications, is the nuisance factor. People using such systems were getting annoyed at the 'smart' decisions taken by the system, which were sometimes badly timed. Conventional homes are predictable; when appliances around you start getting ideas, they may become unpredictable, causing frustration. Recognition of frustration in the user is one valuable skill for AmI applications.

Other AmI applications include virtual guide systems, and virtual teachers. The best tutoring systems have extensive feedback for the student, and they should be able to support, explain, evaluate, motivate, and provide expectations. Also, the social aspect of learning cannot be neglected; social interaction is a powerful catalyst for learning and needs to be harnessed for exploring new ways of teaching (Meltzoff et al., 2009). Autonomous systems that can provide such feedback can be the key to a revolution in education, making high-quality tutoring available to millions of people worldwide through computers. Embodied conversational agents (ECA) is an active research area for such virtual tutoring and guiding systems (Cassell et al., 2002, Ruttkay & Pelachaud, 2004). The aim is to create a virtual agent that is expressive enough to communicate appropriate affective cues to the user, thereby ensuring an improved communication experience. Figure 9 shows two such agents, XFace (Balcı, 2004) and GRETA (Ruttkay & Pelachaud, 2004), respectively.

Applications in Gaming

Future gaming applications will have more input from the user, through increased sensor capabilities in end–user devices. Two types of developments in gaming are relevant through facial expression research, based on analysis and synthesis of expressions, respectively.

The first type of systems will try to understand the users affect through sensors on the computer or the game console, and subsequently adapt their behaviour appropriately. These systems will obviously require real-time processing, which can be challenging. They may have the advantage, however, of adapting to a specific user, which would mean lightweight feature processing. It is also conceivable that the user spends some time calibrating such a system, tuning it to his or her needs.

Multi-user online games are good examples for this category of game applications. The detection of affect and transfer thereof to the virtual agent (or avatar) controlled by the user is desirable for multi–user games in which multiple human players are embodied. Popular examples like World of Warcraft and Second Life boast millions of users.

With current technology, it is possible to have an avatar projecting real facial expressions in Second Life. The eMotion software mentioned earlier runs an expression recognition tool on the client side, and using the user interface of the program, sends automatic facial texture updates to the avatar. These updates correspond to read expressions of the user. Since the Second Life interface is not yet optimized for such input, the link between eMotion and Second Life is not through a clear interface. We may assume that in the future, multi-user games will implement the necessary stubs on the program side to receive affect from

Figure 9. Synthesizing affect on virtual head models Alice (Xface) and Greta. Alice displays anger, while Greta shows happiness here. See text for references

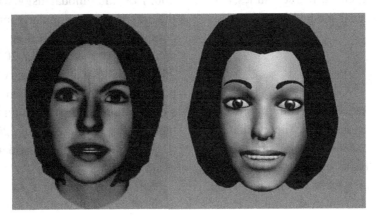

the client, and make it partially available to their virtual characters. Thus, it will be possible to register for example a 'disgust' reaction of the real user, captured on the client side by the affective system, recognize and encode this as 'disgust', and enact it on the avatar simultaneously.

The facial expressions can also serve as novel input modalities to a computer, allowing different gaming experience. The eMotion webpage mentioned before also includes a popular demo (also installed at the NEMO Science Museum in Amsterdam) where you can play a game of pong using facial expressions.

The second group of systems try to incorporate believable non-player characters, with a wide range of expressions. The game-playing experience is enriched by these emotional displays with possibly different intensities, with clearly visible or subtle signs, and with different frequencies of occurrence. The FACS system, for instance, is already used in the game industry to synthesize realistic face expressions (e.g. in the Half-Life 2 game by Valve).

Naturally, there will be systems that combine both aspects. If a camera can be used to register the users disgust on the client side, and that information is conveyed to nearby virtual characters that are participating in the current interaction, these characters can act accordingly and modify their behaviours. For a more realistic gaming environment, it is also useful to have automatic characters that are able to respond to situations with pre–programmed or even learned semantics, and show affect in their facial and bodily expression.

CONCLUSION

There are several limitations of existing approaches to facial expression analysis. The evaluation is often conducted on posed expressions, with a small number of 'basic' emotions considered. Recent work in this area seeks to remedy this by considering natural data. However, manual annota-

tion tools are not sufficiently developed to make annotation fast and cheap. Furthermore, if the temporal dimension and simultaneously recorded multimodal information are taken into account, it becomes apparent that annotation becomes much more difficult. Yet annotation is crucial for training statistical algorithms, as well as for evaluating methods against the golden standard of human judgement. Finally, recording high-resolution faces in isolation helps face detection and facial feature tracking, but it also means that contextual cues are neglected to a large part.

The current approach in social signal processing is to evaluate dynamic facial information in natural contexts. The results of such an approach will eventually influence psychological and neurological research, which predominantly work on static facial expressions to date. A future challenge is to create the tools for annotation and evaluation of dynamic and more granular affective content for psychological and neurological research. Also, it has been made clear that the transmission of human affect is a composite somatory event, and multimodal analysis of affect has much greater potential than unimodal analysis.

The communication of human affect does not solely rely on facial expression, but also on physical appearance, gestures, postures, spatio–temporal dynamics of behaviour, and vocal behaviour. Multimodal analysis takes into account these modalities, and stresses the importance and integration of contextual information (Sebe et al., 2005). For multimodal fusion with audio modality, the prosody is the singularly most used feature to complement visual information for expression analysis (Caridakis et al., 2010). (Zeng et al., 2009) includes a thorough survey of audio-visual methods for affect recognition. Other cues for fusion, while dependent on cultural context, include hand gestures (Yang & Ahuja, 2001), head motion (Cohn et al., 2004) and shoulder gestures (Valstar et al., 2007).

A machine learning system is only as good as its data; if the annotation is erroneous, the learning system will model incorrect correlations. Robust systems that can tolerate a certain level of noise in the data require increasing amounts of training data. Collecting and publishing rich emotional data is difficult, particularly as multimedia information would reveal personal and intimate information, and complex annotations are difficult and expensive to create. A potential solution is adapted by the SSPNet project (http://sspnet.eu), which aims at annotating and analysing existing videos of news and political debates. While alleviating the privacy issues, this approach has to deal with restricted context and imbalanced emotional content. Also, it foregoes the benefit of using auxiliary biosensors in automatically establishing ground truth for emotional content. However, the natural setting of these recordings and the relevance of the particular application makes it a worthwhile challenge.

One additional challenge is the dissociation of facial affect from speech–induced facial movement. This issue is rarely tackled, as most 'neutral' expressions in the available databases have closed mouths. Normal speech causes many deformations, which should not be recognized as emotional expressions.

Getting the appropriate training data is a challenge in many respects. Some affective states (like fatigue) can be induced, but some more complicated configurations are much more difficult to obtain. Humans can distinguish fine nuances of affective displays. A good example (given by Nick Campbell in a talk) is the following: "She was projecting happiness, but I could see she was unhappy". This kind of analysis is not surprising for us, it would be quite surprising if done by, say, a robot. Human-like understanding of affective states remains a grand challenge, especially since the optimal granularity of affect representation is not obvious. The categories we choose for computer classification can mimic linguistic levels, or they can be arbitrary groupings that we don't have words for.

Approaches motivated from a machine learning perspective are mostly interested in short-term correlations. However, long-term within-subject correlations (consistency of pain expression, for instance) are just as important as between-subject correlations, especially for clinical studies. This kind of analysis requires meticulous data collection and evaluation.

The bottom-up (or data-driven) approach can only take us so far in determining affect; we need top-down, semantic information to disambiguate patterns by also taking goals and environmental factors into account. The bottom-up approach essentially treats the problem as a classification task. Given a certain facial image, or a sequence of images, one (or multiple) classifications into affective categories are selected. While the sensory information contains physical, physiological, performance-related and behavioural cues, its relation to semantic indicators like goals, context or workload are not easy to assess, and the latter will have implications on the affective state of the individual. It may be particularly desirable to make inferences about the latter.

In spite of all these challenges, the availability of new tools, faster algorithms, more extensive databases, and the formation of research clusters and associations for affective computing (as well as new journals like IEEE Transactions in Affective Computing) make it a vibrant and rapidly progressing field.

ACKNOWLEDGMENT

This work is supported by the EU NEST project PERCEPT. The work of Nicu Sebe was supported by the FIRB S-PATTERNS project.

REFERENCES

Adolphs, R. (2002). Recognizing emotion from facial expressions: Psychological and neurological mechanisms. *Behavioral and Cognitive Neuroscience Reviews, 1*(1), 21–62. doi:10.1177/1534582302001001003

Afzal, S., Sezgin, T. M., Gao, Y., & Robinson, P. (2009). Perception of Emotional Expressions in Different Representations Using Facial Feature Points. *Proc. Int. Conf. Affective Computing and Intelligent Interaction.*

Alyüz, N., Gökberk, B., Dibeklioğlu, H., Savran, A., Salah, A. A., Akarun, L., & Sankur, B. (2008). 3D Face Recognition Benchmarks on the Bosphorus Database with Focus on Facial Expressions. *Proc. First European Workshop on Biometrics and Identity Management* (pp.62–71).

Balcı, K. (2004). Xface: MPEG-4 based open source toolkit for 3d facial animation. *Proc. Working Conference on Advanced Visual Interfaces,* (pp. 399-402).

Bartlett, M. S., Littlewort, G., Frank, M., Lainscsek, C., Fasel, I., & Movellan, J. (2005). Recognizing Facial Expression: Machine Learning and Application to Spontaneous Behavior. *Proc. IEEE Int. Conf. Computer Vision and Pattern Recognition* (pp. 568–573).

Blair, R. J. R., Morris, J. S., Frith, C. D., Perrett, D. I., & Dolan, R. J. (1999). Dissociable neural responses to facial expressions of sadness and anger. *Brain, 122,* 883–893. doi:10.1093/brain/122.5.883

Blanz, V., & Vetter, T. (1999). A morphable model for the synthesis of 3D faces. *Proc. SIGGRAPH,* (pp. 187–194).

Borod, J. C., Obler, L. K., Erhan, H. M., Grunwald, I. S., Cicero, B. A., & Welkowitz, J. (1998). Right hemisphere emotional perception: Evidence across multiple channels. *Neuropsychology, 12,* 446–458. doi:10.1037/0894-4105.12.3.446

Breazeal, C. (2001). Affective interaction between humans and robots. In Kelemen, J., & Sosík, P. (Eds.), *ECAL, Lecture Notes in Artificial Intelligence, 2159* (pp. 582–591).

Bruce, V., & Young, A. W. (1986). Understanding face recognition. *The British Journal of Psychology, 77,* 305–327.

Calder, A. J., Burton, A. M., Miller, P., Young, A. W., & Akamatsu, S. (2001). A principal component analysis of facial expressions. *Vision Research, 41*(9), 1179–1208. doi:10.1016/S0042-6989(01)00002-5

Caridakis, G., Karpouzis, K., Wallace, M., Kessous, L., & Amir, N. (2010). Multimodal user's affective state analysis in naturalistic interaction. *Journal on Multimodal User Interfaces, 3*(1), 49–66. doi:10.1007/s12193-009-0030-8

Carletta, J. (2006). Announcing the AMI Meeting Corpus. *The ELRA Newsletter, 11*(1), 3–5.

Cassell, J., Sullivan, J., Prevost, S., & Churchill, E. (Eds.). (2002). *Embodied Conversational Agents.* Cambridge, MA: MIT Press.

Cohen, I., Sebe, N., Garg, A., Chen, L. S., & Huang, T. S. (2003). Facial Expression Recognition from Video Sequences: Temporal and Static Modeling. *Computer Vision and Image Understanding, 91*(1-2), 160–187. doi:10.1016/S1077-3142(03)00081-X

Cohn, J., Reed, L. I., Ambadar, Z., Xiao, J., & Moriyama, T. (2004). Automatic Analysis and Recognition of Brow Actions and Head Motion in Spontaneous Facial Behavior. Proc. *IEEE Int'l Conf. Systems, Man, and Cybernetics,* (pp. 610-616).

Cohn, J., & Schmidt, K. (2004). The Timing of Facial Motion in Posed and Spontaneous Smiles. *International Journal of Wavelets, Multresolution, and Information Processing, 2*(2), 121–132. doi:10.1142/S021969130400041X

Cootes, T. F., Edwards, G. J., & Taylor, C. J. (2001). Active appearance models. *IEEE Transactions on Pattern Analysis and Machine Intelligence, 23*(6), 681–685. doi:10.1109/34.927467

Dautenhahn, K., & Werry, I. (2004). Towards interactive robots in autism therapy: background, motivation and challenges. *Pragmatics & Cognition, 12*(1), 1–35. doi:10.1075/pc.12.1.03dau

Ekman, P. (1993). Facial expression and emotion. *The American Psychologist, 48*, 384–392. doi:10.1037/0003-066X.48.4.384

Ekman, P., & Friesen, W. V. (1978). *Facial action coding system: A technique for the measurement of facial movement*. Palo Alto, CA: Consulting Psychologists Press.

Ekman, P., & Rosenberg, E. (Eds.). (2005). *What the Face Reveals: Basic and Applied Studies of Spontaneous Expression Using the Facial Action Coding System (FACS)* (Revised 2nd Edition). New York, NY: Oxford University Press.

El Kaliouby, R., Picard, R., & Baron-Cohen, S. (2006). Affective Computing and Autism. *Annals of the New York Academy of Sciences, 1093*(1), 228–248. doi:10.1196/annals.1382.016

Fasel, B., & Luettin, J. (2003). Automatic facial expression analysis: Survey. *Pattern Recognition, 36*, 259–275. doi:10.1016/S0031-3203(02)00052-3

Gauthier, I., Tarr, M. J., Aanderson, A., Skudlarski, P., & Gore, J. C. (1999). Activation of the middle fusiform 'face area' increases with expertise in recognizing novel objects. *Nature Neuroscience, 2*, 568–573. doi:10.1038/9224

Gross, R., Matthews, I., Cohn, J., Kanade, T., & Baker, S. (2010). Multi-PIE. *Image and Vision Computing, 28*(5), 807–813. doi:10.1016/j.imavis.2009.08.002

Hanjalic, A., & Xu, L. Q. (2005). Affective video content representation and modeling. *IEEE Transactions on Multimedia, 7*(1), 143–154. doi:10.1109/TMM.2004.840618

Hasselmo, M. E., Rolls, E. T., & Baylis, G. C. (1989). The role of expression and identity in the face–selective responses of neurons in the temporal visual cortex of the monkey. *Behavioural Brain Research, 32*, 203–218. doi:10.1016/S0166-4328(89)80054-3

Ji, Q., Lan, P., & Looney, C. (2006). A probabilistic framework for modeling and real-time monitoring human fatigue. *IEEE Transactions on Systems, Man, and Cybernetics-A, 36*(5), 862–875. doi:10.1109/TSMCA.2005.855922

Kanade, T., Cohn, J. F., & Tian, Y. (2000). Comprehensive database for facial expression analysis. *Proc. Fourth IEEE Int. Conf. on Automatic Face and Gesture Recognition* (pp. 46–53).

Kanwisher, N., McDermott, J., & Chun, M. M. (1997). The fusiform face area: A module in human extrastriate cortex specialized for face perception. *The Journal of Neuroscience, 17*, 4302–4311.

Koelstra, S., & Pantic, M. (2008). Non-rigid registration using free-form deformations for recognition of facial actions and their temporal dynamics. *Proc. IEEE Int. Conf. on Automatic Face and Gesture Recognition.*

Lee, S. J., Park, K. R., & Kim, J. (2009). A comparative study of facial appearance modeling methods for active appearance models. *Pattern Recognition Letters, 30*(14), 1335–1346. doi:10.1016/j.patrec.2009.05.019

Littlewort, G. C., Bartlett, M. S., & Lee, K. (2009). Automatic coding of facial expressions displayed during posed and genuine pain. *Image and Vision Computing, 27*(12), 1797–1803. doi:10.1016/j.imavis.2008.12.010

Lyons, M. J., Budynek, J., & Akamatsu, S. (1999). Automatic Classification of Single Facial Images. *IEEE Transactions on Pattern Analysis and Machine Intelligence, 21*(12), 1357–1362. doi:10.1109/34.817413

Meltzoff, A., Kuhl, P., Movellan, J. R., & Sejnowski, T. (2009). Foundations for a New Science of Learning. *Science, 235*(5938), 284–288. doi:10.1126/science.1175626

Milborrow, S., & Nicolls, F. (2008). Locating Facial Features with an Extended Active Shape Model. *Proc. European Conference on Computer Vision, 4*, (pp. 504-513).

Mpiperis, I., Malassiotis, S., & Strintzis, M. G. (2008). Bilinear models for 3-D face and facial expression recognition. *IEEE Transactions on Information Forensics and Security, 3*(3), 498–511. doi:10.1109/TIFS.2008.924598

Nusseck, M., Cunningham, D. W., Wallraven, C., & Bülthoff, H. H. (2008). The contribution of different facial regions to the recognition of conversational expressions. *Journal of Vision (Charlottesville, Va.), 8*(8), 1–23. doi:10.1167/8.8.1

Ortony, A., Clore, G., & Collins, A. (1988). *The Cognitive Structure of Emotions.* Cambridge, UK: Cambridge University Press.

Pavlidis, I., Dowdall, J., Sun, N., Puri, C., Fei, J., & Garbey, M. (2007). Interacting with human physiology. *Computer Vision and Image Understanding, 108*(1-2), 150–170. doi:10.1016/j.cviu.2006.11.018

Pollak, S. D., Messner, M., Kistler, D. J., & Cohn, J. F. (2009). Development of perceptual expertise in emotion recognition. *Cognition, 110*(2), 242–247. doi:10.1016/j.cognition.2008.10.010

Russell, J. A. (1980). A circumplex model of affect. *Journal of Personality and Social Psychology, 39*(6), 1161–1178. doi:10.1037/h0077714

Russell, J. A., & Fernández–Dols, J. M. (Eds.). (1997). *The Psychology of Facial Expression.* Cambridge, UK: Cambridge University Press. doi:10.1017/CBO9780511659911

Ruttkay, Z., & Pelachaud, C. (Eds.). (2004). *From Brows till Trust: Evaluating Embodied Conversational Agents.* Kluwer.

Salah, A. A., Çınar, H., Akarun, L., & Sankur, B. (2007). Robust Facial Landmarking for Registration. *Annales des Télécommunications, 62*(1-2), 1608–1633.

Salter, T. (2009). A Need for Flexible Robotic Devices. *AMD Newsletter, 6*(1), 3.

Sebe, N., Cohen, I., & Huang, T. S. (2005). Multimodal emotion recognition. In *Handbook of Pattern Recognition and Computer Vision.* World Scientific. doi:10.1142/9789812775320_0021

Soyel, H., & Demirel, H. (2007). Facial expression recognition using 3D facial feature distances. *Lecture Notes in Computer Science, 4633*, 831–843. doi:10.1007/978-3-540-74260-9_74

Stegmann, M. B. (2002). *Analysis and segmentation of face images using point annotations and linear subspace techniques.* Technical Report, Informatics and Mathematical Modelling, Technical University of Denmark (DTU). Retrieved 19 September 2009, from http://www2.imm.dtu.dk/~aam/.

Sun, Y., & Yin, L. (2009). Evaluation of spatiotemporal regional features for 3D face analysis. *Proc. IEEE Computer Society Conf. on Computer Vision and Pattern Recognition Workshops.*

Tang, H., & Huang, T. S. (2008). 3D facial expression recognition based on automatically selected features. *Proc. IEEE Computer Society Conf. on Computer Vision and Pattern Recognition Workshops.*

Tian, Y., Kanade, T., & Cohn, J. F. (2001). Recognizing action units for facial expression analysis. *IEEE Transactions on Pattern Analysis and Machine Intelligence, 23*(2), 97–115. doi:10.1109/34.908962

Tong, Y., Liao, W., & Ji, Q. (2007). Facial action unit recognition by exploiting their dynamic and semantic relationships. *IEEE Transactions on Pattern Analysis and Machine Intelligence, 29*(10), 1683–1699. doi:10.1109/TPAMI.2007.1094

Valstar, M., & Pantic, M. (2006). Fully automatic facial action unit detection and temporal analysis. *Proc. Computer Vision and Pattern Recognition Workshop.*

Valstar, M. F., Güneş, H., & Pantic, M. (2007). How to Distinguish Posed from Spontaneous Smiles Using Geometric Features. *Proc. ACM International Conference Multimodal Interfaces,* (pp. 38-45).

Vinciarelli, A., Pantic, M., & Bourlard, H. (2009). Social Signal Processing: Survey of an Emerging Domain. *Image and Vision Computing, 27*(12), 1743–1759. doi:10.1016/j.imavis.2008.11.007

Viola, P., & Jones, M. J. (2004). Robust real-time face detection. *International Journal of Computer Vision, 57*(2), 137–154. doi:10.1023/B:VISI.0000013087.49260.fb

Vural, E., Çetin, M., Erçil, A., Littlewort, G., Bartlett, M., & Movellan, J. (2007). Drowsy driver detection through facial movement analysis. *Lecture Notes in Computer Science, 4796,* 6–19. doi:10.1007/978-3-540-75773-3_2

Whitehill, J., Littlewort, G., Fasel, I., Bartlett, M., & Movellan, J. (2009). Towards Practical Smile Detection. *IEEE Transactions on Pattern Analysis and Machine Intelligence, 31*(11), 2106–2111. doi:10.1109/TPAMI.2009.42

Yang, M. H., & Ahuja, N. (2001). *Face Detection and Gesture Recognition for Human – Computer Interaction.* New York: Kluwer Academic Publishers.

Yang, M. H., Kriegman, D., & Ahuja, N. (2002). Detecting Faces in Images: A Survey. *IEEE Transactions on Pattern Analysis and Machine Intelligence, 24*(1), 34–58. doi:10.1109/34.982883

Yin, L., Chen, X., Sun, Y., Worm, T., & Reale, M. (2008). A High-Resolution 3D Dynamic Facial Expression Database. *Proc. 8th Int. Conf. on Automatic Face and Gesture Recognition.*

Yin, L., Wei, X., Sun, Y., Wang, J., & Rosato, M. J. (2006). A 3D facial expression database for facial behavior research. *Proc. Int. Conf. on Automatic Face and Gesture Recognition,* (pp.211–216).

Zeng, Z., Pantic, M., Roisman, G. I., & Huang, T. S. (2009). A Survey of Affect Recognition Methods: Audio, Visual, and Spontaneous Expressions. *IEEE Transactions on Pattern Analysis and Machine Intelligence, 31*(1), 39–58. doi:10.1109/TPAMI.2008.52

Zhang, Y., & Ji, Q. (2005). Active and dynamic information fusion for facial expression understanding from image sequences. *IEEE Transactions on Pattern Analysis and Machine Intelligence, 27*(5), 699–714. doi:10.1109/TPAMI.2005.93

ADDITIONAL READING

Baron–Cohen, S. Golan, O., Wheelwright, S. & Hill, J.J. (2004). *Mind reading: The interactive guide to emotion.* London: Jessica Kingsley Publishers Ltd.

Coan, J. A., & Allen, J. J. B. (2007). *Handbook of Emotion Elicitation and Assessment.* New York, NY: Oxford University Press.

Cohn, J. F. (2006). Foundations of Human Computing: Facial Expression and Emotion. Presented in *Int. Conf. on Multimodal Interfaces,* (pp.233–238).

Cowie, R., Douglas–Cowie, E., Tsapatsoulis, N., Votsis, G., Kollias, S., Fellenz, W., & Taylor, J. G. (2001). Emotion Recognition in Human–Computer Interaction. *IEEE Signal Processing Magazine*, *18*(1), 32–80. doi:10.1109/79.911197

Davidson, R. J., Scherer, K. R., & Goldsmith, H. H. (Eds.). (2009). *Handbook of Affective Sciences*. Oxford Univ. Press.

Ekman, P. (2003). *Emotions revealed*. New York: Times Books.

Ekman, P., & Friesen, W. V. (1975). *Unmasking the face: A guide to recognizing emotions from facial expressions*. CA: Consulting Psychologists Press.

Fridlund, A. J. (1994). *Human facial expression*. New York: Academic Press.

Gatica-Perez, D. (2009). Automatic nonverbal analysis of social interaction in small groups: A review. *Image and Vision Computing*, *27*(12), 1775–1787. doi:10.1016/j.imavis.2009.01.004

Güneş, H., Piccardi, M., & Pantic, M. (2008). From the Lab to the Real World: Affect Recognition Using Multiple Cues and Modalities. In Or, J. (Ed.), *Affective Computing: Focus on Emotion Expression, Synthesis and Recognition* (pp. 185–218). Vienna, Austria: I–Tech Education and Publishing.

Izard, C. E. (1979). *The Maximally Discriminative Facial Movement Coding System (MAX)*. Newark, DE: University of Delaware, Instructional Resources Centre.

Lewis, M., Haviland-Jones, J. M., & Barrett, L. F. (Eds.). (2008). *Handbook of Emotions*. New York, NY: The Guildford Press.

Mehrabian, A. (1972). *Nonverbal Communication*. Chicago, IL: Aldine Atherton.

Pantic, M. (2009). Machine Analysis of Facial Behaviour: Naturalistic and Dynamic Behaviour. *Philosophical Transactions of Royal Society B*, *364*, 3505–3513. doi:10.1098/rstb.2009.0135

Pantic, M., Pentland, A., Nijholt, A., & Huang, T. (2008). Human–centred intelligent human–computer interaction (HCI2): How far are we from attaining it? *International Journal of Autonomous and Adaptive Communications Systems*, *1*(2), 168–187. doi:10.1504/IJAACS.2008.019799

Pantic, M., & Rothkrantz, L. J. M. (2000). Automatic analysis of facial expressions: The state of the art. *IEEE Transactions on Pattern Analysis and Machine Intelligence*, *22*(12), 1424–1445. doi:10.1109/34.895976

Picard, R. W. (1997). *Affective Computing*. Cambridge, MA: MIT Press.

Picard, R. W., Papert, S., Bender, W., Blumberg, B., Breazeal, C., & Cavallo, D. (2004). Affective learning — a manifesto. *BT Technology Journal*, *22*(4), 253–269. doi:10.1023/B:BTTJ.0000047603.37042.33

Picard, R. W., Vyzas, E., & Healey, J. (2001). Toward machine emotional intelligence: analysis of affective physiological state. *IEEE Transactions on Pattern Analysis and Machine Intelligence*, *23*(10), 1175–1191. doi:10.1109/34.954607

Sander, D., & Scherer, K. R. (Eds.). (2009). *The Oxford Companion to Emotion and the Affective Sciences*. Oxford Univ. Press.

Scherer, K. R. (2000). Psychological models of emotion. In Borod, J. C. (Ed.), *The neuropsychology of emotion* (pp. 137–162). New York, NY: Oxford University Press.

Schmidt, K. L., & Cohn, J. F. (2001). Human facial expressions as adaptations: Evolutionary questions in facial expression research. *Yearbook of Physical Anthropology*, *44*, 3–24. doi:10.1002/ajpa.20001

Thiran, J.-P., Bourlard, H., & Marques, F. (Eds.). (2009). *Multimodal Signal Processing.* Academic Press.

Tian, Y., Kanade, T., & Cohn, J. F. (2005). Facial expression analysis. In Li, S. Z., & Jain, A. K. (Eds.), *Handbook of face recognition* (pp. 247–276). New York: Springer. doi:10.1007/0-387-27257-7_12

Vinciarelli, A., Pantic, M. & Bourlard, H. (2009). *Social Signal Processing: Survey of an Emerging Domain.* Journal of Image and Vision Computing.

Whissell, C. (1989). *The dictionary of affect in language.* New York: Academic Press.

KEY TERMS AND DEFINITIONS

Appearance: The appearance of the face consists of the visual features of the facial image.

Basic Emotions: According to Ekman, these are 'happiness', 'sadness', 'anger', 'fear', 'surprise' and 'disgust', which have universal manifestations on the face, readable by people regardless of cultural background.

Chapter 9
Facial Expression Synthesis and Animation

Ioan Buciu
University of Oradea, Romania

Ioan Nafornita
University of Timisioara, Romania

Cornelia Gordan
University of Oradea, Romania

ABSTRACT

Living in a computer era, the synergy between man and machine is a must, as the computers are integrated into our everyday life. The computers are surrounding us but their interfaces are far from being friendly. One possible approach to create a friendlier human-computer interface is to build an emotion-sensitive machine that should be able to recognize a human facial expression with a satisfactory classification rate and, eventually, to synthesize an artificial facial expression onto embodied conversational agents (ECAs), defined as friendly and intelligent user interfaces built to mimic human gestures, speech or facial expressions. Computer scientists working in computer interfaces (HCI) put up impressive efforts to create a fully automatic system capable to identifying and generating photo - realistic human facial expressions through animation. This chapter aims at presenting current state-of-the-art techniques and approaches developed over time to deal with facial expression synthesis and animation. The topic's importance will be further highlighted through modern applications including multimedia applications. The chapter ends up with discussions and open problems.

INTRODUCTION

In human – to – human interaction (HHI) people mostly use their face and gestures to express emotional states. When communicating with each other, people involve both verbal and non-verbal communication ways: speech, facial expression or gestures (nods, winks, etc). As pointed out by Mehrabian (Mehrabian 1968), people express only 7% of the messages through a linguistic language,

DOI: 10.4018/978-1-61692-892-6.ch009

38% through voice, and 55% through facial expressions. Closely related to HHI, Human-computer interaction (HCI) deals with the ways humans communicate with machines. The term is broad and has an interdisciplinary character concerning various scientific fields, such as computer science, computer graphics, image processing, neurophysiology, and psychology. We should note that human-computer interface differs from brain-computer interfaces as the latter describe the communications between brain cells and machine and mainly involves a direct physical link.

Our psychological need of being surrounded by "human–like" machines in terms of their physical appearance and behavior is the main driving force behind the necessity of developing realistic human-computer interfaces. We would like machines acting like us, interpreting our facial expressions or gestures conveyed by emotions and respond accordingly. During the last decade the endeavor of scientists for creating emotion-driven systems was impressive. Although facial expressions represent a prominent way of revealing an emotional state, emotional states may also be expressed, coupled or associated to other modalities, such as gestures, change in the intonation, stress or rhythm of speech, blood pressure, etc. However, within the context of this chapter, we only consider facial expressions whenever we refer to emotion.

A *fully automatic facial expression analyzer* should be able to handle the following tasks (Krinidis, 2003):

1. Detect (and track) the face in a complex scene with random background;
2. Extract relevant facial features;
3. Recognize and classify facial expressions according to some classification rules.
    4.

Likewise, a *facial expression synthesizer* should:

1. Create realistic and natural expressions;
2. Operate in real time;
3. Require minimum user interaction in creating the desired expression;
4. Be easily and accurately adaptable to any individual face.

This chapter is focusing on the facial expression synthesis part and animation of synthesized expressions. Once the facial expression is synthesized the facial animation comes next, a task intensively employed in computer graphics applications. For instance, in the film industry, moviemakers try to build virtual human characters that are indistinguishable from the real ones. In the games industry, the designed human characters should be interactive and as realistic as possible. Commercial products are available to be used by users to create realistic looking avatars for chatting rooms, e-mails, greeting cards, or tele-conferencing. Face synthesis techniques have also been used for compression of talking head in the video conferencing scenario, such as MPEG – 4 standard (Raouzaiou, 2002).

The purpose of this chapter is to present current state–of–the–art techniques and approaches developed over time concerning facial expression synthesis and animation. These techniques will be elaborated throughout the chapter along with their limitations. The topic's importance is highlighted through modern applications. The chapter ends up with further discussions and open problems.

FACIAL EXPRESSION SYNTHESIS, ANIMATION AND APPLICATIONS

Facial expression synthesis methods roughly may fall under two categories: geometry based approaches where the face geometry is manipulated, and appearance (image) based approaches where face deformation mainly relies on morphing and blending techniques. Geometry based approaches consider the facial geometry extraction and manipulation, and, more precisely, the extraction of geometric parameters of those fiducial points that contribute to face region deformation involved in mimic the expression. Geometry manipulation includes several techniques such as interpolation, parameterization, physics-based modeling (mass-spring, muscle vector, etc.) or finite element method. Appearance based approaches rather rely on representing the face as an array of intensity values that are globally processed.

Facial Expression Descriptors

Each facial expression is the result of several facial muscle activations, so that, while contracted, the facial muscles temporally deform the facial features represented by eyebrows, eyes, nose, mouth and skin texture, leading to changes of the face appearance. When measuring the facial deformation, three characteristics are usually taken into account: location, intensity and dynamics. Location refers to the specific facial region where the facial action that is specific to a particular expression, occurs. The intensity is defined by the magnitude of the geometric deformation of facial features, typically when is fully deformed. We must note that the intensity of a deliberate facial expression can substantially differ from that of a spontaneous one. Generally, a deliberate facial expression possesses an exaggerated intensity. The third characteristic, namely dynamics, conveys information about the temporal evolution of facial expression and the related face surface deformations.

Facial expression measurements and descriptors are required in order to map the facial deformation to a synthetic face. There are several facial expression descriptors proposed in the literature. The most complete system for describing the facial expressions is the so-called Facial Action Coding System (FACS) developed by Ekman and Friesen (Ekman, 1978). The main goal of this system is to encode a comprehensive set of all possible visually distinguishable facial appearances by measuring specific facial muscle movements.

The facial motion is decomposed into a set of component actions called Action Units (AUs). However, only 30 AUs out of the full set of 44 are responsible for the anatomical contraction of a specific facial muscle set, while the remaining 14 AUs are referred to as miscellaneous actions (such as blinking, for instance). FACS is intensively employed to analyze and synthesize facial expressions. Examples of several AUs along with their description and muscles involved are depicted in Table 1.

Although FACS seems to be the most popular system used to animate and classify muscle action, it lacks time information, which is important for generating automatic smooth and intensity increasing expression over time. Therefore, AUs should be independently adjusted to the model.

The Facial Animation Parameters (FAP) that is especially dedicated to animate synthetic faces provide another descriptors set. FAP were defined to be compliant to the MPEG-4 standard compression technique and comprises 2 high level parameters (visemes and expressions) and 66 low-level parameters (Raouzaiou, 2002). One major drawback of FAP is the fact that it only expresses discrete expressions. According to Mehrabian (Mehrabian 1996), the emotion is not limited to isolated categories but can be described in terms of combination of three nearly orthogonal dimensions, namely pleasure-displeasure (P), arousal-nonarousal (A) and dominance-submissiveness (D) leading to the PAD emotional space model for describing universal emotions. The PAD parameters are considered high-level facial parameters. Recently, intermediate (middle) level parameters termed Partial Expression Parameters (PEP) were proposed by Zhang et al (Zhang, 2007) to get smoother control over the facial movements. PEP allows high correlations between different FAPs. Aside from those aforementioned descriptors, early works involved the 6 basic limited emotions descriptor set, i.e. angry, happiness, sadness, disgust, surprise and fear. We should note that each basic emotion can be described in terms of FACS

Table 1. Samples of Action Units (AU) in the Facial Action Coding System

AU	Action description	Facial muscle involved
1	Inner Brow Raiser	Frontalis,pars medialis
2	Outer Brow Raiser	Frontalis,pars lateralis
4	Brow Lowerer	Corrugator supercilii, Depressor supercilii
15	Lip Corner Depressor	Depressor anguli oris
20	Lip Stretcher	Risorius
27	Mouth Stretch	Pterygoids, Digastric
s28	Lip Suck	Orbicularis oris
44	Squint	Orbicularis oculi, pars palebralis

Table 2. The six basic expressions and their corresponding combination of AUs

Expression	AUs
Angry	2,4,7,9,10,20,26
Happiness	1,6,12,14
Sadness	1,4,15,23
Disgust	2,4,9,15,17
Surprise	1,2,5,15,16,20,26
Fear	1,2,4,5,15,20,26

through AUs combinations, as drawn in Table 2 (Ekman, 2002).

Geometry Based Manipulations

In the early 80's, Badler and Platt (Blader, 1981) were the first to apply geometric based manipulation strategies to model and simulate the human skin on a muscle model. A set of muscles is attached to a skin mesh. The contraction of the muscle set generates skin mesh deformation. Waters (Waters, 1987) developed and modeled linear and sphincter muscles, where the latter are associated to the lips and eyes region. His early work has been extended by Terzopoulos and Waters (Terzopoulos, 1990) by introducing a third layer (between the skin and muscle layers) corresponding to a fatty tissue. The model provides smoother deformation control over animation. These models are limited in the sense of lacking natural facial

expression synthesis. Moreover, fine skin deformations such as temporal wrinkles are difficult to be represented, if not impossible. Hoch et al. (Hoch, 1994) proposed a facial model for facial expression animation based on B-splines surface with 13×16 control points. Four action units (AU1 – inner brow raiser, AU2-outer brow raiser, AU4-brow lower, and AU12-lip corner puller) of FACS are chosen for animating the face. Those action units are hard-wired to the model that is adapted to a given input datum consisting of 3D laser-scanner images each comprising 200×200 points determined by hand. The adaptation process is carried out in two phases. First, the model surface is fitted by minimizing the mean square error between the given data points and the surface points. Second, some constraints are considered in order to correctly position the control points in regions where the respective action units apply (i.e. the control points associated with an action unit result in the deformation of the correct region of skin tissue). To look more realistic, the color information of the laser-scanner texture is mapped onto the facial mask. Pighin et al. (Pighin, 2002) have proposed an image-based system which is able to model and animate 3-D face models from images. This technique reconstructs a continuous image function using a set of sample images. Once this function is found, the original samples can be interpolated or extrapolated to produce novel unseen images. The face models are constructed from a set of photographs of a person's face that can be linearly combined to express a wide range of expressions. A texture map is extracted from the photographs using both the face geometry and the camera parameters. Next, a tracking step is accomplished by recovering, for each video frame, the position of the head, its orientation, and the facial expression of a subject. The purpose is to estimate the model parameters through these frames. After capturing multiple views of a subject (with a given facial expression) these photographs are manually marked with a small set of initial corresponding points on the face in the different views (typically, corners of the eyes and mouth, tip of the nose, etc). The 3-D positions of the corresponding points are further used to deform a generic 3D face mesh to fit the face of the particular human subject. Additional corresponding points may be marked to refine the fit. One or more texture maps for the 3D model are finally extracted from the photos. The approach allows either a single view-independent texture map extraction and rendering or the original images can be used to perform view-dependent texture mapping. However, the system is limited, as the authors did not report any results for mapping the expression to different face model.

A complex facial model for creating highly realistic facial models and flexible expressions was developed by Zhang et al (Zhang, 2002).

The facial model is based on facial measurements including information about face shape and face texture. Three views of the person's face are acquired by using a non-contact 3D laser range scanner, each producing separate 3D reconstructions of the visible face regions. The geometry and color information of the facial surface is obtained by scanning a subject using a Minolta VIVID 700 Digitizer and the acquired data are registered into a single coordinate system. A geometric face model is created by editing corresponding triangular meshes. The originally generated triangular mesh consists of over 104 triangles most of them being redundant. The process is time consuming however. To reduce computational cost the mesh is adaptively reduced up to 70 percent without sacrificing the visible detail of the facial surface. Based on the triangular mesh, a physically-based face model that incorporates a multi-layer (i.e., epidermal, dermal, hypodermal) facial skin tissue to simulate the real skin is constructed. The model simulates a set of anatomically motivated facial muscle actuators and a rigid skull. A number of 23 major functional facial muscles are selected from FACS to animate facial expressions. The sets of those muscles involved in animation are as follows: 2 frontalis inner, 2 frontalis major, 2 frontalis outer, 2 corrugator supercilliary, 2 orbicularis oculi, 2 zygomaticus minor, 2 zygomaticus majos, 2 nasalis, 1 orbicularis oris, 2 risorius, 2 depressor anguli and 2 mentalis. Various flexible and realistic facial expressions can be generated using principles of Lagrangian mechanics applied to deform the facial surface. Although the model is a complex one simulating several layers, it cannot cope with temporal deformations such as wrinkles. Moreover, the teeth area is not modeled.

Zhang et al (Zhang, 2006) developed geometry-driven approach for facial expression synthesis. For each facial expression a set of feature point positions is provided which is further used to render the model employing an example-based strategy. The overall flowchart is depicted in Figure 1.

134 facial points are manually marked and the resulting marked images are all aligned with a standard image as illustrated in Figure 2. Each face image is next divided into 14 regions where

Figure 1. Flowchart of geometry-driven expression synthesis system proposed by Zhang et al. (Zhang, 2006). With permission from © 2006 IEEE

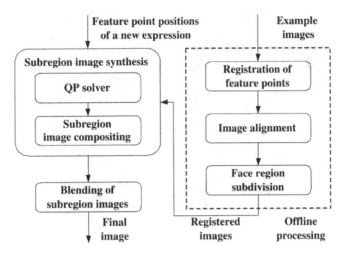

the facial expression synthesis takes place by solving a quadratic programming problem. The animation (motion propagation) is performed by estimating the unknown future location of facial features with the help of a principal components based learning technique. Figure 2 shows the selected feature points and the face subdivision. The final face with synthesized facial expression is obtained by blending those regions. One limitation of the system is the lack of a reliable extrapolation method. Another limitation comes from the blending procedure where image artefacts may become visible. And finally, as many other approaches described in the chapter, the system does not handle out-of-plane head rotations.

Appearance Based Approaches

A self-adaptive mesh is proposed by Yin et al. (Yin, 2001) to compute the deformation of the eyes in a 3D model for eye movement synthesis. Firstly, a Hough transform and deformable template matching combined with color information is used to accurately detect and track the eye features. Once the contours of the iris and eyelids in each frame of the image sequence are extracted the eye features are used to synthesize the real motions

of the eye on a 3D facial model. An extended dynamic mesh (EDM) expressed by a nonlinear second-order differential equation is used to create a realistic eye animation. To make the solution of DM equation more stable and accurate, the conventional dynamic mesh method is modified by introducing a so-called "energy-oriented mesh" (EOM) to refine the adaptive meshes. Thus, the eye model adaptation comprises two major steps: 1) coarse adaptation which applies DM method to make the large movement converge quickly to the region of an object followed by a 2) fine adaptation, where the EOM approach is applied to further adjust the mesh obtained after the first step. The movements are obtained according to the energy minimization principle where the meshes are deformed until an equilibrium state is attained. The method was applied to a real face model consisting of a detailed wireframe model with 2954 vertices and 3118 patches, in which there are 120 vertices for each eye. As reported, the facial expressions rather look unrealistic. The adapted wireframe models in successive frames are texture-mapped by using the first frame of the sequence.

Liu et al. (Liu, 2001) proposed a facial expression mapping method based on the so-called

Figure 2. Left: facial points; Right: face subdivisions (Zhang, 2006). With permission from © 2006 IEEE

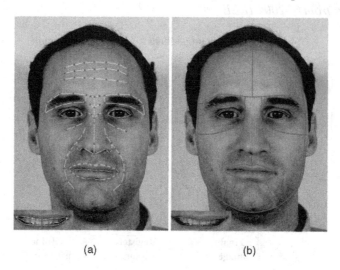

(a)   (b)

"expression ratio image" (ERI). Their method is not only able to exhibit facial feature motion but also to capture subtle changes in illumination and appearance (e.g., facial creases and wrinkles) making the face more expressive and the expression more convincing. This approach was one of the first methods capable of mapping one person's facial expression details to a different person's face. ERI involves the presence of four images: A and A * denoting the images of A's neutral face and expression face, respectively, and B and B*, denoting the image of B's neutral face and unknown image of his face with the same expression as A *, respectively. One drawback of this approach is that it requires the expression ratio image from the performer.

Raouzaiou et al (Raouzaiou, 2002) modeled primary facial expressions by using FAPs. They established the so-called face animation tables (FATs) to specify the model vertices that will be spatially deformed for each FAP as well as the deformation magnitude. The FATs value are MPEG-4 compliant, so that an MPEG-4 decoder can receive a face model accompanied by the corresponding FATs to animate synthetic profiles as illustrated in Figure 3. Figure 4 depicts synthetic expressions built using a 3D model of the POSER

Figure 3. Examples for animated profiles corresponding to anger expression. From Raouzaiou et al, (Raouzaiou, 2002) with permission

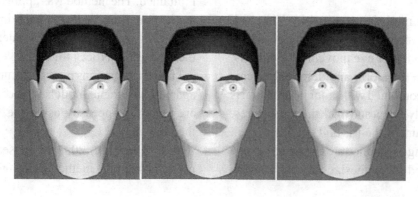

Figure 4. Synthesized archetypal expressions created using the 3D model of the POSER software package: (a) sadness, (b) anger, (c) joy, (d) fear, (e) disgust, and (f) surprise. From Raouzaiou et al, (Raouzaiou, 2002) with permission

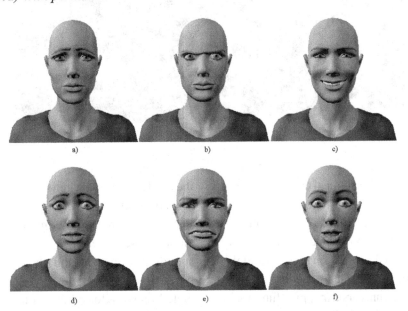

software package available at http://poser.smith-micro.com/poser.html.

Wang and Ahuja (Wang, 2003) derived a higher-order singular value decomposition based approach to decompose the facial expression space. The learned expression subspace model is then mapped to a different identity. However, the technique cannot be applied to synthesize expressions of people with unseen facial characteristics/appearance (such as beard) if no similar images exist in the training set for decomposition. A bilinear decomposition technique is proposed by Abboud and Davoine (Abboud 2004) where appearance parameters are encoded through an Active Appearance Model (AAM), which, in turn, relies on Principal Component Analysis (PCA). The shape and texture of a set of training images are modeled with PCA. The method may lead to moderate results when only a limited number of training samples are available. However, the resulting facial expressions rather look blocky and

unrealistic, as the synthesis generation accuracy highly depends on the size of the PCA learned space. Tewes et al (Tewes, 2005) used elastic graphs to build a Gabor wavelet based flexible object model (FOM) to synthesize nine different facial expressions for video frames. The model graphs are generated by manually locating the nodes of the graph over facial landmarks in the first frame. The nodes are automatically tracked over time using Gabor wavelets phase information. FOM is constructed as a parameterised model of graph deformation by merging raw data extracted from several video frames using PCA and Neural Gas. Smooth transitions are modeled with Principal Curves. In the training phase four persons are employed to construct the FOM. For testing, a person not contained in the training set is chosen. The corresponding background is discarded and an initial graph is superimposed. The graph is then deformed to generate a specific facial expression. The best matching gesture is

Figure 5. Original(b) and synthesized (c) expression of the subject depicted in (a) using the approach proposed by Ghent and McDonald, (Ghent, 2005). With permission from © 2005 Elsevier

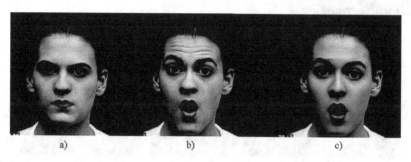

picked up from a set of 9 canonical trained gesture deformations.

Ghent and McDonald (Ghent, 2005) introduce two statistical models named facial expression shape model and facial expression texture model, both derived from FACS. The procedure allows for the generation of a universal mapping function. To map a neutral image of a face to an image of the same subject posing an expression, several radial basis function based neural networks were trained. Figure 5 depicts one person with original and synthesized expression.

Malatesta et al (Malatesta, 2006) extended the work of Raouzaiou et al (Raouzaiou, 2002) by combining MPEG-4 FAPs and action units (AUs) with the help of appraisal theory. The appraisal theory comes from the psychology field and was proposed by Scherer (Scherer, 2001) in order to investigate the connection between the elicitation of an emotion and the response patterning in facial expression. This approach can conduct to intermediate expressions based on sequential checks and derives a cumulative effect on the final combined expression. The theory was directly applied to generate intermediate expressions of hot anger and fear. To generate the cumulative effect the transaction between frames was considered to yield the final expression. Each intermediate expression is derived by the addition of the AUs of the current expression to the AUs of the previous appraisal check. However, as noted by authors, the appraisal method could lead to confusion in

the final expression when subsequent expressions are constituted of conflicting animations. For instance, when one intermediate expression includes raised eyebrows ("novelty high" corresponding to anger) and the next intermediate prediction is "goal obstructive" with the predicted facial deformation as lowered eyebrows, those effects would cancel each other. Deng and Neumann (Deng, 2006) proposed a facial expression synthesis system where the animation is controlled by phoneme-isomap space. The isomap framework is introduced for generating low-dimensional manifolds for each phoneme cluster. Given novel-aligned speech input and its emotion features the system automatically generates expressive facial animation by concatenating captured motion data. The best-matched captured motion nodes are found in the database by minimizing a cost function. The method is a data-driven approach and its computational complexity limits the application for real-time expression synthesis. Deng et al (Deng et al, 2006) further extended the work by proposing an approach where learned co-articulation models are concatenated to synthesise neutral visual speech according to novel speech input. A texture-synthesis-based method is next employed to generate novel expression from a phoneme-independent expression eigenspace model that is finally blended with the synthesized neutral visual speech to create the final expressive facial animation. The system overview is depicted in Figure 6.

Figure 6. System overview proposed by Deng et al. Here both audio and motion are simultaneously captured as input for the novel model. (Deng et al, 2006). In the figure, Mocap refers to facial motion capture. With permission from © 2006 IEEE

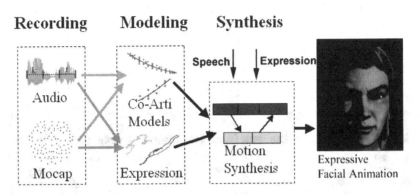

A statistical analysis based approach is proposed by Krinidis and Pitas (Krinidis, 2006) to synthesize facial expressions. The dynamic facial expression model is MPEG-4 compliant, i.e. the statistics is applied to facial animation parameters (FAPs) used by MPEG-4 standard, more precisely to the vectors' displacement. The advantage of this approach is that it permits the analysis of full facial expression animation, starting from a neutral pose to a fully expressive state. When a large face database is available,

Huang and Su (Huang, 2006) propose a facial expression synthesis method based on nonlinear manifold learning for estimating the full facial expression subspace and to create a so-called hallucinated facial expression. The whole process is accomplished in two steps. The first step is related to learning the subspace (manifold) of face images with neutral expression to retrieve the intrinsic parameters of that manifold. The same procedure is applied for face images with happiness expression. The relationship between the two manifolds is learned. The second step concerns the inference issue. More precisely, the parameters of an input face image with neutral expression are obtained and its happy parameters learned from the first step are inferred to reconstruct the happy face image using the happy parameters. The authors reported fairly realistic expressions close to the

ground truth. Lee and Elgammal also employed nonlinear manifold decomposition to extract shape and appearance models for facial expression synthesis (Lee, 2006). An empirical kernel mapping is employed for learning low-dimensional nonlinear manifolds that encode facial dynamics from a larger face database. To achieve accurate shape normalized appearance images a thin−plate spline (TPS) warping is used, where every image is warped with its corresponding shape vector into a new image given shape landmark points. Song et al (Song, 2006) proposed an appearance based method where the subtle changes in face deformations and are captured by decomposing the vector field expressed by Helmholtz-Hodge (HH) equations. Different expression states are treated as 3D vector field of the luminance variation. Three sets of feature points, one for the image S of source neutral, one for the source expression S' and the third one T corresponding to the target neutral expression are formed (manually or automatically). The corresponding images are aligned and the motion vector of the feature points between S and S' is computed. A geometric warping on T is next performed. A pixel triangulation on S, S' and T is performed to build the correspondence between the source and target face image 3D vector field. Finally, a HH decomposition based expression mapping is carried out followed by a

Figure 7. Synthesized facial expression images of a new person (Wang, 2008). From left to right: neutral, anger, disgust, fear, happiness, sadness, surprise. First row: original sample face. Second row: the proposed method. Third row: eigentransformation with shape alignment. Fourth row: direct warping of the original face. With permission from © 2008 Elsevier

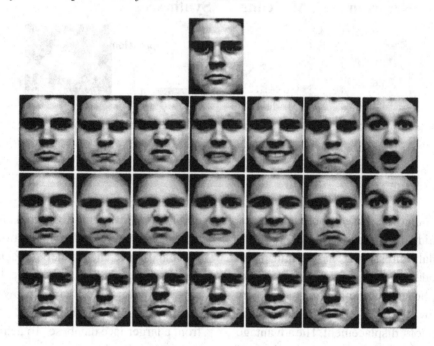

pixel's luminance update according to the novel values. One advantage of the method is its robustness against illumination variation.

The facial expression dynamics expressed over time is described as discrete-time sequences of random feature vectors by Mana and Pianesi (Mana, 2006). They have employed Hidden Markov Models (HMMs) that are trained on a set of different facial expression appearances with different intensities. The model is next used to generate sequences of feature vectors according to the probability lows that are described by the parameters of the model itself. The vectors are further converted to FAPs according to the MPEG-4 standards. The idea of using manifold for generating facial expression is also embraced by Wang and Wang (Wang, 2008). A person- independent facial expression space is introduced and different subjects with different facial expression intensity are aligned using supervised localized preserving

projections. The method not only allows generating basic realistic facial expressions but also mixed expression synthesis. Figure 7 shows the results of the proposed method in comparison with other two approaches.

Sucontphunt et al (Sucontphunt, 2008) developed an interactive system to synthesize 3D facial expressions through 2D portrait manipulation. Pre-recorded facial motion capture database is required for generating fine details. The system exploits the fact that 2D portrait typically relates prominent features of human faces and editing in 2D space is more intuitive than directly working on 3D face meshes. During the editing process the user moves one or a group of 2D control points on the portrait while the rest of the control points are automatically adjusted. The 2D portrait is also used as a query input to reconstruct the corresponding 3D facial expression from the pre-recorded facial motion capture database.

Zhang et al (Zhang 2008) proposed a probabilistic framework based on a coupled Bayesian network (BN) for synthesizing facial expressions through MPEG-4 FAPs while achieving very low bitrate in data transmission. The FAPs and FACS are cast into a dynamic BN while a static BN is used to reconstruct the FAPs along with their intensity. The proposed architecture is suitable for data transmission as 9 bytes / frame can be achieved. Due to the fact that the facial expression is inferred through both spatial and temporal inference the perceptual quality of animation is less affected by the misdetected FAPs when compared to facial expression synthesis using directly the original FAPs, as illustrated in Figure 8.

To capture a large range of variations in expressive appearance, a deep belief network with multiple layers is proposed by Susskind et al (Susskind, 2008). The network is able to learn association specific identities and facial actions in a cleaver way so that, novel combinations of identities and facial actions may be generated by blending them, even for unseen faces (not included in the training process).

The survey of facial expression synthesis we provided herein is not an extensive survey. Rather, we tried to provide a wide spectrum of techniques that we found applicable and promising in this trade. Next, we will try to provide a set of applications relying on the currently available facial expression synthesis technology.

Applications of Facial Expression Synthesis

We categorize the applications of facial expression synthesis in two classes in terms of their physical support: computer generated (cartoon or more

Figure 8. FAP errors (Zhang 2008). The row represents the animation outcome from the Zhang et al. method, while the bottom row shows the results of directly applying the original FAPs. Animation artifacts are visible in this case around the mouth region

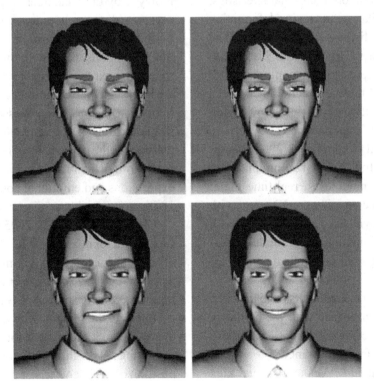

Figure 9. System overview proposed by Chandrasiri et al (Chandrasiri, 2002). With permission from © 2002 IEEE

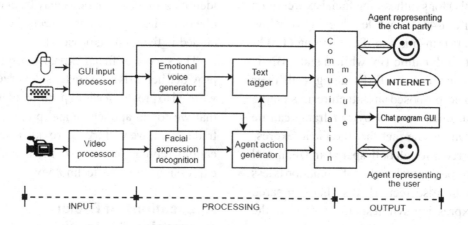

realistic) avatars and social robots. For the first category, applications of facial expression synthesis mainly involve the creation of embodied conversational agents for general communications, either in the form of animated avatars or, more simply, "talking heads". We should note here that, the "talking heads", in their simpler form, do not necessarily imply emotional state characteristics; they may simply imitate mouth region deformation for more or less realistic speech formation. The existing works either deform facial features to imitate the 6 basic expressions or manipulate AUs to animate artificial muscles, while other works carry out the animation process by employing MPEG-4 compliant facial parameters.

Chandrasiri et al (Chandrasiri, 2002) developed a system for Internet chat communication composed of three modules: a real-time facial expression analysis component, a 3D agent with facial expression synthesis and text-to-speech capabilities and a communication module. Figure 9 depicts the system components and their relationship.

The system takes several inputs from the user, such as the current user face with the help of a head-mounted video camera, keyboard and mouse messages. The user face appearance is converted into MPEG-4 compliant FAPs and special tags

for text-to-speech synthesis engines are inserted into the chat message using an emotional voice generator module to carry prosody information. The FAPs are also processed by an agent action generator that decides on the appropriate animation intensity command to be sent over to the agent representing the user. The agent actions are replayed by the local agent representation of the user providing some feedback about his behaviour during the chat conversation. Those agent animation commands along with the tagged chat messages are next transmitted to the chart party over the Internet by the communication module. In the same time, the module processes the data coming from other chat parties and passes it to the agents that decode the user emotional state and representing it through facial deformation with synthesized expressions and emotional content voice. Figure 10 illustrates a chat session example.

Choi and Kim (Choi, 2005) proposed a basic framework for integrating the 3D facial animation of an avatar on a PDA via mobile network. In addition, eye-gaze of the user is incorporated using an eye-tracker approach. Basically, the system first detects the facial area within a given image then classifies the expression into 7 emotional weightings. This information along with the eye position of the user is transmitted to the PDA and

Figure 10. A chat session using the system proposed by Chandrasiri et al (Chandrasiri, 2002). Both agents, the chat window setup and live video window are depicted. With permission from © 2002 IEEE

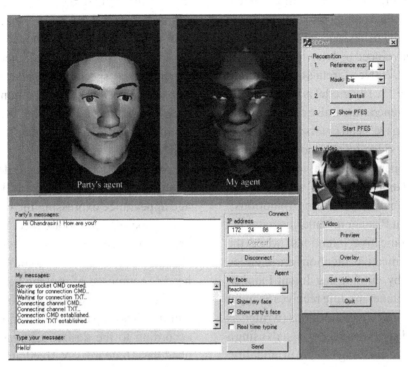

used for non-photorealistic facial expression animation for the PDA avatar. On the other hand, Albrecht et al. (Albrecht, 2005) created photorealistic animations of a talking head capable of expressing a continuum of shades of emotion. The proposed system is able to generate facial expressions with various intensities and also mixed emotions by blending basic emotions. Zhang et al. (Zhang, 2007) proposed PEP to depict the facial expression movements for a Chinese talking avatar, acting as mid-level parameters between FAPs and PAD. The PAD-PEP mapping model and PEP-FAP translation model are then implemented to translate the PAD parameters to PEP parameters and then to FAP parameters for facial expression synthesis. The PAD values are calculated using the method described in (Mehrabian 1996).

Most recently, the work of Catherine Pelachaud and her colleagues greatly contributed to the development of virtual agents expressing emotions

through facial expressions, gaze, body movement, gesture and voice (Pelachaud, 2009). The dynamics of each facial deformation is defined by three parameters: the expression intensity (magnitude) is controlled through a spatial extent; the expression duration (onset, apex and offset) is controlled by a temporal parameter; the deformation acceleration is also controlled. Although impressive, the model is limited to the six basic emotions. Niewiadomski et al. (Niewiadomski et, 2009a) proposed an algorithm for generating multimodal sequential expressions where the expressions enable the recognition of other affective states that are not prototypical expression of the six basic emotions (such as relief, for instance). In their second paper, Niewiadomski et al. (Niewiadomski et, 2009b) evaluate the recognition of expression representing 8 emotional states that are generated over a ECA face. They have reported high recognition rate (a maximum of 93% for angry and a minimum of 41% of embarrassment, often confused with anxiety and tension), suggesting a reliable model in expressing distinctive emotions. A conversational agent embodied in a 3D face named Greta, that tries to achieve a believable behaviour while interacting with a user was developed by Niewiadomski et al. (Niewiadomski et, 2009c). Greta's architecture is depicted in Figure 11. The model is not limited to facial expression generation, it also communicates through gestures, gaze, head or torso movements. User's audio and video information is captured for generating proper model behaviour. An FML-APML XML – language is used to specify the agent's communicative intentions (emotions). The Listener Intent Planner module generates the listener's communicative intentions, while the speaker's communicative intentions are intended to be preformed by the Speaker Intent Planner. The Behaviour Planner module receives as input the agent's communicative intensions (written as FNL-AMPL) and generates a list of signals using a BML tag each corresponding to a given modality: head, torso, face gaze, gesture or speech. Furthermore, signalling through the Behaviour Realizer generates the MPEG4 FAP-BAS files which, in turn, results in an animation through a dedicated player. The modules are synchronized using a central clock and a Psyclone messaging system.

An interesting application of facial expression application is proposed by Vogiatzis et al. (Vogiatzis, 2008) who mapped synthetic facial expressions into an INDIGO robot (http://www.ics.forth.

Figure 11. Greta's architecture

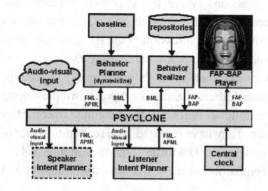

gr/indigo/) that serves as a guide for a museum. The robot's affective component is described in terms of three issues, i.e., personality, emotional state and the mood, while the facial expression is described by different components such as lip-synchronized speech, face idle emotions, emotional expressions, conversational expressions and look-at behaviour. The facial expression synthesis information is converted into MPEG-4 FAPs.

Another robot application is developed by Ge et al (Ge, 2008) who mapped 2D real face image appearance expressing the 6 basic emotions into an expressive robotic face. Unlike the robot proposed by Vogiatzis et al., where facial expressions are displayed on a monitor, the Ge's robot head is composed of moving parts imitating the facial components such as eyebrows, eyes, eyelids and lips. Those parts are moved by servomotors according to the desired expression. The robot head has 16 degrees of freedom. The robot first detects and recognizes the facial expression of a human then imitates it. The input consists of two images, one corresponding to the neutral one and one corresponding to the desired expression. When the human changes his facial expression the difference between the two images is derived and the displacement and velocity information is extracted. This information is further multiplied by a weight vector to reach the desired animation effect on a robot head. The weight vector is added on the face plane of the robot head in its neutral state (default state) forcing the facial parts to move and simulate the human's expression. Figure 12 depicts two examples for "happy" and "surprise" expression, respectively. This application resembles learning by imitation which is observed in chimpanzees and humans through the mirror neuron and pre-motor systems found in frontal lobe.

The work of Cynthia Breazel and her colleagues (Breazel et al., 2009) is, perhaps, the most prominent in the field of emotional robots. Her work focuses in creating social robots that interact with

Figure 12. Human expression imitation by a robot (Ge, 2008). Detected keyframes associated to the video (left), the recognized expression (middle) and the corresponding response of the robot. With permission from © 2008 IEEE

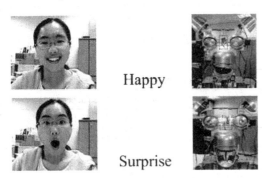

humans and imitate their emotional states. The first robot called Kismet (Breazel, 2002) is augmented with expression performing capabilities. Kismet acts like babies to encourage exaggerated expressions of emotion in people. Her most recent robot Leonardo combines art with state of the art research in social intelligent robots.

RELATED PROJECTS AND SOFTWARES

The importance of the human-computer interaction and, in particular, the development of intelligent and expressive human-like machines is emphasized through large EU projects, such as SEMAINE (http://www.semaine-project.eu/), HUMAINE (http://emotion-research.net/), or dedicated workshops (http://www.enterface.net/). Open source or facial expression oriented freely distributed software tools include Xface (http://xface.itc.it/index.htm) for creating MPEG-4 and keyframe based 3D talking heads or Greta (http://www.tsi.enst.fr/~pelachau/Greta/).

DISCUSSIONS AND CONCLUSIONS

In this chapter we have tried to review the most prominent state-of-the-art techniques for facial expression synthesis and animation prospectively. Table 3 summarizes the approaches described in this Chapter along with their shortcomings and descriptors used.

Applications of this topic to real life, including embodied conversational agents enhanced or humanoid robots with affective components are also briefly discussed.

From the synthesis point of view, both geometry and appearance approaches have their own specific limitations. The problem with the geometry based (and more specifically the physically) approaches is the difficulty of generating natural looking expressions obtained for subtle skin deformation such as wrinkles and furrows. The main advantage of these approaches is that they are, generally, subject independent. On the other hand, because the appearance approaches rely on morphing and warping techniques, modeling requires a large database. These approaches (especially PCA and manifold based techniques) find emotional subspaces using subjects from the database, thus, mapping one expression from a subject in the database to another unseen (not included in the database) subject, sometimes leading to unsatisfactory results.

Apart from the approach dependent drawbacks, all current methods share (more or less) issues that are insufficiently tackled:

- *Open mouth issue.* This issue appears for certain expression, such as happiness or surprise and is more specific to appearance approaches. When going from neutral to surprise, teeth appear, and, consequently, they must be modeled as well. A few works accurately addressed this issue, most works ignoring this aspect (see below).
- *Frontal pose.* Most approaches were developed and tested only to subjects with

Table 3. Summary of facial expression synthesis techniques presented in the chapter

Method	Descriptors and characteristics	Shortcomings
(Blader, 1981)	Set of muscles attached to a skin mesh	Lack of natural expressions
(Waters, 1987)	Sphincter muscles	Does not address fine details as temporal wrinkles
(Terzopoulos, 1990)	Set of muscles attached to a skin mesh plus a third layer (fat tissue)	Does not address fine details as temporal wrinkles
(Hoch, 1994)	B-spline and 4 AUs	Lack of natural expressions
(Pighin, 2002)	3D Face mesh	It requires a set of images and it is face-dependent.
(Zhang, 2002)	FACS	Does not address wrinkles and teeth model
(Zhang, 2006)	134 facial points	Blending artefacts, lack of a reliable extrapolation method
(Yin, 2001)	Extended dynamic mesh (2954 vertices and 3118 patches)	Unrealistic facial expressions
(Liu, 2001)	Expression ratio image	It requires the expression ratio image from the performer.
(Raouzaiou, 2002)	FAPs and FATs	Limited facial deformation
(Wang, 2003)	Statistical method based on singular value decomposition of a training data	Not applicable for images not included in the training data.
(Abboud 2004)	Active Appearance Model	Not applicable for images not included in the training data.
(Tewes, 2005)	Gabor wavelet based flexible object model derived from graph nodes (landmarks)	Its accuracy highly depends on the landmarks location.
(Ghent, 2005)	Texture and shape model derived from FACS	Unrealistic facial expressions
(Malatesta, 2006)	FAPs + AUs	It generates confusion when subsequent expressions are constituted of conflicting animations.
(Deng, 2006)	Eigenspace model	Not applicable for images not included in the training data.
(Krinidis, 2006)	FAPs	Not applicable for images not included in the training data.
(Huang, 2006)	Manifold (learning) model	Large database requirement
(Lee, 2006)	Nonlinear manifold (learning) model	Large database requirement
(Mana, 2006)	HMM and FAPs	It highly depends on the training set
(Wang, 2008)	Manifold (learning) model	Large database requirement
(Sucontphunt, 2008)	3D face meshes	Computational expensive and requires extensive user interaction
(Zhang 2008)	FAPs, FACS and Bayesian Network	Large database requirement
(Susskind, 2008)	Deep Belief Nework	Large database requirement

frontal pose, although some works had dealt with 3D scanned images. Modeling facial expressions along with rotated faces is much difficult and requires high compu-

tational load, making the process unattractive for the current real-time facial expression synthesis models.

- *Illumination problem.* This is a common issue to any face related analysis. The reflection of human skin is approximately specular when the angle between the view direction and lighting direction is around 90^0. The light reflection should be treated seriously, as slight illumination variation (in its direction or intensity) may lead to failure in accurate synthesis of facial expression, particularly when the morphing step is employed. While other face analysis topics, such as face recognition for instance, addressed this issue, not much work was devoted in the literature for facial expression synthesis. Approaches borrowed from the face recognition field (including image gradients or illumination cone model) may help in accurately synthesizing facial expression under uncontrolled illumination variation.

- *Smooth deformation of fine geometric details.* Geometric details are important for human perception and measure the emotion intensity. However, they are difficult to be synthesized and to smoothly deform them is even harder so that the expression is realistically generated.

- *The own-race bias.* This term refers to the tendency of people to be more accurate in perceiving and recognizing differences amongst the faces of their own race than those pertaining to other racial groups. For the particular case of facial expression, several studies indicated major differences in facial expression perception of different race groups. For instance, comparing British and Japanese people asked to decipher non-verbal relationships in photographs, Kito and Lee (Kito, 2006) have found that Japanese participants were generally better at understanding subtle information provided by facial expression to decipher interpersonal relationships. In another study, Elfenbein and Amady

(Elfenbein, 2002) brought evidence that the emotion recognition accuracy was higher when emotions were expressed and perceived by participants from the same "cultural" group. The own race bias concept highly relates to the fourth major and generic objective of the expression synthesizer, i.e., easy and accurate model adaptation to individual faces. Although important for universal facial expression mapping, this issue was not addressed, to our knowledge, by scientists involved in creation of facial expression synthesis models.

- *Generating distinctive (non-ambiguous) synthetic facial expression.* This is a common issue with the human ability of accurately discriminate between some particular emotions. Humans often confuse, for instance, fear and surprise due to the fact that they are perceptually similar and engage common muscle configuration and AUs. *Fear* and *surprise* share 5 common AUs out of 7 (see Table 2). Similar findings were reported when facial expressions have been classified automatically (Buciu et al, 2003). The difficulty of accurately recognizing these two emotions by both humans and machines, and, moreover, the almost common corresponding AUs set consequently leads to problems in generating distinctive associated synthetic facial expression for *fear* and *surprise*.

The first four issues above have been recently addressed by the Digital Emily Project that is a collaboration between the facial animation company Image Metrics and the Graphics Laboratory at the University of Southern California's Institute for Creative Technologies (see http://gl.ict.usc.edu/Research/DigitalEmily/ and Alexander et al (Alexander et al, 2009). The common work employs latest generation techniques in high-resolution face scanning, character rigging, video-based animation and compositing (blending). An actress

Figure 13. High resolution 3D geometry from fourteen of the thirty-three facial scans of the Emily actress's face posing several facial expressions (Alexander et al, 2009). With permission from © 2009 IEEE

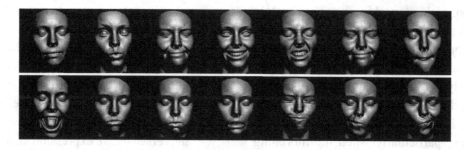

Figure 14. (a) A plaster cast of Emily actress's upper and lower teeth. (b) Tesulting merged 3D model before remeshing. (c) Remeshed model (Alexander et al, 2009). With permission from © 2009 IEEE

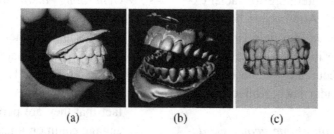

(a) (b) (c)

is first filmed on a studio set speaking emotive lines. The light variation is captured as a high dynamic range light probe image while the face of the actress is three-dimensional scanned in thirty-three facial expressions down to the level of skin pores and fine wrinkles. Animated eyes and teeth was added to the model and a semi-automatic video-based facial animation system was used to animate the 3Dface do to match the performance seen in the original video. The final face is also illuminated using the acquired reflectance maps with a complex skin translucency shading algorithm. The resulting model was generally accepted as being a real face. Figure 13 illustrates several high-resolution scans of the actress' face posing several facial expressions, while Figure 14 depicts the process of generating the model's teeth. It should be noticed that each resulting face mesh contains approximately three million polygons while the artificial teeth mesh is generated using 600.000 polygons, both processes requiring high

computational load and resources. Despite being highly detailed and accurate, the expression scans require some pre-processing before blending into the final model. Mesh artifacts around teeth and eye regions may occur due to irregular edges with poor triangulation.

The applications involving humanoid robots also have limitations. On one hand, emotional robots with higher degree of freedom have to be built. The higher the degree of freedom, the more natural expression is achieved. On the other hand, robots with high degree of freedom may suffer from the uncanny valley issue, defined as the repulsion among humans caused by "too" human-like robots (MacDorman, 2006), leading to creepy robot faces. A fundamental question still remains when mapping a synthetic expression either to an affective robot or a computer generated avatar: what is the minimal level of display in order to generate an emphatic response and avoid thus the frightening effect when exaggerated (deformation) expressions are posed ? How social intelligent robots plan appropriate actions according to stimuli is another challenge. The issue is complex and involves advanced learning strategies that have to be addressed and implemented in the future.

The ultimate goal of human-computer interaction concerning the development of friendly human interfaces is the necessity of having real-time photo-realistic expression synthesis for unseen images. Although current implementations are close to achieving this goal (see Digital Emily Project), to date this complex requirement is still not fully accomplished, in spite of great endeavor provided by a large number of computer scientists and researchers. In addition, the human-computer interface is not limited to realistic facial expression synthesis, but also realistic gestures, eye gazes or natural lip movements, presenting important issues to be carefully addressed.

REFERENCES

Abboud, B., & Davoine, F. (2004) Appearance factorization based facial expression recognition and synthesis. In *IEEE International Conference on Pattern Recognition*, 958 – 965.

Albrecht, I., Schröder, M., Haber, J., & Seidel, H.-P. (2005). Mixed feelings: expression of non-basic emotions in a muscle-based talking head. *Virtual Reality (Waltham Cross)*, *8*(4), 201–212. doi:10.1007/s10055-005-0153-5

Alexander, O., Rogers, M., Lambeth, W., Chiang, M., & Debevec, P. (2009), Creating a Photoreal Digital Actor: The Digital Emily Project, *IEEE European Conference on Visual Media Production* (CVMP).

Badler, N., & Platt, S. (1981). Animating facial expressions. *Computer Graphics*, 245–252.

Breazeal, C. (2002). *Designing Sociable Robots.* MIT Press.

Breazeal, C., Gray, J., & Berlin, M. (2009). An embodied cognition approach to mindreading skills for socially intelligent robots. *The International Journal of Robotics Research*, *28*(5), 656–680. doi:10.1177/0278364909102796

Buciu, I., Kotropoulos, C., & Pitas, I. (2003) ICA and Gabor representations for facial expression recognition. *IEEE International Conference on Image Processing (ICIP 2003)*, September 14-17,Barcelona, Spain, pp. 1054 – 1057.

Chandrasiri, N. P., Barakonyi, I., Naemura, T., Ishizuka, M., & Harashima, H. (2002) Communication over the Internet using a 3D agent with real-time facial expression analysis, synthesis and text to speech capabilities. In *Proceeding of the 8th International Conference on Communication Systems*, 01, 480 – 484.

Choi, S.-M., & Kim, Y.-G. (2005) An affective user interface based on facial expression recognition and eye – gaze tracking. *First International Conference on Affective Computing & Intelligent Interaction*, 3784, 907 – 914.

Deng, Z., & Neumann, U. (2006) eFASE: expressive facial animation synthesis and editing with phoneme-isomap controls. *Proceedings of the 2006 ACM SIGGRAPH/Eurographics Symposium on Computer Animation* (LNCS, 251 – 260).,New York: Springer.

Deng, Z., Neumann, U., Lewis, J. P., Kin, T.-Y., & Bulut, M. (2006). Expressive facial animation synthesis by learning speech coarticulation and expression spaces. *IEEE Transactions on Visualization and Computer Graphics*, *12*(6), 1523–1534. doi:10.1109/TVCG.2006.90

Ekman, P., & Friesen, W. V. (1978). *Facial Action Coding System. Consulting Psychologists Press.* Alto, CA: Palo.

Ekman, P., Friesen, W. V., & Hager, J. C.,(2002). *Facial Action Coding System*. The Manual.

Elfenbein, H. A., & Ambady, N. (2002). On the universality and cultural specificity of emotion recognition: A meta-analysis. *Psychological Bulletin, 128*, 203–235. doi:10.1037/0033-2909.128.2.203

Ge, S. S., Wang, C., & Hang, C. C. (2008). A Facial Expression Imitation System in Human Robot Interaction, *The 17th IEEE International Symposium on Robot and Human Interactive Communication*, 213 – 218.

Ghent, J., & McDonald, J. (2005). Photo-realistic facial expression synthesis. *Image and Vision Computing, 23*(12), 1041–1050. doi:10.1016/j.imavis.2005.06.011

Hoch, M., Fleischmann, G., & Girod, B. (1994). Modeling and animation of facial expressions based on B-splines. *The Visual Computer, 11*, 87–95. doi:10.1007/BF01889979

Huang, L., & Su, C. (2006). Facial expression synthesis using manifold learning and belief propagation. *Soft Computing - A Fusion of Foundations. Methodologies and Applications, 10*(12), 1193–1200.

Kito, T., & Lee, B. (2004). Interpersonal perception in Japanese and British observers. *Perception, 33*, 957–974. doi:10.1068/p3471

Krinidis, S., Buciu, I., & Pitas, I. (2003*). Facial expression analysis and synthesis: A survey.* Proceedings of HCI International, 10th Int. Conference on Human-Computer Interaction, pp. 1432 – 1433, June 22-27, Crete, Greece.

Krinidis, S., & Pitas, I. (2006) Facial expression synthesis through facial expressions statistical analysis. In *Proc. 2006 European Signal Processing Conference.*

Lee, C.-S., & Elgammal, A. (2006) Nonlinear shape and appearance models for facial expression analysis and synthesis. *International Conference on Pattern Recognition, 1*, 497 – 502.

Liu, Z., Shan, Y., & Zhang, Z. (2001). Expressive expression mapping with ratio images. *In International Conference on Computer Graphics and Interactive Techniques (SIGGRAPH)*, 271 – 276.

MacDorman, K. F. (2006). Subjective ratings of robot video clips for human likeness, familiarity, and eeriness: An exploration of the uncanny valley. *Proceedings of the ICCS/CogSci-2006 Long Symposium: Toward Social Mechanisms of Android Science.*

Malatesta, L., Raouzaiou, A., Karpouzis, K., & Kollias, S. (2006). MPEG-4 facial expression synthesis based on appraisal theory, *3rd IFIP Conference* on *Artificial Intelligence Applications and Innovations*, 378 – 384.

Mana, N., & Pianesi, F. (2006) HMM-based synthesis of emotional facial expressions during speech in synthetic talking heads. In Proc. International Conference on Multimodal Interfaces, 380 – 387.

Mehrabian, A. (1968). Communication without words. *Psychology Today, 2*(4), 53–56.

Mehrabian, A. (1996). Pleasure-arousal-dominance: A general framework for describing and measuring individual differences in temperament. *Current Psychology (New Brunswick, N.J.), 14*, 261–292. doi:10.1007/BF02686918

Niewiadomski, R., Bevacqua, E., Maurizio, M., & Pelachaud, C., (2009c) Greta: an interactive expressive ECA system. *AAMAS* (2), pp. 1399-1400

Niewiadomski, R., Hyniewska, S., & Pelachaud, C. (2009a) Modeling emotional expressions as sequences of Behaviors, International conference on Intelligent virtual agents IVA'09, Amsterdam.

Niewiadomski, R., Hyniewska, S., & Pelachaud, C. (2009b) Evaluation of Multimodal Sequential Expressions of Emotions in ECA, International conference on Affective Computing & Intelligent Interaction ACII'09, Amsterdam.

Pelachaud, C., (2009) Modelling Multimodal Expression of Emotion in a Virtual Agent, *Philosophical Transactions of Royal Society B Biological Science*, B, 364, pp. 3539-3548.

Pighin, F., Szeliski, R., & Salesin, D., H. (2002). Modeling and animating realistic faces from images. *International Journal of Computer Vision*, *50*(2), 143–169. doi:10.1023/A:1020393915769

Raouzaiou, A., Tsapatsoulis, N., Karpouzis, K., & Kollias, S. (2002). Parameterized Facial Expression Synthesis Based on MPEG-4. *EURASIP Journal on Applied Signal Processing*, (10): 1021–1038. doi:10.1155/S1110865702206149

Scherer, K. R. (2001) Appraisal considered as a process of multilevel sequential checking. In Scherer, K.R., Schorr, A., & Johnstone, T., (Eds) *Appraisal Processes in Emotion: Theory Methods*, Research. Oxford, New York: Oxford University Press, 92-129.

Song, M., Wang, H., Bu, J., Chen, C., & Liu, Z. (2006) Subtle facial expression modeling with vector field decomposition. In *IEEE International Conference on Image Processing*, 2101 – 2104.

Sucontphunt, T., Mo, Z., Neumann, U., & Deng, Z. (2008) Interactive 3D facial expression posing through 2D portrait manipulation. *Proceeding of Graphics Interface*, 71(10 – 12), 177 – 184.

Susskind, J. M., Hinton, G. E., Movellan, J. R., & Anderson, A. K. (2008). Generating Facial Expressions with Deep Belief Nets. In Kordic, V. (Ed.), *Affective Computing, Emotion Modelling, Synthesis and Recognition*. ARS Publishers.

Susskind, J. M., Littlewort, G., Bartlett, M. S., Movellan, J. R., & Anderson, A. K. (2007). Human and computer recognition of facial expressions of emotion. *Neuropsychologia*, *45*(1), 152–162. doi:10.1016/j.neuropsychologia.2006.05.001

Terzopoulos, D., & Waters, K. (1990). Physically-based facial modeling and animation. *Journal of Visualization and Computer Animation*, *1*(4), 73–80.

Tewes, A., Würtz, R. P., & Von der Malsburg (2005) A flexible object model for recognising and synthesising facial expressions. In Takeo Kanade, Nalini Ratha, & Anil Jain (eds.), *Proceedings of the International Conference on Audio- and Video-based Biometric Person Authentication*,(LNCS, 81-90) Springer.

Vogiatzis, D., Spyropoulos, C., Konstantopoulos, S., Karkaletsis, V., Kasap, Z., Matheson, C., & Deroo, O. (2008) An affective robot guide to museums. *In Proc. 4th International Workshop on Human-Computer Conversation*.

Wang, H., & Ahuja, N. (2003) Facial expression decomposition. In *IEEE International Conference on Computer Vision*, 958 – 965.

Wang, H. & Wang, K. (2008) Affective interaction based on person independent facial expression space. *Neurocomputing, Special Issue for Vision Research*, 71(10 – 12), 1889 – 1901.

Waters, K. (1987). A muscle model for animating three – dimensional facial expression. *Computer Graphics*, *22*(4), 17–24. doi:10.1145/37402.37405

Yin, L., Basu, A., Bernögger, S., & Pinz, A. (2001). Synthesizing realistic facial animations using energy minimization for model-based coding. *Pattern Recognition*, *34*(11), 2201–2213. doi:10.1016/S0031-3203(00)00139-4

Yongmian, Z. Q. J. Z. Z. B. Y. (2008). Dynamic Facial Expression Analysis and Synthesis With MPEG-4 Facial Animation Parameters. *IEEE Trans. on Circuits and Systems for Video Technology*, *18*(10), 1383–1396. doi:10.1109/TC-SVT.2008.928887

Zhang, Q., Liu, Z., Guo, B., Terzopoulos, D., & Shum, H.-Y. (2006). Geometry – driven photo-realistic facial expression shyntesis. *IEEE Trans. on Visualization and Computer Graphics*, *12*(1), 48–60. doi:10.1109/TVCG.2006.9

Zhang, S., Wu, Z., Meng, H. M., & Cai, L. (2007) Facial expression synthesis using PAD emotional parameters for a chinese expressive avatar. *In Proceedings of the 2nd International Conference on Affective Computing and Intelligent Interaction*, 4738, 24 – 35.

Zhang, Y., & Prakash, E., C., & Sung, E. (2002). Constructing a realistic face model of an individual for expression animation. *International Journal of Information Technology*, *8*(2), 10–25.

KEY TERMS AND DEFINITIONS

Embodied Conversational Agents (ECAs): Friendly and intelligent user interfaces built to mimic human gestures, speech or facial expressions.

Facial Action Unit (AUs): A facial action unit is an objective description of facial signals in terms of component motions.

Facial Action Coding System (FACS): A system developed to encode a comprehensive set of all possible visually distinguishable facial appearances by measuring specific facial muscle movements.

Facial Action Parameters (FAPs): Geometrical facial descriptors.

Face Animation Tables (FATs): MPEG-4 compliant values of model vertices used to deform the face geometry.

PAD Parameters: High-level parameters defined as pleasure-displeasure (P), arousal-nonarousal (A) and dominance-submissiveness (D) use to express a continuous facial space model for describing universal emotions.

Partial Expression Parameters (PEP): middle level facial parameters describing the facial motion.

Section 4
Affect in Language–Based Communication

Chapter 10
The Role of Affect and Emotion in Language Development

Annette Hohenberger
Middle East Technical University, Turkey

ABSTRACT

In this chapter, language development is discussed within a social-emotional framework. Children's language processing is gated by social and emotional aspects of the interaction, such as affective prosodic and facial expression, contingent reactions, and joint attention. Infants and children attend to both cognitive and affective aspects in language perception ("language" vs. "paralanguage") and in language production ("effort" vs. "engagement"). Deaf children acquiring a sign language go through the same developmental milestones in this respect. Modality-independently, a tripartite developmental sequence emerges: (i) an undifferentiated affect-dominated system governs the child's behavior, (ii) a cognitive and language-dominated system emerges that attenuates the affective system, (iii) emotional expression is re-integrated into cognition and language. This tightly integrated cognitive-affective language system is characteristic of adults. Evolutionary scenarios are discussed that might underlie its ontogeny. The emotional context of learning might influence the course and outcome of L2-learning, too.

INTRODUCTION

Language is a central aspect of human cognition. In cognitive science with its predominant computational perspective, cognition and language, as its core module, have been viewed as research areas that are strictly separated from emotion (Davidson,

2000; Smith & Kosslyn, 2007, chapter 8; Harris, Berko Gleason, & Aycicegi, 2006; Ochsner & Barrett, 2001; Niedenthal, 2007). Affect and emotion, which are inherently subjective processes and feelings, did not fit into the concept of the human mind that was thought to be governed by universal abstract symbols and rules. The two spheres were therefore considered orthogonal to each other, if not oppositional. Their interplay was

DOI: 10.4018/978-1-61692-892-6.ch010

only poorly understood (Forgas, 2008). Emotion was even defamed as a potentially destructive and subversive power that undermined the functioning of the rational mind (ibid.). However, following the 'cognitive revolution' in the middle of the 20th century, we now witness an 'emotion revolution' (Harris et al., 2006, p. 2258; Caldwell-Harris, 2008) in contemporary times. Emotion is no longer the pariah of cognitive science but is now becoming an increasingly respected partner of cognition.[1]

In this chapter, the role of affect and emotion in language development is surveyed. The intimate link between affective and language development has nowhere been more dramatically established than in the crude historical "experiments" in search for the "proto-language" of mankind. It is historically bequeathed that several emperors, namely the Pharaoh Psammetic, the Staufer King Frederic II, and the Scottish King Jacob IV arranged for rigorous experiments on newborns which they had deprived of any language and human companionship in order to find out what language they would develop. This language should then be considered the human proto-language. These experiments all failed: the poor infants either died (as in Frederic II's case) or uttered only some sparse proto-words (which, however, led Psammetic to conclude that Phrygian must be the proto-language and Jacob that it was Hebrew). Thus, the most basic condition which must be met for any language-learning to be possible at all is human companionship and the willingness to communicate, i.e, "human and humane contact." (Goldin-Meadow, 2003, p. 48; cf. also Hohenberger, 2004) A similar claim has been made for feral children grown up without any social and affective interaction (Kuhl, 2007, p. 116).

Although the link between affect and language is now well established, we still do not know the exact nature of this link. In this chapter, I will present various studies and views on the link between affect and language in infant and child development. In order to provide a neuroscience

backdrop to the present topic, neuropsychological studies are presented to the reader in the appendix.

THE SOCIAL-EMOTIONAL FRAMEWORK OF LANGUAGE DEVELOPMENT

The study of the social origins of language and cognitive development has its roots in the work of Bruner (1975, 1983) and Vygotsky (1962). They argue that all learning, i.e., also language learning, is rooted in social interaction, most notably between parents and their children (cf. also Tamis-LeMonda & Rodriguez, 2008; Paavola, 2006). Recently, the role of social interaction in cognitive and language development has received again much attention (Tomasello, 2003, 2008), in particular its neural underpinnings (Striano & Reid, 2006; Johnson, 2007, 2008; Grossmann & Johnson, 2007; Kuhl, 2007). This shift in focus from a predominantly computationally to a more socially oriented view of brain processes is relevant for our investigation here insofar as the social framing goes together with an affective framing. Johnson and Grossmann argue for the existence of a relatively independent network of brain areas for processing social stimuli, in short, a "social brain". This network comprises various areas that participate in processes such as face processing (including eye gaze processing), perception of emotions (in faces and in speech), perception of biological motion, human goal-directed action, and joint attention (Grossmann & Johnson, 2007). The level of neural processing drives cognitive processes which, under the additional influence of motivational and social factors, lead to social behavior and experience. Together, these three levels constitute the new area of "social cognitive neuroscience" (Lieberman, 2006). "Social developmental cognitive neuroscience" then takes into account the developmental aspect (Zelazo, Chandler, & Crone, 2009). Yet, an explicit mentioning of affect in (developmental) cognitive neuroscience is absent, still. Hence, there is a clear need in the future to add affect to the present view. In which way this could be done I want to exemplify with a recent proposal made by Kuhl (2007) on the role of the social brain in language acquisition.

Kuhl (2007) interprets the role of the "social brain" in terms of "gating" of the more computational aspects of language acquisition (phoneme discrimination, word segmentation, referential lexical learning) in the first year of life and beyond. Without social interaction language understanding and acquisition is impossible. In their own language learning studies Kuhl and her colleagues present evidence that 9-month old American infants learned to discriminate phonemes of a foreign language, namely Chinese, only through live interaction with a real person who played with them and not from TV or from auditory presentation alone (Kuhl, Tsao, & Liu, 2003). This phonemic learning was long-lasting and still showed up even after 33 days following the 4-5 week-long exposure to Chinese. In another experiment by Goldstein, King, and West (2003) the role of mothers' contingency on their infants' vocalization was tested. In a contingent condition mothers reacted responsively with smiling, approaching, and touching their infants when they vocalized. In a non-contingent control condition the same mothers' positive responses were shown to the child on a TV monitor – however, with a temporal delay that corrupted the original contingency. As a result, infants with contingent mothers showed more and more mature vocalizations (cf. Kuhl, 2007). Kuhl presents two possible mechanisms underlying the impact of social interaction on language development. On the first account, which she calls "attention and arousal" account and which I call here tendentiously "affective" account it is a global mechanism of motivation, attention, and arousal that positively affects language learning. Enhanced attention and arousal may lead to higher quantities and quality of language input which infants subsequently encode and remember better. Infant- or child-directed speech (ID, CD

speech), or, "motherese", is one aspect of this first account. Normal children but not children with autism spectrum disorder (ASD) tend to prefer ID/CD over non-ID/CD (Kuhl, 2007, p. 116). ID/CD is phonetically characterized by exaggerated phonemic contrasts and exaggerated pitch contours as well as clear segmentation clues. It is judged as highly affectionate and sensitive speech. On the second account, which she calls "information" account and which I call here tendentiously "cognitive" account, it is the specific information content present in a natural setting that positively affects language learning. For example, social cues such as eye gaze and pointing to a referent may help in word segmentation and later referential word learning. Through "joint attention" to an object of common interest between parent and infant and contingent behavior of the parent the infant learns to appreciate both the communicative intent of her interlocutor as well as the verbal labels of the objects referred to. This situation is referred to as "triadic interaction". In sum, interactivity and contingency are both relevant to successful communication.

The idea of social *alias* affective cognition as gating computational learning leads to an extension of Kuhl's original "Native Language Magnet" (NLM) model (Kuhl, 1993, 1994), now called "Native Language Magnet-Extended" (NLM-extended, Kuhl, 2007). The NLM is a perceptual effect that distorts the space around a language-specific phonetic prototype, attracting the phonetic processing to its area. The phonetic prototype acts like a magnet in guiding perception reliably to its center. Gradual variations that always exist in perception are attenuated and categorical boundaries are built up with the result that incoming noisy phonetic information is mapped onto stable phonemic categories that represent the language's distinctive phonemes. Thus, when the infant becomes a skilled listener of and neurally committed to the sounds of her own mother tongue by the end of the first year, it is through the attracting effect of the language magnet. The recent extension allows for a gating of this effect through social aspects, some of which can reasonably be interpreted as affective. Interestingly, however, Kuhl never speaks of "affect" or "affective", only of "social". Insofar the contribution of affect in the first "attention and arousal" account remains implicit. This ambiguity is certainly worthwhile being clarified in future research.

PARENT-CHILD INTERACTION

The way the primary caregivers interact with their infants and how infants respond and stimulate their caregivers is essential for infants' development. In an evolutionary perspective, a successful mutual adaptation of caregiver and child has crucial consequences for the reproductive success of the species (Preston & de Waal, 2002). If both parents and infants can be affected by each other's emotional state they may co-regulate each other's state and behavior. Although a transactional perspective, taking into account the mutual interactions and adaptations going on between parents and child, is certainly the best framework for child development (Baldwin, 1995; Preston & de Waal, 2002; Paavola, 2006), the bulk of the literature is on the impact of parents on child development. There is, indeed, a vast literature on the relation between parent-child and in particular mother-child interaction and the general cognitive and language development of young children (Bornstein & Tamis-LeMonda, 1989; Tamis-LeMonda, Bornstein, & Baumwell, 2001; Tamis-LeMonda & Rodriguez, 2008; Landry, 2008; IJzendoorn, Dijkstra, & Bus, 1995). In particular a sensitive or responsive[2] interactional style has been associated with positive outcomes. How is sensitive/responsive behavior towards infants and children characterized? Parental sensitivity in the interaction manifests itself mainly in affectively rich expressive behavior (facial, vocal), enjoyable body contact, and contingent and reciprocal interaction with the infant. As we have seen in the previous paragraph, contingent interaction in a setting of joint attention may modulate the gating of information that is crucial for language development (Kuhl, 2007). Responsive and sensitive interaction is therefore crucial in this respect. Child-directed speech (or "motherese") is just one aspect of parents' affective language behavior towards their children.[3]

Tamis-LeMonda and Rodriguez (2008, p. 2) point out three aspects of parenting that foster children's language development: (i) frequency of *children's engagement in routine language learning opportunities*, such as book reading and story-telling (ii) *quality of parent-child interaction*, in particular sensitivity/responsiveness, and (iii) offering *age-appropriate learning materials*, such as books and toys. Among these three, we shall focus on (ii) in the following. The quality of early parent-child interaction has been shown to be one the best predictors for early and later language learning. Rich and varied adult speech informs children about a wide range of objects and events and, importantly, on the affective attitude that their parents have towards them. Children whose parents respond contingently to their verbal utterances have a head-start into vocabulary development (ibid., p. 3).

Parents' Sensitivity to Informational and Affective Content in Their Infants' Vocalizations

However, already long before the occurrence of discernable verbal utterances, parents respond intuitively to infants' vocal signals expressing discomfort, comfort, neutral mood, or joy. Parents' affective response to these early vocalizations is considered as the basis for a secure attachment and affective attunement between the interactants (Papoušek, 1992, p. 239). Components of parental responsiveness are (i) the ability to decode information from infants' signals, (ii) readiness to respond (in terms of latency), and (iii) quality of response. With respect to decodability of information, Papoušek (1989) presented various groups of adults with 50 infant sounds (discomfort, comfort, joy) and asked them to estimate the quality and intensity of the sounds. As a result, she found that "voiced sounds in the infant's presyllabic vocal repertoire effectively transmit both discrete information pertaining to the categorical distinction between comfort and discomfort and graded information pertaining to the relative intensity of affective arousal." (Papoušek, 1992, p. 241) Moreover, adults spontaneously attribute meaning to these early vocalizations. With this inclination they anticipate later emerging meaningful and language-based communication with children. Parents' early and mostly correct intuitions about their offspring's vocalizations are an important driving force for building up successful interactions and for language development. Parents' responses are affect-based as well as content-based. Identifying the content and intensity of their infants' affective vocalizations and responding to them affectively results in affective attunement within the dyad (Friend, 1985; cf. Papoušek, 1992, p. 243). Adults' responsiveness, according to Papoušek, depends on perceptual and behavioral predispositions and not on experience, gender, and age. It has the effect of "scaffolding" a dyadic communicative setting within which the infant's vocalization has its proper structural slot already. Any vocal material the infant utters will wind up in this slot and will be interpreted by the parent as meaningful and communicatively successful "speech act". Thus, infants find themselves already in interactional settings. Depending on their cognitive and language development, they grow into this framework and contribute increasingly more explicit, language-based utterances to the communication.

The Role of Prosodic Contours in Early Language Development

The modulation of speech that adults display in their speech – be it child-directed or not – does not only carry affective information that is readily exploited by the human mirror neuron system (see appendix) but also structural information about the prosodic properties and parts of speech of the native language. In this respect, it is particularly the melodic contours that carry such information. Prosodic contours help to guide infants' attention to basic units of speech (Papoušek, 1992, p. 245). They are thus in the service of parsing. In fact, post-natally and even pre-natally, infants are sensitive to the prosodic information in the speech signal. Thus, Mehler, Jusczyk, Lambertz, Halsted, Bertoncini, and Amiel-Tison (1988) could show that French neonates can already distinguish their native language French from a foreign language that belongs to a different rhythmic class, such as Russian. Further studies have confirmed this early discriminative ability with other languages (Nazzi, Bertoncini, & Mehler, 1998; Nazzi & Ramus, 2003). What makes prosody of major importance in early language acquisition is the fact that it provides cues for segmenting the seamless speech stream into units, in particular words. Later, at around the age of one year, when semantics comes in, these candidate units can be mapped onto meaning and the first words, which are pairs of form and meaning, emerge. The languages of the world can choose from a variety of prosodic properties on which segmentation may rely, such as word stress (English, Dutch, German), syllable structure (French), syllable weight (Japanese), and vowel harmony (Finnish, Turkish) (Cutler, 1999; Cutler, Norris, & McQueen, 1996). Between 6 and 10 months of age, infants set the rhythmic parameters of their native language with which they will subsequently parse any language input, native or foreign.

The Impact of Affective Mother-Child Interaction on Early Communicative and Language Development

Studying the impact of parent-child interaction on early communicative and language development requires good instruments to assess quantitative measures in both areas longitudinally. Paavola (2006) conducted a study on the relation of early mother-child interaction on preverbal communicative behavior and later language behavior of 27 normally developing Norwegian infants and their mothers. In this study, a multitude of behavioral inventories are applied[4]. Among these the CARE (Child-Adult-RElation)-Index (Crittenden, 2004, 1988) is an assessment tool of adult-child interaction that –unlike other attachment measures – can be used from birth onwards. It measures qualitatively and quantitatively various interaction styles of the adult (sensitive, controlling, unresponsive) and the child (cooperative, compulsive/compliant, difficult, passive) on 7 expressive scales: (1) facial, (2) vocal, (3) position and body contact, (4) affective, (5) contingent, (6) controlling, and (7) choice of activity. The main construct of the CARE-Index is sensitivity in play, which is defined as "any pattern of behavior that pleases the infant and increases the infants' comfort and attentiveness and reduces its distress and disengagement." (Crittenden, 2004, p. 6) Paavola (2006) takes a "transactional view" on the communicative dyad, that is, not only parental behavior is important for infants' communicative and language acquisition but also the child contributes to its success. Moreover, the child's communicative and linguistic behavior influences the adults' behavior such that a framework of mutual transaction is established within which positive feedback enhances and negative feedback attenuates the acquisition process. In the beginning sensitive mothers show some degree of directive control also, as exemplified in initiation of communicative acts and elicitation of conversation. In the course of the development, however, the role of the child becomes increasingly important for the developmental outcome: "It is possible that linguistic development becomes increasingly child-driven over time (…)". (Paavola, 2006, p. 77)

Paavola (2006) found that a high degree of sensitivity of the mother was related to a high amount of communication with the child, in terms of number of communication acts and number of verbal responses, i.e., highly sensitive mothers communicated most with their children, medium sensitive mothers somewhat less and unresponsive mothers least. Likewise, high and medium cooperative infants uttered more intentional communicative acts than uncooperative infants. Maternal responses and child intentional communicative acts with 10 months in the MacArthur Communicative Development Inventories (MCDI) could predict the numbers of phrases understood and vocabulary comprehension at 30 months. The child measures could also predict vocabulary production, whereas maternal scores could not. Sensitive mothers were able to fine-tune their communication in that they talked about age-appropriate here-and-now topics rather than talking in displaced speech. They elicited more communication from their infants, their speech acts were more descriptive and less directive. Highly sensitive mothers made the most compliments. The degree of sensitivity was not crucial in the upper and middle range of sensitivity, i.e., infants of highly and also medium sensitive mothers showed equally good performance. It seems that "good enough maternal care" (Paavola, 2006, p. 78) was sufficient for the linguistic thriving of their children. A crucial part of maternal sensitivity is an active role and initiation of interactions as well as elicitation of conversation with the infants.

The Impact of Mother-Child Interaction on Phonemic Discrimination

It is well-known that infants start out with the ability to discriminate any phonemic contrast of the languages of the world until the age of 6 months, however, lose it by 10-12 months of age (Werker & Tees, 1984; Werker, 1993; Pater, Stager, & Werker, 2004; Kuhl, 2004). By the end of the first year they have become competent listeners of their ambient language and neurally committed to processing it (Kuhl, 2000, 2004, 2007). However, it is not known whether, besides language-related factors other, extraneous factors may also exert an influence on the timing of this development. Typically, in group studies, the majority of infants show discrimination at 6 months of age, however, a minority does not show it. Likewise, at 10 months of age, the group on average shows no discrimination anymore, however, a minority still does. In attempt to explain (part of) this inter-individual variation, the impact of mother-child interaction (as measured by the CARE-Index) on early phonemic discrimination in 6- and 10-month old infants was studied (Elsabbagh, Hohenberger, van Herwegen, Campos, Serres, de Schoenen, Aschersleben, & Karmiloff-Smith (submitted). The study was carried out in three European labs, in London, Paris, and Munich, with mono-lingual infants acquiring English, French and German. In the native condition of the language task, our subjects had to discriminate between two syllables, [ba] and [da] (both syllables had been recorded in French, English, and German versions, respectively). In the non-native condition they had to discriminate between [da] and a non-native Hindi [da] (with a retroflex [d]). As reported in Elsabbagh et al. (submitted), we found that overall, 6-month old infants discriminated the native as well as between the non-native contrasts, whereas 10-months olds only discriminated the native contrast but not the non-native one anymore. This result is expected on the background of the vast literature on early sensitivity to phonemic contrasts in infants up to the age of 8-10 months after which only native contrasts are still discriminated (Werker & Tees, 1984; Kuhl, 2004, among many others). When we looked at the relation of phonemic discrimination with mother-child interaction, we found that at 6 months of age, it was the group of infants of low-contingent mothers (low on maternal sensitivity) that discriminated the non-native contrast whereas infants of high-contingent mothers did not. From this finding we concluded that 6-month old infants of highly contingent mothers had already

proceeded so far in their language development that they had already lost their original universal discrimination abilities. In this case, absent discrimination ability is a sign of a more mature language development. We explained this higher maturity of the infants of sensitive mothers in terms of (i) more language input the infants had already received (see Paavola, 2006) and, more importantly, in terms of (ii) contingent interaction. Contingent interaction is also characterized by sensitive verbal and non-verbal interaction. Contingently responsive mothers provide more mutual gaze, turn-taking (verbal and non-verbal) and mutual affect, which may foster the development of communication and language as opposed to the non-contingent behavior.

EMOTIONAL EXPRESSION IN LANGUAGE

A particular area of research is devoted to the relation between language and emotional expression in language, as in affective prosody, and how this relation develops from early childhood onwards.

Bloom's Intentionality Model of Language Acquisition

In taking a functional perspective, Bloom (1998) sees "the convergence of emotion, cognition, and social connectedness to other persons" (p. 1272) at the heart of language development in the second year of life. In her view, children learn to represent the contents of their mind (belief, desires, thoughts) in language for the purpose of relating to other persons, and to communicate to them their own thoughts and feelings. These two aspects, (i) representation of conscious mental contents and (ii) communication, that is, sharing of these conscious mental contents with others, constitute Bloom's and Tinker's (2001) "intentionality" model of language acquisition. Her interactive model of language development rests on the two concepts of "engagement" and "effort". The first concept, "engagement", relates to the child's affective and social directedness and interactions with her communicative partners, that is, the child is engaged into the social world *via* language. The second concept, "effort", relates to the resources she has to spend on the cognitive processing of language, that is, the child has to work out and compute the threefold relations that exist within language. Language itself comprises form (sound, words, and syntax), content (meaning), and use (pragmatics). Figure 1 depicts the two intersecting spheres of effort and engagement, at the core of which is language (L), embedded itself in its three components (form, content, and use).

Effort and engagement stand in a relation of fruitful tension and may, at times, dominate the development more or less. Three principles that relate to emotion, social development, and cognition, govern this dialectic tension, (i) relevance, (ii) discrepancy, and (iii) elaboration (cf. Bloom, 1998, p. 1273):

i. *Emotion and relevance*: According to Bloom, children's language learning is tied to their emotional life, which they want to share with others. They communicate to their social partners what is relevant to them and thereby engage themselves into the social world.

ii. *Social development and discrepancy*: A child's social development is dependent on her being understood by her caregivers. If her language and other communicative expressions are insufficient for conveying her intentional states, the child has to acquire the necessary expressive linguistic means to do so successfully. The discrepancy between what the child expresses linguistically and what her social partners understand and *vice versa*, what the caregivers express and what the child understands, is the motor of language development. This motor stops only when the child has fully mastered all aspects of language.

Figure 1. Redrawing of Bloom's intentionality model of language development in terms of effort and engagement (1998, p. 1273; cf. also Bloom and Tinker 2001, p. 14). L = Language[5]

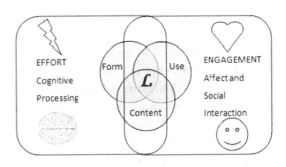

iii. *Cognition and elaboration*: As the child's intentional states become increasingly complex, the linguistic means which represent them also have to become more elaborate. In this sense the child has to invest more resources into the expressive and representative power of the linguistic system.

Bloom and her colleagues studied the relation between the expression of affect and of language in children's spontaneous communication from 9 months to 2 1/2 years of age. This period covers three important language milestones: the first words (FW), the vocabulary spurt (VS), and simple sentences. Subjects varied in their onset of these three milestones and also in their expression of positive, negative, and mixed affect. Importantly, the expression of emotion was a function of the age when the three language milestones were mastered. Early word learners were more often in states of neutral affect, whereas late word learners showed increased emotional expression during that time. Taken together, these complementary findings suggest that children invest their mental efforts either into word learning or into emotional expression. Doing both at the same time – learning words and expressing emotions – seems impossible. Rather, there is a trade-off between the language and emotion which results in the two types of learners.

After equating children for their level of language learning and then looking at their emotional development two findings were revealed: (i) during the second year the expression of emotions was constant, only language increased and (ii) children did not express less emotional content when they learned more words, that is, they did not learn to utter words instead of emotional expressions. The words the children learned during that period were basic words and not emotional words. The above-mentioned trade-off between language and emotional expression can be understood in terms of cognitive load and interference. Uttering words and expressing emotions is both effortful and taps a partially shared pool of resources. Bloom and colleagues found that those words that went along with emotional expressions were among those learned first and used most frequently whereas those words that were uttered without emotional expression were among those learned recently and used less frequently. Taking these two observations together, it can be concluded that the effort spent on learning words interferes with the concurrent expression of emotion. Only words that are highly over-learned can afford a concurrent emotional expression. Often, these emotional expressions were positive, indicating that an objective the child had represented with that word had been achieved and no further effortful mental computations had to be carried out anymore.

Looking into the temporal dynamics of the interaction between affective and language expression on a second-to-second basis, Bloom and colleagues found that the emotional expression was built up and preceded the linguistic expression, e.g., a word. Shortly before the peak in emotional expression the word would be uttered and soon after its completion it would fade again. This fine-grained analysis of the time-course of expression of emotion and language is evidence for both components in the acquisition process – effort and engagement. Children speak about relevant things that are on their mind. In the moment of utterance there is mutual adaptation

between emotional engagement and cognitive effort. What has been found for word learning is even more evident for sentence learning, the third milestone. Sure enough, uttering whole sentences is even more cognitively demanding than uttering a single word at a time. In addition, the child is now challenged with the temporal synchronization of an emotional expression across the sentence or across parts of it, i.e. with phrasal or sentential prosody. The same pattern as found in word learning repeated itself again, namely children who had learned syntax earlier showed more emotional expression whereas late learners of syntax showed little emotional expression.

While the developmental course of emotional and language expression that Bloom and her colleagues unraveled, is unquestionable and can be nicely explained in terms of the dialectics between cognition and social engagement, their functional approach may be considered more controversial. The functionalist view, according to which the development of language can be explained in terms of its communicative function, i.e., the child's language learning in order to communicate successfully with the environment, has encountered some serious criticism. Among the arguments against functionalism the criticisms of circularity of functional argumentation and lack of "dysfunctionality" is most prominently (for a critical discussion of functionalism in linguistics, see Keller, 1997). Bloom argues that the need for communication or the fact that communication is successful can explain why language has the structure it has. However, there is no way in which the presumed function of language – communication – can explain why a sentence has the form it has. There is simply no causal chain from the purpose of communication to the form of language. This relation can be explained better by other, more formal theories of language. Generative grammar with its focus on the architecture of linguistic representations is a better candidate, in this respect. The answer to the puzzle of linguistic structure may lie in "principles of neural organization that may be even more deeply grounded in physical law (Chomsky, 1965, p. 59, as cited in Chomsky 2007, p. 14). Generally, those physical principles will be principles of computational efficiency. The human cognitive ability of recursion that yields hierarchically structured expressions is a better explanation in this respect than the emotionally motivated wish to communicate more complex thoughts to one's social partners. After all, one first needs to have some mechanism that enables communication before one can praise the benefit of communicating. Such a mechanism can only be a cognitive one, though, which, then, can be co-opted for communicative purposes.

A more promising view on the role of emotion for language acquisition, therefore, is the "gating" view (Kuhl, 2007) which holds that social and emotional factors direct the child's attention to language as a part of the "social brain" (Grossmann & Johnson, 2007, among others). Through this gating mechanism language acquisition is not explained but rather constrained. This view implies that overall the social and emotional relevance of communication is a supportive factor for language learning. However, Bloom's findings rather show that emotional and cognitive expression can also hinder each other on a more local time-scale, since they seem to partially tap into the same resource during on-line production. Therefore, it seems important to distinguish carefully global from more specific aspects of the relation between language and emotion as well as comprehension from production.

Infants' Sensitivity to What is Said Versus How It is Said

While Bloom studied the relation between emotional and linguistic expression in production, other researchers have looked at this relationship in comprehension. A communicative utterance always comprises language and paralanguage, among the latter affective prosody, facial expressions, gestures, etc. In normal discourse, both sources of information are congruent with each other. However, they may also conflict as when language ("what is said") and paralanguage ("how it is said") contradict each other. These special cases allow particularly well to study the relation between language and affective expression.

Early studies by Fernald (1989, 1993) and Lawrence and Fernald (1993) on the effect of conflicting messages in children of various ages showed that 9-month old infants regulated their behavior more in terms of paralanguage whereas 18-month old infants relied more on language. They concluded that in the first year of life "the melody [is] the message".

Following up on these seminal investigations, Friend studied such conflicting messages in children of various ages (2000, 2001, 2003) with the "social referencing paradigm". Social referencing typically takes place in a novel and ambiguous situation where the infant refers back to an interacting human in order to acquire cues regarding how to handle the situation. In the experiments reported here, interaction was with a female character on a video monitor. In Friend (2001) 15-16-month old infants were presented with novel toys which they were encouraged or discouraged to play with by means of language or facial and vocal paralanguage, respectively. The language and paralanguage cues were either congruent (+language/+paralanguage; -language/-paralanguage) or incongruent (+language/-paralanguage; -language/+paralanguage).[6] As expected, as a group, infants relied more on paralanguage, that is, if the facial and vocal affect was disapproving, infants hesitated longer to grasp the toy and played for a shorter time with them, even if the verbal message was approving and *vice versa* for the reverse combination of cues. However, on the individual level reliance on language was positively correlated with lexical acquisition, as measured by the McArthur Communicative Developmental Inventory (CDI), that is, the more words the infants knew the more they relied on language. This study tapped into an important transition phase characterized by ample inter-individual variation in language development as well as in behavior regulation. This transition gives way to a subsequent phase where children rely more heavily on language cues, suppressing any affective information from the paralinguistic channel. This subsequent stage was studied in Friend (2003) with 4-year olds in the same social referencing paradigm. She found a general effect of the lexical content of the verbal message such that positive messages led to faster approach of the toy as compared to negative messages, irrespective of the +/- affective information. The effect was pervasive in the group: 54-71% of the subjects were more regulated by language as opposed to paralanguage, as measured by the dependent variables "play with novel toys" and "delay to approach", respectively. However, lexical content had a gradual rather than an all-or-nothing effect on behavior and at least in one of the variables, there was a considerable minority being regulated by paralanguage. Summarizing, this study confirmed the general "lexical bias" in the behavior regulation of older children (4 years). Individual analyses, however, point to differential regulation by language and paralanguage on the micro-level.

This line of studies parallels the findings of Bloom and colleagues, as discussed above. Both in perception and production studies the same developmental pattern emerges: infants (by 9 months of age) first attend to information conveyed through the affective channel. When they start to learn words (by 18 months of age), the lexical channel takes over and pushes back the significance of the affective channel. What is interesting is that both channels stay separate for a protracted period of time. Bloom explains this with the effort that computing both kinds of information requires. It has to be done sequentially before it can be done simultaneously. Only at some later stage can children eventually integrate the information on the two channels. In the perceptual studies at 4 years of age the language channel still dominates the affective channel. From these, two important

questions arise: 1. Is there more evidence for this developmental sequence and 2. When does the integration eventually take place?

Language and Emotion in a Cross-Modal Perspective

Evidence for the same developmental sequence and for the eventual integration of language and affect in children comes from the cross-modal comparison of the expression of language and emotion in spoken and signed languages (Reilly & Seibert, 2003). Sign language offers a unique perspective on the relation of these two systems since the same means – in particular facial gestures – are used for both systems: syntax and emotion. On the one hand, sign languages, beyond certain manual parameters, make use of facial expressions (eyes, eyebrows, facial and mouth gestures) and body leans in order to express syntactic properties, e.g., sentence types (*yes-no* and *wh*-questions, topic, negation, conditionals, relative clauses), scope of syntactic and/or prosodic domains and signing perspective (Sandler & Lillo-Martin, 2006). Less prominently, these features are also used to convey lexical information, e.g., the manual sign HAPPY has an obligatory happy facial expression, as a part of its lexical content. On the other hand, facial and bodily expressions are used for conveying emotional information such as the signer's current affective state, subjective attitude towards and evaluation of the present topic. For example, raised eye-brows syntactically indicate a *yes-no* question, whereas, in a different context, affectively they indicate surprise. While the muscles used to innervate these facial expressions are the same, however, the morphology, i.e., the form of these expressions, the context in which they are used, their scope, and their timing characteristics differs in both domains (Reilly & Seibert, 2003). Syntactic prosody is linguistically constrained. It occurs in the context of clauses, is carried out with a higher muscle tension, and has a strictly defined temporal distribution in the sentence with neatly marked onsets and offsets and characteristic prosodic contours. This is because syntactic prosody is a part of the language core computational system. In adults these two systems – language and emotion – are clearly separable but highly integrated in normal, healthy subjects. The language and emotional systems show a characteristic break-down in lesions. Deaf signers who suffered either a right- or left-hemispheric stroke revealed a double dissociation of affective and syntactic expression. A stroke in the right hemisphere leads to flat emotional facial expressions, however, unimpeded syntactic prosody whereas the reverse pattern holds for a left-hemispheric lesion (Poizner, Klima, & Bellugi, 1990; Corina, Bellugi, & Reilly, 1999). Thus, a deaf patient having suffered a right-hemispheric stroke cannot raise her eyebrows anymore as a sign of surprise but still can raise her eyebrows in a syntactic *yes-no* question. How do children acquire and – most interestingly – integrate both? Reilly and Seibert (2003) discuss the two systems in a dynamical developmental framework that takes factors with different scopes in consideration: "…, these systems interact in a dynamical way, according to both specific (i.e., contextual) and potentially universal (i.e., developmental and biological) factors." (p. 553) The emphasis of the remainder of this paragraph will lie on the acquisition of grammatical and emotional facial expressions in American Sign Language (ASL) and how their use develops in narratives.

Acquisition of grammatical and emotional facial expression in ASL: Deaf infants younger than two years of age sign one-word utterances with prosodic expressions, e.g., HAPPY with a happy face or WHAT with furrowed eyebrows. On closer inspection, however, these holophrases appear to be unanalyzed chunks in which the facial expression cannot be detached from the manual sign, indicating that they have not yet been analyzed separately as a systematic part of the sign or phrase. Also, the timing, scope, and individual characteristics of these facial expressions are often

erroneous. Around 2;6 years, interestingly, the facial expression disappears. Deaf toddlers then produce grammatical constructions which need syntactic prosody, e.g., *wh*-phrases, with correct manual syntax but with totally blank faces (Reilly & McIntire, 1991). Only at older ages than four years the prosody reappears and becomes integrated with the manual component. The correct morphology, scope and timing characteristics have to be learned in a protracted time period over the next couple of years. Summarizing, a non-linear developmental sequence can be stated in the acquisition of syntactic prosody in deaf ASL-acquiring children: (i) initial co-articulation of prosody alongside manual signs in the sense of unanalyzed chunks (<2 yrs), (ii) absence of syntactic prosody (2;6-4 yrs), and (iii) reappearance and integration (> 4 yrs). Reilly and Seibert interpret this developmental sequence in terms of a reanalysis of affective and syntactic resources feeding it: "Initially, (…), both language and emotional expression have access to a general, underlying symbolic function. Children at the one-sign stage draw on early affective and communicative abilities collaboratively with their first signs. However, as language emerges, especially as syntax develops, and the child begins to combine signs, there is a bifurcation of systems such that language and emotion unfold as independently organized and differentially mediated systems, each following its own developmental path." (p. 547)

Acquisition of narrative skills in hearing and deaf children in terms of emotional expression: In narratives, language and emotion must be integrated in order to convey and understand the narrated episodes. Evaluative elements represent the attitude of the narrators towards the story and the characters in it. These evaluations typically give a narrative its meaning. They can be conveyed in various ways: lexically, syntactically, and paralinguistically, as with affective prosody, facial expressions and gestures. Reilly and Seibert studied hearing and deaf children between 3 and 12 years of age with the famous "Frog, where are you?" story (Bamberg & Reilly, 1996). For the hearing children they found that the youngest age group (3-4 yrs) could not really tell the story well. Their productions were structurally weak, however, were full of vocal prosody, stress, vowel lengthening and showed sing-song like intonation contours. There was little facial expression. The role of the affective prosody was to "glue together" the structurally unconnected parts of the story (Reilly & Seibert 2003, p. 549). The school-children (7-8 yrs) told structurally more elaborate stories, however, almost without any paralinguistic evaluation, flat affect and stereotypical. Bamberg and Reilly (1996) conceive of this developmental pattern so far as "a transition from paralinguistic to linguistically conveyed evaluation, that is, a lexicalization of affective expression that appears to occur during the early school years." (Reilly & Seibert 2003, p. 549) As an explanation for the early prevalence of prosodic means and its later ban the authors propose "that paralinguistic expression functions as a support system and stepping stone into the lexicalized expression of evaluation." (p. 549) Only the 10-11-year olds could reintegrate these two systems again and tell structurally complex and affectively rich stories. Summarizing the developmental process of narratives, the now familiar tripartite sequence re-occurs again: (i) narratives with much affective prosody but little structure (3-4 yrs), (ii) lexicalization of affective evaluation, flat emotional expression (7-8 yrs), (iii) integration of affective paralanguage and structurally elaborate language (> 10 yrs).

Would ASL-acquiring deaf children show the same sequence as their hearing counterparts, or, due to the different modality, a different one? Adult signers heavily use paralinguistic means for evaluative purposes in narrations: affective prosody, emotional facial expressions and gestures. This is a modality-specific phenomenon which stands in marked contrast to adult hearing subjects who rely more on linguistically encoded evaluations. The development of signing children,

however, was found to be quite similar to that of their hearing counterparts and all three stages were confirmed, as well. In perspective taking, for example, adult signers make body shifts and facial expressions so as to adopt the position and the facial expression of the story character who they are about to quote directly subsequently. Preschoolers show facial expressions as well, however, their occurrence is incorrectly timed, unspecific for particular characters, and erratic. From 5 years onwards, however, all children use the lexical expression SAY in order to introduce the quotation, which, according to the authors "reflects a linguistic reorganization: direct quotes are introduced lexically before the non-manual behaviors are linguistically integrated with the manually signed quote." (p. 551) Again, only the older children were able to produce the non-manual affective prosody synchronized with the manual lexical signs. This parallel development of narrative skills in hearing and deaf children led the authors to the conclusion that this development was modality-independent. They summarize their findings as follows: "This recurrent pattern – first relying on affective means, then moving on to a manual lexical strategy, and finally integrating both channels such that the facial behaviors are now under linguistic control – appears across structures, from single lexical items to phrasal, clausal, and now discourse level structures. These data provide strong evidence that the child's prelinguistic, emotional abilities are not directly accessible to the linguistic system, even when they continue to convey affective information." (p. 551)

Summarizing the common developmental pattern in the reviewed areas – the role of linguistic and paralinguistic information in early language production and perception, the cross-modal similarities in speaking and signing children's narratives and in the expression of affect in sign language acquisition – there seems to be a recurring universal tripartite sequence of

i. an undifferentiated mixed system dominated by affect over language
ii. a strictly language-dominated system in which affect is lexicalized and language governs behavior
iii. a bifurcation into two mature systems, emotion and language, and a concurrent re-integration of both systems

This development resembles the classical three steps "thesis – anti-thesis – synthesis". It seems to be not only applicable to various domains but also to occur independently of age. Note that in Friend's studies on the role of paralanguage and language on children's behavior regulation these steps occur, roughly, at (i) 9 months, (ii) 15-16 months, and (iii) 4 years. In Reilly and Seibert's study on the expression of emotion in narratives, however, they occur at (i) 3-4 years, (ii) 6-7 years, and (iii) 10-11 years. This décalage suggests that the underlying process is not so much age-dependent, i.e., a matter of (perhaps neuronal) maturation, but one that needs to be recapitulated in different domains at different times. The model that best accommodates these properties is Karmiloff-Smith's *representational redescription* model (1979, 1986, 1992). This model states that in the course of acquiring a skill or cognitive faculty, irrespective of age, subjects entertain different representations as they proceed. Initially, these representations are implicit (e.g., represented sensu-motorically), however, later on, they become more and more explicit, which makes them amenable to linguistic expressions. The earlier levels are not lost; rather they are "redescribed" in a more general, abstract cognitive vocabulary that can be shared by other cognitive systems that can access that level as well. At these higher levels, integration is possible, even with the original "lower"-level format. In the present context, the formal language system having become sufficiently autonomous from the emotional system can be re-integrated with it again. This re-integration seems to have to be achieved for different domains separately, however, in a similar, tripartite, process.

The developmental sequence of an early emotional language phase of young children and the later "ban" on emotional expressions in their narrative productions may also be related to a novel evolutionary account in terms of "self-domestication" of humans in the course of their social-cognitive evolution. In their "emotional reactivity" hypothesis Hare and Tomasello (2005; Hare, 2007) try to explain how humans managed to evolve socially-relevant cognitive abilities that make them uniquely human. This hypothesis holds that the evolution of human social problem solving might have proceeded in two steps: First, the level of emotional reactivity towards con-specifics needed to be lowered, i.e., they had to feel comfortable and be capable of interacting cooperatively in a group; second, and contingent upon the first development, socially relevant cognitive abilities such as action and intention understanding and theory of mind came under selection pressure and evolved. For the development of language abilities a similar two-step process occurred. First, the original, emotion-based call system was abandoned or, more precisely, not selected as a substrate for linguistic computation, i.e., the emotional reactivity was disconnected from our modern language faculty. Once this had happened, the evolutionary pressure acted directly on the cognitive faculties of thought and language until a potent computational language system emerged. In modern humans, thus, emotion and language are clearly different systems, however, systems that still – or again – interact with each other very strongly on various linguistic levels such as prosody and lexical meaning, maybe even syntax. While they are well integrated in adults, the developmental perspective reveals that at some point the two were dissociated – maybe had to become dissociated in order to reach higher levels of performance before becoming reintegrated again in the mature form that we witness today in contemporary adults.

EMOTIONS IN FIRST AND SECOND LANGUAGE LEARNING

Harris et al. (2006; cf. also Caldwell-Harris, 2008) lament that the "emotion revolution" which started in the cognitive science in the 1990'ies has not yet captured psycholinguistics, including first (L1) and second language (L2) learning and bilingualism. They claim that the fact that speakers experience more emotions in their L1 as compared to their L2 is due to the more emotional context of language acquisition and not so much to the time of language acquisition as such. In their "emotional contexts of learning hypothesis" they propose that "words and phrases that are acquired early will have strong connections to the amygdala (LaBar & Phelps, 1998), because early language develops at the same time as emotional regulation systems (Bloom & Beckwith, 1989). Later learned language may have a more purely cortical representation, lacking connections to subcortical areas (Lieberman, 2000)." (Harris et al., 2006, p. 271) The direct connections of words with their associated emotions strengthen their representation and facilitate their processing. As a consequence, an L2 can, in principle, achieve the same "emotionality" if acquired in an equally emotional context as the L1. "Age of acquisition" is not the causal factor, but "emotional context of learning". The L1, on the one hand, is so emotional because it has been acquired in an emotionally rich context of binding to the primary caregivers: "Early age of acquisition thus functions as a proxy for a more emotional context of learning." (Harris et al., 2006, p. 274) Early age and proficiency are systematically confounded with the emotionality of the learning context. The L2, on the other hand, is less emotional because it is acquired later in a large variety of settings, most of which are formal such as learning at school. This hypothesis is compatible with the results of their studies in which they investigated the psycho-physiological reaction, as measured by the skin conductance response (SCR), of subjects belonging to various

bilingual learner groups to emotional words. In study 1 they investigated Turkish-English bilinguals; in study 2 they investigated (i) subjects coming to the US as adults, (ii) subjects coming to the US as children, and (iii) bilinguals born in the USA as children of immigrants. The subjects listened to emotional phrases and neutral words in their L1 and L2, respectively. The results showed that age of acquisition of the L2 influenced the emotional response, however, only for late learners who had better language proficiency in their L1. When L2 had become the stronger language, the electro-dermal responses of the subjects to emotional stimuli in L1 and L2 did not differ.

Harris et al.'s hypothesis requires a different model of language processing and of the mental lexicon. In the classical Levelt model of lexical access (Levelt, Roelofs, & Meyer, 1999; Levelt, 1999), words, are related with abstract conceptual structures which then may have connections to some emotions. The "emotional contexts of learning" hypothesis, however, suggests a direct connection between a word and its associated emotion as well as with the context in which it was learned and is predominantly used. This view is in favor of the connectionist idea of a distributed associative lexicon. Their hypothesis also requires a different language learning model, namely one that is age-independent and which poses the explanatory burden pre-dominantly on the emotional context of learning.

Despite the intriguing arguments from the proponents of the emotional contexts of learning hypothesis, there are counter-arguments against several of their claims. If it were true that it is not the age of acquisition but the emotional context of acquisition that decides on the success of the learning process and the emotionality in the achieved language, then there should also be a non-negligible number of low-proficiency L1 adult speakers who, as children, did not have the luck of having been raised in an ideal emotionally supportive and rich environment. However, also such individuals acquire their native language successfully. Furthermore, there is evidence that L2 learners regularly switch back to their native language in the number domain, e.g., when it comes to counting and carrying out mathematical operations in real-time. However, arithmetic is certainly the least emotionally dependent domain. Why, then, should subjects fall back on their L1 in an area that is unrelated to emotions? Lastly, there is good evidence that a critical period for language learning exists, which is denied by Caldwell-Harris (2008). Even connectionists, on who these authors rely when they argue for distributed lexical representations, nowadays model brain plasticity, that is, the timing of the developmental susceptibility for learning in various sensory domains (Elman et al., 1996). Unless these and possibly other inconsistencies are resolved, the emotional contexts of learning hypothesis is nothing more than – a hypothesis.

DELIMITATION OF LANGUAGE, COGNITION AND EMOTION FROM AN EVOLUTIONARY VIEW

In the traditional view, emotion and cognition (comprising language), have been strictly separated. However, more recent approaches propose a very tight integration, if not inseparability of language, cognition, and emotion (at least for adult processing), as most strongly expressed by Pessoa (2008) and Caldwell-Harris (2008), and of direct mapping between these domains, as in the mirror neuron and embodiment literature (Rizzolatti & Craighero, 2004; Foroni & Semin, 2009, among many others). However, whether we espouse a separatist view or an integrational, embodied view, may depend on the level of our analysis. As Ochsner and Barrett (2001) point out, a separation of cognition and emotion seems to make sense for researchers that study high-level phenomena, such as phenomenal experience or behavior, e.g., there are distinct feelings connected with the experience of emotional or neural processing. This clear separation cannot be maintained, however, at lower levels of analyses such as information processing and neural processing. As an example, Ochsner and Barrett refer to the evaluative/monitoring function of the anterior cingulate cortex (ACC). This brain structure is implied in the decision whether a current action should be continued or changed. Whether this action is a purely cognitive one, such as retrieving a word meaning, or an emotional one, such as evading a predator, makes the same functioning either cognitive or emotional. The activation of the ACC does not tell us straightforwardly what kind of computation is carried out, in contrast to, e.g., the amygdala, whose activation is a better sign of affective computation (in this case, fear). Given this ambiguity at least at the lower levels of information and neural processing, it is not at all clear which criteria should be used in order to distinguish between cognition and emotion: experiential, behavioral, computational, or neural criteria? (Ochsner & Barrett, 2001, p. 65) Ochsner and Barrett ask critically whether only processes that are accompanied by conscious experiencing of feelings should be called emotional or also those that only show the involvement of a brain area known to be involved in affective computation despite the absence of any experiential emotional state. Hence, would a measured level of arousal be sufficient to define a state as affective? This ambiguity is far from being resolved. It is important, however, to frame it in a theoretical approach that has the capacity of integrating the various domains. It seems as if the emerging discipline of "social cognitive neuroscience" is the most suitable and promising framework for this task (Ochsner & Barrett, 2001; Lieberman, 2007). If, as has been attempted here, a developmental perspective is taken, then the framework is called "developmental social cognitive neuroscience" (Zelazo, Chandler, & Crone, 2009). These two novel research areas certainly have a very promising future.

The paradigm of embodied cognition that was initially put forward to explain action and intention understanding, memory, and language in general, has recently also been used to explain the impact of emotion in first and second language acquisition. The claim of embodied cognition is that emotional words are acquired in emotional contexts (Harris et al., 2006) and that these contexts are (partially) relived or simulated somatically, as in motor resonance, when we process them (Foroni & Semin, 2009). However, it is not clear at all whether motor resonance and simulation contribute to lexical processing. As argued above, conceptual and lexical representations must be clearly demarcated. The proposed grounding seems to take place at the conceptual level where numerous multi-modal systems interface with each other and jointly contribute to the pre-verbal conceptual representation of a word, among them the motor system. In this respect, the exact time-course of the processing of these various sources of information needs to be investigated in more detail. In Foroni and Semin (2009) motor resonance sets in only after 250 ms of stimulus presentation and unfolds at least during a period of 2 seconds. Such a long dwell-time for a single word is not viable in normal language processing where up to four syllables are processed within one second and where simply no time is available for such extended reverberation processes. It is more likely that motor resonance is an optional post-lexical process that may take place when the conceptual structure is accessed in the later course of lexical access of the perceived word. It is an open question whether it can then still contribute to word comprehension. This scenario does not preclude the attested role of motor resonance in influencing later affective evaluations and prompting actions. However, Gallese (2008) counters the criticism against this "late motor imagery hypothesis." (p. 325) He adduces findings from an ERP-study on single word processing (Pulvermüller, Härle, & Hummel, 2000) that detects modality-specific activation of somatotopic brain areas after a delay of ~200ms

after word onset. He evaluates this delay as short enough to support lexical, and not just post-lexical, processing. Niedenthal (2007, p. 1005) shares this criticism. She argues that the reaction times found in the brain's modality-specific systems are on an appropriate time-scale whereas older accounts that argued with activation of muscles and viscera may not. If the output of these more subtle brain-internal computations need not have to surface at the level of overt behavior, but may remain confined to the neural interface-level of pre-motor representations, these may still count as grounded, embodied representations. The view that the pre-motor cortex, which supports action as well as language representations, is the site of simulation whereas the motor cortex is the site of execution may indeed be acceptable to both views – the classical cognitivist and the recent embodied view. If the pre-motor cortex is an interface, indeed, it may be called "cognitive" as well as "embodied" – it depends on which side of the interface one is looking at. The theoretical discussion has actually already proceeded beyond a strict dichotomy between these paradigms. Thus, Dove (2009) pleads for "representational pluralism". It may neither be feasible nor advisable to try to ground every concept in perception. For an abstract notion such as "democracy" it may not be possible to show how the conceptual and lexical processing is causally determined by simulation and re-enactment of whatever situations people associate with it.

The grounding of language in the body and in emotional states is still a relatively recent proposal whose viability cannot be evaluated conclusively at this point. However, it touches on some very basic and important topics in the evolution of human cognition and language as well as in language development. For the evolution of language, we know that affective vocalizations, which are also abundant in the animal kingdom, are supported by sub-cortical brain regions, whereas human language is processed pre-dominantly in the left hemisphere of the neo-cortex. Ancient affective cries and calls, though vocally based, have not evolved into modern human language. This is because they are under involuntary, sub-cortical control. If a predator is recognized, the individual must signal the threat to its con-specifics as fast as possible. Language, however, needs to be under voluntary, neo-cortical control. Forming a non-verbal message and communicating it to others is a deliberate act of the mind. Therefore, spoken language presumably evolved from the gestural system of sign language (Corballis, 2002, 2010; Rizzolatti & Arbib, 1998; Rizzolatti & Craighero, 2004). This is because the hands (also the fore-limbs, head and torso), are under voluntary control. The first language thus was a sign language. In terms of Hare and Tomasello's "emotional reactivity hypothesis" (Hare, 2007; Hare & Tomasello, 2005), this step in the evolution of language would then be comparable to the selection of a cognitive ability once the emotional reactivity had been down-regulated. To be more precise, in this case, the whole communication system was shifted to another brain circuitry: from sub-cortical to cortical control. The transition from sign to spoken language was a later process that was presumably supported by the co-articulation of sounds along with hand and mouth gestures (Rizzolatti & Arbib, 1998; Arbib, 2005). Once the imitative capabilities to reproduce the sounds of the concurrent hand or mouth actions without actually having to carry out the actions had become potent enough, language shifted from gestural to spoken language. Hence, the crucial achievement was to free the concurrent mouth gesture from its grounding in the body such that it could become a symbol in an emerging abstract linguistic system. This achievement cannot be appreciated high enough. Insofar the discussion of embodied cognition is misconceived. It is well taken that eventually language is rooted in the action system, however, isn't it more significant that it emancipated itself from it? Actually, proponents of embodied cognition as well as of traditional linguistic theories could be equally

content if the significance of both systems, the body and the mind, could be acknowledged with equal rights. Non-reductive philosophical theories of supervenience or emergence seem best suited to mediate in this dispute (Kim, 2006; Stephan, 2006). That emotional prosody, gesturing, and facial expressions, are part of skillful speaking and signing, is owed to the reintegration of the discrete digital linguistic system and the analog emotional system, after their separation. Language, according to Goldin-Meadow (2003), has to accommodate both functions: the systemic and the imagistic function. The imagistic function is what Reilly and Seibert (2003) refer to as the evaluative, affective stance taken in narratives. In spoken languages this division is labor is usually accomplished across the modalities such that gestures, facial expressions and other paralinguistic devices are relegated to the gestural modality while the systemic function is fully covered by the auditory modality (except prosody). In sign languages, the gestural modality can accomplish both functions: the systemic function we call "sign language" and the imagistic function we call "gestures" or "pantomimes". As we have seen, during acquisition, deaf children acquiring a sign language have to understand this division in spite of a common gestural channel in which they are expressed. This functional divergence is often accomplished through temporal abandoning of one function, namely the emotional gestural function, while the linguistic system achieves dominance, before it becomes reintegrated (Reilly & Seibert, 2003).[7] The ability of "stripping off" emotion from language by lexicalizing them is actually an important achievement in human evolution and in human development. In fact, the literature reviewed here hints at such a process (Friend, 2001, 2003; Reilly & Seibert, 2003). Counterintuitively, the language of school children appears less grounded and less emotional than the language of adults! This surprising finding is not in line with a recent trend in cognitive science to stress the mutual penetration between emotion and cognition but is well in line with Hare and Tomasello's "emotional reactivity" hypothesis which proposes that an emotional down-regulation or self-domestication must have happened some time during the evolution of humans which paved the way for a following selection of genuine cognitive abilities that boosted human's unique cognitive, social, and cultural abilities – perhaps also language.

Speaking of culture, the intimate relation between language and emotion is most clearly expressed in the area of art. Poetry and music are powerful forms of language use that humans in all cultures and times enjoy(ed) producing and perceiving. While the fashions are changing over time, the bond between language and emotion remains constant. Singing children's songs and listening to children's rhymes and poetry probably belong to the most precious memories of any adult person. A baby falling asleep to the soothing sound of a lullaby requires no less than a human brain that is exquisitely adapted to the processing of language and emotion, embedded in a body capable of resonating with the conveyed emotional state.

CONCLUSION

After reviewing a broad range of areas where language, cognition, and emotion interact, the main conclusion to be drawn is that these different systems interact strongly, at times to a degree that they cannot reasonably be separated anymore. However, when a developmental (and evolutionary) perspective is taken, their tight integration appears as the result of a characteristic tripartite sequence of consecutive steps: (i) an undifferentiated affect-dominated system governs the infant's and child's behavior, (ii) a cognitive and language-dominated system emerges in the course of which emotions are lexicalized, behavior is mainly driven by explicit language, and affect expression in the linguistic behavior

is strongly attenuated, (iii) emotional expression is re-integrated into language and cognition and the characteristic tight and skillful coupling of both systems as in adult behavior is observed. The distinct cognitive and linguistic system in (ii) appears to have evolved either from the undifferentiated emotion-dominated system in (i) or has selected a different system for its evolution, despite its roots in or remaining connections with the former emotion system. As it became more and more independent, it offered the possibility of re-organization of the affective system as well and allowed for a division of labor between the two. At the same time, it offered the opportunity of re-integration of the two systems. As far as the evolution of this tripartite process is concerned, many aspects of it still remain elusive, however, as far as ontogeny is concerned, the picture is much clearer, as the process can be studied empirically. Besides this substantive conclusion there is another, methodological conclusion, to be drawn here, which perhaps is of even higher significance, namely that of taking a developmental perspective. Only such a dynamical perspective reveals the strands of adult behavior, their (speculative) phylogeny in evolution and their ontogeny in infants and children. We have seen that what looks like inseparable and fully intertwined processes might have developed from an undifferentiated domain to two differentiated and then again re-integrated domains or has chosen a different neural substrate and developmental pathway as in the shift from the vocal call system to sign and then spoken language. Developmental processes taking place in these domains can be looked at neuro-scientifically and/or behaviorally, within one modality (speech) and across modalities (sign). A review of these areas and evaluation of the implications for our understanding of how language, cognition, and emotion interact in the human mind, brain, and body was presented in this chapter. However, the complexity of the subject matter prohibits drawing any pre-mature conclusions; hence at this stage the proposed tripartite scenario aims at stimulating future discussion and research.

REFERENCES

Arbib, M. A. (2005). From monkey-like action recognition to human language: An evolutionary framework for neurolinguistics. *The Behavioral and Brain Sciences*, *28*, 105–167. doi:10.1017/S0140525X05000038

Aziz-Zadeh, L., Sheng, T., & Gheytanchi, A. (2010). Common premotor regions for the perception and production of prosody and correlations with empathy and prosodic ability. *PLoS ONE*, *5*(1), e8759. .doi:10.1371/journal.pone.0008759

Baldwin, D. A. (1995). Understanding the link between joint attention and language. In Moore, C., & Dunham, P. J. (Eds.), *Joint attention: Its origins and role in development* (pp. 131–158). Hillsdale, New Jersey: Erlbaum.

Bamberg, M., & Reilly, J. S. (1996). Emotion, narrative and affect. In Slobin, D. I., Gerhardt, J., Kyratzis, A., & Guo, J. (Eds.), *Social interaction, social context and language: Essays in honor of Susan Ervin-Tripp* (pp. 329–341). Norwood, New Jersey: Erlbaum.

Bastiaansen, J. A. C. J., Thioux, M., & Keysers, C. (2009). Evidence for mirror systems in emotions. *Philosophical Transactions of the Royal Society B*, *364*, 2391–2404. doi:10.1098/rstb.2009.0058

Bloom, L. (1998). Language development and emotional expression. *Pediatrics*, *102*(5), 1272–1277.

Bloom, L., & Beckwith, R. (1989). Talking with feeling: Integrating affective and linguistic expression in early language development. *Cognition and Emotion*, *3*, 315–342. doi:10.1080/02699938908412711

Bloom, L., & Tinker, E. (2001). The intentionality model and language acquisition: Engagement, effort, and the essential tension in development. *Monographs of the Society for Research in Child Development*, *66*(4), i–viii, 1–91.

Bornstein, M. H., & Tamis-LeMonda, C. S. (1989). Maternal responsiveness and cognitive development in children. In Bornstein, M. H. (Ed.), *Maternal responsiveness: Characteristics and consequences. New directions for child development, no. 43* (pp. 49–61). San Francisco: Jossey-Bass.

Brand, R. J., Baldwin, D. A., & Ashburn, L. A. (2002). Evidence for 'motionese': Modifications in mothers' infant-directed action. *Developmental Science*, *5*(1), 72–83. doi:10.1111/1467-7687.00211

Brass, M., & Heyes, C. (2005). Imitation: is cognitive neuroscience solving the correspondence problem? *Trends in Cognitive Sciences*, *9*(10), 489–495. doi:10.1016/j.tics.2005.08.007

Bruner, J. S. (1975). The ontogenesis of speech acts. *Journal of Child Language*, *2*(1), 1–19. doi:10.1017/S0305000900000866

Bruner, J. S. (1983). *Child's talk: Learning to use language*. New York: Norton.

Cahill, L., & McGaugh, J. L. (1998). Mechanisms of emotional arousal and lasting declarative memory. *Trends in Neurosciences*, *21*(7), 273–313. doi:10.1016/S0166-2236(97)01214-9

Caldwell-Harris, C. L. (2008). Language research needs an "emotion revolution" AND distributed models of the lexicon. *Bilingualism: Language and Cognition*, *11*(2), 169–171. doi:10.1017/S1366728908003301

Carr, L., Iacoboni, M., Dubeau, M.-C., Mazziotta, J. C., & Lenzi, G. L. (2003). Neural mechanisms of empathy in humans: A relay from neural systems for imitation to limbic areas. *Proceedings of the National Academy of Sciences of the United States of America*, *100*(9), 5497–5502. doi:10.1073/pnas.0935845100

Cato, M. A., Crosson, B., Gokcay, D., Soltysik, D., Wierenga, C., & Gopinath, K. (2004). Processing Words with Emotional Connotation: An fMRI Study of Time Course and Laterality in Rostral Frontal and Retrosplenial Cortices. *Journal of Cognitive Neuroscience*, *16*(2), 167–177. doi:10.1162/089892904322984481

Chakrabarti, B., Bullmore, E., & Baron-Cohen, S. (2006). Empathizing with basic emotions: Common and discrete neural substrates. *Social Neuroscience*, *1*(3-4), 364–384. doi:10.1080/17470910601041317

Chomsky, N. (1965). *Aspects of the theory of syntax*. Boston, MA: MIT Press.

Chomsky, N. (2000). *New horizons in the study of language and mind*. Cambridge: Cambridge University Press.

Chomsky, N. (2007). Biolinguistic explorations: Design, development, evolution. *Journal of Philosophical Studies*, *15*(1), 1–21. doi:10.1080/09672550601143078

Corballis, M. C. (2002). *From hand to mouth. The origins of language*. Princeton, Oxford: Princeton University Press.

Corina, D. P., Bellugi, U., & Reilly, J. (1999). Neuropsychological studies in linguistic and affective facial expressions in deaf signers. *Language and Speech*, *42*(2-3), 307–331. doi:10.1177/00238309990420020801

Crittenden, P. M. (1988). Relationships at risk. In Belsky, J., & Nezworski, T. (Eds.), *Clinical implications of attachment* (pp. 136–174). Hillsdale, NJ: Erlbaum.

Crittenden, P. M. (2004). *CARE-Index: Coding Manual*. Unpublished manuscript, Miami, FL.

Cutler, A. (1999). Prosodic structure and word recognition. In Friederici, A. D. (Ed.), *Language comprehension: A biological perspective* (pp. 41–70). Berlin, Heidelberg: Springer.

Cutler, A., Norris, D. G., & McQueen, Ja. M. (1996). Lexical access in continuous speech: Language-specific realisations of a universal model. In T. Otake and A. Cutler (Eds.), *Phonological structure and language processing: Cross-linguistic studies* (pp. 227-242). Berlin: Mouton de Gruyter.

Davidson, R. J. (2000). Cognitive neuroscience needs affective neuroscience (and vice versa). *Brain and Cognition*, *42*(1), 89–92. doi:10.1006/brcg.1999.1170

Davidson, R. J., & Irwin, W. (1999). The functional neuroanatomy of emotion and affective style. *Trends in Cognitive Sciences*, *3*(1), 11–21. doi:10.1016/S1364-6613(98)01265-0

De Gelder, B., & Vroomen, J. (2000). Perceiving emotion by ear and by eye. *Cognition and Emotion*, *14*(3), 289–311. doi:10.1080/026999300378824

De Vignemont, F., & Singer, T. (2006). The empathic brain: how, when and why? *Trends in Cognitive Sciences*, *10*(10), 435–441. doi:10.1016/j.tics.2006.08.008

Decety, J., & Ickes, W. (2009). *The social neuroscience of empathy*. Cambridge: MIT Press.

Decety, J., & Jackson, P. L. (2004). The functional architecture of human empathy. *Behavioral and Cognitive Neuroscience Reviews*, *3*(2), 71–100. doi:10.1177/1534582304267187

Decety, J., & Jackson, P. L. (2006). A social-neuroscience perspective on empathy. *Current Directions in Psychological Science*, *15*(2), 54–58. doi:10.1111/j.0963-7214.2006.00406.x

Dove, G. (2009). Beyond perceptual symbols: A call for representational pluralism. *Cognition*, *110*, 412–431. doi:10.1016/j.cognition.2008.11.016

Elman, J., & Karmiloff-Smith, A. Bates, Elizabeth, Johnson, Mark, Parisi, Domenico, & Plunkett, Kim (1996). *Rethinking innateness. A connectionist perspective on development*. Cambridge, MA: MIT Press.

Elsabbagh, M., Hohenberger, A., Van Herwegen, J., Campos, R., Serres, J., de Schoenen, S., Aschersleben, G., & Karmiloff-Smith, A. (submitted). *Narrowing perceptual sensitivity to the native language in infancy: exogenous influences on developmental timing.*

Falck-Ytter, T., Gredebäck, G., & von Hofsten, C. (2006). Infants predict other people's action goals. *Nature Neuroscience, 9*(7), 878–879. doi:10.1038/nn1729

Fernald, A. (1989). Intonation and communicative intent in mothers' speech to infants: is the melody the message? *Child Development, 60*(6), 1497–1510. doi:10.2307/1130938

Fernald, A. (1993). Approval and disapproval: Infant responsiveness to vocal affect in familiar and unfamiliar languages. *Child Development, 64*(3), 657–674. doi:10.2307/1131209

Fodor, J. A. (1975). *The language of thought.* New York: Crowell.

Fogassi, L., & Ferrari, Pier F. (2007). Mirror neurons and the evolution of embodied language. *Current Directions in Psychological Science, 16*(3), 136–141. doi:10.1111/j.1467-8721.2007.00491.x

Forgas, J. P. (2008). Affect and cognition. *Perspectives on Psychological Science, 3*(2), 94–101. doi:10.1111/j.1745-6916.2008.00067.x

Foroni, F., & Semin, G. R. (2009). Language that puts you in touch with your bodily feelings. The multimodal responsiveness of affective expressions. *Psychological Science, 20*(8), 974–980. doi:10.1111/j.1467-9280.2009.02400.x

Friend, M. (2000). Developmental changes in sensitivity to vocal paralanguage. *Developmental Science, 3,* 148–162. doi:10.1111/1467-7687.00108

Friend, M. (2001). The transition from affective to linguistic meaning. *First Language, 21,* 219–243. doi:10.1177/014272370102106302

Friend, M. (2003). What should I do? Behavior regulation by language and paralanguage in early childhood. *Journal of Cognition and Development, 4*(2), 162–183. doi:10.1207/S15327647JCD0402_02

Gallese, V. (2001). The "Shared Manifold" hypothesis: from mirror neurons to empathy. *Journal of Consciousness Studies, 8*(5-7), 33–50.

Gallese, V. (2008). Mirror neurons and the social nature of language: The neural exploitation hypothesis. *Social Neuroscience, 3*(3-4), 317–333.

Gallese, V., Fadiga, L., & Fogassi, L., & Rizzolatti, Giacomo. (1996). Action recognition in the premotor cortex. *Brain, 119*(2), 593–609. doi:10.1093/brain/119.2.593

Gallese, V., & Keysers, C., & Rizzolatti, Giacomo. (2004). A unifying view of the basis of social cognition. *Trends in Cognitive Sciences, 8*(9), 396–403. doi:10.1016/j.tics.2004.07.002

Gazzola, V., Aziz-Zadeh, L., & Keysers, C. (2006). Empathy and the somatotopic auditory mirror system in humans. *Current Biology, 16*(18), 1824–1829. doi:10.1016/j.cub.2006.07.072

Glenberg, A. M., & Robertson, D. A. (1999). Indexical understanding of instructions. *Discourse Processes, 28*(1), 1–26. doi:10.1080/01638539909545067

Glenberg, A. M., & Robertson, D. A. (2000). Symbol grounding and meaning: a comparison of high dimensional and embodied theories of meaning. *Journal of Memory and Language, 43*(3), 379–401. doi:10.1006/jmla.2000.2714

Goldin-Meadow, S. (2003). *The resilience of language. What gesture creation in deaf children can tell us about how all children learn language.* New York, Hove: Psychology Press (Taylor and Francis).

Grossmann, T., & Johnson, M. H. (2007). The development of the social brain in human infancy. *The European Journal of Neuroscience, 25*(4), 909–919. doi:10.1111/j.1460-9568.2007.05379.x

Grossmann, T., Striano, T., & Friederici, A. D. (2005). Infants' electric brain responses to emotional prosody. *Neuroreport, 16*(16), 1825–1828. doi:10.1097/01.wnr.0000185964.34336.b1

Grossmann, T., Striano, T., & Friederici, A. D. (2006). Crossmodal integration of emotional information from face and voice in the infant brain. *Developmental Science, 9*(3), 309–315. doi:10.1111/j.1467-7687.2006.00494.x

Hare, B. (2007). From non-human to human mind. What changed and why? *Current Directions in Psychological Science, 16*(2), 60–64. doi:10.1111/j.1467-8721.2007.00476.x

Hare, B., & Tomasello, M. (2005). Human-like social skills in dogs? *Trends in Cognitive Sciences, 9*(9), 439–444. doi:10.1016/j.tics.2005.07.003

Harris, C. L., Berko Gleason, J., & Aycicegi, A. (2006). When is a first language more emotional? Psychophysiological evidence from bilingual speakers. In Pavlenko, A. (Ed.), *Bilingual minds. Emotional experience, expression and representation* (pp. 257–283). Clevedon: Multilingual Matters.

Hauk, O., Johnsrude, I., & Pulvermüller, F. (2005). Somatotopic representation of action words in human motor and premotor cortex. *Neuron, 41*(2), 301–307. doi:10.1016/S0896-6273(03)00838-9

Hohenberger, A. (2004). S.Goldin-Meadow (2003). The resilience of language. What gesture creation in deaf children can tell us about how all children learn language. New York, Hove.: Psychology Press (Taylor and Francis). *Linguist List 15-683.*

Iacoboni, M., Molnar-Szakacs, I., Gallese, V., Buccino, G., Mazziotta, J. C., & Rizzolatti, G. (2005). Grasping the intentions of others with one's own mirror neuron system. *PLoS Biology, 3*(3), 529–535. doi:10.1371/journal.pbio.0030079

Kaplan, J. T., & Iacoboni, M. (2006). Getting a grip on other minds: Mirror neurons, intention understanding, and cognitive empathy. *Social Neuroscience, 1*(3-4), 175–183. doi:10.1080/17470910600985605

Karmiloff-Smith, A. (1979). Micro- and macrodevelopmental changes in language acquisition and other representational systems. *Cognitive Science, 3*(2), 91–118. doi:10.1207/s15516709cog0302_1

Karmiloff-Smith, A. (1986). From meta-processes to conscious access: Evidence from children's metalinguistic and repair data. *Cognition, 23*, 95–147. doi:10.1016/0010-0277(86)90040-5

Karmiloff-Smith, A. (1992). *Beyond modularity. A developmental perspective on cognitive science.* Cambridge, MA: MIT Press.

Keller, R. (1997). In what sense can explanations of language change be functional? In Gvozdanovic, J. (Ed.), *Language change and functional explanations* (pp. 9–19). Berlin: Mouton de Gruyter.

Keysers, C., & Gazzola, V. (2010). Social neuroscience: Mirror neurons recorded in humans. *Current Biology, 20*(8), R353–R354. doi:10.1016/j.cub.2010.03.013

Kim, J. (2006). Emergence: Core ideas and issues. *Synthese, 151*(3), 547–559. doi:10.1007/s11229-006-9025-0

Kuhl, P. K. (1993). Early linguistic experience and phonetic perception: implications for theories of developmental speech perception. *Journal of Phonetics, 21*(1-2), 125–139.

Kuhl, P. K. (1994). Learning and representation in speech and language. *Current Opinion in Neurobiology, 4*(6), 812–822. doi:10.1016/0959-4388(94)90128-7

Kuhl, P. K. (2000). A new view of language acquisition. *Proceedings of the National Academy of Sciences of the United States of America, 97*(22), 11850–11857. doi:10.1073/pnas.97.22.11850

Kuhl, P. K. (2004). Early language acquisition: Cracking the speech code. *Nature Reviews. Neuroscience, 5*(11), 831–843. doi:10.1038/nrn1533

Kuhl, P. K. (2007). Is speech learning 'gated' by the social brain? *Developmental Science, 10*(1), 110–120. doi:10.1111/j.1467-7687.2007.00572.x

Kuhl, P. K., Tsao, F.-M., & Liu, H.-M. (2003). Foreign-language experience in infancy: effects of short-term exposure and social interaction on phonetic learning. *Proceedings of the National Academy of Sciences of the United States of America, 100*(15), 9096–9101. doi:10.1073/pnas.1532872100

LaBar, K., & Phelps, E. (1998). Arousal-mediated memory consolidation: Role of the medial temporal lobe in humans. *Psychological Science, 9*, 490–493. doi:10.1111/1467-9280.00090

Lamm, C., Nusbaum, H. C., Meltzoff, A. N., & Decety, J. (2007). What are you feeling? Using functional magnetic resonance imaging to assess the modulation of sensory and affective responses during empathy for pain. *PLoS ONE, 12*, e1292. .doi:10.1371/journal.pone.0001292

Landry, S. H. (2008). The role of parents in early childhood learning. In R. E. Tremblay, R.G. Barr, R. de Peters, & M. Boivin (Eds.), *Encyclopedia on Early Childhood Development* [online] (pp. 1-6). Montreal Quebec: Centre of Excellence for Early Childhood Development. http://www.child-encyclopedia.com/documents/LandryANGxp.pdf. (Accessed 25/07/2010).

Lawrence, L.L., & Fernald, Anne (1993). *When prosody and semantics conflict: infants' sensitivity to discrepancies between tone of voice and verbal content*. Poster session presented at the biennial meeting of the Society for Research in Child Development, New Orleans, LA.

Levelt, W. J. M. (1999). Models of word production. *Trends in Cognitive Sciences, 3*(6), 223–233. doi:10.1016/S1364-6613(99)01319-4

Levelt, W. J. M., Roelofs, A., & Meyer, A. S. (1999). A theory of lexical access in speech production. *The Behavioral and Brain Sciences, 22*, 1–75. doi:10.1017/S0140525X99001776

Liberman, A. M., & Mattingly, Ignatius G. (1985). The motor theory of speech perception revised. *Cognition, 21*, 1–36. doi:10.1016/0010-0277(85)90021-6

Liberman, A. M., & Whalen, D. H. (2000). On the relation of speech to language. *Trends in Cognitive Sciences, 4*(5), 187–196. doi:10.1016/S1364-6613(00)01471-6

Lieberman, M. D. (2007). Social cognitive neuroscience: A review of core processes. *Annual Review of Psychology, 58*, 259–289. doi:10.1146/annurev.psych.58.110405.085654

Liebermann, P. (2000). *Human language and our reptilian brain: the subcortical bases of speech, syntax, and thought*. Cambridge, MA: Harvard University Press.

Liu, H.-M., Kuhl, Patricia K., & Tsao, F.-M. (2003). An association between mothers' speech clarity and infants' speech discrimination skills. *Developmental Science, 6*, F1–F10. doi:10.1111/1467-7687.00275

Mehler, J., Jusczyk, P., Lambertz, G., Halsted, N., Bertoncini, J., & Amiel-Tison, C. (1988). A precursor of language acquisition in young infants. *Cognition, 29*, 143–178. doi:10.1016/0010-0277(88)90035-2

Mukamel, R., Ekstrom, A. D., Kaplan, J., Iacoboni, M., & Fried, I. (2010). Single-neuron responses in humans during execution and observation of actions. *Current Biology, 10*(8), 750–756. doi:10.1016/j.cub.2010.02.045

Nazzi, T., Bertoncini, J., & Mehler, J. (1998). Language discrimination by newborns: Towards an understanding of the role of rhythm. *Journal of Experimental Psychology. Human Perception and Performance, 24*(3), 756–766. doi:10.1037/0096-1523.24.3.756

Nazzi, T., & Ramus, F. (2003). Perception and acquisition of linguistic rhythm by infants. *Speech Communication, 41*(1-2), 233–243. doi:10.1016/S0167-6393(02)00106-1

Niedenthal, P. M. (2007). Embodying emotion. *Science, 316*(5827), 1002–1005. doi:10.1126/science.1136930

Ochsner, K., & Barrett, L. F. (2001). The neuroscience of emotion. In Mayne, T., & Bonnano, G. (Eds.), *Emotion: Current Issues and Future Directions* (pp. 38–81). New York: Guilford.

Oztop, E., & Kawato, M., & Arbib, Michael. (2006). Mirror neurons and imitation: A computationally guided review. *Neural Networks, 19*(3), 254–271. doi:10.1016/j.neunet.2006.02.002

Paavola, L. (2006). Maternal sensitive responsiveness, characteristics and relations to child early communicative and linguistic development. *ACTA UNIVERSITATIS OULUENSIS B Humaniora 73.* Doctoral dissertation, University of Oulu, Finland.

Papoušek, M. (1989). Determinants of responsiveness to infant vocal expression of emotional state. *Infant Behavior and Development, 12*, 505–522. doi:10.1016/0163-6383(89)90030-1

Papoušek, M. (1992). Early ontogeny of vocal communication in parent-infant interactions. In H. Papoušek, Uwe Jürgens, & Mechthild Papoušek (Eds.), *Nonverbal vocal communication. Comparative and developmental approaches* (pp. 230-261). Cambridge: CUP and Paris: Edition de la Maison des Sciences de l'Homme.

Pater, J., Stager, C., & Werker, J. (2004). The perceptual acquisition of phonological contrasts. *Language, 80*(3), 361–379. doi:10.1353/lan.2004.0141

Pessoa, L. (2008). On the relationship between emotion and cognition. *Nature Reviews. Neuroscience, 9*, 148–158. doi:10.1038/nrn2317

Petitto, L. A. (1987). On the autonomy of language and gesture: Evidence from the acquisition of personal pronouns in American Sign Language. *Cognition, 27*, 1–52. doi:10.1016/0010-0277(87)90034-5

Pickering, M., & Garrod, S. (2007). Do people use language production to make predictions during comprehension? *Trends in Cognitive Sciences, 11*(3), 105–110. doi:10.1016/j.tics.2006.12.002

Poizner, H., Bellugi, U., & Klima, E. S. (1990). Biological foundations of language: Clues from sign language. *Annual Review of Neuroscience, 13*, 283–307. doi:10.1146/annurev.ne.13.030190.001435

Pourtois, G., Debatisse, D., Despland, P., & de Gelder, B. (2002). Facial expressions modulate the time course of long latency auditory brain potentials. *Brain Research. Cognitive Brain Research, 14*(1), 99–105. doi:10.1016/S0926-6410(02)00064-2

Preston, S., D., & de Waal, F. B. M. (2002). Empathy: It's ultimate and proximate bases. *The Behavioral and Brain Sciences, 25*, 1–72.

Prinz, W. (1997). Perception and action planning. *The European Journal of Cognitive Psychology, 9*(2), 129–154. doi:10.1080/713752551

Pulvermüller, F. (2005). Brain mechanisms linking language and action. *Nature Reviews. Neuroscience, 6*(7), 576–582. doi:10.1038/nrn1706

Pulvermüller, F., Härle, M., & Hummel, F. (2000). Neurophysiological distinction of semantic verb categories. *Neuroreport, 11*(12), 2789–2793. doi:10.1097/00001756-200008210-00036

Reilly, J. S., & McIntire, M. L. (1991). *WHERE SHOE: The acquisition of wh-questions in ASL. Papers and Reports in Child Language Development* (pp. 104–111). Stanford University, Department of Linguistics.

Reilly, J. S., & Seibert, L. (2003). Language and emotion. In Davidson, R., Scherer, K., & Goldsmith, H. (Eds.), *Handbook of affective sciences* (pp. 535–559). New York: Oxford University Press.

Rifkin, J. (2009). *The empathic civilization. The race to global consciousness in a world in crisis.* Cambridge: Polity Press.

Rizzolatti, G., & Arbib, M. (1998). Language within our grasp. *Trends in Neurosciences, 21*(5), 188–194. doi:10.1016/S0166-2236(98)01260-0

Rizzolatti, G., & Craighero, L. (2004). The mirror-neuron system. *Annual Review of Neuroscience, 27,* 169–192. doi:10.1146/annurev.neuro.27.070203.144230

Sandler, W., & Lillo-Martin, D. (2006). *Sign language and linguistic universals.* Cambridge: Cambridge University Press.

Schirmer, A., & Kotz, S. (2003). ERP evidence for a sex-specific Stroop effect in emotional speech. *Journal of Cognitive Neuroscience, 15*(8), 1135–1148. doi:10.1162/089892903322598102

Singer, T., Seymour, B., O'Doherty, J., Kaube, H., Dolan, R. J., & Frith, C. D. (2004). Empathy for pain involves the affective but not sensory components of pain. *Science, 303*(5661), 1157–1162. doi:10.1126/science.1093535

Smith, E. E., & Kosslyn, S. M. (2007). *Cognitive psychology. Mind and brain.* New Jersey: Prentice Hall.

Stephan, A. (2006). The dual role of 'emergence' in the philosophy of mind and in cognitive science. *Synthese, 151*(3), 485–498. doi:10.1007/s11229-006-9019-y

Tamis-LeMonda, C. S., Bornstein, M. H., & Baumwell, L. (2001). Maternal responsiveness and children's achievement of language milestones. *Child Development, 72*(3), 748–767. doi:10.1111/1467-8624.00313

Tamis-LeMonda, C. S., & Rodriguez, E. T. (2008). Parents' role in fostering young children's learning and language development. In R.E. Tremblay, R.G. Barr, R. de Peters, and M. Boivin (Eds.), *Encyclopedia on Early Childhood Development* [online] (pp. 1-10). Montreal Quebec: Centre of Excellence for Early Childhood Development. http://www.ccl-cca.ca/pdfs/ECLKC/encyclopedia/TamisLemondaRodriguezANGxpCSAJELanguage.pdf. Accessed 25/07/2010.

Tomasello, M. (2003). *Constructing a language: A usage-based theory of language acquisition.* Cambridge, MA: Harvard University Press.

Tomasello, M. (2008). *Origins of human communication.* Cambridge, MA: MIT Press.

Tzourio-Mazoyer, N., de Schonen, S., Crivello, F., Reutter, B., Aujard, Y., & Mazoyer, B. (2002). Neural correlates of woman face processing by 2-month-old infants. *NeuroImage, 15*(2), 454–461. doi:10.1006/nimg.2001.0979

van Ijzendoorn, M. H., Dijkstra, J., & Bus, A. G. (1995). Attachment, intelligence, and language: A meta-analysis. *Social Development, 4*(2), 115–128. doi:10.1111/j.1467-9507.1995.tb00055.x

Vygotsky, L. S. (1962). *Thought and language.* Cambridge, MA: MIT Press. doi:10.1037/11193-000

Walker-Andrews, A. S. (1997). Infants' perception of expressive behaviors: differentiation of multimodal information. *Psychological Bulletin, 121,* 1–20. doi:10.1037/0033-2909.121.3.437

Walker-Andrews, A. S., & Grolnick, W. (1983). Discrimination of vocal expression by young infants. *Infant Behavior and Development, 6,* 491–498. doi:10.1016/S0163-6383(83)90331-4

Werker, J. F. (1993). Developmental changes in cross-language speech perception: implications for cognitive models of speech processing. In G. Altman and R. Shillcock (Eds.), *Cognitive models of speech processing. The second Sperlonga Meeting* (pp. 57-78). Hillsdale, NJ: Erlbaum.

Werker, J. F., & Tees, R. C. (1984). Cross-language speech perception: Evidence for perceptual reorganization during the first year of life. *Infant Behavior and Development, 7*, 49–63. doi:10.1016/S0163-6383(84)80022-3

Zelazo, P. D., Chandler, M., & Crone, Eveline (Eds) (2009). *Developmental social cognitive neuroscience.* New York, Hove: Psychology Press.

KEY TERMS AND DEFINITIONS

Emotional Context of Learning Hypothesis: According to Harris et al. (2006), it is the emotional context of early L1 or later L2 learning that is decisive for the success of language learning. If language is learned in an emotional context, additional brain areas like the amygdala will support and thus foster linguistic representation and processing.

Emotional Reactivity Hypothesis: According to Hare and Tomasello (2005), human cognitive abilities arose through a two-step evolutionary process. First, humans learned to suppress their strong emotional reactivity towards their conspecifics for the sake of cooperation. This first step amounts to a kind of "self-domestication". In the second step, which is contingent upon the first step, higher cognitive abilities such as theory of mind, language, and problem solving, became available for selection.

Intentionality Model of Language Acquisition: According to Bloom and Tinker (2001), infants acquiring a language wish to share their thoughts about the world with their social partners. (The "aboutness" of thoughts is called "intentional".) In order to do so infants make (i) a cognitive effort to learn the language and become (ii) socially and affectively engaged with their partners.

Modality: Here, modality refers to the medium through which language is conveyed. Spoken languages use the acoustic-vocal modality; sign languages the visual-gestural modality.

Motherese: also called **infant-** or **child-directed speech (ID, CD speech):** Motherese refers to a special speech register used in interaction with infants and young children. It is characterized by exaggerated intonation and phonemic contrasts, clear segmentation clues, strong affective vocal and facial expression, among others. Motherese is thought to support language development though its efficiency is still a matter of debate.

Native Language Magnet (-Extended): According to Kuhl (1993), infants in their first year of life build up phonemic prototypes of their native language. Incoming matching sounds are attracted to these prototypes that function like perceptual magnets. Recently, Kuhl (2007) extended the earlier version of this concept to include a **gating** of this process through social aspects. Information processing in the brain is canalized through social (and emotional) factors: A socially and affectively supportive environment is deemed to be beneficial for cognitive and language development.

Paralanguage: Non-verbal, vocal aspects of language, such as affective prosody. Paralanguage is mostly processed unconsciously along with the core "verbal" aspects of language (form and meaning).

Prosody: Supra-segmental, intonational aspects of language such as temporal structure, loudness, roughness, and pitch. Prosodic contours can span parts of speech and thus help segmenting the speech stream. Prosody also exists in sign languages in the form of non-manual markers such as facial expressions and bodily movements. Prosody serves core linguistic functions (e.g., syntax) as well as affective functions.

Social Brain: Network in the brain for processing social stimuli. It comprises the processing of faces, emotion, biological motion, human goal-directed actions, and joint attention (Grossmann & Johnson, 2007). Mirror neurons are involved in the processing of goal-directed actions.

Social Referencing: In a novel and potentially frightening situation, children tend to refer back to their caregivers in order to resolve the emotional ambiguity of the situation. The "social referencing paradigm" exposes children to such emotionally charged situations and then observes their reactions.

ENDNOTES

[1] Similarly, the concept of empathy is currently being revived. Rifkin (2009) even heralds an "empathic civilization", i.e., a global society whose members strive for mutual understanding and cooperation on the basis of an enlarged consciousness that includes the self and others. It is noteworthy that emotion, empathy and related topics emerge in the scientific and the societal discourse at the same time. This concurrence reflects the depth and scope of the ongoing paradigm shift in science and society.

[2] Often, in the literature, the two terms "sensitivity" and "responsiveness" are used interchangeably. If a distinction is to be made, then responsiveness is related to the contingency and frequency of the mother's response toward her child whereas sensitivity is related to the qualitative appropriateness of her response in terms of the child's developmental level and situational needs (Paavola, 2006, p. 19).

[3] Recently, a parallel of motherese has been argued for in the motor domain. Brand, Baldwin, & Ashburn (2002) observed that sensitive parents modify their actions when manipulating objects so as to highlight the objects' properties and affordances for the child. This sensitive enhancement has been called "infant-directed action (IDA)" or "motionese".

[4] The CARE-Index as an instrument for assessing mother-child interaction was applied at 10 months of age. In addition, maternal and infant communicative acts, maternal verbal responsiveness and infant intentionality were measured. At 12 months of age, the MacArthur Communicative Development Inventories (MCDI) and the Communication and Symbolic Behaviour Scales (CSBS) were measured. Finally, at 30 months of age, the Reynell Developmental Language Scales III were measured.

[5] Three of the added icons in this redrawing are standard graphics items from the word program. The icon of the brain is taken from www.schulbilder.org/gehirn-obenansicht-t4300.jpg (accessed 25/07/2010).

[6] A positive language stimulus was, e.g., "Nice play" and positive paralinguistic stimulus were a smiling face and approving voice. A negative language stimulus was, e.g., "Don't touch" and negative paralinguistic stimuli were a frowning face and disapproving voice.

[7] A similar discontinuous developmental pattern has been reported for the acquisition of pronouns in American Sign Language (Petitto, 1987). Sign language pronouns are identical to deictic pointing gestures, however, are subject to linguistic constraints which have to be acquired. While in the beginning, pointing gestures occur frequently, at some time in the language acquisition process they vanish completely. During this time the children work out the linguistic pronominal system. Afterwards, deictic pointing reoccurs, along with but functionally segregated from true linguistic pronouns.

[8] Mukamel et al. (2010) found mirror neurons in a wider variety of brain areas than previ-

ously thought, e.g., in the hippocampus. They also found "anti-mirror neurons" that are excited during action execution but inhibited during action perception. The significance of these new findings needs to be followed up by future research.

9 Ironically, this view converges with Fodor's (1975) "language of thought" or "mentalese" hypothesis, namely the idea that human thought is structured syntactically, much like language.

10 Already very young infants have clearly differentiated expectations how animate agents and inanimate objects behave. Thus, Falck-Ytter, Gredebäck, and von Hofsten (2006) could show in an eye-tracking study that 12-month olds, but not yet 6-month-olds, anticipate the movement of a human hand towards a spatial target with their eyes pro-actively, whereas they do not show such anticipatory eye-movements if objects move to this spatial target by themselves. The authors argue that this difference is evidence for the emerging mirror neuron system during the second half of the first year of life.

APPENDIX

AFFECT IN LANGUAGE DEVELOPMENT FROM A NEUROSCIENCE PERSPECTIVE

ERP Studies on the Processing of Emotional Prosody in Infants

Language as part of the "social brain" in the sense of Grossmann and Johnson (2007) is one expressive channel for affect. In this paragraph we will be concerned with the emotional-affective tone of a verbal message which is carried by the speech prosody. Emotional prosody is characterized by its temporal structure, amplitude (loudness), roughness, and pitch (fundamental frequency) (Grossmann, Striano, & Friederici, 2005). From previous research it is known that adults distinguish reliably between neutral, happy and angry prosody, as expressed by characteristic ERP components. Thus, the difference between neutral *vs.* happy messages is captured by the higher amplitude of the P200 for happy messages, whereas the difference between neutral *vs.* happy and angry messages is captured in the N400 (as summarized in Grossmann et al., 2005). The follow-up question that could only recently be addressed since the use of ERP in infant research has become feasible is how infants process emotional prosody (Grossmann et al., 2005, 2006). Previously, the processing of emotional prosody could only be studied behaviorally. Based on these early studies, Walker-Andrews (1997) proposed a developmental sequence in which children learn to discriminate emotional expressions, first on the basis of multimodal, then prosodic, and finally facial, cues. Although the auditory system develops earlier than the visual system, prosody alone is not enough to distinguish the conveyed emotion initially. When 5-month old infants are habituated to a congruent combination of facial and vocal cues (happy/sad face plus happy/sad voice) they dishabituate if subsequently the prosody changes (happy/sad face plus sad/happy voice), thus creating an incongruity between facial and vocal information; 3-month olds can only detect the change if a sad voice changes to a happy one (Walker-Andrews & Grolnick, 1983). Grossmann et al. (2005, 2006) recently studied infants' understanding of emotional prosody with the ERP paradigm. ERP had already proven successful in the study of facial emotional expressions in adults. Schirmer and Kotz (2003) could show that a stronger negative ERP component was present when 7-month old infants looked at angry as compared to happy faces.

In a first ERP study, Grossmann et al. (2005) asked whether (i) 7-month old infants would discriminate neutral *vs.* emotional prosody (happy and angry) and (ii) among the emotional prosody, whether they would discriminate happy *vs.* angry prosody of semantically neutral German verbs. They found a stronger negative shift at 300-600 ms post stimulus following angry as opposed to happy and neutral words and a stronger positive slow wave at around 500 ms following angry and happy as opposed to neutral stimuli, however only at left temporal sites. Their results confirmed the earlier results on facial emotional processing where infants likewise responded stronger to angry as opposed to happy faces. In both cases, the processing of verbal and visual emotional information, the higher amplitude of the negative component was thought to reflect a higher allocation of attention to the negative stimuli. The ERP results confirm a more generally found "negativity bias" that has been reliably found in adults also. Taken together, these findings converge with an evolutionary viability explanation: it is much more important to detect and react to potentially threatening, negative stimuli in the environment than to positive ones. The stronger positive slow wave to both angry and happy as opposed to neutral prosody reflects a heightened sensory response to emotionally laden as opposed to neutral words in the associative auditory cortex, more specifically, in the left superior temporal sulcus. This early sensitivity to prosodic cues may underlie the finding that vocal affect, sometimes also called "paralanguage", can facilitate the recognition and learning of spoken words (see above, the studies of Friend).

In a second ERP study, Grossmann, Striano, and Friederici (2006) asked how multisensory emotional information (face and voice) is integrated in young infants. As is known from previous studies, adults readily integrate both modalities, even when they are asked explicitly to ignore one – either the facial or the vocal information. When judging faces in the presence of incongruent vocal affect, adults showed a bias towards the incongruent voice (likewise for evaluation of the voice in the presence of incongruent facial affect) (de Gelder & Vroomen, 2000). In an ERP study by Pourtois, de Gelder, Vroomen, Rossion, and Crommelick (2000), subjects first saw an angry or a sad face followed by a congruent or incongruent vocal affective stimulus which they were supposed to evaluate. The congruent condition resulted in a stronger N100 in the auditory cortex, which suggests that the facial information strengthened the auditory processing. In a second experiment, Pourtois, Debatisse, Despland, and de Gelder (2002) compared happy *vs.* fearful faces and voices, respectively. They found that congruent face-voice pairs led to a positive ERP component that had an earlier peak as compared to incongruent pairs. The site of this effect was the anterior cingulate cortex, a region that is known to play a role in error monitoring. From these results, the authors concluded that emotionally congruent information is processed faster than incongruent information. Against the backdrop of these findings in adults, Grossmann et al. (2006) conducted an ERP study with 7-month old infants on the processing of congruent/incongruent visual and vocal affective stimuli. Subjects saw pictures of a woman with a happy or angry face and concurrently heard semantically neutral words spoken with a happy or angry voice. Incongruent voices led to a more negative component as compared to congruent voices, already 350 ms after stimulus onset and with a peak at 500 ms over frontal and central electrodes on both hemispheres. Specifically, the angry voice presented with the happy face had higher negative amplitude than the happy voice presented with the angry face. Also, congruent voices led to higher positive amplitude as compared to congruent voices after 600-1000 ms over central and parietal electrodes. The authors concluded that already 7-month old infants recognize identical affect across modalities, in accordance with behavioral studies. This recognition is presumably supported by infants' memory of happy and angry faces. Since before the age of 10 months they are more likely to be exposed to happy faces, infants more strongly expect a happy voice, so that they are more surprised when they rather hear an angry voice. This reasoning could explain the above result that their response was stronger to a happy face/angry voice than to an angry face/happy voice. In this context, a study by Tzourio-Mazoyer, de Schonen, Crivello, Reutter, Aujard, and Mazoyer (2002) deserves mentioning. They found that 2-month olds activated a similar neural network as adults when viewing faces (right-lateral fusiform face area, bilateral inferior occipital and parietal areas), however, they also showed activation in one additional area, namely Broca's area. The authors speculated that this co-activation of face and language regions in young infants reflects social aspects of language in face-to-face communication and possibly serves to facilitate early language acquisition, as discussed above.

The Human Mirror Neuron System: Human Action, Emotion, Empathy, and Language

In this section, I will give an overview over studies on the adult human mirror neuron system in order to provide a relevant neuro-scientific frame for the main developmental topic of this chapter. The discovery of the mirror neuron system by Rizzolatti and his collaborators was one of the major discoveries in the neurosciences in the 1990ies. The mirror neuron system had first been found in monkeys, and later also in humans (for an overview, see Rizzolatti & Craighero, 2004). Mirror neurons are a special class of neurons that fire when a subject perceives a goal-directed action as well as when the subject plans and produces the action herself. In the monkey, this property of mirror neurons could be proven through single cell recordings (Gallese, Fadiga, Fogassi, & Rizzolatti, 1996, among others). In humans, the evidence is mostly indirect and stems from fMRI studies (as summarized by Rizzolatti & Craighero, 2004). Mirror neurons are located in a variety of areas in the brain, in humans most notably in the left inferior frontal gyrus (IFG) that also comprises Broca's area, the classical area for language (production), in the adjacent premotor cortex and in the inferior parietal cortex. Only recently, single cell recordings have been reported in patients to be surgically treated for epilepsy (Mukamel, Ekstrom, Kaplan, Iacoboni, & Fried, 2010).[8] The primary function of mirror neurons has first been related with understanding of goal-directed transitive actions (actions directed at a goal-object) and later also with understanding of intentions (Iacoboni, Molnar-Szakacs, Gallese, Buccino, Mazziotta, & Rizzolatti, 2005). In humans, the mirror mechanism further suggests itself as an explanation of imitation (Meltzoff & Prinz, 2002; Brass & Heyes, 2005; Oztop, Kawato & Arbib, 2006). Theories of imitation presuppose some common representational format between perception and action, a "common code" (Prinz, 1997), and it is this commonality that the mirror neuron system can naturally account for. After the discovery of mirror neurons for perception and production of goal-directed, intentional behavior, their involvement in other cognitive areas such as social cognition, emotion and empathy, theory of mind, and language, has been investigated, too (Arbib, 2005; Bastiaansen, Thioux, & Keysers, 2009; Carr, Iacoboni, Dubeau, Mazziotta, & Lenzi, 2003; Decety & Ickes, 2009; Fogassi & Ferrari, 2007; Gallese, Keysers, & Rizzolatti, 2004; Gallese, 2008; Rizzolatti & Arbib, 1998; Rizzolatti, Fogassi, & Gallese, 2006). The universality, immediacy, and intuitiveness with which humans understand the emotional states of others and empathize with them led to the search for dedicated neural networks supporting those (Carr et al., 2003; deVignemont & Singer, 2006; Singer, Seymour, O'Doherty, Kaube, Dolan, & Frith, 2004; Lamm, Nusbaum, Meltzoff, & Decety, 2007). One system that has been invoked for emotion and empathy is the mirror neuron system (Preston & de Waal, 2002; Decety & Jackson, 2004, 2006; Decety & Ickes, 2009; Gallese, 2001, 2008; Kaplan & Iacoboni 2006). Emotions, according to Rizzolatti et al. (2006), allow for a seemingly direct mapping between the sensory input, i.e., the observation of an emotion, and the experience of that emotion in the perceiver. The mirror neuron system thus forms the basis for empathy in the case of reading another person's affective state and for mind reading in the case of discerning the intentions of others through observation of their goal-directed behavior and emotional display. The relation between action and emotion understanding and empathy, however, is highly intricate and far from being fully understood. Pieces of a still to be uncovered mosaic are emerging, though. Kaplan and Iacoboni (2006) argued that intention understanding in the observation of human action is informed by contextual information (whether a grasping action is carried out in the context of a meal or cleaning up) as well as by specific information about the grasping type (precision *vs.* whole hand grip). Furthermore, they showed that signal changes in the relevant right posterior inferior frontal gyrus (right posterior IFG) correlated with subjective ratings in some subscales of the Interpersonal Reactivity Index (IRI), namely the fantasy scale measuring cognitive aspects of empathy and empathic concern measuring affective aspects of empathy, respectively. From these results they deduce "a central role of the human mirror neuron system in social competence." (Kaplan & Iacoboni, 2006, p. 182). In another fMRI study, Carr et al. (2003) monitored the brain activity of subjects whose task was to imitate or just observe emotional facial expressions. They found a similar network of active areas in imitation and observation consisting of the premotor face area, the dorsal sector the pars opercularis of the IFG, superior temporal sulcus (STS), the insula and the amygdala. Rather than claiming that empathy is a mirror system itself, they emphasize the link between emotion understanding and empathy with the mirror system of action understanding. By simulating the action which leads to the emotional (face) expression, the observer can empathize with that emotion. This "empathic resonance occurs via communication between action representation networks and limbic areas provided by the insula." (Carr et al. 2003, p. 5502) For the understanding of emotional facial expressions, "embodied" approaches have been put forward. Either mimicry or internal simulation is invoked as a mechanism for understanding others' emotions. A direct account in terms of facial mimicry – which may, however, remain subliminal – is proposed by Niedenthal (2007). She reports behavioral studies measuring activation of facial muscles corresponding to emotions in subjects looking at pictures that evoke various emotions: anger was related to a subliminal activation of the corrugator supercilii ("frowning"), disgust to the levator labii ("grimacing"), and joy to the zygomatic major ("smiling"). Other studies showed that reading words that are related to positive and negative emotions, e.g., "to smile" or "to frown", and that involve typical facial expressions, leads to motor resonance *via* the subliminal activation of the corresponding muscles (zygomatic major and corrugator supercilii) (Foroni & Semin, 2009). This effect is stronger for verbs than for adjectives that are more abstract and less directly related to facial expressions ("funny", "annoying"). The effect vanishes if motor resonance is inhibited as when subjects have to hold a pencil between their lips so that the muscle cannot engage in motor resonance when the emotional word is being processed. Not only the conscious perception of emotion words but also their unconscious processing induced by subliminal presentation evokes motor resonance. Motor resonance was shown to further influence evaluative judgments of cartoons. Thus, subjects whose "smile" muscles are not disabled, reading the word "smile" on a computer screen subsequently rate cartoons funnier as compared to subjects whose "smile" muscles are inhibited. Foroni and Semin (2009) as well as Niedenthal (2007) take these results as evidence for the "embodiment of language" in general, and for the "indexical hypothesis of language comprehension" of Glenberg and Robertson (1999, 2000), in particular. Somatic responses involved in the processing of emotion words lead to simulation of the emotional experience in the perceiver and thus contribute to the understanding of the meaning of those words. How exactly the concepts of facial mimicry and motor resonance are related to the mirror neuron mechanism in the brain is not fully clear, yet. A more indirect account in terms of internal embodied simulation (and not just overt facial mimicry) that makes the hidden inner states of the observee accessible to the observer is proposed by Bastiaansen et al. (2009). They call this link the "Rosetta stone" (2009, p. 2397) that helps translate observable (facial) actions of others into their hidden internal states, i.e., their emotions and intentions. This link could exist between the premotor cortex and IFG. Since premotor areas do not activate motor actions (such as facial expressions), this more indirect account seems less embodied and somewhat more cognitive than the more direct account of Niedenthal, Foroni and Semin. However, common to both approaches is the claim that it is the modality-specific, perceptual systems of the brain that support the simulation of the affect and that simulation is not so much a matter of the muscles and viscera (Niedenthal, 2007, p. 1005).

Chakrabarti, Bullmore, and Baron-Cohen (2006) showed that a cluster of mirror-neuron areas, namely left dorsal inferior frontal gyrus and premotor cortex, correlated positively with the "Empathy Quotient" (EQ), a measure of trait empathy, across a variety of emotional conditions (happy, sad, angry and surprised facial expressions). Thus, the mirror neuron system mediates between the perception and recognition of actions and emotions. Also de Vignemont and Singer (2006) stress the link between empathy and action understanding. They propose that "empathy provides a more precise and direct estimate of other people's future actions because shared emotional networks also directly elicit the activation of associated relevant motivational and action systems." (p. 439). This is an epistemological function. A social function of empathy is that it facilitates social communication and social coherence. The link between the presumed mirror neuron system for emotion and communication points to a possible connection between the mirror neuron system and language. Already long before the discovery of mirror neurons, it had been proposed in the "motor theory of speech perception" that the sounds of language are perceived in terms of their motor gestures (Liberman & Mattingly, 1985; Liberman & Whalen, 2000). After the discovery of mirror neurons, a mirror mechanism was proposed for the relation between language perception and production, too (Arbib 2005; Gallese 2006; Oztop, Kawato, and Arbib 2006; Rizzolatti and Arbib 1998). In a similar vein, simulation of language production during comprehension has been invoked as a mechanism for explaining the ease of mutual understanding in communication (Pickering & Garrod, 2007). While these studies focused on the inherent mirror qualities of the language system, the relation between emotion and language in the scope of a mirror mechanism became a research topic subsequently. Not only direct observation of (visual) emotional displays, as discussed above, informs us about the affective state of others, but also properties of language. Here, language is conceived of in terms of human social cognition and not so much as an autonomous mental faculty of the human mind (in the sense of Chomsky, 2000, 2007, among many others). In such an "embodied view" on language, the support of human social communication and action by the language circuits in the brain are in focus (Gallese, 2008; Niedenthal, 2007). Crucial in this respect is the re-assessment of the role of Broca's are (BA 44), which is one part of the left ventral premotor cortex. Previously, it had been reserved for language (production) functions only; however, nowadays it is considered to play a major role in action understanding and production also. Broca's area generally supports the construal of complex hierarchical representations that may serve the planning and production of action sequences, musical themes, and sentences alike. The notion of "syntax" thus becomes generalized and comprises various domains of cognition, not just language.[9] Mirror neurons provide a mechanism that establishes a direct relation between the sender and receiver of a communicative message, be it an observed action or communication. They solve two problems at the same time: the "parity" and the "direct comprehension" problem (Rizzolatti et al., 2006). Parity means that the meaning is the same for the sender and the receiver and direct comprehension means that there is a direct, hard-wired mapping of the percept (visual action scene, emotional expression) onto its meaning, "without any cognitive mediation" (Rizzolatti & Craighero, 2004, p. 183). Turning to the relevance of the mirror neuron account for language, Gallese (2008) proposes an "embodied" view that grounds the processing of language in the human action system. He points out how such an embodied language is instantiated on various levels: the vehicle level of motor articulation, the content level of meaning, and even the syntactic level of recursive phrase structure. In his "neural exploitation hypothesis" he claims that neural circuits that originally evolved for the perception and control of motor actions were later exploited by the newly emerging language faculty. Thus, language (and thought) inherited crucial properties, among them "mirror" properties, from these evolutionarily older action systems. Much like stringing together individual actions to form an "action sentence", we are now also stringing words together to form sentences. A crucial "relay" mechanism might be provided by the "auditory mirror neuron system". Shortly after the discovery of visual mirror neurons another population of mirror neurons was found (in the monkey brain) that respond to the production of an action and also to the perception of the specific sounds that accompanied actions and instantiate action effects, e.g., cracking a peanut, tearing a sheet of paper, or opening a can (Rizzolatti & Craighero, 2004; Gallese, 2008; Gazzola et al., 2006; Aziz-Zadeh et al., 2010). Some of these actions and corresponding sounds involve the hand and some of them the mouth. The left temporo-parietal premotor circuit is organized in a somatotopic way, i.e., hand actions/sounds activate dorsal premotor hand areas (BA6) and mouth actions/sounds activate left ventral premotor mouth areas (BA 44) (Gazzola et al., 2006). This somatotopic organization is also supported by the effector-specific "word nets" that Pulvermüller and colleagues found for action words related to those effectors. They showed in a number of studies that during the processing of action words that imply certain body parts such as "lick", "pick", and "kick" (pre-)motor areas of the brain, namely for the mouth, hands, and legs, are co-activated along with the classical language areas. Likewise, during the processing of visual words such as "see", areas in the occipital lobe are co-activated (Hauk, Johnsrude, & Pulvermüller, 2004; Pulvermüller, 2005, among many others). Since the auditory mirror neuron system is left-lateralized, as expected from its relation with language, it may also be connected to the left-hemispheric multi-modal mirror system that comprises the visual modality, thus forming a supra-modal interface between human action and language in perception and production (Gazzola et al., 2006, p. 1827).

Emotional resonance, as suggested by the "embodied" or simulation account of emotion understanding, has been related to observational learning (Niedenthal, 2007). If the emotional expression of the observed other person is mirrored in the observer, the corresponding emotional experience may be relived and thus an empathic understanding may be reached. Not only through observational learning, but also through instructed learning, i.e., through language, reexperience of an emotion may be triggered. As Niedenthal (2007, p. 1004) points out, a child being told not to put her fingers into an electrical outlet, otherwise she will experience a painful electric shock, must be able to reexperience the linguistically conveyed emotion (here, pain).

Few neuro-imaging studies have so far investigated the production of emotional words. Cato et al. (2004) showed in an fMRI study that (silently) generating emotional words with positive and negative meaning activates dedicated areas in the rostral frontal and retrosplenial/posterior cingulate cortex as compared to emotionally neutral words. The rostral, frontal area presumably supports "the generation of words with emotional connotation", whereas the role of the retrosplenial/posterior cingulate cortex is "the evaluation of an external stimulus with emotional salience" (Cato et al., 2004, p. 173). More common are studies that investigate the brain areas active in the production of syllables with specific affective prosody. These studies tap into the relation between affective aspects of language and empathy.

As the mirror neuron system is presumably in the service of understanding others, several neuro-imaging studies on the perception (and production) of human action and action-related sounds also assessed individual empathy levels of the subjects. The hypotheses (i) that there should be a relation between the activation of the mirror neuron system and empathy, as measured in questionnaires in general, and, more specifically, (ii) that higher empathy ratings should go along with higher levels of activation in the mirror neuron areas were confirmed in several studies (Gazzola et al., 2006; Aziz-Zadeh et al., 2010; Kaplan et al., 2006). The property of language most intimately related to the expression of affect is prosody. As prosody is related to language and to emotion, for both of which mirror neuron systems had been found, it was conjectured that there may exist a mirror system for prosody, too. A candidate system would be the auditory mirror system as discussed above. In a combined behavioral and fMRI study, Aziz-Zadeh et al. (2010) assessed subjects' brain activity while they judged the emotional quality of audio-clips with happy, sad, question, and neutral intonation. Also, subjects had to utter non-sense syllables ('dadadadada') with emotional prosody in the scanner. In the behavioral part, they tested again subjects' own production of affective prosody (that was subsequently rated for their prosodic quality) and had subjects rate another set of audio-clips with affective prosody. In order to assess their empathy, subjects filled in a two questionnaires. The fRMI study showed that common areas were active during perception and production of emotional (as well as linguistic) prosody, namely areas in the left premotor cortex (left inferior frontal gyrus (IFG), left dorsal premotor cortex). This is evidence for a prosodic mirror system. IFG and premotor areas have links to auditory areas. Through this dorsal pathway the interface between perceived and articulated language might be constituted. Moreover, there were correlations between the amount of activation of brain areas for emotional prosody and empathy scores as well as between prosodic perceptual abilities and empathy scores. Also prosody production inside and outside the scanner were found to be correlated. From these findings Aziz-Zadeh et al. concluded: "This data support the notion that components of empathy to emotional stimuli may rely on simulation processes carried out, in part, by motor-related areas (…). Thus, in order to understand someone else's prosodic intonation, we may simulate how we would produce the given intonation ourselves, which in turn may be a component of the process involved in creating empathic feeling for that individual." (2010, p. 6)

Motor resonance might equally contribute to and facilitate lexical learning in young children. Contexts in which young children learn words are those where they interact with others and with objects that have certain characteristics, internal, and external. These properties are revealed during the interaction, e.g., emotions, motives, and goals of the human play partners on the one hand, and physical properties, affordances, and action effects of the objects, on the other hand.[10] The tight connection between emotions and language is witnessed in language acquisition where initially, in the first year of life, the speech melody that carries the affective prosody, is the main message to the child (Papoušek, 1992). Young children are more susceptible to this information in the speech stream than to the lexical information, initially. When they acquire language, however, they have to learn to integrate the emotional information and the lexical information – a not at all trivial task (see section on "Parents' sensitivity to informational and affective content in their infants' vocalizations" above).

Chapter 11
Problems Associated with Computer–Mediated Communication:
Cognitive Psychology and Neuroscience Perspectives

Gülsen Yıldırım
Informatics Institute, METU, Turkey

Didem Gökçay
Informatics Institute, METU, Turkey

ABSTRACT

In this chapter, the authors examine some of behavioral problems frequently observed in computer-mediated communication and point out that a subset of these behavioral problems is similar to those of patients with brain lesions. The authors try to draw an analogy between the lack of affective features in text-based computer-mediated communication (CMC) versus the functional deficits brought along by regional brain damage. In addition, they review the social psychological studies that identify behavioral problems in CMC, and merge the literature in these different domains to propose some requirements for initiating conceptual changes in text-based CMC applications.

INTRODUCTION

Humans solve real life problems through an intricate interplay between emotion and cognition. In general, cognitive processing demands conscious involvement of the individual, but emotional processing employs automatic survival mechanisms as well. In daily situations, communication usually occurs through face-to-face (FtF) interaction. This type of interaction contains adequate environmental context for generation of subjective judgments automatically, using the emotional circuitry in our brains. For example, individuals are capable of evaluating the real intent or meaning behind

DOI: 10.4018/978-1-61692-892-6.ch011

a sentence, not only by judging the content in semantics (which is accomplished by cognitive procedures), but also by judging facial expressions, prosody in speech and sensory inputs received from the surrounding environment. A sentence which is neutral according to semantic content can be conceived as a happy or a fearsome event, if extra information regarding subjective ratings of the present situational cues is provided by the emotional circuitry.

On the other hand, computer- mediated communication (CMC) became an indispensable part of our lives. For more than two decades, CMC applications have been evolving continuously (Antheunis et al., 2010). Starting the journey with primitive and asynchronous text-based communication tools, the latest generation of CMC applications such as social network sites is very different from the initial examples of CMC applications in terms of both media richness and the largeness of the communities using those applications (Antheunis et al., 2010). For instance, social network sites are different from conventional CMC applications as they support both offline-online and asynchronous-synchronous communication, the audiovisual content and "one-to-many communication" (Antheunis et al., 2010; Ross et al., 2009). In addition, users of the social network sites can interact with each other in all passive, active and interactive strategies in order to collect more information about the individuals of the target of the social attraction (Antheunis et al., 2010).

Although CMC eases our lives, it also brings along some problems. The anonymous and socially disconnected medium of CMC applications cause people to exhibit behaviors which are otherwise prohibited to be performed in natural social environments (Short et al., 1976; Siegel et al., 1986). In addition, CMC ranks far behind FtF communication in terms of media richness causing less social presence, reduced social norms and control (Daft & Lengel, 1986). Because of these reasons, people communicating through CMC, whether in a text-based environment or not,

exhibit a multitude of negative behaviors such as flaming (Siegel et al., 1986; Moor et al., 2010), fearlessness (Maksimova, 2005), and inability to self-monitor (Sproull & Kiesler, 1991; Short et al., 1976; Zhao et al., 2008). Furthermore, there is a lack of awareness in this type of miscommunication (Kruger et al., 2005) as well as inability to evaluate social cues (Lo, 2008; McKenna et al., 2002; Bargh et al., 2002).

Interestingly, similar behavioral problems also exist in patient populations with damage to the limbic system and its anatomic correlates. In this study, we investigated the behavioral problems in CMC from both socio-psychology (Section 2) and cognitive neurology perspectives (Section 3) by examining the literature. We found striking behavioral similarities between the users of, mainly, text-based communication platforms and patients with deficits of the limbic system (amygdala, OFC and septal nuclei). These similarities and the fundamental concepts about limbic system are provided in Section 3. In light of the problems of CMC and corresponding anomalies in the human brain, we will present a preliminary perspective to help to interpret problems associated with text-based CMC and emphasize the immediate need for the enhancement of the affective dimension in platforms that depend primarily on text.

In our review, we mainly concentrated on text-based CMC for the following reasons. First, although CMC applications evolve continuously, the most rigid, in other words resistant to change, part of these applications are text-based CMC applications. Therefore, understanding behavioral problems in text-based CMC is essential, especially when the exponential increase in the number of individuals using these environments is considered. Second, text based communication is the main component of, roughly, all CMC applications, regardless of the multimedia features supported by the applications. For that reason, text-based communication requires attention constantly as a core component. Third, even though the number of CMC environments operating with multimedia channels increase day by day, especially with the success of social network sites, the studies conducted on the next-generation CMC environments are limited for now.

THE SOCIO-PSYCHOLOGICAL EVALUATION OF CMC

In this section, we present the studies and theoretical approaches in an attempt to explain the reasons underlying some of the fundamental problems in CMC: the lack of social cues and self-monitoring, flaming, anonymity, and exaggerated truth bias. Although one may find lots of studies that approach the social and psychological problems in CMC in different perspectives like the effect of personality in CMC usage (Swickert et al., 2002; Ross et al., 2009) and changes in group behavior in CMC (Siegel et al., 1986), we tried to encapsulate only the topics which are strongly connected to the proposed neuroscientific approach.

In the first part, social presence theory and cues-filtered-out is examined to clarify the absence of social cues, flaming and lack of self-monitoring. In addition, opposing or complementing views for the cues-filtered-out is presented. In the following part, identity creation and self-disclosure on the Internet are presented in order to underline one of the most important problems of Internet, and so of CMC, anonymity as well as the lack of self-monitoring. In the third part, we mention the difficulty of developing trust on the Internet in order to make clear the concept of underestimated and exaggerated truth bias. In the last part of this section, we present the studies, and thus, the proved facts about transmission of emotional cues and in particular, flaming.

Social Presence, Media Richness and Cues-Filtered-Out

Social presence theory states that parties involved in communication must be aware of each other

(Short et al., 1976). When people stop considering other social actors in interaction, their social attitude changes; they stop monitoring themselves as individuals, and thus, altering their behavior based on social norms (Zimbardo, 1970). Consequently, their evaluation of the opposite party according to social norms decreases. Therefore, the absence of social presence leads to inefficient social communication due to the inhibition of the interpersonal situations and social rules in extreme cases.

On the other hand, there is a strong relationship between the codes and channels available in the communication medium, which is in fact media richness, and the attention paid to the existence of other people (Riva, 2002). In the case of fewer codes or channels, users pay less attention to the social presence of others. Accordingly, FtF communication ranks highest with respect to the quality and diversity of information carried during communication and CMC ranks far behind FtF communication in terms of media richness (Bos et al., 2002). Therefore, social presence, and thus, the social norms and control, is much less in CMC environments (Daft & Lengel, 1986).

The social presence theory is the fundamental concept which explains the "cues-filtered-out" in CMC (Culnan & Markus, 1987). Based on the social presence theory, 'the cues-filtered-out' means that, in CMC, individuals are isolated from social cues and rules required to identify both personal and interpersonal situations, resulting in depersonalization, disinhibition, and misinterpretation in CMC (Kiesler et al., 1984; Sproull & Kiesler, 1991). Once social cues are excluded from the communication medium, social identities are curtained in such a way that the social presence of communicating parties disappears and more open and free communication styles arise (Sproull & Kiesler, 1991). This context, then, encourages individuals to break social rules and engage in swearing or flaming.

To emphasize the effect of the absence of social cues in a more detailed manner, Kiesler et al. assess CMC environments according to the following technical and cultural characteristics (Kiesler et al., 1984, 1125):

a. Lack of social context: In FtF communication, due to the existence of the corporal body, individuals handle the information exchanged during communication with the help of social cues such as "head nods, smiles, eye contact, distance, tone of voice, and other nonverbal behavior." Such regulating feedback that assists in the in-depth exploration of the meaning and evaluation of communication are absent in CMC. This characteristic also reduces the cues for "dramaturgical" assessment, such as head position, tone of speaking, and touching, which helps us in coordination of communication. In addition, as there is no way to interpret the social hierarchy, especially in text-based CMC environments, in which computer communication is blind to "status and position cues" in terms of both "contextual" ways (i.e., "the way clothes communicate") and "dynamic" ways (i.e., communication through facial expression, touch, etc.).

b. Accepted norms driving CMC usage: Most importantly, communication via computers is depersonalizing. The medium through which we interact terminates individuality with the common and anonymous standards it imposes, which results in "more uninhibited text and more assertiveness in return." As for common standardization, the widely used language in CMC (i.e., the abbreviations people use within computer chat mediums, the technical terminology infiltrated into our conversations or the use of emoticons) and CMC medium standards like the pressure of instantaneous communications can be considered. For instance, instantaneous communication, like in the case of chat or email, forces individuals to engage in rapid information transitions that could lead to

a decrease in quality of information and, consequently, miscommunication.

Along with the studies supporting the cues-filtered-out concept (e.g., Zhao et al., 2008), the ones opposing or complementing it have also been published. The most widely cited theoretical approaches that try to explain the miscommunication and the effects of the absence of social cues in CMC are social information processing perspective (Walther, 1992; Walther & Burgoon, 1992), social identity model of deindividuation (Lea & Spears, 1995), and miscommunication as a chance theory (Anolli, 2002). These approaches will be introduced in the following along with a summary in Table 1.

According to the social information processing (SIP) perspective (Walther, 1992; Walther & Burgoon, 1992), individuals have the capability to adopt given communication circumstances independent from the constraints provided, such as language and textual display. Although it takes time to learn usage specifications of the communication medium, individuals are capable of finding alternative ways to sustain relational content and impression management in the absence of social cues in CMC.

On the other hand, the social identity model of deindividuation (SIDE) tries to cover the absence of social cues and regulating feedbacks in CMC with the invisible social norms and identity (Lea & Spears, 1995). According to SIDE, the processes driven by the unseen social regulations become more important in the absence of social cues in CMC. Therefore, individuals are forced to regulate their behaviour with respect to hidden social norms within the uncertain environment of CMC.

The miscommunication as a chance theory (MaCHT) (Anolli, 2002) focuses on the advantage of the lack of social cues. According to MaCHT, the miscommunication that arises in CMC provides individuals with the opportunity to communicate freely. This degree of freedom may lead to the discovery of new communicative

Table 1. Summary of theoretical approaches for miscommunication in CMC

Theory	Explanation	Corresponding Publication
Cues-filtered-out	Based on the social presence theory, CMC lacks social cues required to identify the interpersonal situations	Kiesler et al., 1984
Media Richness	Due to the insufficient media richness, CMC lacks social norms and control.	Daft & Lengel, 1986
Social Information Processing (SIP)	Individuals have ability to adopt the absence of social cues and find alternative ways to handle relational and impression management in the interaction with others.	Walther, 1992
Social Identity Model of Deindividuation (SIDE)	Hidden social norms will be more important in the absence of regulating social cues such that individuals tune their behavior according to these hidden social norms to interact with the others effectively.	Lea & Spears, 1995
Miscommunication as a CHance Theory (MaCHT)	The miscommunication and absence of social cues in CMC provides a free way of communication for the individuals. Under the existence of such constraints, individuals may find compensatory ways to communicate and obtain results that FtF communication may not allow.	Anolli, 2002

tools to improve the efficiency of interaction such that the results not observed in FtF communication may be explored. For instance, the creation of a relationship in CMC for a person with low social skills is given as a result that supports MaCHT.

To summarize, we tried to present explanations to clarify the problems of the absence of social cues, flaming and lack of self-monitoring in CMC. The inadequate characteristics of CMC like the paucity of rich media may result in the absence of self presence which results in disinhibition, and consequently flaming. In addition, the CMC medium in which the social cues are filtered out causes depersonalization, disinhibition, and misinterpretation. Although, there are opposing arguments such as the ability of individuals to adopt to weak communication mediums (SIP), the existence of invisible social norms to regulate interpersonal relationships (SIDE), and the benefits of free communication environment which the drawbacks of CMC medium produces (MaCHT), the disadvantages brought by the cues-filtered-out is likely to dominate the evaluation of CMC environments.

Although the cues-filtered-out in CMC has been evaluated for more than two decades ago (Kiesler et al., 1984; Sproull & Kiesler, 1991), most of the claims are still valid today. Since that time, only the variety of CMC applications and the

multimedia content they support, consequently the media richness, have changed. Fortunately, today, we have a chance to engage in video conferences or communicate in an enhanced audiovisual environment. Certainly, the inventions of technology such as the realization of large-bandwidth usage have an important effect on enabling rich multimedia applications of CMC. However, we would like to mention in this chapter the paucity of innovative approaches in CMC applications to overcome the constraints and behavioral problems in the communication medium. Ever since the cues-filtered-out was highlighted, only minor functional but not conceptual changes have been observed in the widely used text-based CMC applications like email.

Identity Creation, Self-Disclosure, and Anonymity

Many studies have examined the motivations behind people's use of the Internet to identify the Internet's effect on our social lives and to understand the shift in some traditional human behaviors. Among the many motivations behind Internet usage, the fact that the Internet serves as a domain for identity recreation stands out. Needless to say, identity recreation for the sake of better self-presentation to a larger audience in contrast to FtF interaction is commonly observed in CMC environments (Yurchisin et al., 2005; Ellison et al., 2006; Zhao et al., 2008; McKenna et al., 2002; Bargh et al., 2002). Moreover, Yurchisin and her colleagues (2005) found that one of the main reasons people use Internet dating sites is because they wish to (re)create themselves, thereby giving expression to the selves what they wish to be, although seeking friendship or romance partners is thought to be the main motivator. Therefore, in this section, we will try to enhance the idea of identity recreation via CMC environments, and introduce some of the characteristics, such as anonymity, which facilitate this behavior. We will first introduce the notion of self-concept and identity creation to give a brief idea of the fundamental concept of this section. Then, we will provide plenty of studies on identity creation in CMC environments to present the reader with the new ways the Internet offers to create and present identities.

Schouten (1991, p. 413) defines self-concept as "the cognitive and affective understanding of who and what we are." In other words, self-concept is all of the explicit and implicit symbols, feelings, and thoughts we use for self-creation and self-understanding. Self-concept is "what comes to mind when we think of ourselves" (Oyserman, 2001, p. 499).

Identity is defined as a social product of self-concept, which is developed through social context and shaped to fit the characteristics of the participated social environment. Hence, identity construction occurs according to relationships with others and the way others view us (Oyserman, 2001; Schau & Gilly, 2003; Yurchisin et al., 2005; Ellison et al., 2006; Zhao et al., 2008; McKenna et al., 2002; Bargh et al., 2002). The individuals evaluate and tend to redefine their identities when they encounter a triggering event. In other terms, identity construction is a continually ongoing dynamic interplay of the social context and cognitive processes (Oyserman, 2001). Markus and Nurius (1986) put forward the concept of

possible selves to identify the dominant factors in this interplay, which leads the winning decision of the identity recreation process. They have shown that possible selves have a remarkable impact on identity recreation.

Markus and Nurius (1986) categorize self-concept in two divisions: now (or "here-and-now" - Markus & Nurius, 1986, p. 961) and possible selves. The way we perceive ourselves at the present time refers to 'now selves'. The selves that are not currently realized, but are hoped or feared for, are called possible selves: "hoped-for" and "feared" possible selves (Markus & Nurius, 1986, p. 957). In other words, what we want to be or not be (like) has a significant influence on our identity recreations: "possible selves can be viewed as cognitive bridges between the present and future, specifying how individuals may change from how they are now to what they will become" (Markus & Nurius, 1986, p. 961).

In addition, the identity recreation process is affected by others' feedbacks (Yurchisin et al., 2005). In the recreation process, feedbacks from, and thus, the validation of others, together with the hoped-for selves play an important role in identity recreation.

Online applications, in which individuals introduce themselves to someone or an audience, seek friendships or social interactions, meet their offline social network partners became part of our social worlds. Hence, the process of online identity creation and recreation is an important issue of our social lives. Some of the prominent online environments in which recreation is frequently observed are personal Web sites (Schau & Gilly, 2003), Internet dating forums (Yurchisin et al., 2005; Ellison et al., 2006; Gibbs et al., 2006; Whitty, 2008), and even social network sites (Zhao et al., 2008). The most fundamental reason for identity recreation on the Internet is stated to be anonymity (Yurchisin et al., 2005; McKenna et al., 1999; McKenna et al., 2002).

Possibly, the most remarkable CMC applications in which self-presentation, self-disclosure and, thus, continuous progress of identity recreation can be observed are Internet dating sites. This is not a surprising fact, as, with the help of the profile matching tools these sites offer, individuals have a chance to communicate with lots of possible partners with whom they probably share similar interests and motivations. It is also reported that social network sites which are today's hot interaction domains with large audiences are also fertile grounds to find romance partners (Lee & Bruckman, 2007) although their main purpose is to serve as an online meeting point for the offline social networks.

There are several studies about self-presentation strategies (Gibbs et al., 2006; Whitty, 2008) and the identity construction characteristics (Yurchisin et al., 2005; Ellison et al., 2006) of individuals on Internet dating sites. These studies tell us a lot about the behavioral characteristics of users in self-presentation more generally on the Internet. To summarize, individuals who overemphasize the importance of physical looks in attraction find the online dating experience more comfortable, probably due to the absence of a corporal body, and the opportunities to be creative in terms of self-presentation and identity construction (Whitty, 2008). Those individuals are extremely strategic in self-presentation on Internet dating sites. Needless to say, the amount and depth of self-disclosure differs from FtF interactions (Whitty, 2008), which also results in the fact that individuals encounter more misrepresentation issues in online romantic relationships than in FtF interactions. Furthermore, the amount of misinterpretation varies according to the degree of involvement (Ellison et al., 2006). The perceived success of online dating sites is evaluated by the dimensions of disclosure, such as amount, intent, valance, and honesty (Gibbs et al., 2006). However, the users of these sites consider that honesty has a negative effect on the success of online dating sites (Gibbs et al., 2006), which explains one of the motivations underlying deception. In a survey of one online dating site's participants conducted by Gibbs et. al. (2006), 86% of participants found that others misrepresented their physical appearance, and 49% reported this misrepresentation by others was about their relationship goals. Finally, Internet dating sites are used not only to create friendships or romantic relationships, but also to recreate identities according to the hoped-for selves (Yurchisin et al., 2005; Ellison et al., 2006).

In contrast to the claims stated above, some of the relationships maintained via the Internet tend to be close and lasting, which provides support for the argument that the Internet provides new ways for identity creation. In order to explain this phenomenon, McKenna et al. (McKenna et al., 1999; McKenna et al., 2002; Bargh et al., 2002) focused on the correlation between intimacy and self-presentation on the Internet. McKenna and her colleagues (2002) assume that the Internet eases the formation of relationships and intimacy due to the following characteristics:

- The anonymity of the Internet reduces the risks of ridicule and disapproval which is facilitated by identity recreation (McKenna et al., 1999). This eases the inclusion of self-disclosure in communications, and therefore promotes intimacy in the relationships.
- The absence of presenting selves physically eases concerns about self-disclosure, particularly in relation to physical appearance, anxiety in social interactions, etc.
- People tend to be attracted by others who are found to be similar, and the Internet forms a playground for people to find "similar others."
- As self-disclosure is facilitated, relationships and intimacy are formed faster than the ones acquired offline.

However, the authors also state that the above assumptions are valid only for those who are lonely or have difficulties in forming relationships offline due to anxiety in social interactions. They suppose that, although socially skillful people attach more importance to relations in offline conditions, such as FtF encounters rather than Internet friendships, those who hesitate to disclose themselves in offline circumstances feel more comfortable in self-disclosure on the Internet, and thus, form more intimate and lasting relationships via the Internet. According to the authors' results, people of the given profile above form close and lasting relationships via the Internet, and those relationships develop faster than relationships in the offline environment. They also make these relationships a part of their real lives so they become a social reality. In fact, relationships established online by the majority of the subjects canvassed in their initial experiment lasted more than two years. It was also found that the Internet, as the medium for the initial impressions, did not affect the quality of the communication and the attractiveness of the relationship that followed. For example, from the first meeting on the Internet, an increasing satisfaction was observed that was different from initial FtF meetings.

The evolving applications of CMC such as social network sites deal with anonymity and self-disclosure situations in a different manner. According to Zhao et al. (2008), some online environments, such as Facebook, are "anchored" to the users' real offline lives. Users register in those environments with true information about their reality, such as their name, e-mail, location, etc. Moreover, individuals from offline social networks who know about the true identity of their network partners exist in those environments. Since presenting a false identity in such an environment may result in blaming, isolation and, in extreme cases, punishment by the offline social relations, the existence of "anchored relationships" in online environments avoids anonymity. Consequently, contrary to the anonymous environments of both the online (chat rooms, MUDs, dating sites, etc.) and offline (bars, clubs, etc.) worlds, in "nonymous" (the opposite of anonymous - Zhao et al., 2008, p. 1818) online environments, people tend

to declare "real selves" instead of creating false identities. Nonymous environments are persistent guards that inhibit deviant behaviors on the Internet, as these environments are connected to real offline social lives and, therefore, users are forced to make declarations aligned with their true identities. The results of three experiments conducted by Zhao and his colleagues (2008) show that Facebook users follow more implicit strategies than explicit ones while constructing their identities: "they show rather than tell" while presenting their selves to the large Facebook audience. Users prefer to present themselves implicitly with visual posts (pictures, photographs etc.) or "enumerative" entries (declaring hobbies, interests, etc.), rather than using explicit ways, such as filling up "about me" parts, which require more narrative descriptions.

Moreover, the results prove that Facebook users present their hoped-for selves instead of creating false identities. As Facebook is a nonymous and anchored online environment, the presented selves consist of real selves. However, like other virtual applications, Facebook lacks the corporal body that is useful for transferring regulating features such as gender, appearance, attractiveness, language usage, ethnic origin, etc. in FtF communication. Therefore, in the absence of such regulating features, the users have a chance to manipulate reality by presenting only the socially attractive parts of their existence, which results in the presentation of hoped-for selves.

In conclusion, the Internet, and particularly intensely CMC environments, provides individuals the opportunity to present their identities in a different way because of the anonymous characteristic of these environments. The anonymity of the Internet reduces the risks of disclosing the self and eases the inclusion of self-disclosure in communications. Especially, for an individual with low social skills, the absence of presenting the self physically, in other words anonymously, diminishes concerns about self-disclosure and, thus, these individuals feel more comfortable in communication via anonymous environments. However, anonymity also causes misrepresentation and deception, and the socio-psychological requirements of human nature provide a ground to exaggerate, and sometimes abuse, this possibility. Therefore, in order to create more realistic applications there is an emerging need for extra features and tools based on the experience of nonymous environments like social network sites, so individuals can be given the chance to identify more with the identities of those with whom they interact.

Truth Bias

Truth bias is simply our assumption of how truthful the opposite party is. Individuals bear higher truth bias towards the others they know closely: "trust needs touch" (Handy, 1995). Therefore, individuals need intimacy which may be provided by socially rich mediums.

Rocco (1998) reports that once trust was formed in a medium with enriched social cues like telephone where affective factors like voice, prosody, accent etc. are simultaneously processed, it can be preserved in a socially poor text-based media such as email. Supportingly, Bos et al. (2002) showed that chat gave the worst satisfaction result in means of trust when compared with video, audio and FtF communications. Interestingly, although communications in audiovisual channels were as satisfactory as the case of FtF communication, trust gained via these channels was improved much slower than the one in FtF condition.

Therefore, developing trust in online environments can be much more difficult than FtF experiences. However, it has also been observed in CMC that truth bias increases with respect to the richness of the utilized media or the enhancements of the graphical visual displays (Wilson et al., 2006). Additionally, it has also been observed that the deception rates of people do not change along the same lines with truth bias. When users have been questioned regarding the trustworthi-

ness of a message received from the opposite party, the rates by which they decided that the received message is trustworthy has been much higher than the estimated truth bias (Maksimova, 2005). Hence, truth bias is also found to be modulated not by the actual media richness provided in the communication environment, but by the perception of it by the users. For instance, once a picture is sent in a message as an attachment, the receiver may stop questioning the content of the picture and choose to believe that a deceptive picture is trustworthy. In these types of scenarios, the truth bias may increase miscommunication and misinterpretation.

Expression of Emotions in CMC

Expression and interpretation of emotions in communication are vital processes in our offline social lives. However, peers communicating through CMC are usually prone to make wrong emotional judgments. Lo (2008) proved that the actual emotion and intent of the sender could not be extracted from the pure text content without emoticons. In addition, the paucity of the CMC environments in terms of transmission of social cues hardens the communication of emotions, and therefore result in more misinterpretation and miscommunication issues frequently observed in CMC. For instance, Harris and Paradice (2007) found that emotion in CMC is conveyed mainly through implicit phrases. Individuals prefer to use indirect phrases to mention emotions (e.g., "That's impossible, you can't do that to me" - Harris and Paradice, 2007, 2083) rather than direct and accurate ones (e.g., "I'm angry", - Harris and Paradice, 2007, 2083) to avoid presenting emotion explicitly. This finding explains the hesitation for direct emotion communication via CMC in order to avoid miscommunication and misinterpretation. On the other hand, the same authors report that the existence of emotional phrases in the emails affects the perceived emotion levels in the receiver, supporting the idea that the tools which facilitate better emotional communication are needed in CMC.

In order to facilitate emotional expressions, and thus the emotional communication in CMC, individuals use emoticons which can be described as the graphical representations of facial expressions usually in a humored sense. Emoticons are as easily recognized as facial expressions reported by Ekman and Friesen (1969) (Walther & D'Addario, 2001). Emoticons facilitate the communication of moods or mental states of individuals (Constantin et al., 2002). and make the interpretation of textual messages more clear and hence, substitute the non-verbal displays (i.e. facial expressions or eye gaze) in FtF (Walther & D'Addario, 2001, Derks et al., 2008). Individuals tend to use more emoticons in social interactions than task-oriented contexts (Derks et al., 2008).

The existence of emoticons plays a prominent role in the interpretation of the messages. Emoticons empower the meaning of the verbal part of a message (Rezabek & Cochenour, 1998). Emoticons also affect the degree of perceived emotions in emails (Harris & Paradice, 2007) but only in the case of positively valanced emails. Although, emoticons usually help to strengthen the content, they do not convey a meaning alone; they rarely enrich the semantic content. The contribution of emoticons to the context transmitted is limited by the narrative content and the meaning extracted from verbal content overwrites the sense of emoticons (Walther & D'Addario, 2001).

One of the widely discussed topics in CMC is flaming which can be defined as an extreme form of negatively valenced expression. From the perspective of the social presence theory, flaming, which can also be defined as sending messages that contain threats and insults, is a result of loss of personality (Short et al., 1976). In addition, it is known that the anonymity of the interacting parties reinforces flaming (Siegel et al., 1986). Unfortunately, the level of flaming gives an idea about the effect of anonymity in CMC: flaming is found more often in CMC than in FtF (Dyer et al.,

1995). More precisely, Gaunt (2002) has reported that flaming is observed to occur four times more frequently in text-based CMC in comparison to FtF communication.

As for another explanation for flaming, changes in the interpretation of positively and negatively valenced content are frequently observed in CMC. For instance, in the case of negative content, whether or not the message contains emoticons, the negative meaning of the message comes forward (Walther & D'Addario, 2001). Additionally, in interactions with low emotional cues transmitted, negative emotions tend to increase (Kato et al., 2007). In fact, this behaviour may explain one of the reasons underlying flaming: flaming is not only a result of anonymity but also a result of the medium with weak capabilities for transmission of emotional cues.

According to Derks, Fischer, and Bos (2008), there is not much evidence to support the idea that CMC is less emotional in terms of talking, expressing and interpreting emotions, than FtF communication. However, the claims and results given above clearly states that: (i) although emotional communications is handled very commonly in CMC, the existing CMC environments do not have necessary tools and features for a plausible emotion transmission; (ii) the use of emoticons somehow fills the gap of insufficient emotional cue transfer but it is still primitive form; (iii) flaming is not only a result of anonymity but also a result of the medium with weak capabilities for transmission of emotional cues. Therefore, all these facts emphasize the emergent need for affective designs.

In the following section, we present the correlation between the behavioral problems which are summarized throughout the previous section, and the lessons learned from brain damages. In fact, we aim to convince the reader about the emerging need of affective and intelligent CMC applications by showing the similarities of these concepts. There is a high correlation between the behavioral problems stated above and some of brain anomalies studied in neuroscience. CMC has usually been compared to FtF which is unavoidable as FtF is our native communication medium. However, in this chapter, we tried to express a new way of analysis by comparing the behavioral problems in CMC with the characteristics of a brain functioning properly.

THE COGNITIVE NEUROSCIENCE PERSPECTIVE FOR CMC

The Fundamental Neuroscientific Concepts

Limbic system is located in the central part of the brain, consisting of cingulate cortex, parahippocampal cortex, hippocampus, amygdala, septal nuclei, and hypothalamus. Through its bidirectional connections to the prefrontal, temporal and occipital cortices, the limbic system helps emotional and cognitive processes to work in synchronization. Episodic memory, attention, visual perception, fear conditioning are some cognitive processes modulated directly by the limbic system (Phelps, 2006). On the other hand, prefrontal cortex is the area of the brain within which higher cognitive functions such as executive function, working memory, decision-making, social behavior, and goal-directed behavior are localized. The functions that are directly related to social behavior are localized in the orbitofrontal (OFC), ventromedial and dorsolateral cortices of the prefrontal cortex (Mah et al., 2004). Amygdala and OFC, which are shown in Figure 1, are two key players in this big picture (Kringelbach & Rolls (2004)). Amygdala takes an important role in the evaluation of social cues in the surrounding environment and attaining a subjective rating whereas OFC participates in self-monitoring and attaining an objective reward-based rating, in a multitude of abstract versus concrete modalities spread out by spatial location on the OFC.

Figure 1. Emotions and subjective evaluation at the neurological level. (Adapted from Kringelbach & Rolls (2004))

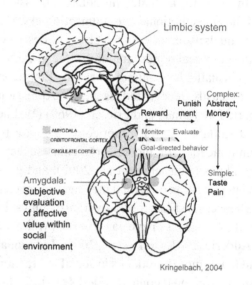

Several social adaptation and behavioral problems are observed in patients with amygdala and/or OFC lesions. Because amygdala and OFC lesions are rarely found in humans, the lesion literature benefits quite a lot from animal studies. For example, when bilateral amygdalectomy is performed on monkeys in a colony in the Caribbean islands, they no longer seemed to be restricted by social mores, they embarked in socially inappropriate behavior, acted fearless in presence of higher ranking monkeys and soon are killed by other monkeys. There are several studies regarding development of fearlessness in monkeys with damaged amygdalae (Kalin et al., 2004; Skuse et al., 2003) In addition, observation of socially disinhibited behavior in monkeys with amygdala lesions makes researchers believe that amygdala may have a role in inhibiting inappropriate social behavior (Amaral, 2002). It is also known that monkeys with damage to septal nuclei become extremely aggressive even in completely natural and neutral environments.

In humans, when there is damage to amygdala, people fail to identify facial expressions, especially the expression of fear (Adolphs, 1995; Adolphs,

2005). However, it is also a fact that amygdala does not participate in fear perception in an isolated way. Awareness facilitated through participation of hippocampal areas as well as insular cortex and existence of autonomic responsivity are key factors in fear conditioning (Critchley et. al., 2002). On another front, experiments reveal that humans with amygdala lesions fail to evaluate trustworthiness and show a high tendency to trust even strangers due to increased truth bias (Adolphs, 1998). Also, amygdala lesion patients are shown to be deficient in interpreting social cues and fail to capture the emotional content in social situations (Phelps, 2006). On another front, in humans, amygdala and OFC are believed to have balancing roles; because in impulsive aggressive behavior disorders, where this balance is tipped, exaggerated amygdala activation is observed in conjunction with reduced OFC activity (Coccaro et al, 2007).

The best example for social behavioral problems introduced by OFC lesions is inarguably the utilization behavior reported by Lhermitte (1986). Utilization behavior can be explained simply as the impulsive use of tools made available to an individual without hesitation and questioning their appropriateness in the existing social context. For example, in a congress, Lhermitte invited his patient with OFC damage to the stage while a large crowd of people were present in the audience. The patient briefly looked at the presented tools at the desk. He immediately wrote something using the pen and paper, tried to wear the two glasses at the same time and urinated to the provided duck in front of all the onlookers without hesitation. The most important functionality attributed to the OFC is thought to be self-monitoring. In patients with OFC damage, there is a self-monitoring deficit, which, in turn, presents itself as lack of feelings of shame or guilt. It has been reported that behavioral therapies which consist of providing feedback to the patients by having them watch their behavior from video recordings at a later time seem to be of use, at least to reduce the intensity of the inappropriate social behaviors (Beer et al., 2006).

Behavioral Problems in CMC and Brain Damages

We can group the communication problems in, especially, text-based CMC with respect to the properties of the sender and receiver parts in the communication. The behavioral problems in each party and related brain analogies are given in Table 2.

Text-based CMC degrades social presence which in turn makes the sender act fearless just like patients with amygdala damage. Disinhibition, flaming and aggressive behavior are other behavioral disorders connected to fearlessness exhibited on the sender side. In addition, the sender takes advantage of the absence of the social normative pressure in the text-based CMC environment, and attempts impulsive behavior which is

Table 2. The summary of behavioral problems in CMC and the corresponding analogy in brain regions

Behavioral Problem	Localization in brain	Party Affected in CMC
Lack of social cues	Amygdala, OFC	Receiver, Sender
Lack of self-monitoring	OFC	Sender
Aggression	Septal nuclei	Sender
Fearlessness	Amygdala	Sender
Disinhibition, flaming	Amygdala, OFC	Sender
Exaggerated truth bias	Amygdala	Receiver
Utilization	OFC	Sender

prohibited under normal environmental settings. This is mainly because the sender does not recognize himself as an individual, which in turn causes him to skip self-monitoring his behavior in this type of communication. Uninterrupted availability and ease of the accessibility of the communication channel triggers utilization behavior in the sender, due to expectations of immediate satisfaction similar to that of patients with OFC damage.

Because of the absence of social cues in text-based CMC, the receiver cannot evaluate the received message correctly from a subjective viewpoint. In addition, the receiver can be deceived easily because of the ease of manipulation of the truth bias. Usually, the receiver is prone to interpret the received message with a higher truth value than normally expected. These types of mistakes in the judgment of the social environment are deficits observed in patient populations with amygdala damage as explained above.

NEW ASPECTS FOR THE DESIGN OF CMC APPLICATIONS

Although most of the problems stated in the earlier sections of this chapter have been known for more than two decades, up to now, only minor practical but not major conceptual improvements have been implemented in the widely used text-based CMC applications. In this statement, the innovation brought by the social network sites is not accounted for, because we categorize these media as another form of CMC which is very different form text-based CMC, primarily due to the nonymous environment and the anchored relationships (see Identity Creation, Self-Disclosure, and Anonymity part for further information). So in this chapter, the limitations of CMC are predominantly discussed within the context of text based environments.

We believe that although solutions for the problems mentioned in the earlier sections may not be entirely possible, reformative and innova-

tive designs may produce better results in terms of the communication and perception of affect in CMC. Some of the studies we examined also support this view. For instance, Lee & Bruckman (2007) evaluates the current interface in social network sites and states that:

User-interface design choices in social computing software can have a profound effect on non-trivial activities like finding a life partner. For example, is a friends list alphabetical, or is the order determined by the user? This may seem at first glance like a low-level detail, but we have found that people pay attention to such details and use them to convey a surprising amount of meaning. (p. 377)

Another suggestion of intelligent interface design arises from the study of Lour and his colleagues (2010):

We suggest avoiding the use of "flaming" emoticons in IM because these may cause unexpected negative emotions between the communicators even if the original intention was to just kid around... The use of neutral emoticons in unnecessary circumstances should be avoided since it has no significant difference as compared to the use of pure text messages. (p. 894)

The above examples suggest very simple, but remarkable and innovative solutions for the problems targeted. The following examples are given in order to clarify what we mean by a more affective and intelligent design for CMC applications:

- Anonymity: Individuals can be given the chance to identify more with the identities of those with whom they interact. If the identity is not known, data accumulated with the behavioral characteristics of the opposing party could be presented. In addition, feedbacks from the other users in the interaction network could be used to evaluate or rank the anonymous character of the individual.

- Effective Tools for Emotion Transmission: The existing CMC environments do not have necessary tools and features for a plausible emotion transmission. The use of emoticons somehow fills the gap of insufficient emotional cue transfer but they are primitive forms. Emoticons could be re-analyzed and a sufficient set of emotional cues could be transferred into graphical user interfaces defining a new pseudo-language for emotional communication. On the other hand, the emotional engagement techniques in game or movie business can be adapted to text-based CMC environments.

- Self-monitoring: Mood detection could be done using affective text processing techniques. This information could be provided to the sender through simple feedback indicators or warnings as well as the feedbacks from the interaction network of the sender. In order to allow for better self-monitoring, the messages can be buffered and sent to the receivers only after a review and approval phase imposed on the sender.

- Media Richness: Enhancing the media channels in CMC applications or supporting text with audiovisual data (i.e. voice-mail) is necessary to overcome other problems like the lack of social cues, or weak transmission of emotions.

Finally, there are some important points to be mentioned considering the analysis given in Table 2, which will be valuable for future design considerations. First, the roles of peers as sender and receiver are changing dynamically in real-time CMC platforms like chat. Therefore, all the problems must be considered for each peer independent of the present role. Second, there are commonalities in terms of the causes and effects of behavioral problems, which mean that

a solution for one of the problems may also end another problem.

CONCLUSION

In this chapter, we presented a group of social problems frequently observed in text-based CMC such as misinterpretation of messages and exaggerated truth bias caused by lack of social cues, or reduced self-monitoring, flaming and aggressiveness caused by anonymity. According to the literature review about socio-psychological problems in CMC, decoding of the underlying social and emotional cues can be evaluated as a missing component of CMC at the site of the receiver. On the other hand, at the site of the sender, due to the anonymity and reduced social presence, lack of self-monitoring and impulsivity are major factors that cause negative behaviors such as flaming and aggressiveness. When a neuroscientific perspective is brought along, these behavioral deficits are no different than those of patients with brain damage. When locations of the brain which subserve roughly the functional profile of these behaviors are severed, similar behavioral problems are observed in patients as well.

CMC has usually been compared with FtF communication because FtF is our native communication medium. However, in this chapter, we tried to express a new perspective in which affective features of communication is compared across healthy versus severed brain areas. Implications and appropriateness of this type of comparison will become evident in emerging designs of affective text-based CMCs hopefully in the near-term future.

REFERENCES

Adolphs, R., Gosselin, F., Buchanan, T. W., Tranel, D., Schyns, P., & Damasio, A. R. (2005). A Mechanism for Impaired Fear Recognition after Amygdala Damage. *Nature, 433*, 68–72. doi:10.1038/nature03086

Adolphs, R., Tranel, D., & Damasio, A. R. (1998). The Human Amygdala in Social Judgment. *Nature, 393*, 470–474. doi:10.1038/30982

Adolphs, R., Tranel, D., Damasio, H., & Damasio, A. R. (1995). Fear and the Human Amygdala. *The Journal of Neuroscience, 15*, 5879–5891.

Amaral, D. G. (2002). The Primate Amygdala and the Neurobiology of Social Behavior: Implications for Understanding Social Anxiety. *Biological Psychiatry, 51*, 11–17. doi:10.1016/S0006-3223(01)01307-5

Anolli, L. (2002). MaCHT—miscommunication as chance theory: toward a unitary theory of communication and miscommunication. In Anolli, L., Ciceri, R., & Riva, G. (Eds.), *Say not to say: new perspectives on miscommunication* (pp. 3–42). Amsterdam: IOS Press.

Antheunis, M. L., Valkenburg, P. M., & Peter, J. (2010). Getting acquainted through Social Network Sites: Testing a model of online uncertainty reduction and social attraction. *Computers in Human Behavior, 26*, 100–109. doi:10.1016/j.chb.2009.07.005

Bargh, J. A., McKenna, K. Y., & Fitzsimons, G. M. (2002). Can you see the real me? Activation and expression of the "true self" on the Internet. *The Journal of Social Issues, 58*(1), 33–48. doi:10.1111/1540-4560.00247

Beer, J., John, O. P., Scabini, D., & Knight, R. T. (2006). Orbitofrontal Cortex and Social Behavior: Integrating Self-Monitoring and Emotion-Cognition Interactions. *Journal of Cognitive Neuroscience, 18*, 871–879. doi:10.1162/jocn.2006.18.6.871

Bos, N., Olson, J., Gergle, D., Olson, G., & Wright, Z. (2002). Effects of Four Computer-Mediated Communications Channels on Trust Development. *Proceedings of the SIGCHI* (pp.135 – 140).

Coccaro, E. F., McCloskey, M. S., Fitzgerald, D. A., & Phan, K. L. (2007). (in press). Amygdala and Orbitofrontal Reactivity to Social Threat in Individuals with Impulsive Aggression. *Biological Psychiatry*. doi:10.1016/j.biopsych.2006.08.024

Constantin, C., Kalyanaraman, S., Stavrositu, C., & Wagoner, N. (2002). *To be or not to be emotional: Impression formation effects of emoticons in moderated chatrooms.* Paper presented at the communication technology and policy division at the 85th annual convention of the Association for Education in Journalism and Mass Communication (AEJMC). Miama, Fl.

Critchley, H. D., Mathias, C. J., & Dolan, R. J. (1995). Fear Conditioning in Humans: The Influence of Awareness and Autonomic Arousal on Functional Neuroanatomy. *The Journal of Neuroscience, 15*(10), 6846–6855.

Culnan, M. J., & Markus, M. L. (1987). Information technologies. In Jablin, F. M., Putnam, L. L., & Roberts, K. H. (Eds.), *Handbook of organizational communication: an interdisciplinary perspective* (pp. 420–443). Newbury Park, CA: Sage.

Daft, R. L., & Lengel, R. H. (1984). Information richness: A new approach to managerial behavior and organization design. *Research in Organizational Behavior, 6*, 191–233.

Derks, D., Bos, A. E., & von Grumbkow, J. (2008). Emoticons and online message interpretation. *Social Science Computer Review, 26*, 379–388. doi:10.1177/0894439307311611

Derks, D., Fischer, A. H., & Bos, A. E. (2008). The role of emotion in computer-mediated communication: A review. *Computers in Human Behavior, 24*, 766–785. doi:10.1016/j.chb.2007.04.004

Dyer, R., Green, R., Pitts, M., & Millward, G. (1995). What's the flaming problem? CMC-deindividuation or disinhibiting? In Kirby, M. A. R., Dix, A. J., & Finlay, J. E. (Eds.), *People and Computer X*. Cambridge, UK: Cambridge University Press.

Ekman, P., & Friesen, W. V. (1969). The repertoire of nonverbal behavior: Categories, origins, usage, and coding. *Semiotica, 1*, 49–98.

Ellison, N., Rebecca, H., & Gibbs, J. (2006). Managing Impressions Online: Self-Presentation Processes in the Online Dating Environment. *Journal of Computer-Mediated Communication, 11*(2), 415–441. doi:10.1111/j.1083-6101.2006.00020.x

Gaunt, N. (2002). Beyond the Fear of Cyber-strangers: Further Considerations for Domestic Online Safety. In Hosking, J. (Ed.), *Netsafe: Society* (pp. 107–118). Safety and the Internet.

Gibbs, J. L., Ellison, N. B., & Heino, R. D. (2006). Self-presentation in online personals: The role of anticipated future interaction, self-disclosure, and perceived success in Internet dating. *Communication Research, 33*(2), 1–26. doi:10.1177/0093650205285368

Handy, C. (1995). Trust and the virtual organization. *Harvard Business Review, 73*(3), 40–50.

Harris, R. B., & Paradice, D. (2007). An investigation of the computer-mediated communication of emotion. *Journal of Applied Sciences Research, 3*, 2081–2090.

Kalin, N. H., Shelton, S. E., & Davidson, R. J. (2004). The Role of the Central Nucleus of the Amygdala in Mediating Fear and Anxiety in the Primate. *The Journal of Neuroscience, 24*, 5506–5515. doi:10.1523/JNEUROSCI.0292-04.2004

Kato, Y., Sugimura, K., & Akahori, K. (2001). An affective aspect of computermediated communication: analysis of communications by E-mail. *Proceedings of ICCE/SchoolNetM: 2* (pp. 636–642).

Kiesler, S., Siegel, J., & McGuire, T. W. (1984). Social psychological aspects of computer-mediated communication. *The American Psychologist, 39*, 1123–1134. doi:10.1037/0003-066X.39.10.1123

Kringelbach, M. L., & Rolls, E. T. (2004). The functional neuroanatomy of the human orbitofrontal cortex: evidence from neuroimaging and neuropsychology. *Progress in Neurobiology, 72*(5), 341–372. doi:10.1016/j.pneurobio.2004.03.006

Kruger, J., Epley, N., Parker, P., & Ng, Z. (2005). Egocentrism over e-mail: Can we communicate as well as we think? *Journal of Personality and Social Psychology, 89*(6), 925–936. doi:10.1037/0022-3514.89.6.925

Lea, M., & Spears, R. (1995). Love at first byte? Building personal relationships over computer networks. In Wood, J. T., & Duck, S. (Eds.), *Understudied relationships: Off the beaten track* (pp. 197–233). Beverly Hills, CA: Sage.

Lee, A., & Bruckman, A. (2007). Judging You by the Company You Keep: Dating on Social Networking Sites. *Proceedings of the 2007 International ACM Conference on Supporting Group Work* (pp. 371-378).

Lhermitte, F., Pillon, B., & Serdaru, M. (1986). Human anatomy and the frontal lobes. Part I: Imitation and utilization behavior: A neuropsychological study of 75 patients. *Annals of Neurology, 19*, 326–334. doi:10.1002/ana.410190404

Lo, S. (2008). The nonverbal communication functions of emoticons in computer-mediated communication. *Cyberpsychology & Behavior, 11*(5), 595–597. doi:10.1089/cpb.2007.0132

Luor, T., Wub, L., Lu, H., & Tao, Y. (2010). The effect of emoticons in simplex and complex task-oriented communication: An empirical study of instant messaging. *Computers in Human Behavior, 26*, 889–895. doi:10.1016/j.chb.2010.02.003

Mah, L., Arnold, M. J., & Grafman, J. (2004). Impairment of Social Perception Associated with Lesions of the Prefrontal Cortex. *The American Journal of Psychiatry, 161,* 1247–1255. doi:10.1176/appi.ajp.161.7.1247

Maksimova Y. (2005). *Deception and its Detection in Computer-mediated Communication.* Iowa State University Human Computer Interaction Technical Report, ISU-HCI-2005-006.

Markus, H., & Nurius, P. (1986). Possible selves. *The American Psychologist, 41,* 954–969. doi:10.1037/0003-066X.41.9.954

McKenna, K. Y. A., & Bargh, J. A. (1999). Causes and consequences of social interaction on the Internet: A conceptual framework. *Media Psychology, 1,* 249–269. doi:10.1207/s1532785xmep0103_4

McKenna, K. Y. A., Green, A. S., & Glenson, M. E. J. (2002). Relationship formation on the Internet: What's the big attraction? *The Journal of Social Issues, 58*(1), 9–31. doi:10.1111/1540-4560.00246

Moor, P. J., Heuvelman, A. & Verleura, R. (2010) Flaming on YouTube. Computers *in Human Behavior.* Article in Press for June 2010.

Oyserman, D. (2001). Self-concept and identity. In Tesser, A., & Schwarz, N. (Eds.), *The Blackwell Handbook of Social Psychology* (pp. 499–517). Malden, MA: Blackwell.

Phelps, E. A. (2006). Emotion and Cognition: Insights from Studies of the Human Amygdala. *Annual Review of Psychology, 57,* 27–53. doi:10.1146/annurev.psych.56.091103.070234

Rezabek, L. L., & Cochenour, J. J. (1998). Visual cues in computer-mediated communication: Supplementing text with emotions. *Journal of Visual Literacy, 18,* 210–215.

Riva, G. (2002). The sociocognitive psychology of computer-mediated communication: the present and future of technology-based interactions. *Cyberpsychology & Behavior, 5*(6), 581–598. doi:10.1089/109493102321018222

Rocco, E. (1998). Trust breaks down in electronic contexts but can be repaired by some initial face-to-face contact. *Proceedings CHI '98 (Los Angeles CA, 1998) ACM Press* (pp. 496-502).

Ross, C., Orr, S. O., Sisic, M., Arseneault, J. M., Simmering, M. G., & Orr, R. R. (2009). Personality and motivations associated with Facebook use. *Computers in Human Behavior, 25,* 578–586. doi:10.1016/j.chb.2008.12.024

Schau, H. J., & Gilly, M. C. (2003). We are what we post? Self-presentation in personal web space. *The Journal of Consumer Research, 30*(3), 385–404. doi:10.1086/378616

Schouten, J. W. (1991). Selves in transition: Symbolic consumption in personal rites of passage and identity re-construction. *The Journal of Consumer Research, 17,* 412–425. doi:10.1086/208567

Short, J., Williams, E., & Christie, B. (1976). *The Social Psychology of Telecommunications.* NY: John Wiley.

Siegel, J., Dubrovsky, V., Kiesler, S., & McGuire, T. W. (1986). Group process and computer-mediated communication. *Organizational Behavior and Human Decision Processes, 37,* 157–187. doi:10.1016/0749-5978(86)90050-6

Skuse, D., Morris, J., & Lawrence, K. (2003). The Amygdala and Development of the Social Brain. *Annals of the New York Academy of Sciences, 1008,* 91–101. doi:10.1196/annals.1301.010

Sproull, L., & Kiesler, S. (1991). *Connections: new ways of working in the networked organizations.* Cambridge, MA: MIT Press.

Swickert, R. J., Hittner, J. B., Harris, J. L., & Herring, J. A. (2002). Relationships among Internet use, personality and social support. *Computers in Human Behavior, 18,* 437–451. doi:10.1016/S0747-5632(01)00054-1

Walther, J. B. (1992). Interpersonal effects in computer mediated interaction: a relational perspective. *Communication Research, 19,* 52–90. doi:10.1177/009365092019001003

Walther, J. B., & Burgoon, J. K. (1992). Relational communication in computer-mediated interaction. *Human Communication Research*, *19*, 50–88. doi:10.1111/j.1468-2958.1992.tb00295.x

Walther, J. B., & D'Addario, P. (2001). The impacts of emoticons on message interpretation in computer-mediated communication. *Social Science Computer Review*, *19*, 324–347. doi:10.1177/089443930101900307

Whitty, M. T. (2008). Revealing the 'real' me, searching for the 'actual' you: Presentations of self on an internet dating site. *Computers in Human Behavior*, *24*(4), 1707–1723. doi:10.1016/j.chb.2007.07.002

Wilson, J. M., Straus, S. G., & McEvily, B. (2006). All in due Time: Development of Trust in Computer-mediated and Face-toFace Teams. *Organizational Behavior and Human Decision Processes*, *99*, 16–33. doi:10.1016/j.obhdp.2005.08.001

Yurchisin, J., Watchravesringkan, K., & McCabe, D. B. (2005). An Exploration of Identity Re-creation in the Context of Internet Dating. *Social Behavior and Personality*, *33*(8), 735–750. doi:10.2224/sbp.2005.33.8.735

Zhao, S., Grasmuck, S., & Martin, J. (2008). Identity construction on Facebook: Digital empowerment in anchored relationships. *Computers in Human Behavior*, *24*, 1816–1836. doi:10.1016/j.chb.2008.02.012

Zimbardo, P. G. (1970). The Human Choice: Individuation, Reason, and Order versus Deindividuation, Impulse and Chaos. In A. WJ. Levine (Eds), *Nebraska Symposium on Motivation* (pp. 237-307). Lincoln: University of Nebraska press.

KEY TERMS AND DEFINITIONS

Computer-Mediated Communication (CMC): Term describes communication of individuals via two or more computers. Text-based messaging (e.g., chat, email), MUDs (Multi User Dungeons – the general term used to refer multiplayer online fantasy role playing games), internet dating sites, social network sites are some examples of CMC applications.

Depersonalization: This term defines an anomaly in which self-awareness weakens.

Disinhibition: Disinhibition is a term in psychology used to explain the condition in which the individual feels the lack of social moderation and looses self-control. Within the scope of this chapter, disinhibition is mostly used to recall the case of abuse and flaming.

Face-to-Face (FtF): Direct communication of individuals in which corporal body and non-verbal social cues exits. There must be no inclusion of transferring or telecommunication tools such as computers and telephone in communication. In FtF, individuals handle the information exchanged during communication with the help of social cues such as "head nods, smiles, eye contact, distance, tone of voice, and other nonverbal behavior." (Kiesler et al., 1984, 1125).

Chapter 12
The Influence of Intimacy and Gender on Emotions in Mobile Phone Email

Yuuki Kato
Tokyo University of Social Welfare, Japan

Douglass J. Scott
Waseda University, Japan

Shogo Kato
Tokyo Woman's Christian University, Japan

ABSTRACT

This chapter focuses on the roles of interpersonal closeness and gender on the interpretation and sending of emotions in mobile phone email messages[1]. 91 Japanese college students were shown scenarios involving either a friend or an acquaintance describing situations intended to evoke one of four emotions: Happiness, sadness, anger, or guilt. The participants' rated their emotions and composed replies for each scenario. Analysis revealed that in the happy and guilt scenarios, emotions experienced by the participants were conveyed to their partners almost without change. However, in the sad and angry scenarios, the emotions sent to the partners were weaker than the actual emotions experienced. Gender analysis showed that men were more likely to experience and express anger in the anger scenario, while women were more likely to experience and express sadness in the anger scenario. In addition, more women's replies contained emotional expressions than did the men's messages.

INTRODUCTION

While modern technology continues to expand our communication options, much of our daily communications rely on one of our oldest tools: Written text. As a distance communication medium, written communications offer numerous benefits including smaller file sizes, faster transfer speeds, and lower costs. There are limitations as well, although researchers are divided on the degree to which these limitations impact our communications. The following section will consider the positive elements of text-based mediated

DOI: 10.4018/978-1-61692-892-6.ch012

communications and some of the challenges to using these methods.

As infants, we are introduced to communication through face-to-face interaction. These early exchanges are essential to our developing communication ability and continue throughout our lives. Face-to-face communications involve a combination of verbal and nonverbal cues which are we use to create understanding. One way these cues are used is to judge the emotional state of our communication partner (Krauss & Fussell 1996; Kraut 1978; Patterson 1994). Our long experience with such interactions makes us proficient at judging other people's characteristics, such as familiarity, gender, emotions, and temperament (Cheng, O'Toole, & Abdi 2001). So how our communication efforts affected when a significant portion of this information (e.g. non-verbal cues) is unavailable to us?

Text-based communications lack much of the non-verbal communication cues we are accustomed to in face-to-face interactions (Short, Williams, & Christie 1976; Sproull & Kiesler 1991). Both sender and receiver rely on the written word to convey not only their meaning, but also their emotional intent (Kato, Kato, & Scott 2007). Research has shown that the transmission of emotions is difficult and misunderstandings can easily happen (Hancock 2007; Kato & Akahori 2006; Kato, Kato, & Scott 2007). Studies also suggest that low degrees of emotional cues transmitted between communication partners in email messages can cause misunderstandings (Kato, Kato, & Akahori 2007). Such emotional misunderstandings in computer-mediated communications (CMC) can, if left unchecked, develop into serious human-relations problems (see for example Green, Pitts, & Millward, 1995; Lea, O'Shea, Fung, & Spears, 1992; Morahan-Martin 2007; Siegel, Dubrovsky, Kiesler, & McGuire, 1986).

Kruger and his colleagues noted that the lack of nonverbal cues such as gesture, emphasis, and intonation can make it difficult to convey emotion and tone in email messages (Kruger, Epley, Parker & Ng 2005). Kruger et al. conducted several studies on email writers' estimates of how well they can communicate in email messages. The studies' findings confirmed that email writers were largely unaware of email's limitations that would inhibit their ability to convey emotion or tone (e.g. sarcasm or humor). The authors characterize these findings as egocentrism—using one's own perspective in lieu of another's—and believe it to be the cause of email miscommunications as "the greater the difference between the communicator's own interpretation of the stimuli and the stimuli available to the audience, the greater the miscalibration" (Kruger et al. 2005, p. 933). Egocentrism may be a necessarily element in communication but "…successful communication depends on an accurate assessment of one's clarity (Keysar & Henly 2002), [thus] overconfidence of that clarity reduces the quality of communication" (Kruger et al. 2005, p. 934). These studies suggest that if writers remain unaware of email's limitations, they may experience a variety of communication problems.

Even trivial misunderstandings in email exchánges can produce unpleasant emotions (Kato & Akahori 2004a, 2004b). Unpleasant emotions may cause communication partners to distrust one another damaging their interpersonal relationship. Kato, Kato, & Akahori (2007) focused on the relationships between the emotions experienced by senders and receivers and the degree of emotional cues contained in the email messages. The researchers investigated the influence the degree of emotional cues transmitted between the sender and receiver had on the emotions which were experienced. They found that while positive emotions were directly expressed and easily understood, negative emotions proved to be more difficult to interpret (Kato, Kato, & Akahori 2007). The results of the current study, described below, address this final point, that is, why are negative emotions more challenging to interpret?

Young people may be particularly susceptible to the potential problems of text-based communications as they tend to be early adopters and heavy users of new technologies (Jones 2002). This phenomenon seems common in many countries and examples from Japan and America are presented here. The overall mobile phone ownership rate by household in Japan was 85.3% at the end of 2005 (Ministry of Internal Affairs and Communications, Japan 2006). Mobile phone use by Japanese young people in general, and college students in particular, is nearly universal; even back in 2003, Ito noted that mobile telephone use by college students was over 97% (Ito, Okabe, & Matsuda 2003). Mobile phone email makes up a large percentage of this use. The Japanese Ministry of Internal Affairs and Communications reported in their 2006 white paper on information and communications in Japan (2006) that email is the most widely used function of mobile phones. This report pointed out that 57.7% of the users of mobile phones used email by the end of 2005. As one point of comparison, all participants of the current study owned mobile phones and 97.8% said that they use mobile phone email every day or several times each week.

Email is frequently used in Japan when voice communications are difficult or socially unacceptable. It is this type of social prohibition that promotes the use of mobile phone email. For instance, making and receiving voice calls on public transportation is limited (and in some areas, prohibited) and train, bus, and subway companies make frequent announcements reminding passengers to silence or turn off their phones. Many passengers accept this prohibition and turn to mobile telephone email to enable them to keep in contact while riding on the train or subway (see Okabe & Ito 2006 for a detailed discussion of this phenomenon, including its historical development).

In contrast to their Japanese counterparts, American young people are using computers to access the Internet and communicate with their friends. According to a Pew Internet Project Data Memo (Jones 2009), 93% of American young peo-

ple between the ages of 12 and 17 were accessing the Internet. Their top four online activities were gaming (78%), email (73%), instant messaging (68%), and social networking (65%) (Jones 2009). Mobile phone use by American teens has increased over the past five years. Lenhart noted in 2009 that a Pew Internet & American Life Project study in 2004 showed 45% of young people between the ages of 12 and 17 had mobile telephone. Five years later, a similar study showed that number had increased to 71% (Lenhart 2009).

Heavy use of text-based communications—both mobile and computer-based—by young people carries the potential for a variety of miscommunications and emotional problems. The authors are studying the characteristics of emotional transmission in text-based communications with the goal of preventing emotional misunderstandings like those described above. Previous research on emotional transmission focused on how well the emotion produced by mediated-communication users was conveyed to their communication partner (Hancock 2007; Kato, Kato, & Akahori 2007; Kato, Kato, & Scott 2007). One barrier to this process is the disconnect between the sender's intended emotion and the actual message they compose. That is, the sender may be angry, but doesn't want to project that emotion too strongly or directly to the receiver. Such traits are particularly common among Japanese people. Japanese language and culture emphasize toning down or suppressing one's true feelings to avoid complicating or damaging interpersonal relations (Matsumoto & Kudo 1993). Given the importance of in-groups and out-groups in Japanese culture, the current study focuses on the emotional experience, intended emotional transfer, and message contents to two types of receivers: Close friends and acquaintances.

The current study also considers the role of gender in the reading and writing of mobile phone email messages. Colley, Todd, Bland, Holmes, Khanom, and Pike's study (2004) compared email and conventional letters to friends to see if there were gender differences in the style and content of these two methods. The authors had thought they would find more emotional and relational features of women's written communications (e.g. Rubin & Greene 1992) and the more humorous and offensive nature of men's written communications (e.g. Herring 1994, as cited in Colley et al. 2004). What they found was that "(w)omen used the less formal stylistic conventions of e-mails to signal excitability in different ways to their male and female friends, whereas men ended their communications in a more relational way to their female than their male friends" (Colley et al. 2004, p. 369).

Some work on gender communication in text-based communications has been done in Japan. Scott (2008) looked at Japanese college students' hand-written communication logs as part of a qualitative study. He noted several gender differences, notably that the women's log entries were far longer (over three times) than the men's, that the men's log entries tended to be short and practical notations, and that women's entries were more context-oriented and contained greater elements of reflection (Scott 2008).

Two hypotheses guide the current study. The first hypothesis is

H1: Participants will experience and transmit emotions more strongly to close friends than to acquaintances.

To test this hypothesis, the authors presented the participants with identical scenarios from both a close friend and an acquaintance. Unlike Colley et al. and Rubin and Greene, this study did not specify the recipient's gender; such an approach is intriguing for future research.

Our second hypothesis states that

H2: Messages sent to a friend will contain more emotional cues than messages sent to an acquaintance.

To test this hypothesis, the authors will analyze the emotions which the senders experienced and the email contents they actually sent in response to four basic emotional scenarios: Happiness, sadness, anger, and guilt. It is thought that anger contributes to the creation of emotional trouble, and guilt can lead to avoiding emotional problems. It is also thought that emotions which mobile phone email users want to convey to their partners will change with the degree of intimacy they have with their partner.

RESEARCH METHOD

The participants of the current study were 91 Japanese undergraduate students (56 men, 35 women, ranging in age from 18 to 27 with an average of 19.3 years old) who were studying information processing at a four-year university. All participants owned their own mobile phone. When asked about their mobile phone email use, 89 participants (97.8%) responded that they used mobile phone email every day or several times each week. This heavy reliance on mobile phone email is congruent with the data presented in the previous section on Japanese young people's widespread use of mobile phones.

Scenarios intended to evoke four target emotions (i.e. happiness, sadness, anger, and guilt) were given to the participants. Examples of the messages used for the close friend scenarios are listed in Table 1. The participants were presented with two messages from both close friends and acquaintances for each emotional scenario resulting in a total of eight scenarios. The underlined portions of the scenarios in Table 1 (i.e. "a close friend") were replaced by "acquaintance" to create the second set of scenarios.

In this experiment, a questionnaire was given to the participants to determine the following two emotional aspects:

Table 1. Scenarios presented to the participants (originals were in Japanese)

Happiness	You studied hard for a test. A close friend of yours went to see the results. You received a mobile phone email from them saying you passed the exam!
Sadness	You studied hard for a test. A close friend of yours went to see the results. You received a mobile phone email from them saying you failed the exam!
Anger	A close friend of yours sent you a mobile phone email explaining that they forgot to tell you the test time had been changed and you missed an important exam!
Guilt	You missed a class and a close friend of yours agreed to meet you and give you the class notes. You forgot about the meeting and you received a mobile phone email from them saying they waited for you but you never showed up!

1. Degree of emotions participants experienced when they read each scenario (hereafter called their "emotional state"), and
2. The degree of emotions participants wanted to convey to their communication partner in their response to each scenario (hereafter called their "intended emotion").

These questionnaires measured four basic emotions without limiting the choices to the emotional focus of each scenario; that is, participants were asked to rate their responses to all four emotions for all four scenarios.

This study is limited to a small number of emotions. Although there are many possible emotions from which to choose, they can be classified into certain fundamental ones. In a previous study on computer- and mobile phone-based communications in a business context (Scott, Coursaris, Kato, & Kato 2009), the authors used Izard, Libero, Putnam, & Haynes's 12 emotions: Interest, enjoyment, surprise, sadness, anger, disgust, contempt, fear, guilt, shame, shyness, and inward hostility (Izard, Libero, Putnam, & Haynes 1993). Since the current study included two levels of intimacy with the communication partner, such a lengthy list of emotions seemed too unwieldy for this analysis. A more concise list was offered by Ekman (1992) which contained six basic emotions: Joy, sadness, anger, surprise, fear, and dislike. For the current study, the authors further limited this list to four basic emotions: Happiness, sadness, anger (which correspond to positive, negative and

hostile emotions as used in Kato, Kato, Scott, & Sato 2008), and guilt.

The data collection procedure was straightforward. First, the eight scenarios and related questionnaires were distributed and explained to the participants. Each questionnaire used a five-point scale (1 = strongly disagree, 5 = strongly agree) about the emotional aspects described in the scenarios listed in Table 1. Participants rated the degree to which they experienced each of these four emotions when reading the scenario using the "emotional state" questionnaire (e.g. "You experienced happiness when reading the mobile phone email from your partner."). Similarly, they rated the degree to which they wanted to convey the target emotions in their email response in the "intended emotions" questionnaire (e.g. "You want to convey happiness to your partner in your email response." Analysis of these data are described in detail in the following section.

After completing the emotional state questionnaire, the participants were asked to write an email response for each scenario before starting the intended emotions questionnaires. This was done to simulate the writing of an actual message in hopes of eliciting more natural emotional responses from the participants. For the purposes of this study, participants' responses were written on paper and collected at the end by the researchers. This was done, in part, because of the logistical complications in having students send actual email messages to the researchers, and to enhance participant anonymity. However, the authors are currently working on a mobile phone-based data collection system that would allow participants to use mobile devices to complete questionnaires and anonymously send actual messages as part of a study. Details of this system will be published in the near future. The total time for data collection was about 1 hour and 30 minutes.

RESULTS

Emotional Questionnaire Data (Combined)

As described above, two sets of data were collected from each participant: The participant's emotional state upon reading the scenario presented, and their intended emotions when writing their email response to their close friend or acquaintance. These self-evaluations of their emotional responses were collected and analyzed and the results are presented below. A third set of data—participants' actual message contents—was also collected and those results are presented later in this section.

In the happy and sad scenarios, the mean of the emotional states and intended emotions showed significant differences depending on the degree of closeness to the communication partner in each scenario as shown in Figure 1. Repeated ANO-VAs of 2x2 were conducted using two factors: "Emotional states and intended emotions" and "close friends and acquaintances." Figure 1 shows that emotional states and intended emotions are

significantly higher in scenarios involving close friends (happiness, $F(1,90) = 6.64$, $p < 0.05$; sadness, $F(1,90) = 20.97$, $p < 0.01$). And, compared with the emotional states, intended emotions fell in both the happy and sad scenarios (happiness, $F(1,90) = 55.34$ $p < 0.01$; sadness, $F(1,90) = 11.96$ $p < 0.01$). Moreover, there was a significant difference for intended emotions to fall rather than emotional states in the scenario of sadness compared with happiness as seen in Figure 1.

These data show that for the happy and sad scenarios, participants experienced significantly greater emotions when the scenario involved a close friend rather than an acquaintance, and that they wanted to convey a significantly greater degree of that emotion to their close friend.

The mean of the emotional states and intended emotions for anger and guilt are shown in Figure 2. This figure is displayed according to the degree of closeness the participants had with their communication partners. In the anger scenario, the mean of the emotional states and intended emotions showed significant differences depending on the degree of closeness to the communication partner in each scenario.

In order to confirm statistically the tendencies implied in these graphs, repeated ANOVAs of 2x2 were conducted using two factors "emotional states and intended emotions" and "close friends and acquaintances." The data sets were slightly reduced as deficit values were excluded, thus a final data set of 87 was used in the anger scenario and 88 in the guilt scenario. Figure 2 shows

Figure 1. Writers' emotional states and intended emotions for happy and sad scenarios

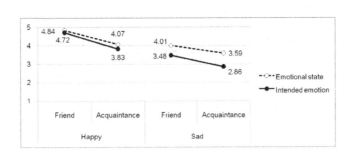

Figure 2. Writers' emotional states and intended emotions for anger and guilt scenarios

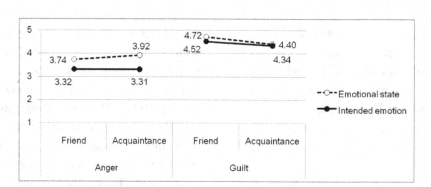

that intended emotions in the anger scenario fell compared with the emotional states ($F(1,86) = 23.41, p < 0.01$, with a significant main effect of factor "emotional states and intended emotions." Figure 2 also shows there was a significant difference for emotional states and intended emotions to be higher for close friends ($F(1,87) = 5.09, p < 0.05$, with the significant main effect of factor "close friends and acquaintances").

The analysis of these last two figures was extended as the emotions of anger and guilt included in the current study are not necessarily produced in isolation. Often, these emotions are produced with the emotion of sadness as described in a separate article (Kato, Kato, Scott, & Sato 2008). Therefore, as part of the analysis of the emotions of anger and guilt presented here, we felt it was

necessary to also investigate the tendency of the emotion of sadness.

The mean of the emotional states and intended emotions of sadness in both the anger and guilt scenarios is shown in Figure 3 according to the degree of intimacy with the communication partner. Repeated ANOVAs of 2x2 were conducted using two factors: "Emotional states and intended emotions" and "close friends and acquaintances." Compared with the emotional states, intended emotions fell in the anger scenario ($F(1,86) = 8.28, p < 0.01$, with the significant main effect of factor "emotional states and intended emotions"), compared with the intended emotions, emotional states fell in the guilt scenario ($F(1,87) = 13.00, p < 0.01$, with a significant main effect of the factor "emotional states and intended emotions"). In addition, the tendency for emotional states and

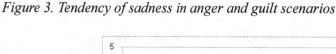

Figure 3. Tendency of sadness in anger and guilt scenarios

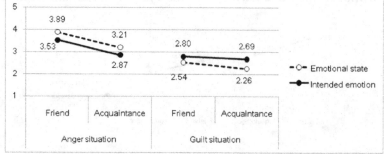

intended emotions to be higher was seen for close friends in the anger scenario ($F(1,86) = 26.86$, $p < 0.01$, with the significant main effect of factor "close friends and acquaintances").

From Figure 2, we saw a tendency to weaken the degree of the emotion of anger expressed to the communication partner. On the other hand, in the guilt scenario, the tendency to convey the emotion of the guilt which participants actually experienced directly to the partners was seen. In the anger scenario shown in Figure 3, the emotion of sadness is suppressed when conveyed, and in the guilt scenario, the tendency to convey sadness more strongly than actually experienced was seen. From these results, it is thought there is a difference between the anger scenario and the guilt scenario.

In addition, as influenced by the degree of intimacy with communication partners, in the anger scenario the tendency to convey the emotion of sadness to a close friend more than an acquaintance was seen. In the guilt scenario, there was a tendency to convey the emotion of guilt to a close friend more. From these results, we conclude that there is a tendency to convey an emotion more to a close friend in both the anger and the guilt scenarios, though the particular emotion expressed (e.g. sadness in the anger scenario and guilt in the guilt scenario) may be different.

Emotional Questionnaire Data (Gender)

The previous section described the results of the combined data of all participants, men and women. The following section considers the relationship between gender and emotion.

Figures 4, 5, and 6 show the results of repeated ANOVAs of 2x2x2 that were conducted using three factors: "Emotional states and intended emotions," "close friends and acquaintances," and "participants' gender." No significant results or tendencies regarding gender differences were observed for the happy, sad, or guilt scenarios. In these cases, men's and women's experiences with the scenarios and email responses showed no statistically significant differences.

However, in the anger scenarios (Figure 4), one significant difference was observed. In the scenario of anger, men experienced anger more than the women in the study. Moreover, men choose to convey the anger they experienced to their partners more than women ($F(1,85) = 4.12$, $p < 0.05$).

As was done in the combined analyses, the factor of sadness in the anger (Figure 5) and guilt (Figure 6) scenarios was investigated. In the scenario of anger, women experienced sadness to a greater extent than men. In addition, women tended to convey sadness to their partners more ($F(1,85) = 2.67$, $p < 0.10$) in the anger scenario.

Figure 4. Anger scenario: Emotional state and intended emotion by gender

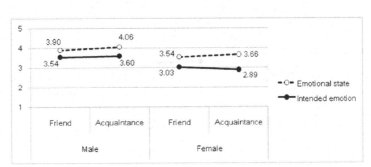

Figure 5. Tendency of sadness in the anger scenario

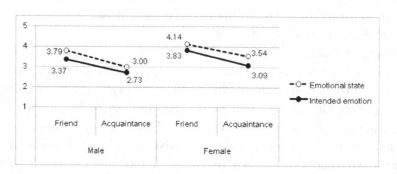

The gender analysis of the emotional state and intended emotion data revealed that it was anger, the negative emotion in the current study, that was the area where difference could be observed. Men were more likely than women to experience anger when reading the anger scenario and elected to convey their emotions more directly to their communication partner. When the factor of sadness was added to the analysis, it was found that women were more likely to experience sadness in an anger scenario and were more likely than the men to express those feelings.

Content Analysis of Mobile Phone Messages (Combined)

As described above, participants were asked to write out their replies to both close friends and acquaintances for each scenario. These messages were collected, input, and analyzed for three elements: Number of characters, emotional cues, and greetings. Emotional expressions and greetings are included in the index of social presence (Murphy 2004). Garrison & Anderson (2003) note that these elements are considered a socio-emotional utterance which promotes social presence (Sato 2007). The importance of social presence was mentioned above (Short et al. 1976) and is helpful in order to prevent emotional trouble in communications that lack nonverbal information, such as mobile phone email interactions.

In 364 copies of email replies (91 participants x two scenarios x two degrees of intimacy), the number of characters were counted, emoticons and language like "I am glad" were included as emotional expressions, and the existence of greetings, such as "hello" and "thank you," were

Figure 6. Tendency of sadness in the guilt scenario

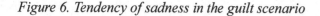

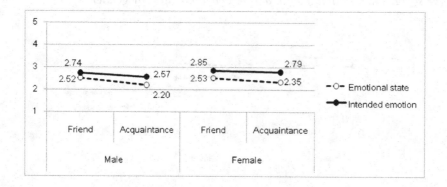

Table 2. Total characters in email responses by degree of intimacy

	Close Friends	Acquaintances
Happy	21.18	17.34
Sad	21.73	17.71
Anger	20.52	17.81
Guilt	25.34	22.43

counted. The result of the total number of characters is shown in Table 2.

The results of the number of characters in all scenarios is shown in Table 2. In order to confirm statistically these apparent differences, repeated ANOVAs of 4x2 were conducted using two factors: The "happy, sad, anger, and guilt scenarios" and "close friends and acquaintances." A data set of 87 was used as invalid or empty responses were excluded.

These data reveal a statistically significant main effect for "close friends and acquaintances" ($F(1,87) = 26.25$, $p < 0.01$) in all scenarios with messages to close friends being significantly longer. This result indicates that intimacy with the communication partner is a significant factor in email message length for these scenarios.

Figure 7. Emotional expressions and greetings for each emotion to friends and acquaintances

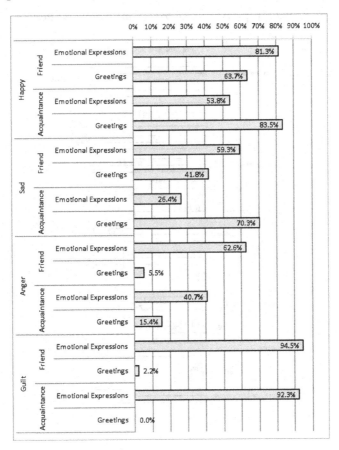

These data also reveal a statistically significant main effect for "the happy, sad, anger, and guilt scenarios" $(F(3,261) = 11.25, p < 0.01)$. It is worth noting that happy, sad, and anger scenarios had similar average message lengths. However, a Bonferroni test confirmed significant differences between the "happy, sad, and anger scenarios" and "the guilt scenario" with the guilt scenario having significantly more characters $(p < 0.01)$. This difference may be attributable to the sense of responsibility the participants may have felt vis-à-vis their communication partner; this difference may warrant additional investigation.

This section describes the basic emotional expressions and greetings that were included in the participants' written responses and are shown in Figure 7. The number in each bar in Figure 7 expresses the percentage of email messages containing emotional expressions. In the happy and the sad scenarios, the tendency for emotional expressions to be included more in the email replies to close friends was seen. On the other hand, there was a tendency for more greetings in the email replies to acquaintances. Moreover, the tendency for two indicators (i.e. emotional expressions and greetings) to be included was seen more in the happy scenario compared with the sad scenario. In the anger scenario, the tendency for emotional expressions to be included more in the email replies to close friends was seen. On the other hand, the tendency for greetings to be included more was seen in the email replies to acquaintances. In Figure 7, emotional expressions were seen in almost all the replies in the guilt scenario.

Just as with the data presented above, more messages to close friends contained emotional cues than did the messages to acquaintances. This was especially true for the sad scenario where

Figure 8. Emotional cues in email responses by degree of intimacy and gender

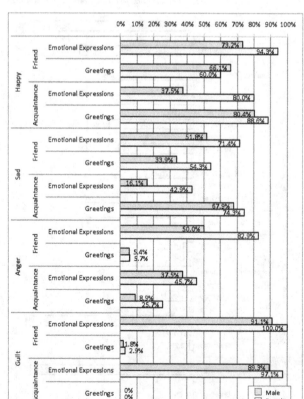

less than half as many replies to acquaintances contained emotional cues as did replies to close friends (59.3% vs. 26.4%). However, while slightly more messages to friends had emotional cues, nearly all messages to both close friends and acquaintances in the guilt scenario contained some degree of emotional cues (94.5% vs. 92.3%).

The overall lack of greetings is typical of the informal nature of email messages. In these scenarios, as the topic becomes more negative, the writers seem to further dispense with formalities and enter directly into the message contents. However, a more detailed analysis—including interview data—will need to be done to test this theory.

Content Analysis of Mobile Phone Messages (Gender)

Content data were further analyzed by gender to see if men's and women's email responses showed any significant differences. Table 3 shows message length data for both men and women for all four emotional scenarios.

In both happy and sad scenarios, women's email responses contained more characters than did the men's messages. In addition, the difference of women's and men's message length was bigger in sadness than in happiness (interaction effect: Scenario (emotion) x gender, $F(1,87) = 7.08$, p < 0.01). In both anger and guilt scenarios, women's

message contain significantly more characters than men (Main effect: Gender, $F(1,87) = 12.19$, p < 0.01). These findings echo the results of another study where the women participants wrote significantly longer entries than did their male colleagues (Scott 2008).

Figure 8 shows the percentage of email replies that contained emotional cues for both men and women participants.

These data show that more women's email messages contained emotional expressions to both close friends and acquaintances than did the men's replies for all four emotional scenarios. This difference was particularly pronounced in happy scenario messages to acquaintances (80.0% vs. 37.5%) and anger scenario messages to friends (82.9% vs. 50.0%). Other notable cases of large differences were sad scenario replies to acquaintances (42.9% vs. 16.1%), happy scenario replies to friends (94.3% vs. 73.2%), and sad scenario responses to friends (71.4% vs. 51.8%). Thus, more women's messages included emotional cues than men's messages for happy and sad scenarios to both friends and acquaintances. There seems to be no clear difference in these results that would favor close friends and acquaintances implying that the sender's relationship with the recipient is less of an issue than is the sender's gender.

The results for messages including greetings is similar to those for emotional cues with more women's replies containing greetings than their

Table 3. Total characters in email responses by degree of intimacy and gender

		Close Friends	**Acquaintances**
Happiness	Men	19.70	15.56
	Women	23.46	20.09
Sadness	Men	17.87	15.06
	Women	27.71	21.80
Anger	Men	16.96	15.08
	Women	25.54	21.63
Guilt	Men	20.45	18.58
	Women	32.74	28.26

male counterparts. The two exceptions are greetings to friends in the happy scenario (66.1% vs. 60.0%) and greetings to acquaintances in the guilt scenario where no participant—man or woman—sent a reply with a greeting. In contrast to the emotional cue data, the gender differences for greetings are less pronounced; the one case of greatest difference being messages to friends in the sad scenario (54.3% for women vs. 33.9% for men). While the current data preclude a more detailed analysis, these results show promising differences that warrant a more fine-grained analysis in a future study.

DISCUSSION AND CONCLUSION

This chapter described a study of Japanese young people's emotional reactions to four sets of emotional scenarios. The participants were Japanese college students who rely on mobile phones for their daily communications. Email messages designed to evoke four target emotions (i.e. happiness, sadness, anger, and guilt) were presented to the participants who rated their emotional responses to each scenario, wrote out a reply, and rated the degree of emotion they intended to convey to their communication partner. The data were collected and analyzed and those results are summarized below.

The first hypothesis (H1) was that participants would experience greater emotions when reading email from close friends than acquaintances and that they would transmit stronger emotions to their friends. In the happy and sad scenarios, both parts of the hypothesis were supported: Participants rated their emotional state upon reading the close friend scenario higher than the acquaintance scenario, and intended to convey their emotions more strongly to their friend. However, the situation for the anger and guilt scenarios was complicated, only partly supporting the hypothesis. While participants experienced stronger emotions when reading their close friend's message in the guilt

scenario, the situation was reversed in the anger scenario. And while the participants wanted to convey their angry emotions more strongly to a friend, their estimated emotions for the guilt scenario were nearly identical for both friends and acquaintances. Therefore, the relationship between interpersonal closeness and emotional states and intended emotions seems dependent on the emotional context of the communication.

The overall participant response to the scenarios can be summarized in two main sets, depending on the emotional context: The first is for the happy and guilty scenarios. In these situations, the emotions experienced by the participants tended to be expressed directly to their communication partner almost without change. However, in the sad and angry scenarios, the emotions the participants experienced when reading the scenarios were not transmitted to their communication partner with the same intensity. The resulting messages tended to weaken or downplay the writer's actual emotional experience. This second result is important for understanding and ultimately developing strategies to minimize emotional miscommunication in text-based mediated communications. It is also a point of interest for potential cross-cultural comparisons. While in this study, Japanese participants downplayed their emotional reactions, we wonder how email writers from other cultures might respond. This is a promising area for future research.

The degree of sadness experienced in the anger and guilt scenarios was also examined. Sadness experienced in the anger scenario was suppressed when conveyed to the communication partner although when the partner was a close friend, the participants did express their feelings more strongly. In contrast, in the guilt scenario, the participants showed a tendency to express sadness more strongly than they actually experienced it. These results imply that participants' responses to their emotional state were to avoid sending too strong of a negative message to their partner, whether that was to diminish the sadness they felt, or overstate their emotions when they were the ones who caused a problem.

As noted in the introduction, in a communication that produces positive emotions (e.g. happiness), previous research showed there is a tendency to directly convey the emotion of happiness the participants experienced to their partner. However, in response to communications where negative emotions (e.g. sadness) are produced, writers tend to express their feelings more weakly in the message than they actually experienced. These findings can help explain the results of our previous studies (Kato, Kato, & Akahori 2006; Kato, Kato, & Akahori 2007) that suggested that while positive emotions were effectively conveyed to the partner, negative emotions in messages were more easily misunderstood. Based on the results of the current study, since negative emotions were weakly conveyed to the partners, the partners may have received insufficient information to correctly judge the writer's emotions resulting in the miscommunication.

The combined results were separated by gender to see if the participant's gender influenced the degree of emotions they experienced and the degree to which they wanted to convey those emotions to their communication partner. The gender analysis of the emotional state and intended emotion data revealed that the anger scenario yielded several significant results. Namely, men were more likely than women to experience anger when reading the anger scenario message and they chose to convey those emotions more directly than women to their communication partner. When sadness was added to the analysis, it was found that women were more likely to experience sadness in the anger scenario and were more likely than men to express those feelings.

The second hypothesis (H2) supposed that more messages to close friends would contain emotional cues as opposed to replies to acquaintances. As described above, the data support this hypothesis. All scenarios showed more replies with emotional content to close friends than to

acquaintances. This was particularly striking in the sad scenario (59.3% vs. 26.4%), but the happy (81.3% vs. 53.8%) and anger (62.6% vs. 40.7%) scenarios were also quite clear. The guilt scenario results showed a slight (2.2%) difference in favor of replies to friends, but this difference seems negligible. What is more important is the far greater inclusion of emotional cues in the guilt scenario messages to both friends and acquaintances which is described in greater detail below.

In addition, the message contents were also analyzed for length. The combined analysis of these data showed that messages were significantly longer when the communication partner was a close friend. One unexpected result was the length of the guilt scenario responses. Responses to the guilt scenarios were significantly longer than the responses to the other three scenarios (i.e. happy, sad, and anger). Happy, sad, and anger scenarios had similar average message lengths. The longer message length in the guilt scenario may be attributable to the sense of responsibility the participants may have felt for inconveniencing their communication partner.

In addition, compared with a close friend, there were more greetings to an acquaintance. From these results, it is thought that (1) responders felt able to ask a close friend for sympathy, while (2) replies to an acquaintance seemed to require more formality—social courtesies like greetings. The factor of intimacy is considered to be a psychological distance. When the distance is shortened, emotional expressions and emotional exchanges increase. However, emotional expressions are restricted in mobile phone email. As such, unexpected troubles may be produced in even intimate relationships because of the limited emotional expressions peculiar to mediated communications. However, to the partner who is not intimate, there seems to be fewer emotional expressions and more exchanges of polite remarks and matter-of-fact contents. Therefore, it is thought that at the time of the uncommon emotional communication with the acquaintance, and the everyday exchange with a close friend, emotional troubles may break out.

Content analysis can explain the results obtained from analysis of these questionnaires. Comparison of the number of characters showed that there was a tendency for the guilt scenario to have more characters than the anger scenario. Moreover, in the guilt scenario, emotional expressions were seen in almost all the reply emails. That is, it is thought that the emotion of guilt is conveyed to the partner by writing reply mail including emotion cues with more numbers of characters in the guilt scenario. On the other hand, it is thought that the emotion of anger is suppressed and conveyed to the partner by writing the reply mail which does not include emotion expression with the smaller number of characters in the anger scenario. From these results, Japanese participants suppress and convey the anger when their partner has responsibility, and Japanese participants convey the emotion of guilt firmly, when they have responsibility. That is, it is considered the care which does not give the partner displeasure by suppressing the emotion of anger. Furthermore, it is considered the care which tries to reduce a partner's displeasure by conveying the emotion of guilt clearly. However, when the emotion of anger is suppressed and conveyed, a recipient may misunderstand the sender's emotion of anger. It is a future subject to examine whether the emotion of anger is conveyed clearly or it is suppressed and conveyed for smoother text communication.

As with the emotional response data, the message content data were also separated by gender and analyzed. In both happy and sad scenarios, women's email responses contained more characters than did the men's messages. This was especially true for the sad scenarios.

The inclusion of emotional cues showed clear gender differences. More women's email messages contained emotional expressions to both close friends and acquaintances than did the men's replies for all four emotional scenarios. The differences in the happy and sad scenario replies to both friends and acquaintances were quite clear. It seems that the sender's relationship with the recipient is less important than is the sender's gender.

Similarly, more women's messages contained greetings than did the men's messages with two minor exceptions. While the gender differences for greetings were less clear than for the emotional cues, they were evident in most scenarios and in two cases (i.e. sad scenario replies to acquaintances and anger scenario replies to acquaintances), showed a considerable gap. These two types of content analysis are limited in their scope but show that this is a promising area for future research.

This study focused on how Japanese young people communicate the experience of various emotions in email messages to close friends and acquaintances. The current study's research design had several weaknesses that should be improved upon in future studies. For instance, only four emotions were included in this study. Given more time and resources, including a greater range of emotions could enhance the nuance of the findings. Also, participants wrote their replies using pencil and paper. While this was sufficient in the current study, future projects will use a mobile phone-based system being developed by the authors. This system (MIDAS or Mobile Input Data Access System) will enable users to read actual mobile phone email, answer questionnaires, and compose and send their responses on their mobile phone all while preserving participant anonymity. Finally, the message content analysis did not include the more fine grained analyses of content used by Colley and her colleagues. This shortcoming should be addressed in a future study.

Future research will also include a study of American young people's transmission of emotional content enabling a cross-cultural comparison of the results. Two primary differences in these populations is their media of choice and cultural differences in the approach to interpersonal communications. As noted above, Japanese young people rely on mobile telephones for most of their email communications. Mobile phones have certain limitations that could affect the nature of the communications, for instance, slower typing speed compared to a full keyboard, smaller device screen limiting the amount of text visible at one time, the tendency for mobile telephone messages to be shorter than computer-based email messages, and the tendency for mobile communications to be accessed in a variety of public and private places whereas the location of accessing computer email tends to be more limited. The second difference, culture, presents the most interesting contrast in such a study. It was explained in the first section that Japanese culture encourages the suppression of one's true feelings. Western cultures in general, and American culture in particular, tend to encourage people to "get things off your chest," and to "say what you mean, and mean what you say," even exhorting those who may be reticent to voice their opinions in public to follow Maggie Kuhn's advice and "speak your mind, even if your voice shakes" (About.com 2010). How people from such a cultural background will approach the task of expressing various emotions in text messages will be a fertile area for future research.

REFERENCES

About.com. (2010). *Women's History: Maggie Kuhn Quotes*. Retrieved March 27, 2010 from http://womenshistory.about.com/cs/quotes/a/maggie_kuhn.htm

Ben-Ami, O., & Mioduser, D. (2004). The affective aspect of moderator's role conception and enactment by teachers in a-synchronous learning discussion groups. *Proceedings of World Conference on Educational Multimedia, Hypermedia and Telecommunications (ED-MEDIA) 2004*, 2831-2837.

Cheng, Y., O'Toole, A., & Abdi, H. (2001). Classifying adults' and children's faces by sex: Computational investigations of subcategorial feature encoding. *Cognitive Science, 25*, 819–838. doi:10.1207/s15516709cog2505_8

Colley, A., & Todd, Z. (2002). Gender-linked differences in the style and content of e-mails to friends. *Journal of Language and Social Psychology, 21*, 380–392. doi:10.1177/026192702237955

Colley, A., Todd, Z., Bland, M., Holmes, M., Khanom, N., & Pike, H. (2004, September). Style and Content in E-Mails and Letters to Male and Female Friends. *Journal of Language and Social Psychology, 23*(3), 369–378. doi:10.1177/0261927X04266812

Dyer, R., Green, R., Pitts, M., & Millward, G. (1995). What's the flaming problem? CMC - deindividuation or disinhibiting? In Kirby, M. A. R., Dix, A. J., & Finlay, J. E. (Eds.), *People and Computers, X*. Cambridge: Cambridge University Press.

Ekman, P. (1992). An argument for basic emotions. In Stein, N. L., & Oatley, K. (Eds.), *Basic emotions: cognition & emotion* (pp. 169–200). Mahwah: Lawrence Erlbaum.

Garrison, D. R., & Anderson, T. (2003). *E-Learning in the 21st Century: A Framework for Research and Practice*. London: Routledge Falmer.

Hancock, J. T. (2007). Digital deception: Why, when and how people lie online. In Joinson, A. N., McKenna, K., Postmes, T., & Reips, U. (Eds.), *The Oxford Handbook of Internet Psychology* (pp. 289–301). Oxford: Oxford University Press.

Ito, M., Okabe, D., & Matsuda, M. (Eds.). (2005). *Personal, portable, pedestrian: Mobile phones in Japanese life*. Cambridge, MA: MIT Press.

Izard, C. E., Libero, D. Z., Putnam, P., & Haynes, O. M. (1993). Stability of emotion experiences and their relations to traits of personality. *Journal of Personality and Social Psychology, 64*, 847–860. doi:10.1037/0022-3514.64.5.847

Jones, S. (2002). The Internet goes to college: How students are living in the future with today's technology. *Pew Internet and American Life Project*. Retrieved March 18, 2010 from http://www.pewinternet.org/~/media//Files/Reports/2002/PIP_College_Report.pdf.pdf.

Jones, S. (2009). *Generations online in 2009. Pew Internet and American Life Data Memo* [Online]. Retrieved March 16, 2010 from http://www.pewinternet.org/~/media//Files/Reports/2009/PIP_Generations_2009.pdf.

Kang, M., Kim, S., & Park, S. (2007). Developing an emotional presence scale for measuring students' involvement during e-learning process. *Proceedings of World Conference on Educational Multimedia, Hypermedia and Telecommunications (ED-MEDIA) 2007*, 2829-2831.

Kato, S., Kato, Y., & Akahori, K. (2006). Study on emotional transmissions in communication using bulletin board system. *Proceedings of World Conference on E-Learning in Corporate, Government, Healthcare, and Higher Education (E-Learn) 2006*, 2576-2584.

Kato, S., Kato, Y., Scott, D. J., & Akahori, K. (2008). Analysis of anger in mobile phone Emil communications in Japan. *Waseda Journal of Human Sciences, 21*(1), 29–39.

Kato, S., Kato, Y., & Tachino, T. (2007). Lesson practice which took in the lesson preliminary announcement using the mobile phone. *Poster-Proceedings of ICCE, 2007*, 21–22.

Kato, Y., & Akahori, K. (2006). Analysis of judgment of partners' emotions during e-mail and face-to-face communication. *Journal of Science Education in Japan, 29*(5), 354–365.

Kato, Y., Kato, S., & Akahori, K. (2007). Effects of emotional cues transmitted in e-mail communication on the emotions experienced by senders and receivers. *Computers in Human Behavior, 23*(4), 1894–1905. doi:10.1016/j.chb.2005.11.005

Kato, Y., Kato, S., & Scott, D. J. (2007). Misinterpretation of emotional cues and content in Japanese email, computer conferences, and mobile text messages. In Clausen, E. I. (Ed.), *Psychology of Anger* (pp. 145–176). Hauppauge, NY: Nova Science Publishers.

Kato, Y., Kato, S., Scott, D. J., & Sato, K. (2008). Emotional strategies in mobile phone email communication in Japan: focusing on four kinds of basic emotions. *Proceedings of World Conference on Educational Multimedia, Hypermedia and Telecommunications (ED-MEDIA) 2008*, 1058-1066.

Kato, Y., Kato, S., Scott, D. J., & Takeuchi, T. (2008). Relationships between the emotional transmissions in mobile phone email communication and the email contents in Japan. *Proceedings of World Conference on E-Learning in Corporate, Government, Healthcare, and Higher Education (E-Learn) 2008*, 2804-2811.

Keysar, B., & Henly, A. S. (2002). Speakers' overestimation of their effectiveness. *Psychological Science, 13*, 207–212. doi:10.1111/1467-9280.00439

Krauss, R. M., & Fussell, S. R. (1996). Social Psychological models of interpersonal communication. In Higgins, E. T., & Kruglanski, A. W. (Eds.), *Social Psychology: Handbook of Basic Principles* (pp. 655–701). NY: The Guilford Press.

Kraut, R. E. (1978). Verbal and nonverbal cues in the perception of lying. *Journal of Personality and Social Psychology, 36*, 380–391. doi:10.1037/0022-3514.36.4.380

Kruger, J., Epley, N., Parker, P., & Ng, Z. (2005). Egocentrism over e-mail: Can we communicate as well as we think? *Journal of Personality and Social Psychology, 89*(6), 925–936. doi:10.1037/0022-3514.89.6.925

Lea, M., O'Shea, T., Fung, P., & Spears, R. (1992). "Flaming" in computer-mediated communication: Observations, explanations, implications. In M. Lea (Ed.), *Contexts of Computer-Mediated Communication*, pp. 89-112. NY: Harvester Wheasheaf.

Matsumoto, D., & Kudo, T. (1993). American-Japanese cultural differences in implicit theories of personality based on smile. *Journal of Nonverbal Behavior, 17*(4), 231–243. doi:10.1007/BF00987239

Ministry of Internal Affairs and Communications. Japan (2006). *White Paper 2006: Information and Communications in Japan.* [Online]. Retrieved June 1, 2007 from http://www.johotsusintokei.soumu.go.jp/whitepaper/eng/WP2006/2006-index.html

Morahan-Martin, J. (2007). Internet use and abuse and psychological problems. n A. N. Joinson, K. McKenna, T. Postmes, & U. Reips (Eds.), *The Oxford Handbook of Internet Psychology*, pp. 331-345. Oxford: Oxford University Press.

Murphy, E. (2004). Recognizing and promoting collaboration in an online asynchronous discussion. *British Journal of Educational Technology, 35*(4), 421–431. doi:10.1111/j.0007-1013.2004.00401.x

Okabe, D., & Ito, M. (2006). Keitai in public transportation. In Ito, M., Okabe, D., & Matsuda, M. (Eds.), *Personal, Portable, Pedestrian: Mobile Phones in Japanese Life* (pp. 205–217). Cambridge, MA: MIT Press.

Patterson, M. L. (1994). Strategic functions of nonverbal exchange. In Daly, J. A., & Wiemann, J. M. (Eds.), *Strategic Interpersonal Communication* (pp. 273–293). Hillsdale, NJ: Erlbaum.

Rubin, D. L., & Greene, K. (1992). Gender typical style in written language. *Research in the Teaching of English, 26*, 7–40.

Sato, K. (2007). Impact of social presence in computer-mediated communication to effective discussion on bulletin board system. *Proceedings of World Conference on Educational Multimedia, Hypermedia and Telecommunications (ED-MEDIA) 2007*, 722-731.

Scott, D. J. (2008). Gender Differences in Japanese College Students' Participation in a Qualitative Study. [Association for the Advancement of Computing in Education]. *AACE Journal, 16*(4), 385–404.

Scott, D. J., Coursaris, C. K., Kato, Y., & Kato, S. (2009). The Exchange of Emotional Content in Business Communications: A Comparison of PC and Mobile E-mail Users. In M. Head and E. Li (Eds.) *Advances in Electronic Business: Vol. 4 - Mobile and Ubiquitous Commerce.* Hershey PA: IGI Global Publishing. pp. 201-219.

Siegel, J., Dubrovsky, V., Kiesler, S., & McGuire, T. W. (1986). Group processes in computer-mediated communication. *Organizational Behavior and Human Decision Processes, 37*, 157–187. doi:10.1016/0749-5978(86)90050-6

Tachino, T., Kato, Y., & Kato, S. (2007). An approach to utilize ubiquitous device for game-based learning environment. *Proceedings of DIGITEL, 2007*, 209–211.

Thompsen, P. A., & Foulger, D. A. (1996). Effects of pictographs and quoting on flaming in electronic mail. *Computers in Human Behavior, 12*(2), 225–243. doi:10.1016/0747-5632(96)00004-0

Yamamoto, M., & Akahori, K. (2005). Development of an e-learning system for higher education using the mobile phone. *Proceedings of World Conference on Educational Multimedia, Hypermedia and Telecommunications (ED-MEDIA) 2005*, 4169-4172.

ENDNOTE

[1] Drafts of this chapter were presented at E-Learn 2008 and ED-MEDIA 2009. Copyright by AACE. Reprinted with permission.

Section 5
Emotions in Human–Computer Interaction

Chapter 13
A Scientific Look at the Design of Aesthetically and Emotionally Engaging Interactive Entertainment Experiences

Magy Seif El-Nasr
Simon Fraser University, Canada

Jacquelyn Ford Morie
University of Southern California, USA

Anders Drachen
Dragon Consulting, Copenhagen

ABSTRACT

The interactive entertainment industry has become a multi-billion dollar industry with revenues overcoming those of the movie industry (ESA, 2009). Beyond the demand for high fidelity graphics or stylized imagery, participants in these environments have come to expect certain aesthetic and artistic qualities that engage them at a very deep emotional level. These qualities pertain to the visual aesthetic, dramatic structure, pacing, and sensory systems embedded within the experience. All these qualities are carefully crafted by the creator of the interactive experience to evoke affect. In this book chapter, the authors will attempt to discuss the design techniques developed by artists to craft such emotionally engaging experiences. In addition, they take a scientific approach whereby we discuss case studies of the use of these design techniques and experiments that attempt to validate their use in stimulating emotions.

INTRODUCTION

Virtual 3D environments can be developed to evoke emotions similar to what people feel within their everyday lives. For example, in the 1960s

DOI: 10.4018/978-1-61692-892-6.ch013

Eleanor Gibson conducted a perceptual study known as the visual cliff experiment (E. J. Gibson & Walk, 1960). She developed an environment with surfaces of two different heights: a raised surface next to one positioned a few feet below it. A black and white checkered cloth was then draped over the two surfaces. Then, a large sheet of heavy clear plastic was placed atop the entire setup ensuring the top surface was physically level and continuous, yet, the surfaces below the plastic created the perception that the floor dropped sharply. Babies who learned to crawl (typically from six months on) were placed on one side of this setup and were called by their mothers who were on the opposite side. The babies showed no hesitation as they set out across the shallow side, but when they reached the 'drop,' they showed emotional stress even though they could feel with their hands that the plastic surface was continuous. The act of crawling presumably gave them enough visual knowledge of how physical space works that they would not crawl over the illusive drop.

Fred Brooks and colleagues at the University of North Carolina (Meehan, Insko, Whitton, & Brooks, 2002) replicated a similar setup within a virtual environment. With 3D modeling tools they constructed a sunken room surrounded by a ledge that was experienced with a stereo head mounted display. The stereo view reinforced the illusion that the sunken room was located about ten feet below the participant's position. The visitor was instructed to drop a ball onto a target within the pit room and to do this he or she had to walk to and lean over the edge of the ledge. There was a small section of molding on the floor that the feet touched, which served to provide physical corroboration that there was a real ledge in the virtual space. Even seasoned VR veterans had difficulty over-coming the feeling that the pit was real. One of our co-authors experienced this space. She described a visceral gut reaction to being on the edge and looking down. Physiological signals collected from the participants during the experiment showed that the virtual cliff provoked the same physiological responses as the traditional visual cliff or a corresponding real space.

In addition to stimulating emotions such as fear of heights, virtual environments can also be developed and designed to evoke a myriad of emotions and affect. In order to discuss these, we first introduce the concept of emotional affordances. In the late 1970s, perceptual scientist J. J. Gibson (J. J. Gibson, 1979) outlined a concept wherein elements in an environment are considered in the possibilities for actions they provide. He termed such possibilities affordances. Gibson's work led him to develop a theory of ecological psychology, in which behavior is mediated by the affordances present. While Gibson's work focuses on concrete perceptual possibilities for action, we use an expanded definition, called emotional affordances, that includes a wide range of affective elements that could provide opportunities for emotional reaction (Morie et al. 2005). The addition of affective elements requires a broader definition of perception. Perception is usually thought of as conscious reactions to stimuli. The affordances we use can, and often does, fall below the levels of conscious perception. Such subconscious stimuli still afford mental and physical reactions, as intense, sometimes even more so, than reactions from stimuli of which we are aware (as with the visual cliff (E. J. Gibson & Walk, 1960)) (Bornstein, 1992). Gibson's affordances are extrinsic; they allow for external behavior (physical actions or reactions). Emotional affordances are intrinsic; they allow for internal actions or reactions. If a perceptual affordance is a perceptual cue to the function of an object that causes an action, then an emotional affordance is a sensory cue to the function of a stimulus that causes an emotional reaction.

Emotional affordances must be designed to seem natural to the situation. They can serve various purposes beyond eliciting emotions, including subtly guiding the participant along a desired path through the virtual environment (J. Morie et al., 2003). Clive Fencott (Fencott, 1999) describes affordances for virtual environments in terms of three basic perceptual opportunities—sureties, shocks and surprises. He further breaks down these opportunities into attractors, connectors, and retainers. Fencott's work was the first to include both perceptual and emotional affordances. These affordances can be viewed as a continuum to illustrate the complementary and overlapping domains of perception and emotion. All affordances are user contingent; in an interactive game environment, they are essentially triggers that result in an action (physical response) or a reaction (emotional response) from the participant. This affordance continuum – from perceptual actions to emotional reactions – is illustrated in Figure 1.

Artists and designers have mastered the skill of developing virtual environments with such emotional affordances – environments that engage the participants in a deep emotional level and evoke emotions, such as fear, empathy, and others. In fact, if one takes a virtual roller coaster ride at Universal Studio, one would feel similar, if not the same, emotions stimulated during that the ride as in a real roller coaster ride. An example of this experience is the Simpson's virtual roller coaster ride, which was experienced by one of the co-authors and described as a successfully designed ride that elicited many of the same emotions as a real roller coaster ride and has, in fact, deceived many participants into thinking they are in a real roller coaster while they didn't even leave the room.

Developing such an emotionally evocative interactive virtual environment involves a large number of techniques that engage participants at both emotional and cognitive levels. These techniques include, but are not limited to, visual effects, environmental composition, color choices, light-

ing and design, audio work, character implementation, and effective story. In this chapter, we take a scientific approach to discussing these techniques. While there are many resources where designers discuss design techniques to elicit emotions, these resources are not scientific in nature. They do not set out to prove or evaluate the design techniques used. In this book chapter, we will discuss both a set of successful design techniques for eliciting arousal and measurement methods for validating the arousal level elicited. In addition, we discuss two case studies: one on the use of lighting for eliciting emotions and the other on the use of an amalgam of sensory modalities for stimulating arousal. Both case studies were validated through arousal identification devices and quantitative analysis methods.

Identifying and measuring emotions is an inexact science. There are many approaches discussed in the literature, including self-report measures, or more objectives methods such as the use of biometric or physiological sensory data. There are systems built on new and emerging measurement devices, which are increasingly demanded by companies that need to evaluate their products for their perceived emotional engagement. In this book chapter, we discuss these approaches and devices as well as discuss their validity. In the case studies discussed, we focus on arousal rather than specific complex or simple emotional states due to the lack of validated analysis techniques that can reliably identify emotions at the time we ran our experiments.

Figure 1. Continuum of affordances from perceptual to emotional

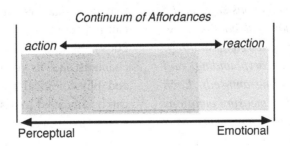

Therefore, this chapter provides the reader with the following contributions: (1) an understanding of the myriad emotions and affect that can be elicited within an interactive entertainment product through a discussion of design techniques used by designers and artists and case studies that validate some of these techniques scientifically and (2) a listing and explanation of methods that can be used to identify and measure different types of emotions and arousal, including devices and analysis methods developed.

The chapter proceeds by first discussing and defining emotions and methods for identifying them. We then discuss the two case studies discussing the design details and methods to evoke emotions and methods to measure the elicited emotional reactions.

DEFINING AND IDENTIFYING EMOTIONS

Emotions work through neuro-chemical transmitters, which influence areas of the brain, successively guiding behavior and modifying how information is perceived and decisions are made (Norman, 2004). There is, however, an ongoing debate about how emotions can be defined, represented and measured, with empirically based studies only recently beginning to converge towards a consensus.

As there seems to be no empirical solution to the debate on which component is sufficient or necessary to define emotions, at present the most favored solutions is to say that emotions are best treated as a multifaceted phenomenon consisting of the following components: behavioral reactions (e.g. approaching), expressive reactions (e.g. smiling), physiological reactions (e.g. heart pounding), and subjective feelings (e.g. feeling amused). Each instrument that is claimed to measure emotions in fact measures one of these components. As a consequence, both the number of reported instru-

ments and the diversity in approaches to measure emotions is abundant. Today's instruments range from simple pen-and-paper rating scales to dazzling high-tech equipment that measures brain waves or eye movements. (Desmet, 2003).

Emotions and arousal form a vital component of the experience of interacting with interactive entertainment, motivating the cognitive decisions made during gameplay (Holson, 2004, April 10; Ravaja & Kivikangas, 2008; Ravaja, Saari, Salminen, Laarni, & Kallinen, 2006). Emotions are important to understanding and predicting user behavior and also in determining the quality of the user experience within interactive entertainment applications such as digital games. Because of this, during the last decade there has been an increase in the amount of research dedicated to the assessment of emotional responses during interactions with digital applications. In the wider human-computer interface community, **emotion** and **affect assessment** is a growing research domain under the wider context of user experience research, focusing on improving interaction quality by bringing it closer to human-to-human communication. This development mirrors the continuing rapid expansion of interactive entertainment applications from a marginal leisure activity to a direct competitor of traditional forms, such as movies, books, sports and music, e.g., (Grodal, 2000; L. E. Nacke, 2009).

The assessment of emotion in the context of digital interactive entertainment is generally focused on the individual user experience, and generally oriented towards assessment during the period of interaction, although it is recognized that other factors, such as prior experiences, can impact the user's experience (L. E. Nacke, 2009). Emotions can be expressed via several channels, such as voice, speech, facial responses and physiological responses. Various features can be analyzed to assess the emotional state of a participant; using a variety of techniques both subjective and objective. Psycho-physiological measures and qualitative methods such as interviews, self-reporting, observational analysis and behavioral analysis, are the most common. The latter subjective and qualitative methods are notably used when the usage of time- and resource-consuming psycho-physiological measures such as fMRI, EEG and EMG are not possible (Drachen, Canossa, & Yannakakis, 2009; Isbister & Schaffer, 2008; Pagulayan, Keeker, Wixon, Romero, & Fuller, 2003). In general, there is a lack of non-cumbersome, real-time tools for measuring arousal and other emotions during interaction periods. Psycho-physiological measures with established validity can provide real-time assessments, and have been used in research or medical contexts. However, these often require specialized equipment and laboratory environments. In addition, the expenditures of time and resources needed for industry-based evaluation are major roadblocks inhibiting successful evaluations of digital entertainment applications. This is true for both evaluating individual emotional components of the user experience as well as modeling and assessing user cognition and emotions during the interaction period. Recent innovations, however, led to several companies producing simplified mobile equipment for in game user-experience interaction experience assessment, usable in real-life settings, e.g. Emotive, OCZNia and EmSense. It remains an open question whether this type of technology can be suitably validated to be able to serve as the basis of scientific studies as well as those of simpler industry-based consumer research. That being said, there currently exists a wide range of more sophisticated testing methods for evaluating emotion and affect. In this section, we will briefly review these approaches. A more in-depth review is beyond the scope of this book chapter, and readers are referred to individual articles for more details.

Dimensional Models of Continuous Emotion

Paralleling the work on developing methods for measuring emotion, models and theories for identifying and classifying emotions was also being developed. Wundt (1896) was one of the earliest psychologists to use classification as a means of grouping feelings. In this case a three-dimensional model containing three fundamental axes: Pleasure-displeasure, arousal-composure and tension-resolution. This was one of the earliest examples of dimensional theories of emotion, which hypothesized that all emotions can be located in a dimensional space defined by orthogonal axes (usually 2D or 3D, up to n-dimensional). Emotions were not considered as discrete phenomena, but rather continuous.

One of the most influential dimensional models – the circumplex model - in emotion assessment was developed by Russel (1980 and 2003). In this model, emotions are divided along two axis formed by valence (negative to positive) and arousal/bodily activation (low-high). Emotional categories defined by everyday language such as joy, depression and anger can be located within the dimensional space, correlating with specific ratios of valence and arousal. There have been several adaptations of the model (e.g. Watson & Tellegen, 1985; Posner et al., 2005). Additionally, Cowie (2000, 2001) used a valence/activation model, similar to the valence/arousal space, to model and evaluate emotions based on speech. Although dimensional spaces do not provide direct verbal description, it is possible to map points or areas which can be labeled categorically according to the specific emotion. These dimensional models are the de facto standard in psycho-physiological research, contrasted by theories of basic emotions (Nacke, 2009).

Psycho-Physiological Player Testing

Psycho-physiological measures are controlled measures of emotion, generally utilized in a laboratory environment. They are used by e.g. psychologists and HCI-experts to identify emotions; and are used widely in Human Factors for studying mental effort and stress (Wilson, 2001).

Psycho-physiological signals can be divided into those originating from the peripheral nervous system, such as heart rate and galvanic skin response, and those originating from the central nervous system, such as brain waves, measured e.g. via ElectroEnchephaloGrams (EEG). The actual meaning of psycho-physiological measures and data is dependent on the context and research approach (Ravaja, 2004), and thus, the interpretation of these measures in the context of digital interactive entertainment requires more study and validation before consistent results can be ensured.

There are two overall ways of conducting psycho-physiological testing: Tonic testing or phasic testing (Nacke, 2009; Lim et al., 1997; O'Donnel, Creamer, Elliot, & Bryant, 2007). In tonic testing, the technology is used to accumulate psycho-physiological data over a specific time period (i.e. averaged across the time period). In phasic measurement, a higher resolution view of the data is allowed, e.g. automated scoring of events.

Experience using psycho-physiological research suggests that it is possible to quantitatively measure some emotional states using these measures, which, thus, permits one to invasively or covertly assess physical reactions of users. Different types of psycho-physiological measures operate differently and are not independently reliable indicators of even well-characterized feelings. Therefore, these methods are usually applied in tandem, or at least cross-correlated across empirical studies, to increase the reliability of measurements. This process is important to identify which patterns of physiological responses reflect which emotional responses. Importantly,

the many-to-one relation between psychological processing and physiological responses (Oatley, Keltner, & Jenkins, 2006) allow for specific psycho-physiological measures to be linked with difference psychological effects, e.g. cognition or emotion. Therefore, attention has been given to the correlation of patterns of physiological measurement with subjective characterizations of emotion (Cacioppo, Tassinary, & Berntson, 2007; L. Nacke, Lindley, & Stellmach, 2008).

There is, however, an increasing body of evidence supporting these approaches. For example, Ravaja et al. (2006) reported that tonic measures of facial EMG and EDA have been shown to be associated with positive and negative affect responses or arousal during interaction (playing) with digital games.

The key psycho-physiological measurement techniques used in emotional assessment and affective computing include cardiovascular measures, EMG, fMRI, EEG, EDA, and respiratory measures.

Cardiovascular Measures

The cardiovascular system includes the organs regulating blood flow in the body and offers a variety of measuring options to determine valence or arousal (Oatley et al., 2006), including: heart rate (HR), which is known to correlate with arousal (Anttonen & Surakka, 2005). Additional differentiation is possible with finger temperature. Blood Volume Pressure (BVP) has been used to show a correlation between greater dilation in the blood vessels and decreasing arousal (Ward & Marsden, 2003). Heart Rate Variability (HRV) is the interval between consecutive heartbeats. The variability of the heart rate, which can be determined from an ElectroCardioGram (ECG), occurs due to the synergistic action of the two branches of the autonomous nervous system. This strives towards a balance via neural, mechanical, hormonal and other physiological mechanisms to maintain cardiovascular parameters in the optimal ranges, to facilitate optimal reaction to changing conditions externally and internally. HRV is generally used as a metric for assessing the positive and negative valence of experiences (Anttonen & Surakka, 2005), and as an indicator of mental workload (Rowe, Sibert, & Irwin, 1998). For example, Rani et al. (Rani, Sims, Brackin, & Sarkar, 2002) correlated HRV with stress, finding that HRV is low under stress, and high during relaxation. Additionally as shown by Rowe et al. (1998), HRV decreases with mental effort. The normalized HRV correlates with subjective ratings of effort, but not with task difficulty (using a normalized HRV).

Finally, HR, HRV and Respiratory Sinus Arrhythmia (RSA) (Gentzler et al., 2009) can be computed from measuring the electrical activity of the heart (ECG). And ECG is externally recorded using skin electrodes and is non-invasive, normally translating the electrical activity into line tracings (Mandryk, Atkins, & Inkpen, 2006).

Electromyography (EMG)

EMG is a measurement technology for recording the electrical activation of muscles (Fridlund & Cacioppo, 1986). Using EMG permits assessment of covert (non-visual) activity of facial muscles (Ravaja, 2004). The correlation between EMG activity and emotion is based in the work of e.g. Ekman (Ekman, 1992), who noted that basic emotions are reflected in facial expressions. This discovery formed the basis for investigating physiological responses of facial muscles as a means of evaluating emotional processing. The empirical backing supporting the posited relationship between facial muscle activity and pleasant/unpleasant emotions is substantial, e.g. (Bradley & Lang, 2007; Ravaja & Kivikangas, 2008).

Facial electromyography is one of the major indices of hedonic valence (Ravaja, 2004), i.e. EMG activity increases with the contractions of the facial muscle groups, which are responsible for positive and negative emotional expressions

(Ravaja & Kivikangas, 2008). For example, increased activity of the cheek muscle region is associated with positive emotions and negative emotions are associated with activity of the brow muscle regions. Similarly, activity of the periocular muscle area has been shown to be associated with positive, high-arousal emotions, permitting mapping of emotions in the valence dimensions of the circumflex model of affect (Mandryk & Inkpen, 2004; Ravaja, 2004; Ravaja & Kivikangas, 2008; Russell, 1980).

EMG remains one of the best validated measures of emotion in interactive entertainment. For example, Ravaja & Kivikangas (Ravaja & Kivikangas, 2008) demonstrated the relationship between phasic facial EMG and EDA responses to different in-game events, with self-reported emotions elicited by these events. EMG is perhaps particularly applicable in situations involving gameplay because of the inherent focus of players on the game playing activity, which minimizes facial activation due to confounding factors. Irrespective of the reason, EMG is the dominant measure of arousal during gameplay. However, as for any other psycho-physiological measure, in order to correctly assess level of arousal, additional measures need to be utilized to cross-validate results.

Measurement of Electrodermal Activity (EDA)

EDA is commonly known as skin conductance, or galvanic skin response, and is the measure of the electrical conductivity of the skin. Due to activation of the central nervous system when people experience physical arousal, sweat is produced from the eccrine glands which measurably change the conductivity of the skin. The sweat glands used for measurement are typically those in the palms of the hand or the soles of the feet, as the glands are more concentrated in these areas and quickly respond to changes to physiological stimulation as opposed to slower responses such as temperature changes in the human body (Stern, Ray, & Quigley, 2001). Research using picture stimuli have shown EDA to be highly correlated with self-reported emotional arousal (Lang, 1995), reflecting emotional responses and cognitive activity (Boucsein, 1992). Finally, EDA is one of the most straight forward and low-cost psycho-physiological measures (Mandryk et al., 2006; Ravaja, 2004).

Electroencephalography (EEG)

EEG is used to measure the arousal dimension of human emotions, using signals from the brain. EEG measures brain waves, usually described in terms of frequency bands (Oatley et al., 2006). These are commonly referred to as alpha (8-13 Hz), beta (14-30 Hz), theta (4-7 Hz) and delta (under 4 Hz). Sometimes wavelengths of 36 Hz or more are used in studies, referred to as gamma-frequency, and can be related to the formation of percepts and memory (Miltner et al., 1999). Alpha band power is indicative of a relaxed stage, where there is limited arousal and cognitive load, and little attentional demand, i.e. permits evaluation of the state of arousal (Pfurtscheller, Zalaudek, & Neuper, 1998; Ray & Cole, 1985). Beta activity relates to a state of attention and alertness, associated with cognitive and information processing (Ray & Cole, 1985). Theta activity appears to be connected with creative processes, intuition, emotions and sensations (Aftanas & Golocheikine, 2001). Delta waves are prominent during deep sleep and can according to Cacioppo et al. (Cacioppo et al., 2007), be associated with unconscious processes. Thanks to the relationship between psychological processing and physiological responses, these measures of brain activity can be linked to psychological structures such as attention, cognitive demand, and arousal. A primary challenge of EEG measurement is that the mechanisms and timing of temporal synchronization of brain activity with exact emotional responses are as yet not well known (Sander, Grandjean, & Scherer, 2005).

EEG is in practice measured as the voltage recorded between two electrodes on the scalp. In order to acquire a signal, EEG requires the users to wear scalp electrodes (usually positioned on a headcap), and can therefore feel intrusive; however, experience indicates that users quickly forget that the electrodes are present during gameplay (L. Nacke et al., 2008).

Functional Magnetic Resonance Imaging (fMRI), Positron Emission Tomography (PET) and Functional Near-infrared Spectroscopy (fNIR)

Functional imaging is generally conducted in order to understand the activity of a given brain region in its relationship to a particular behavior state, or its interaction with inputs from the activity of another region of the brain. fMRI and PET are limited in their practical application because of the size and cost of the equipment as well as requirements on shielding, and a predilection to motion artifacts, making them difficult to utilize in studies focusing on real-time active gameplay. PET scans also require participants to ingest a radioactive tracer in the case of PET. A few studies have emerged using fMRI, e.g. (Mathiak & Weber, 2006), who used fMRI toward brain correlates of natural behavior during video game play. An advantage of fMRI is that the technique provides a better spatial resolution than e.g. EEG, which may make it useful for detecting complex emotions.

Introduced during the last decade, the fNIR technique has gained attention in HCI research because it is portable and more affordable than fMRI (Hirshfield et al., 2009). This method is used to evaluate which regions of the brain that are activated, and functions via the application of near-infrared light (specific wavelengths within the optical window) to find the ratio of oxygenated and deoxygenated hemoglobin in the blood flow of the brain. The method is, therefore, useful for studying the hemodynamic changes due to cognitive and emotional brain activity. Unlike, fMRI, which can detect activity through the brain, fNIR penetrates a shorter distance into the skull, yet it can be used in a similar capacity to EEG. fNIR studies of emotion and cognition have focused on specific areas of the brain (Broadman's areas), showing that specific regions play a critical role in sustained attention, problem solving etc. (Cabeza & Nyberg, 2000). The technology is still new and immature. However, its advantages over fMRI and PET give it future potential for emotion studies during active gameplay.

Unlike the simpler psychophysiological techniques, fMRI, PET, fNIR, EEG and EMG requires the participants to be attached to bulky equipment, and it is therefore not suitable for long-term studies, unlike e.g. HR which can be examined over extended time periods as sensors can be integrated into wearable devices such as watches. Most equipment for EDA measures provides wearable sensors, but not complete participant mobility.

Eye Tracking:

Eye tracking is based on measuring the fixations (dwell times) and saccades (fast movements) of human gazes (Duchowski, 2007). Eye tracking is used for inferring cognitive processes arising from the relationship between eye fixations and attentional focus (Sennersten, 2008). This measure is particularly applicable for the exploration of virtual environments. Combined with other measures, this may give a means of factoring out those EMG signals, for example, that may indicate facial muscle movement due to cognitive processes and not emotions.

In summary, Table 1 shows the different measures, affect (arousal/valance/emotions) that they can measure as well as the applicability of the device.

Table 1. Overview of psycho-physiological measures and the emotional entity they measure

Measure	Abbreviation	Emotional entity measured	Applicability
Heart Rate	HR	Arousal	Simple and cheap, e.g. using pulse watches
Blood Volume Pulse	BVP	Arousal	Relatively inexpensive, signal requires denoising, requires specialized equipment
ElectroCardioGram	ECG (EKG)	Arousal	Requires externally positioned skin electrodes and specialized equipment, time consuming, useful to obtain HR-related signals
Heart Rate Variability	HRV	Valence	Relatively inexpensive, signal requires denoising, requires specialized equipment
ElectroMyoGraphy	EMG	Valence	Requires specialized equipment, time consuming and expensive
ElecetroEncephaloGram	EEG	Valence/arousal	Requires specialized equipment, time consuming and expensive
Functional Magnetic Resonance Imaging	fMRI	Valence/arousal	Complex and expensive, bulky equipment, but high resolution
Positron Emission Tomography	PET	Valence/arousal/complex emotions	Complex and expensive, bulky equipment, but high resolution
Functional Near-infrared Spectroscopy	fNIR	Valence/arousal/complex emotions	Portable and cheaper than fMRI, but lower detection depth
ElectroDermalActivity	EDA	Arousal	Easy to employ, signal denoising often necessary, cheap sensors available on the market
Respiratory Sinus Arrhythmia	RSA	Arousal	Relatively inexpensive, requires specialized equipment

Qualitative Measures

Semi-quantitative and qualitative approaches, such as subjective self-reports through surveys, interviews and think-aloud protocols, traditionally form the basis for user-feedback gathering and evaluation of digital interactive entertainment, combined with objective analysis via observational video analysis increasingly coupled with psycho-physiological measures (L. E. Nacke, 2009). Surveys developed to evaluate emotions in digital interactive entertainment have generally focused on the enjoyment-aspects of user experience; however, recent developments have included dimensions such as tension, frustration or negative affect (IJsselsteijn, Poels, & de Kort, 2008; Poels, Kort, & IJsselsteijn, 2007). Using surveys during natural breaks in the gameplay action is usually the preferred method of deployment (Kim et al., 2008). Self-reported emotions have been successfully correlated with psycho-physiological measures, e.g. (Merkx, Truong, & Neerincx, 2007; L. Nacke et al., 2008; Ravaja & Kivikangas, 2008).

Subjective reporting via surveys, interviews and focus groups are – depending on the openness and closedness of the questions being asked – generalizable, convenient, uncomplicated to administer, providing data that can be statistically treated. There are substantial drawbacks, however. First of all, surveys are hard to develop in a manner that ensures unbiased results. Also, respondents may not all clearly understand the questions (Kuniavsky, 2003). Furthermore, surveys are not conducive to locate complex patterns, and respondent data may not correspond to the actual experience of interacting with an application, for example due to a bias caused by time (Marshall & Rossman, 1999). Additionally, respondents may not be trustworthy, consciously or unconsciously biasing their replies to e.g. make themselves look better than they are; or may try to answer what they think the researcher wants to hear rather than what they actually feel/experience. Finally, people

being interviewed may be biased, because they are aware they are being recorded. In essence, subjective self-report data are cognitively mediated, and may not reflect what is actually occurring (Kuniavsky, 2003).

Think-aloud techniques, on the other hand, provide a popular technique in the evaluation of productivity applications. However, they are progressively harder to utilize in conjunction with digital interactive entertainment applications because they disturb the user, thus impacting on immersion/engagement. This has not prevented the method from being employed for usability evaluation of games (Medlock, Wixon, Terrano, Romero, & Fulton, 2002; Pagulayan et al., 2003).

Observations and Analysis of Nonverbal Behavior

Taking video recordings of users interacting with computers is one of the oldest practices in HCI. The data include using video to code gestures, body language as well as verbal language. Data are analyzed using methods, such as protocol analysis (verbal or non-verbal), cognitive task analysis and discourse analysis, or coding of user actions (Drachen & Heide-Smith, 2008; Fisher & Sanderson, 1996). The major drawback of such approach is the time commitment required for coding of gestures, verbal communication, body language as indicators of user experience and emotion. This coding process also places substantial emphasis on the skill of the researcher in coding the data correctly. Personal bias and inter-rater reliability are typical problems that need addressing. The time commitment is substantial, with the analysis of the recorded material taking up to 100 times the period of time actually recorded (Fisher & Sanderson, 1996). The issues and challenges related to objective analysis of observational data has been a major factor in the popularity of self-report, subjective data in the study of user-computer interaction. Current work on automated coding and logging of user-initiated events in virtual environments may assist in bridging the gap between self-report and objective data (Drachen et al., 2009; Kim et al., 2008).

While there are many methods that have been explored in previous work for measuring emotions and affect, there are pros and cons to each one. In the case studies we outline in this chapter, we decided to use more objective methods, and thus we chose physiological sensors. Due to this decision, our studies only discuss arousal rather than simple or complex emotions. Thus, we will only show how the design methods discussed in section 3 were used to stimulate arousal. In the future, we would like to address the measurement of simple and complex emotions and valence as part of our studies.

TECHNIQUES TO ELICIT EMOTIONS

Developing a successful experience will depend on devising several patterns that evoke specific affective states from participants. This process is more of an art than a science. Designers, cinematographers, dramateurs, and directors use an amalgam of techniques and tricks to evoke emotions and deliver and emotionally effective experience. These techniques range from narrative-based techniques to cinematographic or visual patterns.

In his book, *The Visual Story*, Bruce Block (Block, 2001) discusses many techniques that rely on the use of color features, such as contrast and affinity of color in terms of its warmth or coolness, saturation, and brightness. He discusses how cinematographers can, through carefully changing these properties in time, increase or decrease arousal. In addition, film theory documents the use of several color-based techniques to increase dramatic tension and evoke emotional responses from the audience (Birn, 2000; Block, 2001; Calahan, 1996; Thomas & Johnston, 1981; Thompson, 2001). For example, the use of high contrast scenes, as seen in Film Noir movies, was used to increase tension and arousal. These

techniques are quite similarly used within visual interactive environments. For example, one can see the interplay between contrast and color within *Bioshock* (2K Games, 2007) and *Assassin's Creed* (Ubisoft, 2007).

Within an interactive experience, the plot structure, characters, and pacing also play an important role in evoking and sustaining emotions in the immersed players. Writer and game expert David Freeman (Freeman, 2003) discusses different narrative and writing techniques – developing plot and character – as a way of enhancing participants' emotional experience within interactive entertainment products.

In this section we will give examples of artistic design and narrative techniques used in eliciting emotions within entertainment experiences, most, if not all, work within interactive products as well. Visual aesthetics and design, narrative, environment design, reward systems, identification with the character, use of symbols, agency, engagement and fun, are all tools used to elicit and intensify the dramatic experience. A discussion of all of these techniques is beyond the scope of this chapter, but we cover examples of many basic methods here.

Color and Lighting

As outlined in many film books, movies use several color and lighting techniques to create a desired effect based on the director's style (Birn, 2000; Block, 2001; Brown, 1996; Calahan, 1996; Crowther, 1989; Gillette, 1998; Knopf, 1979; Knoph, 1979; Thompson, 2001). In this section, we will discuss several color patterns that we formulated based on a qualitative study of over thirty movies, including *The Cook, The Thief, His Wife and Her Lover* (1989), *Equilibrium* (2002), *Shakespeare in Love* (1998), *Citizen Kane* (1941), and *The Matrix* (1999). According to our study, the techniques used can be divided into shot-based color techniques: color techniques used in one shot, and scene-based color techniques: techniques used on a sequence of shots.

An example shot-based color technique is the use of high brightness contrast in one shot. High brightness contrast denotes high difference between brightness in one or two areas in the scene and the rest of the scene. This effect is not new; it was used in paintings during the Baroque era and was termed Chiaroscuro— an Italian word meaning light and dark. This kind of composition has also been used in many movies to increase arousal. Perhaps the most well known examples of movies that use this kind of effect are film noir movies, e.g. *Citizen Kane* (1941), *The Shanghai Gesture* (1941), *This Gun For Hire* (1942). Another variation on this technique is contrast between warm and cool colors, which can be seen in many Color Noir movies. These kinds of patterns are usually used in peak moments in an experience, such as a turning point. Lower contrast compositions usually precede these heightened shots, thus developing another form of contrast, contrast between shots.

In addition to color and brightness contrast, filmmakers have also used affinity of color to elicit emotional responses (Birn, 2000; Block, 2001; Brown, 1996; Calahan, 1996; Crowther, 1989; Gillette, 1998; Knopf, 1979; Thompson, 2001). Movies, such as *The Cook, The Thief, His Wife, and Her Lover* sustain an affinity of highly saturated warm colors for a period of time. The temporal factor is key to the effect of this approach; this is due to the nature of the eye. The eye tries to balance the projected color to achieve white color. Hence, when projected with red color, the eye tries to compensate the red with cyan to achieve white color. This causes eye fatigue, which in turn affects participant's stress level, thus affecting arousal. This technique can also be seen in games, such as *Devil May Cry*.

In contrast, designers have used de-saturated colors to project low energy scenes, thus decreasing arousal. For example, *Equilibrium* (2002) and *The English Patient* (1996) both use low saturation cool colors to increase detachment and decrease arousal.

Of course the perception of contrast, saturation, and warmth of color of any shot within a continuous movie depends on colors used in the preceding shots. Several movies used contrast between shots to evoke emotions (Alton, 1995; Block, 2001). For instance, filmmakers have used warm saturated colors in one shot then cool saturated colors in the other, thus forming a warm/cool contrast between shots to affect arousal (in this case decrease arousal). By graphically analyzing the movie, *The Cook, The Thief, His Wife, and Her Lover*, we can visualize these techniques. We can then graphically plot the frequency of pixels against color properties (saturation, warmth, and brightness) over the individual frames making up this section of the movie.

Figure 2-a illustrates color dropping from high saturation to low saturation as time progresses. As shown the drop is significant (more than 40% of the saturation value), which shows a high saturation contrast between shots. Similarly, Figures 2-b and 2-c show brightness contrast (shift from low brightness color to high brightness), and warmth contrast (shift from high warmth to low warmth) over time. This sequence tends to decrease arousal. While moving from less saturated to more saturated or cool to warm or bright to dark, seems to escalate arousal. After reviewing other movies, we deduced that the change of contrast over time should affect arousal linearly.

Thus, there are established patterns that designers use to manipulate color and lighting to stimulate emotions. These patterns constitute the use of contrast and affinity of colors within one shot or through a series of shots. These patterns can be seen in many movies and interactive experiences, including games, virtual rides, etc. One of the case studies discussed below will further evaluate these patterns and explore if arousal was stimulated through contrast and affinity through time.

Environment Design

Environment design is another element that designers extensively use to layout the space and emotional experience for their participants.

Figure 2. Saturation, brightness, and warmth over time

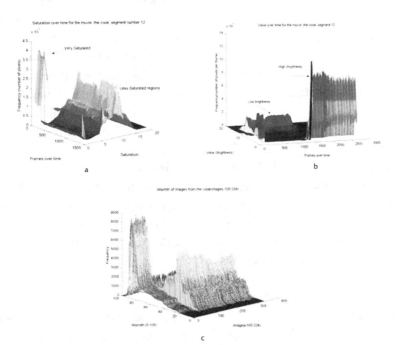

Through the placements of objects, shape and materials of the space, and environmental lighting, designers can create rich atmospheres that elicit desired emotional responses. Architects, for example, often increase the amount of light coming into a space or a building (through windows or skylights), or extend the height of a ceiling (through vaults) to establish a sense of openness, airiness and expansive space (Fitchen, 1961; Millet, 1996). Elements within an environment are also selected and placed to evoke specific responses, whether those objects and furnishings are of a medieval castle or a 1960s modern dining room. The chosen elements evoke certain associations and feelings, based in part, on our knowledge and previous experiences with those items. While people's experience are widely varied, it is safe to assume that a Victorian parlor replete with knick-knacks, ornaments, beaded cushions and flowery fabrics will have a very different impact on a person than the frugal elegance of a Zen garden.

Narrative

There are numerous theories and techniques published on narrative and its influence on emotions within different media. Experiments on using film to induce emotions have found that there are certain emotions that can be evoked through films. For example, Gross and Levenson found that they can successfully elicit amusement, disgust, and sadness, but it was harder to elicit anger, contentment, and fear. They found that contentment films elicit high degree of happiness, while anger films elicit other emotions like disgust, and fear films elicit tension and interest (Gross and Levenson, 1995). Thus, there is no question that films can elicit emotions and affect. However, the question is how filmmakers, and consequently game and interactive narrative designers, can make use of these theories and techniques to embed emotions in their designs.

In this section, we describe tacit knowledge collected through years of training in acting, directing, screenwriting, and animation, particularly, Joseph Campbell's (J. Campbell, 1972) and Propp's (Propp, Wagner, & Scott, 1968) work on storytelling, and Boal's on acting theories (Boal, 1979, 2002).

Plot Structure and Magnitude

Aristotle defined quality of plot using five basic principles: completeness, magnitude, unity, structure, and universality (Aristotle, 1967). He defined the structure of a plot as the order of events in time, where each event constitutes an important part of the plot, and which, if removed cause the plot to lose its meaning. He also identified several plot components, including events leading to astonishment, recognition, reversal (twist), or suffering. In this section we focus on plot structure and magnitude.

The order of events and their dramatic progression in time are important factors affecting plot quality (Baid, 1973). Dramatic tension in a typical film or a play escalates through time until it reaches a peak (the crisis point) after which it is released. The shape of dramatic tension through time can be visualized as an arc, and thus called the Dramatic Arc (Baid, 1973; Styan, 1960). This relationship is non-monotonic, however. As Benedetti describes, a play is composed of scenes and scenes are composed of beats (the word beat here defines the smallest unit of action that has its own complete shape with a goal and an action), each has its own arc with a turning point where tension reaches its maximum point after which it is released (Benedetti, 1994). Therefore, one can imagine the shape of drama as a nonlinear function with many local maxima points representing turning points in beats, but one global maximum point marking the crisis point of the performance. Choosing and ordering events to form this structure define the quality of a plot.

Another factor that is used to evoke emotions is the amount of time spent within each event (such as the pauses), which Aristotle calls Magnitude (Aristotle, 1967). To illustrate this concept

consider a scene where a character opens a door leading to an unknown place. One way to animate this scene is to show the character opening the door and walking in. As an alternative way is to show the character as he slowly reaches for the door, gradually opens it and then hesitantly walks in. Slowing the pace of the scene, in this way creates a different dramatic quality to the scene. Therefore, orchestrating the pacing and magnitude of each event is as important to engagement as plot structure. These techniques are already explored in many game narratives. Examples include *Prince Persia IV* (Ubisoft, 2009), *Assassin's Creed* (Ubisoft, 2007).

Ticking Clock

The concept of the ticking clock has been used as a dramatic device in many productions. Dramatists use dialogue, visual, and audio events to project possible future events. For example, in the movie the *Saw* (2004) a killer traps two people in a room and gives them until 6:00p to find a way out. The director interjected shots of the ticking clock at various points during the movie to create an anticipation of a death event. This dramatic instrument is very effective at creating anticipation, one form of pleasure (Blythe & Hassenzahl, 2004) as noted earlier. Examples of this instrument can be seen in *Nick of Time* (1995) and *Ninth Gate* (1999).

Character Arc

Boorstin (Boorstin, 1990) describes the vicarious eye with which the audience identifies emotionally with a character and his actions. Freeman defines a method which screenwriters use to illicit this type of engagement, called Character Arc (Freeman, 2003), which is a method of defining character's growth through time. An example is the birth of the hero as described by Joseph Campbell (D. Campbell, 1999), where a character struggles and reluctantly becomes the hero in the middle or end of the story.

There are more techniques that artists use including the use of audio, infrasound, scent, biofeedback, and haptics which can not be discussed here due to space limitations.

CASE STUDIES

Case Study: Validating the Color and Lighting Techniques

To validate the effect of the patterns discussed above on arousal, we conducted several experiments testing each pattern individually within a 3D interactive environment. For this purpose we developed a simple interactive 3D environment. The environment is composed of six rooms where participants are only allowed to navigate through the environment, thus no object manipulation was required.

In this environment all walls and ceilings were designed with white texture to allow maximum control using colored light. In computer graphics, the final color of objects within a 3D scene is calculated by adding light color to the color of the texture. Since we want to control all the colors projected, we decided to use white textures for all textures used in the environment, thus all colors are determined by the light colors. For each room, we strategically placed eight lights to cover all surfaces of the room. We implemented

several algorithms that dynamically control the saturation, lightness, warmth, and contrast of these lights depending on the pattern used.

To validate if there was an influence on arousal with time, we monitored participant's physiological responses using the SenseWear® PRO$_2$ Armband, a wearable body monitor that enables continuous collection of low-level physiological factors. It includes several sensors that continuously gather heat flux, skin temperature, near body temperature, and galvanic skin response data from the body. However, it does not include a heart rate monitor. We used the Triax Elite (shown in Figure 3 (right)) for that purpose. It is composed of a stopwatch and a heart rate monitor strap that displays heart rate, current running pace, and pace target information for interval training. We were able to collect readings from these devices and feed it through MATLAB for further data analysis.

We ran 19 experiments, one experiment for each pattern identified. For each experiment we gathered readings from 20-24 participants. We asked participants to volunteer for more than one experiment if they can. If they signed up for more than one experiment, we asked that when they sign up for times to perform the experiment that experiments should be at least one week apart. We think a one week period is enough time to eliminate bias of prior exposure to one experiment on the results collected in the other experiment. Participants were male graduate and undergradu-

Figure 3. Typical data and playback screen from a portion of a participant's time in the interactive experience, DarkCon

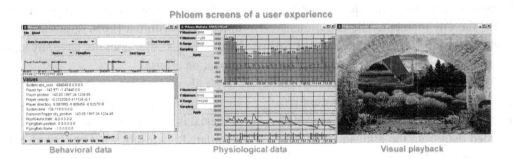

ate students between the ages of 18-30 from the Information Science and Technology, Electrical Engineering, and Computer Science departments of The Pennsylvania State University. Students were recruited from classes taught in Computer Science, Information Sciences and Technology and Electrical Engineering. We specifically targeted male students due to fluctuations on female hormonal state which may affect arousal, and thus interfere with the results.

All nineteen experiments followed the same procedure. In accordance to IRB regulations, before they started the experiment, participants were given consent forms and a brief introduction of the entire experiment. We also asked them to take a color blindness test, to check if they can differentiate between colors. Once they are done with the test, participants were asked to wear the *BodyMedia* device around their arm and the heart rate device around their chest. They were then asked to navigate within a 3D environment that does not exhibit any of the patterns depicted above. This was done to allow them to relax and get acquainted with the controls and the environment.

After one-two minutes of interacting within this environment, we asked them to navigate through a similar environment, but where we embedded the algorithm recreating one of the patterns discussed above. We simultaneously recorded their physiological measures while they navigated and interacted within the environment. After navigating through the environment the participants were asked to fill out a questionnaire which was used as a self report. This procedure was repeated for all the patterns discussed above. We used a different pool of people for each pattern to alleviate the bias of knowing the environment. The experiments were conducted over a period of three weeks.

The response data from the armband i.e. the EDA, HF and body temperature for each input parameter (i.e. the color pattern of saturation, warmth, lightness and contrast) was recorded. This recorded data from the armband, the heart rate monitor, and the time stamp from which the participant started viewing the environment was matched. The response data was normalized by subtracting the mean of the EDA, Heat Flux and Temperature for each participant from the raw data.

Assuming the physiological parameters have a linear response to the color pattern, we used a linear prediction models discussed in more detail in the appendix. This approach can be used to test the hypothesis of whether individual visual parameters affect physiological response variables. If the mean-squared error on a test set is size-ably smaller than the variance of the output sequence for some amount of delay/ latency between the causal inputs and the target output, it indicates that there exists a linear correlation between the two sequences. If it is not then a linear correlation doesn't exist. Using this method, we can deduce with some confidence that there is a linear relationship between the participants' arousal and the pattern used.

We ran subjects through 6 environments set up with high saturation with 6 different colors (red, green, yellow, orange, blue, and cyan). The hypothesis is that arousal will increase as a function of time within a high saturated environment. Results shown confirm this result. Specifically, results for the high saturated red environment are depicted in Table 2 for EDA, HF, and body temperature; similar results were found for other colors tested. As shown in the table the variances of the color patterns were more than the error test values, this indicates that there is a linear correlation between the expected response (linear increase in arousal through time) and the physiological response. The low error rate also indicates that all participants had the same reaction, an increase in arousal as time passes within a 100% saturation. As shown by the results color does not have any significant impact on arousal.

We also tested this environment with linearly changing saturation from 0% to 100%. The hypothesis is that arousal will also be linearly stimulated as a result. We tested it with 6 different environments with different colors. The data

Table 2. Physiological Data Analysis of Red Environment

		GSR	Heat Flux	Temperature
Red	Variance	2.40E-04	6.963	0.0207
	Error Test	7.19E-05	4.1778	0.0124

Table 3. Physiological Data Analysis

		GSR	Heat Flux	Temperature
Red	Variance	1.94E-04	2.1555	0.0070
	Error Test	1.79E-04	2.7814	0.0006

analysis results are shown in Table 3. Similar to the results above, the low error rate indicates that participants all went through the same experience. The variance is more than the error which indicates a linear co-relation between the physiological reaction and the change in saturation, which validates our hypothesis.

We ran another experiment to validate the pattern that arousal will increase within an increase of brightness over time. The data analysis results are shown in Table 4. The low error rate show that participants all went through the same experience. The variance is more than the error which indicates a linear co-relation between the physiological reaction and the change in lightness, which validates our hypothesis.

We ran another experiment to explore the relationship between arousal and change in contrast. We setup the environment with all lights set to white color. We then adjusted the lightness of lights in the corners to create local contrast. Contrast here is measured as the difference in lightness between the lights in the center of the room and the ones in the back and around the corner of the room. We varied the contrast from low, moderate, to high contrast and then from high to medium to low. The data analysis results are shown in Table 5. These results show that participants all went through the same experience. The variance is more than the error which indicates a linear co-relation between the physiological reaction and the change in contrast, which validates our hypothesis.

These experiments and results validate the relationship between arousal increase/decrease as a result of manipulation of lighting and texture colors over time. However, we did not attempt to deduce valence component of emotions within this experiment. An interesting future direction is to explore the relationship between these patterns and valence or emotions. We anticipate that these patterns will have specific influence on arousal and valence but may not induce specific emotional states, still, this needs to be validated.

Table 4. Physiological Data Analysis

		GSR	Heat Flux	Temperature
Lightness	Variance	8.47E-05	7.9099	0.0279
	Error Test	2.74E-05	4.5431	0.0021

Table 5. Physiological Data Analysis

		GSR	**Heat Flux**	**Temperature**
change in	Variance	3.79E-05	5.4548	0.0023
Contrast	Error Test	1.91E-05	3.2385	0.00033

Case Study: The SEE Project's DarkCon Scenario

Following the design concepts discussed above, we present a project, The Sensory Environments Evaluation (SEE) project (2003-2005), as a case study. The SEE project was undertaken with the purpose of developing techniques that could evoke affective responses at specific moments of an interactive, game-like system from players of that game. In addition to developing an emotionally evoking interactive game-like experience, we also conducted a series of experiments to determine if the design patterns developed were effective (i.e. were correlated to the arousal states of the participants during the interactive experience). Results showed high correlations between design patterns developed and emotional responses desired. In this section, we will discuss the design patterns and experiments conducted referencing design techniques and experimental designs and analysis methods discussed above, when appropriate. The details of the experiments themselves are beyond the scope of this chapter; interested readers are referred to (J. F. Morie, Tortell, & Williams, 2007) for more details.

Since the sponsor of the SEE project was the United States Army Research Office, we developed a military, albeit game-like scenario. We built a fully immersive, old-style virtual reality recon mission, which we called *DarkCon*, as it took place at night. The player's 'mission' was to determine if abandoned buildings in an area of Eastern Europe were inhabited by refugees or paramilitary forces. The ostensible goal was to drop a signaling device at the location if the recon

scout, the player, could confirm through observation, that the "rebels" were holding this area.

For this project, we developed an emotionally evocative space through the use of many sensory modalities, including not only visual and audio, as discussed above, but also a device that makes use of the sense of smell, which is a well known evocateur of emotional response (Proust, 1971). The device provided four distinct odors to be released throughout the scenario, to which we assigned a valence (fresh odors were positive, unpleasant ones negative). We also used a head-mounted display (HMD), full three-dimensional spatialized (surround) sound, and kinesthetic inputs through a custom-designed infrasound floor (with ten subsonic transducers). All these modalities served to create an extremely immersive experience that in effect, isolated the participant from the external everyday world, allowing them to be fully engaged within the virtual space and its series of intense and changing emotions.

Sensory modalities are the main techniques used in SEE to stimulate emotions. Although we discussed above several techniques, including narrative, these were not part of our design. In fact, there was no narrative, per se, in the *Dark-Con* scenario except the journey and choices the participant chooses to make. There were also no developed characters in this particular experience. The only people encountered are rebels who can spot you and kill you with no interaction. Thus, our discussion in this section will be constrained to the sensory stimulation design patterns developed within this project and their influence on evoking desired emotions or arousal states.

DarkCon's Use of Sensory Patterns to Evoke Emotions

The *DarkCon* environment is rich with both perceptual and emotional affordances. For example, the culvert in which the journey begins is dark, confined and claustrophobic. It is filled with strange, unidentifiable sounds. The floor of the culvert has detritus: shoes in the mud, flotsam and jetsam deposited by flood waters, a suitcase here, an abandoned photo album there. An abandoned baby doll squeaks if it is stepped on. These objects evoke speculations of who was here and might have left these things. Small creatures hide in the dark and their sounds, along with deep rumbles from the trucks passing overhead, add to the sense of unease. A flickering red light in the dark space corresponds to an intermittent electrical sizzling sound, coupled with a deep rhythmic mechanical sound of a generator housed within an alcove. The red light, its irregular flashing, and the deep sounds combine to create a sinister feeling. All these objects were very strategically placed within the environment to evoke emotions. Thus, we will call this design choice as *environment design*, see section 3, whereby a designer places specific objects, lights, and sounds to stimulate emotions while participants walk through the space. This type of design has been used in many games and interactive experiences, such as the Horror House experience in Universal Studios.

Another method we used in *DarkCon* to heighten arousal states involved the use of a custom-built infrasound floor. This 12 x 16 foot floor had ten subsonic transducers placed at intervals underneath. Audio frequencies between 4 and 20 hertz (below the threshold of normal hearing) could be sent to the transducers (speakers) in the floor, producing not so much a sound, as a sensation, often subliminal. This resulted in a more kinesthetic response. We increased the level (decibel) to heighten the emotional response being experienced, and lessened it to the point of no infrasound to produce a calmer state by contrast.

This 'emotional score' pervaded the entire experience, much like a soundtrack in a film. Both the infrasound and the spatialized audio incorporated techniques such as entrainment (synching the user's heartbeat up to specific rhythms) and the modulations of low frequency sounds (to intensify or mediate the participant's arousal state).

Perceptual cues such as loud sounds and flashing lights served to attract the subject's gaze towards an important event in the landscape, so it was noticed. There were also startle mechanisms (Fencott's shocks) in the scenario such as when the participant walks under a bat colony living in the culvert, disturbing them so that they fly abruptly and loudly off through the darkness.

As the participant makes his way through the culvert, rats scatter and trucks passing on the road overhead cause rocks to jostle and tumble off the ancient stone walls. Just before the exit, hissing pipes are juxtaposed with a blood-stained wall, and if one looks carefully, bullet casings can be seen littered in the muddy floor.

Contrast in the environment design and use of audio and visuals is important as noted in the lighting case study above. Outside the culvert all is calm (the infrasound score cuts off here), and the fresh smell of a riverbank is evident (a contrast to the fetid, muddy odors within the tunnel). A full moon is rising, illuminating the countryside, so one can see the complex of old buildings across the river. But a jeep and a truck cross the bridge over the river, carrying cargo. There is a real danger of being seen. There is only one place that can give the scout cover – an overturned rusty car, half buried in the mud at the edge of the river. From this vantage point it is obvious to the careful observer that a sentinel with a high-powered rifle is stationed on the roof of the largest building, watching the countryside, and the tension starts to rise again. Staying hidden, the scout can also see a man in the barbed wire encased compound, grinding the surface of a military vehicle. Sounds of a radio and loud arguing emanates from the building. Now it is apparent that this is a rebel hideout and it is up to you, as the scout, to drop the signaling device near the building to call in an airstrike. This is where another emotional affordance comes into play: the sound of a heartbeat, increasing in tempo. This sets up the phenomenon of entrainment, whereby one's own heartbeat ends to synchronize with what is heard, again increasing tension. The heartbeat and the infrasound score ramp up, rising to a crescendo as the sentinel or the grinder sees you and dogs come snarling out at you, chains rattling.

At the start of the design process, we determined which types and degrees of emotional response we want to include, and where those need to occur. We then orchestrated multi-modal sensory stimuli, using the design concepts and emotion inducing techniques such as those described here and the previous section. Visual design, including lighting, color and contrast are extensively employed. Audio design is paramount to setting the mood, and enhancing the visual schemas. This, coupled with a secondary technique of coercive narrative that helps steer the actions and behavior of a player within the environment, makes possible predictable patterns of emotional response within the game experience.

Evaluating the Stimulated Arousals Through the Embedded Design Patterns

Studies where the subject self report emotional response via surveys or other instruments tend to be much less reliable and direct that in situ measurements. Therefore, to aid in determining whether our design approach really elicited strong responses, participants were outfitted with two physiological measurements: skin conductance (EDA) and a standard EKG module, provided through (initially) a BioRadio wireless device, and later via a BioPack system[1]. Real time monitoring of these systems allowed us to see the intensities of arousal states experienced by the players during their session. We were also able to playback a full

recording of what they saw and heard throughout the experience with a concurrent display of the physiological signals. A typical screen from this playback and monitoring system, called Phloem, shown in Figure 3.

This process permitted us to also annotate the biometric data, in preparation for final analysis, an example of which can be seen in the two images in Figure 4.

In addition, we used two questionnaires at the beginning and end of the session: the Immersive Tendencies Questionnaire (Witmer & Singer, 1998) and the Simulator Sickness Questionnaire (SSQ) (Kennedy, Lane, Berbaum, & Lilienthal, 1993) before entering the environment, and afterwards a modified Presence questionnaire (Witmer & Singer, 1998), along with a second SSQ test. The Immersive Tendencies, along with the Presence questionnaire provide a rough measurement of immersion or engagement. The Simulator Sickness test was necessary to ensure that any physical discomfort a participant experienced due to the simulator, or motion sickness, was excluded from the arousal data.

While we were unable, with our measurements, to determine the actual valence of the arousal states (with the exception of those tests that were done with specifically valenced smell triggers), we were able to confirm the exact moments in the game where these states happened, and they did correspond to the actual sections, events or encounters during the game where we designed them to occur.

It should be noted that the task was set up to be nearly impossible to complete successfully. When a participant was close enough to the abandoned building where there were many clues to indicate the rebels had control, he or she was always discovered, and either shot, set upon by dogs, or blown up by a landmine. This was done deliberately to cause an extreme state of heightened arousal- a flight or fight, panic-type situation in the player.

The *DarkCon* experiments for the SEE Project provided valuable information that supported the

Figure 4. Annotated arousal data from a DarkCon experience showing peaks and troughs both inside the culvert (above) and outside (below)

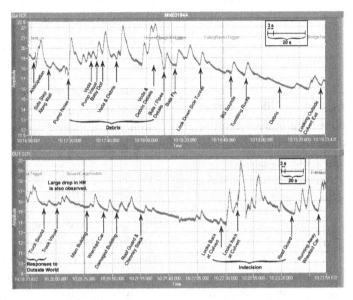

validity of our design approach to eliciting emotions in an interactive game-like experience. We assumed that most of these arousal states were of negative valence, as that was the purpose of most of the sensory stimuli utilized in the scenario. It can be seen from the sample annotated data sheets shown in Figure 4, that peaks tended to correspond to the designed triggers. Two moments where the arousal state eased were at the exit from the culvert, designed to be a calmer area with a running stream and relative quiet after the tunnel, and when the scout was hidden behind a wrecked car, 'safely' observing the situation around him.

The amount of data derived from the biometric measurement device was extensive and a challenge to process. It was subject to a great deal of noise from the participant being able to move about over the extent of the infrasound floor in the traditional virtual reality mode in which this environment was implemented. So, while this modality allowed us much more flexibility in creating techniques to elicit emotional responses, it was more difficult to both process and analyze. Nonetheless, this work can be seen as an interesting effort to both

design and measure emotions within interactive experiences.

CONCLUSION

In this book chapter we discussed several methods that artists use in various interactive and non-interactive media to elicit emotions from the audience to provide the audience with an emotionally rich experience. We believe these techniques are very important, but what is more important is understanding their use and validating them scientifically. This book chapter discussed various techniques for assessing and measuring users' emotions while playing or participating within an interactive experience. We discussed two case studies that attempt to embed several artistic design techniques to evoke emotions and validate these techniques through objective measurements of arousal. This chapter starts to scratch the surface on what we believe as an important area of understanding emotional affordances as tools for developing more engaging emotionally rich interactive experiences. We believe more studies as the ones discussed here is needed to move this field forward.

REFERENCES

Aftanas, L., & Golocheikine, S. A. (2001). Human anterior and frontal midline theta and lower alpha reflect emotionally positive state and internalized attention: high-resolution EEG investigation of meditation. *Neuroscience Letters*, *310*(1), 57–60. doi:10.1016/S0304-3940(01)02094-8

Alton, J. (1995). *Painting with Light*. Berkeley: University of California Press.

Anttonen, J., & Surakka, V. (2005). *Emotions and heart rate while sitting on a chair.* Paper presented at the CHI '05: Proceedings of the SIGCHI conference on Human factors in computing systems.

Aristotle,. (1967). *Poetics* (Else, G. F., Trans.). Ann Arbor: University of Michigan Press.

Baid, C. E. (1973). *Drama*. New York: W. W. Norton & Company.

Benedetti, R. (1994). *Actor at Work* (6th ed.). Englewood Cliffs, NJ: Prentice-Hall.

Birn, J. (Ed.). (2000). *Digital Lighting & Rendering*. Indianapolis: New Riders.

Block, B. (2001). *The Visual Story: Seeing the Structure of Film, TV, and New Media*. New York: Focal Press.

Blythe, M. A., & Hassenzahl, M. (2004). The Semantics of Fun: Differentiating Enjoyable Experiences. In Blythe, M. A., Overbeeke, K., Monk, A. F., & Wright, P. C. (Eds.), *Funology: From Usability to Enjoyment (Human-Computer Interaction Series)*. MA: Kulwer Academic Publishers.

Boal, A. (1979). *Theatre of the Oppressed*. New York, NY: Urizen Books.

Boal, A. (2002). *Games for Actors and Non-Actors* (2 ed.). London: Routledge.

Boorstin, J. (1990). *Making Movies Work: Thinking Like a Filmmaker*. LA, CA: Silman-James Press.

Bornstein, R. F. (1992). Perception without Awareness: Retrospect and Prospect. In *Perception without Awareness: Cognitive, Clinical and Social Perspectives*. New York, New York: BoGuilford.

Boucsein, W. (1992). *Electrodermal Activity*. New York: Plenum Press.

Bradley, M. M., & Lang, P. J. (2007). Emotion and motivation. In Cacioppo, J. T., Tassinary, L. G., & Berntson, G. G. (Eds.), *Handbook of Psychphysiology*. New York, NY: Cambridge University Press. doi:10.1017/CBO9780511546396.025

Brown, B. (1996). *Motion Picture and Video Lighting*. Boston: Focal Press.

Cabeza, R., & Nyberg, L. (2000). Imaging cognition II: An empirical review of 275 PET and fMRI studies. *Journal of Cognitive Neuroscience*, *12*(1). doi:10.1162/08989290051137585

Cacioppo, J. T., Tassinary, L. G., & Berntson, G. G. (2007). *Handbook of Psychophysiology* (3rd ed.). Cambridge University Press. doi:10.1017/CBO9780511546396

Calahan, S. (1996). *Storytelling through lighting: a computer graphics perspective.* Paper presented at the Siggraph Course Notes.

Campbell, D. (1999). *Technical Theatre for Nontechnical People*. New York City, NY: Allworth Press.

Campbell, J. (1972). *The Hero with a Thousand Faces*. New Jersey: Princeton University Press.

Crowther, B. (1989). *Film Noir: Reflections in a Dark Mirror*. New York: Continuum.

Desmet, P. M. A. (2003). Measuring emotion; development and application of an instrument to measure emotional responses to products. In Blythe, M. A., Overbeeke, K., Monk, A. F., & Wright, P. C. (Eds.), *Funology: from usability to enjoyment.* Dordrecht, Boston, London: Kluwer Academic Publishers.

Drachen, A., Canossa, A., & Yannakakis, G. (2009). *Player Modeling using Self-Organization in Tomb Raider: Underworld.* Paper presented at the IEEE Computational Intelligence in Games (CIG).

Drachen, A., & Heide-Smith, J. (2008). Player Talk - The functions of communication in multiplayer Role Playing Games - Players and Media. *ACM Computers in Entertainment, 6*(3).

Duchowski, A. T. (2007). *Eye tracking methodology: Theory and practice* (Second ed. ed.). Berlin: Springer.

Ekman, P. (1992). An argument for basic emotions. *Cognition and Emotion, 6*(3/4), 169–200. doi:10.1080/02699939208411068

Fencott, C. (1999). *Content and Creativity in Virtual Environment Design.* Paper presented at the 5th International Conference on Virtual Systems and Multimedia.

Fisher, C., & Sanderson, P. (1996). Exploratory Data Analysis: Exploring Continuous Observational Data. *Interaction, 3,* 25–34. doi:10.1145/227181.227185

Fitchen, J. (1961). *The Construction of Gothic Cathedrals: A Study of Medieval Vault Erection.* Oxford: Oxford University Press.

Freeman, D. (2003). *Creating Emotions in Games.* IN: New Riders.

Fridlund, A. J., & Cacioppo, J. T. (1986). Guidelines for human electromyographic research. *Psychophysiology, 23,* 567–589. doi:10.1111/j.1469-8986.1986.tb00676.x

Gibson, E. J., & Walk, R. D. (1960). The "Visual Cliff". *Scientific American, 202,* 67–71.

Gibson, J. J. (1979). *The Ecological Approach to Visual Perception.* New York, New York: Houghton Mifflin.

Gillette, J. M. (1998). *Designing with Light* (3rd ed.). Mountain View, CA: Mayfield.

Grodal, T. (2000). Video games and the pleasures of control. In I. Mahwah (Ed.), *D. Zillmann & P. Vorderer (Eds.), Media entertainment: The psychology of its appeal.* NJ: Lawrence Erlbaum Associates.

Hayes, M. H. (1996). *Statistical Digital Signal Processing and Modeling.* New York: Wiley.

Hirshfield, L. M., Solovey, E. T., Girouard, A., Kebinger, J., Jacob, R. J. K., Sassaroli, A., et al. (2009). *Brain measurement for usability testing and adaptive interfaces: an example of uncovering syntactic workload with functional near infrared spectroscopy.* Paper presented at the In Proceedings of the 27th international conference on Human factors in computing systems (CHI).

Holson, L. M. (2004, April 10). Out of Hollywood, rising fascination with video games. *The New York Times on the Web.*

IJsselsteijn, W. A., Poels, K., & de Kort, Y. A. W. (2008). *The game experience questionnaire: Development of a self-report measure to assess player experiences of digital games.* Eindhoven, The Netherlands: FUGA technical report, TU Eindhoven.

Isbister, K., & Schaffer, N. (2008). *Game Usability: Advancing the Player Experience.* Morgan Kaufmann.

Kennedy, R. S., Lane, N. E., Berbaum, K. S., & Lilienthal, M. G. (1993). Simulator sickness questionnaire: an enhanced method for quantifying simulator sickness. *The International Journal of Aviation Psychology, 3*(3), 203–220. doi:10.1207/s15327108ijap0303_3

Kim, J. H., Gunn, D. V., Schuh, E., Phillips, B., Pagulayan, R. J., & Wixon, D. (2008). *Tracking real-time user experience (true): a comprehensive instrumentation solution for complex systems.* Paper presented at the Proceedings of twenty-sixth annual SIGCHI conference on Human factors in computing systems (CHI 2008).

Knopf, D. C. A. (1979). *The Book of Movie Photography.* London: Alfred Knopf, Inc.

Knoph, D. C. A. (1979). *The Book of Movie Photography.* London: Alfred Knopf.

Kuniavsky, M. (2003). *Observing the user experience. A practitioners guide to user research.* San Francisco: CA: Morgan Kauffman publishers.

Lagrange, M., Marchand, S., Raspaud, M., & Rault, J.-B. (2003). *Enhanced Partial Tracking Using Linear Prediction.* Paper presented at the DAFx, London.

Lang, P. J. (1995). The emotion probe: studies of motivation and attention. *The American Psychologist, 50,* 372–385. doi:10.1037/0003-066X.50.5.372

Lim, C. L., Rennie, C., Barry, R. J., Bahramali, H., & Lazzaro, I., manor, B., Gordon, E. (1997). Decompos-ing skin conductance into tonic and phasic measurements. *International Journal of Psychophysiology, 25*(2), 97–109. doi:10.1016/S0167-8760(96)00713-1

Mandryk, R. L., Atkins, S. M., & Inkpen, K. M. (2006). *A continious and objective evaluation of emotional experience with interactive play environments.* Paper presented at the CHI 2006.

Mandryk, R. L., & Inkpen, K. M. (2004). *Physiological indicators for the evaluation of co-located collaborative play.* Paper presented at the CSCW.

Marshall, C., & Rossman, G. B. (1999). *Designing Qualitative Research.* Thousand Oaks, CA: Sage.

Mathiak, K., & Weber, R. (2006). Toward brain correlates of natural behavior: fmri during violent video games. *Human Brain Mapping, 27*(12), 948–956. doi:10.1002/hbm.20234

Medlock, M., Wixon, D., Terrano, M., Romero, R. L., & Fulton, B. (2002). *Using the rite method to improve products: A definition and a case study.* Paper presented at the Proceedings of UPA Conference.

Meehan, M., Insko, B., Whitton, M., & Brooks, F. P. J. (2002). Physiological Measures of Presence in Stressful Virtual Environments. *ACM Transactions on Graphics, 21*(3), 645–652. doi:10.1145/566570.566630

Merkx, P. A. B., Truong, K. P., & Neerincx, M. A. (2007). *Inducing and measuring emotion through a multiplayer first-person shooter computer game.* Paper presented at the Proceedings of the Computer Games Workshop 2007.

Millet, M. S. (1996). *Light Revealing Architecture.* New York: Wiley.

Miltner, W. H. R., & Braun, C.Arnold. M., Witte, H., Taub, E. Coherence of gamma-band EEF activity as a basis for associative learning. *Nature, 397,* 434–436. doi:10.1038/17126

Morie, J., Iyer, K., Valanejad, K., Sadek, R., Miraglia, D., Milam, D., et al. (2003). *Sensory design for virtual environments.* Paper presented at the SIGGRAPH Conference 2003.

Morie, J. F., Tortell, R., & Williams, J. (2007). Would You Like To Play a Game? Experience and in Game-based Learning. In Perez, H. O. R. (Ed.), *Computer Games and Team and Individual Learning* (pp. 269–286). Oxford, UK: Elsevier Press.

Morie, J. F., Williams, J., Dozois, A., & Luigi, D.-P. (2005). The Fidelity of Feel: Emotional Affordance in Virtual Environments. *Proceedings of the 11th International Conference on Human-Computer Interaction.*

Nacke, L., Lindley, C., & Stellmach, S. (2008). *Log who's playing: psychophysiological game analysis made easy through event logging.* Paper presented at the Proceedings of Fun and Games, Second International Conference.

Nacke, L. E. (2009). *Affective Ludology. Scientific Measurement of User Experience in Interactive Entertainment.* Sweden: Bleking Technical University.

Norman, D. A. (2004). *Emotional Design.* New York, NY: Basic Books.

O'Donnell, M., Creamer, M., Elliott, P., & Bryant, R. (2007). Tonic and Phasic Heart Rate as Predictors of Psttraumatic Stress Disorder. *Psychosomatic Medicine, 69*, 256–261. doi:10.1097/PSY.0b013e3180417d04

Oatley, K., Keltner, D., & Jenkins, J. M. (2006). *Understanding Emotions.* Wiley-Blackwell Publishers.

Pagulayan, R., Keeker, K., Wixon, D., Romero, R. L., & Fuller, T. (2003). User-centered design in games. In *The human-computer interaction handbook: fundamentals, evolving technologies and emerging applications.* L. Erlbaum Associates Inc.

Pfurtscheller, G., Zalaudek, K., & Neuper, C. (1998). Event-related beta synchronization after wrist, finger and thumb movement. *Electroencephalography and Clinical Neurophysiology, 109*, 154–160. doi:10.1016/S0924-980X(97)00070-2

Poels, K., Kort, Y. d., & IJsselsteijn, W. (2007). *It is always a lot of fun!: exploring dimensions of digital game experience using focus group methodology.* Proceedings of the 2007 conference on Future Play.

Propp, V., Wagner, L. A., & Scott, L. (1968). *Morphology of the Folktale (American Folklore Society Publications).* Austin, TX: University of Texas Press.

Proust, M. (1971). *The Past Recaptured* (Mayor, A., Trans.). New York: Random House.

Rani, P., Sims, J., Brackin, R., & Sarkar, N. (2002). Online Stress Detection using Psychophysiological Signal for Implicit Human - Robot Cooperation. *Robotica, 20*, 673–686. doi:10.1017/S0263574702004484

Ravaja, N. (2004). Contributions of psychophysiology to media research: Review and recommendations. *Media Psychology, 6*, 193–235. doi:10.1207/s1532785xmep0602_4

Ravaja, N., & Kivikangas, J. M. (2008). *Psychophysiology of digital game playing: The relationship of self-reported emotions with phasic physiological responses.* Paper presented at the Proceedings of Measuring Behavior 2008.

Ravaja, N., Saari, T., Salminen, M., Laarni, J., & Kallinen, K. (2006). Phasic emotional reactions to video game events: A psychophysiological investigation. *Media Psychology, 8*, 343–367. doi:10.1207/s1532785xmep0804_2

Ray, W. J., & Cole, H. (1985). EEG alpha activity reflects attentional demands, and beta activity reflects emotional and cognitive processes. *Science, 228*(4700), 750–752. doi:10.1126/science.3992243

Rowe, D. W., Sibert, J., & Irwin, D. (1998). *Heart Rate Variability: Indicator of User State as an Aid to Human - Computer Interaction.* Paper presented at the Conference on Human Factors in Computing Systems.

Russell, J. A. (1980). A circumplex model of affect. *Journal of Personality and Social Psychology, 39*(6), 1161–1178. doi:10.1037/h0077714

Sander, D., Grandjean, D., & Scherer, K. R. (2005). *A systems approach to appraisal mechanisms in emotion, Neural Networks.* Elsevier.

Sennersten, C. (2008). *Gameplay (3D Game Engine + Ray Tracing = Visual Attention through Eye Tracking)*. Blekinge Tekniska Högskola.

Stern, R. M., Ray, W. J., & Quigley, K. S. (2001). *Psychophysiological Recording*. New York: Oxford University Press.

Styan, J. L. (1960). *The Elements of Drama*. Cambridge: Cambridge University Press.

Thomas, F., & Johnston, O. (1981). *The Illusions of Life: Disney Animation*. New York: Abbeville Press Publishers.

Thompson, D. B. K. (2001). *Film Art: An Introduction* (6th ed.). New York: Mc Graw Hill.

Ward, R. D., & Marsden, P. H. (2003). Physiological responses to different WEB page designs. *International Journal of Human-Computer Studies*, *59*(1-2), 199–212. doi:10.1016/S1071-5819(03)00019-3

Witmer, B. G., & Singer, M. J. (1998). Measuring Presence in Virtual Environments: A Presence Questionnaire. *Presence (Cambridge, Mass.)*, *7*(3), 225–240. doi:10.1162/105474698565686

KEY TERMS AND DEFINITIONS

Affective Design: Designing to induce or evoke emotions or affect.

Interactive Environments: Environments where users interact with objects or entities within, e.g. games or 2D interfaces.

Visual Design: Design of visual details such as lighting, textures, or 3D architectures.

Narrative and 3D Environments: Plot and discourse of telling a story within a 3D environment

ENDNOTE

[1] The BioRadio is a wireless physiological monitoring device used for medical research. It is made by Cleveland Medical Devices, Chicago, IL. The BioPack physiological monitoring system consists of the base module MP150, to which multiple sensor modules can be connected. It is from BioPack Systems, Goleta, CA.

APPENDIX

Linear Prediction Model

In the linear prediction (LP) model, also known as the autoregressive (AR) model, the current sample $x(n)$ is approximated by a linear combination of past samples of the input signal (Lagrange, Marchand, Raspaud, & Rault, 2003). We are looking for a vector a, of d coefficients, d being the order of the LP model. Provided that the a vector is estimated, the predicted value $\hat{x}$ is computed simply by FIR filtering of the p past samples with the coefficients using Equation:

$$\hat{x}(n) = \sum_{i=1}^{p} a_i x(n - i)$$

The main challenge in linear prediction modeling is to use an estimation method that suits the specific need. There are two methods: the autocorrelation method and covariance method. We used the co-variance method of the linear prediction model to estimate if there was a linear relation between the physiological response and expected response using the input pattern, such as change in saturation, warmth over time. As shown above, most patterns describe a linear relationship between color properties over time such as warmth, contrast, or saturation. Thus, we can use the linear prediction model to validate if such linear relationship exists by treating the color properties change over time as output and physiological responses of all participants as input. This will also validate if all participants shared the same response. For patterns that are not defined as a linear relationship between the color properties change over time and arousal, we defined an expected response and treated this as the function to test for linear co-relation.

The covariance method model for linear prediction uses the p order samples to train and design a filter to test predict the $p+1$ sample. The best designed filter would be the order for which we get minimum error. We calculate the mean square error from the difference between the predicted value and the given data value with this method.

We used the covariance method (Hayes, 1996) of least squares linear prediction to design a causal linear estimator for an output or target sequence based on an input (evocative) sequence. We can build an estimation filter using the response data recorded from the participants. The participants were divided into a test and a training set of equal number. The physiological response of the training set and the input color pattern are used to design a filter that is applied on the test set physiological response. The $p+1$ response of the test set is estimated and compared to the recorded $p+1$ value of the response.

Chapter 14
Bringing Affect to Human Computer Interaction

Mahir Akgün
Pennsylvania State University, USA

Göknur Kaplan Akıllı
Middle East Technical University, Turkey

Kürşat Çağıltay
Middle East Technical University, Turkey

ABSTRACT

The current chapter focuses on affective issues that impact the success of human computer interaction. Since everybody is a computer user now and interaction is not only a technical activity, users' affective processes cannot be ignored anymore. Therefore, the issues related to these affective processes that enable efficient, effective and satisfactory interaction with computers are explored. An extensive literature review is conducted and studies related with affective aspects of human computer interaction are synthesized. It is observed that there is a need to adapt computers to people and affect is an important aspect of this trend. Likewise, human characteristics have to be reflected to the interaction. The findings of this chapter are especially important for those people who are planning to bring affect into the computerized environments.

INTRODUCTION

As its name implies, Human Computer Interaction (HCI) deals with human physical and cognitive activities that are enacted during the interaction with computers. Even from the very beginning of its history, theories of HCI have been heavily influenced by those in cognitive psychology (Carroll, 1997; Hartson, 1998). Thus, it is not surprising to see that the combined influence from 1950s cognitive revolution and a focus on the individual differences with a neglect of social processes (Voss, Wiles, Carretero, 1995; Nussbaum, 2008) that reigned over cognitive psychology have found its reflections on HCI field. For instance, De Greef and Neerincx (1995) emphasize the significance of the properties such as users' cognitive limitation, ease of learning and cognitive cost of using a system for designing computer-based systems. Scaife and Rogers (1996) focus on the participants'

DOI: 10.4018/978-1-61692-892-6.ch014

ongoing cognitive processes, while interacting with graphical representations in computer-based systems. Papanikolaou et al. (2006) present an experimental study that aims to model the interaction on a web-based learning environment with regard to the cognitive styles, while in Cegarra and Hoc's (2006) study, the notion of cognitive styles is introduced upon establishing a balance between task requirements and cognitive resources in computer-assisted troubleshooting diagnosis. Dalal and Casper (1994) add concepts such as user satisfaction, user confidence and trust in the design to the notion of cognitive style as essential elements of the effectiveness of computer-based systems.

However, as Voss et al. (1995, p.174) indicated, the recent decade has witnessed the "sociocultural revolution" in psychology focusing on acquisition of intellectual skills through social interaction with a growing interest in the role of affective, social and organizational issues. Beside the increase in the number of the studies that are criticizing the lack of consideration of human affective processes in HCI, there has also been an outburst of studies investigating the psychology of emotion (Gross, 1999). Diaper (2004) criticizes the negligence to examine human affective processes in HCI inspired by psychology:

Notwithstanding the need in HCI to consider affective, social, organizational, and other such issues, most of the psychology in HCI and in current approaches to task analysis focuses on human cognition, and it is human cognition that is the main ingredient of user models in HCI. The point to recognize is that cognitive psychology of people is much more complicated than, for example, the information-processing abilities of computer systems and that this creates a fundamental problem for task analysis. If an analyst cannot understand the operation of a basic system component (such as the human element), then it is not impossible to predict how the various things

in a system will interact and produce the behavior of the system (p.21).

In line with Diaper's (2004) concern, Lisetti and Schiano (2000) emphasize the importance of affective states for many cognitive processes and further propose that questions such as "is the user satisfied, more confused, frustrated, or simply sleepy?" are indispensable for effective HCI designs. They add that

[w]hile making decisions, users are often influenced by their affective states: for example, reading a text while experiencing a negatively valenced emotional state often leads to a very different interpretation than reading the same text in a positive state. A computer interface aware of the user's current emotional state can tailor the textual information to maximize the user's understanding of the intended meaning of the text (Lisetti and Schiano, 2000, p.199).

Similarly, Norman (2004) emphasizes the importance of emotions for HCI and how cognition and emotions are intertwined, along with his regret for investigating only the cognitive aspect throughout years, despite his early identification of emotion as being one of the twelve challenges of cognitive science in the 1980s (Norman, 1980). He further contended that study of emotion is important, since it would likely to provide researchers with critical findings for the study of cognition. The designated critical role of wide range of emotions enacted on every computer-related, goal-directed activity is now better understood, whether it is as simple as sending an e-mail or more complicated as creating a three-dimensional computer-aided design model (Brave & Nass, 2008).

As this brief literature review revealed, there seems to be a major transformation in HCI, where there seems to be a convergence among theorists and researchers who argue the impossibility of having a thought or performing an action without the engagement of one's own emotional systems, or briefly, without emotion and affect (Izard 2007, 2009; Lewis, 2005; Phelps, 2006; Picard, 1997; Russell, 2003; Picard, 2010). In order to provide better understanding concerning the role of affect and emotions on cognitive processes from HCI perspective, the authors analyzed the existing literature to present emotions and the relationship between cognition and emotion as well as affect, which is followed by the conclusion comprising a humble set of suggestions for affective design and projections on the trends and future of the field.

EMOTIONS

Insomuch as William James asked the question of what emotion is in 1884, a vast number of different definitions for emotion had been produced (Kleinginna & Kleinginna, 1981; Larsen & Frederickson, 1999). Yet, the attempts to generate a widely acceptable definition of emotion have failed (Panksepp, 2003). Nevertheless, the idea that emotion is a reaction given to the actions driven by an individual's needs, goals, or concerns and that emotions have many aspects involving feelings, experience, physiology, behavior and cognition are generally accepted by most of the researchers (Ortony, Clore, & Collins, 1988; Brave & Nass, 2008; Izard, 2009). Izard (2009) defines two broad types of emotions, which are "basic emotions" such as joy, anger, disgust, etc. and "emotion schemas" such as shame, anxiety, etc., which are dynamic interactions of emotion with perceptual and cognitive processes to influence mind and behavior (p. 8). He claims that basic emotions can also be assumed as fundamental in the sense that "they are fundamental to human evolution, normative development, human mentality, and effective adaptation" (p. 8). Similar to Ortony, Clore and Collins' (1988) statement that while some emotions, (e.g. disgust), require much less cognitive processing, others involve much more (e.g. shame) cognitive processing; Izard (2009) agrees that emotion schemas involve higher-order

cognition and culture-related cognitive components (Tangney, Stuewig & Mashek, 2007), once the language acquisition occurs. Regardless of this difference in the levels of cognitive processing, emotions always involve some degree of cognition. Ekman (1999), who stresses the influence of emotions on thoughts, describes certain characteristics, which differentiate 'basic emotions' from other affective phenomena. One of these characteristics is 'distinctive universal signals' such as distinctive facial expressions. According to Ekman (1971, 1992) the existence of common facial expressions across cultures supports the notion of the universality of facial displays of emotions, which led him to propose six basic, universal emotions: surprise, anger, fear, disgust, sadness and enjoyment (Ekman 1993), which are referred to as primary emotions (Damasio, 1994).

On the contrary, Ortony, Clore and Collins (1988) refuse Ekman's proposal for a set of 'basic' emotions. According to them, there are more than six emotions, which are distinct and equally basic. They state that some emotions (e.g. fear, anger, sadness, and enjoyment) can be found in all cultures but this does not make them basic emotions similar to the fact that "toe nails might be found in all cultures too, but that would not be sufficient to render them anatomically basic" (Ortony, Clore, & Collins, 1988, p. 25). While they refuse the notion of six basic emotions, they support the idea that some emotions are more basic than others. The reason behind this idea is that "some emotions have less complex specifications and eliciting conditions than others." (Ortony, Clore, & Collins, 1988, p. 28). Eliciting conditions are specified in terms of variables, which can modulate the intensity of emotions, such as the global variables affecting all emotions and the local variables that influence a certain subset of emotions. Based on these variables, O'Rorke and Ortony (1994) provide the following emotion types (see Table 1).

Considered as activation mechanisms for emotions, appraisal processes help providing a cognitive framework for emotions (Ellsworth & Scherer, 2003). As Table 1 shows, where appraisal of an event leads to joy and distress, the appraisal of a prospective event results in hope, satisfaction, relief, fear and disappointment. Similarly, where appraisal of an object causes love and hate; appraisal of the agent's action leads to 'attribution emotions' such as pride, admiration, reproach and shame. While shame occurs when people disapprove of their own actions and at- tribute the negative effects of their actions to themselves, reproach occurs when people disapprove of others' actions and attribute the negative effects of the actions to others. Therefore, as Lazarus (1999) stated, cognitive appraisal processes play a key role in emotion. He further contends that although cognition, motivation and emotion are always associated and interdependent, within the trilogy of mind, there is a real difference between emotion and the other two functions,

Table 1. Emotion Types

Emotion Types		
Group	Specification	Types(name)
well-being	Appraisal of event	pleased (joy)
		displeased (distress)
Fortunes-of-others	Presumed value of an event affecting another	pleased about an event desirable for another (happy-for)
		pleased about an event undesirable for another (gloating)
		displeased about an event desirable for another (resentment)
		displeased about an event undesirable for another (sorry for)
Prospect-based	Appraisal of a prospective event	pleased about a prospective desirable event (hope)
		pleased about a confirmed desirable event (satisfaction)
		pleased about a disconfirmed undesirable event (relief)
		displeased about a confirmed undesirable event (fears-confirmed)
Attribution	Appraisal of an agent's action	approving of one's own action (pride)
		approving of another's action (admiration)
		disapproving of one's own action (shame)
		disapproving of another's action (reproach)
Attraction	Appraisal of an object	liking an appealing object (love)
		disliking an unappealing object (hate)
Well-being/ attribution	Compound emotions	admiration + joy -- gratitude
		reproach + distress -- anger
		pride + joy -- gratification
		shame + distress -- remorse

cognition and motivation: "Thought without motivation is emotionless" (p.10). Lazarus (1999) claims that thinking can occur without emotion, but emotion is not independent from meaning. In addition, emotion occurs after the previous emotional state in the continuous flow of cognitive, motivational and emotional processes. In other words, from Lazarus's point of view (1999), cognition is always involved in emotion.

On the other hand, Lewis and Granic (1999) claim that the relationship between cognition and emotion is not linear. The relationship begins with the interpretation of the event encountered, followed by the appraisal process, and the consequences of the evaluation process give rise to emotions. The emotions people have after the first appraisal leads to a new appraisal process and its consequences are enhanced by emotions, whereby emotions are continuously enhanced by changes in appraisal, which shows that the relation between cognition and emotion is a two-way causal relation. They further suggest that the increase in the number of appraisal chains evokes simultaneous coordination of cognitive and emotional processes, which means that cognitive and emotional processes become synchronized through a recursive loop. Briefly, Lewis and Granic (1999) assert that cognition and emotion are inseparable.

Attribution theory goes one-step beyond the appraisal theories of emotion. Appraisal theories propose that people evaluate whether or not they achieved the pre-determined goal as a first step. The interpretation of the performance leads to outcome-dependent emotions, which are classified as failure-dependent emotions (displeased and unhappy) and success-dependent emotions (satisfaction, happiness, and "feeling good"). As a second step, people make an attribution to the outcome, which triggers the attribution-dependent emotions. Attribution of a resulting failure to the ability makes people feel "incompetent," whereas attribution to "task difficulty" leads to the emotion of surprise. Finally, determining the dimension of the attribution gives rise to another kind of emotion. During the attribution process, cognitive processes are activated especially in the course of evaluating the performance and determining the dimension of the attribution. Figure 1 shows the cognitive (attributional) model of achievement behavior.

Another important concept where attribution and cognition meet in the same line is the concept of 'self'. The meaning of 'self' is very crucial in terms of cognition. In order to realize one's own action, to evaluate its consequences, and to attribute a responsibility of the action; an individual must be capable of owning his or her behavior (Lewis, 1999). Being capable of taking responsibility for behaviors requires self-evaluation, through which certain cognitive processes are enacted. The results of self-evaluation lead to emotions, the type of which depends on the direc-

Figure 1. The cognitive (attributional) model of achievement behavior (Reprinted from Försterling, 2001, p.119)

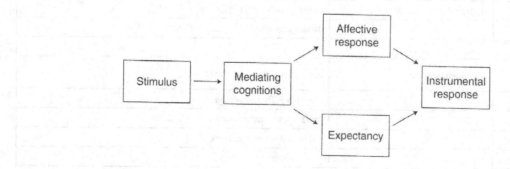

tion of the attribution. In line with O'Rorke and Ortony (1994)'s study, taking the responsibility for an action is an occasion of internally directed attribution, which, in turn, causes feelings of shame; whereas refusing to accept the responsibility is an occasion of externally directed attribution, which does not cause any feelings of shame.

Although emotions are often elicited with appraisal processes, Izard (2009) states that there are also other factors influencing emotions such as images, memories and thoughts, as well as noncognitive factors such as changes in neurotransmitters and levels of hormones (Izard, 1993). He further acknowledges that especially cognitive aspects of emotions are influenced by individual differences, learning, and social and cultural contexts (Izard, 2009, p. 9). This acknowledgment is important, since it is an indication of a possible compromise to one of the classic debates in emotion theory whether emotions are innate or learned. Along with Izard's previous studies (e.g. 1992), researches such as Neese (1990), Tooby and Cosmides (1990) and Ekman (1994) at the evolutionary side of this debate argue that all emotions, regardless of their complexity levels, are evolved in response to a specific environmental concern and inherited from our ancestors. On the other hand, theorists such as Averill (1980), Ortony and Turner (1990), Schweder (1994) and Wierzbicka (1992) argue that emotions are learned social constructs with a few exceptions that are considered as pre-emotions rather than emotions, which raises the probability of varying kinds of emotions across cultures transferred from generation to generation based on common social structures not on biology. However, recently these two sides might be finding a middle ground that there are different forms of emotions, such as basic emotions stemming from evolution and biology and more complex emotions involving various cognitive components that differ across individuals and cultures (Izard 2007, Panksepp 2007).

HUMAN-LIKE INTERFACES

Consistent with the purpose of HCI to create human-like computer interfaces enabling the transparent, seamless, and fluid interaction; users expect properties of human-human interaction (HHI) to be also valid for computer interfaces. Suchman (1987) mentions the term "sociability of computers" and points out that properties of HHI (e.g., dialogue, conversation, etc.) should be considered while describing the interaction between people and machines. Regarding this view, she stated "…the artifact should not only be intelligible to the user as a tool, but that it should be *intelligent* – that is, able to understand the actions of the user, and to provide for the rationality of its own. (p. 17)" Along the lines of this development in HCI, Lisetti and Schiano (2000) point out a conspicuous trend from 'adapting people to computers' to 'adapting computers to people' approach, which occurred in terms of interface design methods. The paradigm of utilizing design-centered approaches focusing on the efficiency of the interface without regarding the user profile shifted towards the use of user-centered approach concentrating on the users' characteristics in interface design. Furthermore, researchers and designers have long been discussing the appropriateness of reflecting human characteristics via the computer interface. Many studies have shown that people apply social rules regulating their interactions with other people to their interaction with machines and more specifically computers. For example, Fogg and Nass (1997) showed that users who received flattery from a computer perceived the interaction more enjoyable and had much greater interest for continuing working with the computer than those who received plain computer feedback. Klein, Moon and Picard (2002) echoed the same results.

Social Norms

Media equation research that employs the standpoint, where 'media equals to real life' is one of the important views, which shapes the human-like interfaces. The body of research focuses on social rules and norms, such as politeness, reciprocity, flattery and assignment of roles; price; and criticism (Reeves & Nass, 1996). This is in accord with the CASA paradigm that stands for "Computers Are Social Actors," which is coined by Nass, Steuer and Tauber (1994) based on their finding that people tend to treat computers as social actors. CASA studies demonstrate that the social rules and dynamics guiding human-human interactions are applied equally well to human-computer interaction. Nass, Steuer and Tauber (1994) showed that the nature of users' interactions with computers was indeed social and this was not because of a conscious belief that computers are human-like. It was because users treat computers as if they were human during their interaction despite their knowledge that computers have no human motivations such as feelings. Furthermore, Nass and Moon (2000) revealed that people tend to rely on social categories and apply social rules to computers unconsciously.

Social norms have important impact on both arousal of emotions and appropriateness of emotional expressions to a given situation (Shott, 1979). Studies investigating the role of apologies in interpersonal interaction offer important findings on the relation between politeness and emotions. While Brown and Levinson (1987) consider it as an act of negative politeness, Bharuthram (2003) regards an apology as an issue of social norms. For instance, when an agent performs a 'blameworthy' act, which causes her/his disapproval of the action afterwards; the feeling of shame (Ortony, Clore, & Collins, 1988) or regret for this undesirable event is explained by using apologies, which are admissions of 'blameworthiness' (Leech, 1983; Schlenker & Darby, 1981). Similarly, when an agent feels reproach upon disapproval of others' 'blameworthy' actions (Ortony, Clore, & Collins, 1988), which causes feelings of anger; apology is offered to the agent as a way to alleviate his/her anger (Leech, 1983; Schlenker & Darby, 1981).

Apologetic Feedbacks

The projection of these relationships in HCI found implementations in many studies investigating the effect of apologetic feedbacks on user performances. Using human-centered interfaces instead of traditional computer-centered interfaces, Nielsen (1998) and Tzeng (2004) present error messages including emotional expressions such as apologies for failure in execution of a command and sympathy for a user's possible frustration. Nielsen (1998) argued that when a user encounters a problem and receives an error message, it should include a simple apologetic statement that the reason of the error is the limitation of the interface to execute the command for the intended task, not user's action. However, most of the error messages embedded in computer interfaces are short and inhuman, which glaringly unfold the nature of computer-centered design in case of a problem while interacting with the interface (Tzeng, 2004).

Investigating the effect of apologetic feedbacks on computer users' perception of their performance, Tzeng (2004) showed that the subjects in apologetic feedback groups did not perceive their performance and ability as better than those in non-apologetic groups. He further demonstrated that computer users might not expect computers to be polite; yet apologetic statements make subjects feel better about their interaction with the program. Based on the idea that participants' politeness orientations might have an influence on their perceptions of apologetic computer error messages, Tzeng (2006) conducted another study investigating users' perceptions about online systems containing three different error messages, each of which includes different politeness strategies. He elicited users' politeness orientations and asked them to interact with websites, each of which contains pre-determined problems. Upon encountering problems, users are provided with certain error messages representing three different politeness strategies, which were positive politeness strategy (i.e. joke), negative politeness strategy (i.e. a simple apology), and a mechanical message for the error (i.e. the page is temporarily unavailable). The findings revealed that users, who use polite expressions while dealing with social events, preferred apologetic messages significantly more than both other mechanical or joke messages and other users, who are less oriented to polite expressions

Inspired by Hatipoglu's (2004) findings pointing to the difference between the type and form of apologies used in e-mails and in spoken and written languages, a more current study by Akgun, Cagiltay and Zeyrek (in press) investigated the similarities and differences between the apologies used in Human-Human Interaction (HHI) and those preferred by the users during their interaction with the computer (HCI). Designing a genuine problem state caused by computer's inability to carry out a requested task, they elicit users' preferences for types of apology messages for the designated problem. The feedback from users were consistent with Nass, Steuer and Tauber's (1994) CASA paradigm that the social dynamics of HHI can be applied equally well to HCI. In the light of these findings, they further investigated the effect of different apologetic error messages on self-appraisal of performance and the interaction effect of message type and mood state on self-appraisal of performance. The results showed that even though the use of apologetic error messages in the computerized environment did not influence users' self-appraisals of performance; the interaction effect of message type and mood state on self-appraisal of performance was significant, i.e. the influence of apologetic messages on self-appraisal of performance depended on participants' mood state. Forgas (1999) found that the individuals in negative affect demonstrated greater politeness than those in positive affect while making requests, which showed that the level of politeness use depends on individuals' affective state. In light of his findings, Akgun et al. (in press) concluded that the use of apologetic

error messages to influence users' self-appraisals of performance in a computerized environment may not be enough by itself, thus, users' affective state should also be considered.

Emotionally Supportive Interactions

Based on the idea of the importance of human emotional expressions in interpersonal communications regarding individuals' relationships with others (Mongrain & Vettese, 2003), interactive computer systems with emotionally supportive interactions have been built to respond to users' negative emotional experiences, such as frustration. There are many studies aiming at how to improve human-computer interaction by investigating the ways to relieve users' negative emotional states caused by a computer application, such as frustration, confusion, and anger. User frustration with information and computing technology is a pervasive problem caused by factors such as crashing of computers and poor user interfaces (Lazar et al., 2005). Lazar and colleagues (2005) investigated whether there were commonalities between student and workplace user frustration during their interaction with computers. Their study showed that there are three important factors influencing the frustration levels of users; the time lost, the time to fix, and the importance of the task and that these three factors were relevant for both students and work place users. This means that the more time is wasted, while dealing with a task of higher importance, the higher the frustration level of both student and work place user gets. Another important finding of the study was that when the participants were asked to write down the specific causes of frustration, the most cited cause was the way computer error messages was presented. In another study, Klein, Moon and Picard (2002) investigated whether an interactive affect-support agent helps users to recover from their negative emotional states. The agent, which was text-based, used 'active listening (e.g. "Hmmm. It sounds like you felt really frustrated playing this game. Is that about right?"), empathy (e.g., "Sorry to hear things didn't go so well"), and sympathy statements (e.g., "It sounds like you didn't have the best experience, then. That's not much fun"). The researchers' prediction was that alleviating users' frustration would make users feel more positive towards the task and therefore make them continue to interact with the system for longer. Similar to Picard's (2000) previous finding that participants' interaction with an emotion-support agent yield to significantly longer playtime than those interacted with similar agents that ignored their emotions; they demonstrated that after interacting with the affect-support agent, users interacted with the system significantly longer in comparison to the two control groups. This is in line with Hone's (2006) finding that text-based agents can be effective in reducing user frustration. In addition, Hone (2006) also examined the effect of embodied agents and found that embodied agents providing emotional feedbacks can be more effective than text-based agents for reducing users' frustration caused by the computer. Correspondingly, Brave, Nass and Hutchinson (2005) investigated whether an embodied agent showing empathy had an influence on users. The results indicated that users found an emphatic agent more caring, more likable, more trustworthy, and more submissive than agents lacking emphatic emotion.

Emphatic Agents

Other recent studies investigating the use of different emphatic agents with different modalities also reported similar results. For instance, Nguyen and Masthoff (2009) investigated the effect of empathy by concentrating on different ways of expressing empathy and the modality of delivering such content. They designed 2 (modality: animated vs. no-visual) x 3 (intervention: non-empathy vs. empathy vs. empathy and expressivity) between-subjects study. In the animated conditions, human-like computer animated agent

with a synthesized voice was employed, whereas in the no-visual conditions, the agent has no visual representation and a voice. Animated agents used several facial expressions such as happy, neutral, concerned and sad as well as a variety of hand, arm, finger, body and head movements. In the empathy interventions, the agent used polite and friendly expressions (e.g. "I see you didn't like this test. Hopefully, you will find the next task more interesting and enjoyable. Would you mind if we continue?"), actively asked questions to understand the subjects' current mood state (e.g. "I can see you didn't perform as well as expected. How do you feel right now?"), and employed such expressions to convey a sense of sympathy and empathy to the subjects (e.g. "I am sorry to hear that things did not go better, but that is completely normal"). Lastly, in empathy and expressivity conditions, the agent also facilitated the subjects to express their feelings freely. The results showed that the level of intervention (empathy and expressivity; empathy; and non-empathy) has no significant effect on alleviating the subjects' negative mood state. Similarly, the findings indicated no difference between different interventions at each level of modality. However, similar to Brave, Nass and Hutchinson' (2005) study, they also found that giving empathic feedback led to a more positive attitude toward the system, including greater likeability, trustworthiness, perceived caring, and enjoyment to interact with regardless of the modality of delivering such content, although the difference was somewhat more profound when the system was represented by a human-like agent. Another study by Liu and Picard (2005) employing a wearable computer designed for acquiring health-related information from users also generated similar results that it was more preferred by users when the computer used empathetic language in its interactions with users. Different from Nguyen and Masthoff's (2009) study, comforting users through expressed empathy via computer agents during interactions have been shown to be important in alleviating user frustration and deemed to have important healthcare applications. In search for the most effective outcome for comforting users, Bicmore and Schulman (2006) examined two different conditions, which were allowing users to freely express their feelings, but having the agents provide imperfect empathic responses versus greatly restricting how users can express themselves, but having the agents provide very accurate empathic feedback. Once the identical mood induction procedure used for both conditions to induce mild anxiety, the intervention by the agent set in motion. While, in the former condition the agent used a high expressivity dialogue script, which prompts users to express themselves more freely and replies with "Really? That is the interesting to hear" with a neutral facial display, in the latter condition, the agent used a high emphatic accuracy script which provided users with appropriate emphatic feedback with a related facial display. They found that an agent with greater empathic accuracy was more efficacious at evoking positive affect and comforting users, even at the cost of restricting user input.

Multimodal Communication

Apart from text-based embodied agents, considering different input channels of affective information, studies investigating various aspects of multimodal communication, such as, appearance, movements of body and face, voice (speech and paralinguistics), touch and smell, etc. (Larsen & Frederickson, 1999) are also begun to appear in the literature. For instance, Fabri (2007) designed a virtual messenger, which was basically a chat tool with a 3D animated avatar, which produces the facial expressions in relation to the emoticons used within the text-based part of the interface. He showed that the use of expressive avatars were more effective and contributed to users' experiences positively. Similarly another study by (Graf, 2005) showed that using a digital character

with multimodal abilities conversing with the user in augmented reality had positive impact on users. He further contended that using a virtual figure in such environments might help building a relation between the user in the real world and presentation content in the virtual space avoiding frustration and contributing empathy. As for the auditory input, Tajadura and Vastfjall (2006) put forward the ignored role of sound in affective responses with a brief literature review. They further showed the importance of voice in image dominant multimedia applications by demonstrating the effects of two types of ecological sounds on emotions, specifically self-representation sounds, such as heart beating and breathing, and embodied activity sounds, such as footsteps. Creed and Beale (2006) conducted experiments mixing face expressions with speech in an animation and investigated the effects of mismatches on subjects' perceptions of emotional expressions. They found that while subjects recognized emotions in static facial expressions easily, they had difficulty in audio only expressions. Furthermore, in animations with appropriately matched audio and video, positive affects (e.g. happy) recognized more than negative ones (e.g. concerned), whereas mismatching of facial expressions and speech had a significant influence on subjects' perceptions of the emotional expressions. In mismatching animations, both visual and auditory representations of positive affects rated higher, despite the fact that neither visual nor auditory channel was found to be dominant over the other.

Lastly, Bianchi-Berthouse, Cairns, Cox, Jennett and Kim (2006) conducted a study, where they trained a system to accurately recognize emotions from bodily expressions even across different cultural backgrounds. They also showed that incorporation of full-body movements in the control of the game produced reports of higher sense of engagement by users.

CONCLUSION

As mentioned in previous sections, numerous researchers pointed out the relationships between emotions and cognitions using different theoretical perspectives. From appraisal theorists' point of view (e.g. Ellsworth & Scherer, 2003; and Scherer, 2003), emotions include patterns of perception and of interpretation. Emotions arise from attending and interpreting the environment and have an influence on thinking. From this perspective, it can be stated that emotion is construed as inherently private and information-based structures, which means that emotions occur at the individual level. On the other hand, others support the idea that emotion is an observable property of social action. For instance, Boehner et al. (2007) suggest that "emotion is an intersubjective phenomenon, arising in encounters between individuals or between people and society, an aspect of the socially organized life world we both inhabit and reproduce." (p.6). The design implication of this statement would be the importance of considerations of sociocultural factors such as social and cultural context, learning, and individual differences contributing emotions, in line with the debate of origins of emotions. Regarding the consensus that there are different forms of emotions, such as basic emotions stemming from evolution and biology and more complex emotions involving various cognitive components that differ across individuals and cultures (Izard 2007; Panksepp 2007; Pelachaud, 2009), it might be possible to define general HCI design principles for basic emotions, while designers should be on watch for more context- and culture-driven designs when emotions requiring higher cognitive processing are in question. Moreover, with the rise of distributed cognition and situated cognition accounts, which place a great emphasis on the role of social interaction in cognitive processes, the relationship between cognition and emotion is being investigated in connection with social action. Being a relatively new territory in HCI,

it is expected that this trend will also influence the studies, which are bringing affect into the computerized environments. The design implication of this change calls into attention the issue of designing interactions for massively multiple users rather than individuals.

Design Suggestions

Based on the reviewed literature, we may come up with some basic design suggestions:

- Follow user-centered design methods, especially the participatory design approach, is the best development approach for creating these types of environments.
- Apply emotions to computer messages, for example write simple apologetic statements for errors.
- Consider sociocultural factors such as social and cultural context, learning, and individual differences contributing emotions, in line with the debate of origins of emotions.
- Follow general HCI design principles for basic emotions.
- Create systems that can recognize and interpret user emotions.

TRENDS AND FUTURE

Even though, several studies presented before mention the importance of considering social norms in HCI, they examined the effects of using social rules governing interpersonal communication on the interaction between users and computer interfaces. Using social rules in the computerized environments could not be equated to constructing electronic environments in which emotions are socially constructed in interaction with other users via computer interfaces. However, with the development of Web 2.0 and Web 3.0 technologies, social networking and collaborative learning environments are becoming popular more and more each day, which signals the importance of multimodal designs utilizing multiple modes of communication channels for affective information and emotions. However, while creating multimodal designs, designers should be alert about choosing compatible modes rather than mismatching them (see Creed & Beale, 2006). This development also triggers the anticipated changes in the role of computer interfaces from assisting users to complete their tasks effectively and efficiently to providing users with an environment that brings them together for different purposes, which may also lead to socially constructed emotion. Since new technologies provide an environment for social interaction among individuals, but not only between the computer and individuals, a new term has appeared to represent the interaction between individuals via technology: Human-Human-Computer Interaction (HHCI) (Twidale, 2005). The design implication of this change is the issue of designing interactions for massively multiple users rather than individuals, namely the issue of HHCI design.

REFERENCES

Akgun, M., Cagiltay, K., & Zeyrek, D. (in press). The Effect of Apologetic Error Messages and Mood States on Computer Users' Self-Appraisal of Performance. *Journal of Pragmatics.*

Averill, J. R. (1980). A constructivist view of emotion. In R. Plutchik & H. Kellerman (Eds.), *Emotion: Theory, research and experience: Vol. I. Theories of emotion* (pp. 305-339). New York: Academic.

Bharuthram, S. (2003). Politeness phenomena in the Hindu sector of the South African Indian English speaking community. *Journal of Pragmatics*, *35*, 1523–1544. doi:10.1016/S0378-2166(03)00047-X

Bianchi-Berthouse, N., Cairns, P., Cox, A., Jennett, C., & Kim, W. W. (2006). On posture as a modality for expressing and recognizing emotions. In Christian Peter, Russell Beale, Elizabeth Crane, Lesley Axelrod, Gerred Blyth (Eds.) *Emotion in HCI: Joint Proceedings of the 2005, 2006, and 2007 Intl. Workshops.* Stuttgart: Fraunhofer IRB Verlag.

Bickmore, T., & Schulman, D. (2007). Practical Approaches to Comforting Users with Relational Agents CHI 2007 April 28-May 3, 2007 • San Jose, CA, USA

Boehner, K., DePaula, R., Dourish, P., & Sengers, P. (2007). How emotion is made and measured. *International Journal of Human-Computer Studies*, *65*, 275–291. doi:10.1016/j.ijhcs.2006.11.016

Brave, S., & Nass, C., & Hutchinson. (2005). Computers that care: Investigating the effects of orientation of emotion exhibited by an embodied computer agent. *International Journal of Human-Computer Studies*, *62*, 161–178. doi:10.1016/j.ijhcs.2004.11.002

Brave, S., & Nass, C. (2008). Emotion in human-computer interaction. In Sears, A., & Jacko, J. (Eds.), *The human computer interaction handbook: Fundamentals, evolving technologies and emerging applications* (2nd ed., pp. 77–92). Hillsdale, NJ: Lawrence Erlbaum Associates.

Brown, P., & Levinson, S. C. (1987). *Politeness: Some universals in language usage.* Cambridge: Cambridge University Press.

Carroll, J. M. (1997). Human-computer interaction: Psychology as a science of design. *International Journal of Human-Computer Studies*, *46*, 501–522. doi:10.1006/ijhc.1996.0101

Cegarra, J., & Hoc, J. M. (2006). Cognitive styles as an explanation of experts' individual differences: A case study in computer-assisted troubleshooting diagnosis. *International Journal of Human-Computer Studies, 64*, 123–136. doi:10.1016/j.ijhcs.2005.06.003

Creed, C., & Beale, R. (2006). Multiple and extended interactions with affective embodied agents. In Christian Peter, Russell Beale, Elizabeth Crane, Lesley Axelrod, Gerred Blyth (Eds.) *Emotion in HCI: Joint Proceedings of the 2005, 2006, and 2007 Intl. Workshops.* Stuttgart: Fraunhofer IRB Verlag.

Dalal, N. P., & Casper, G. M. (1994). The design of joint cognitive systems: The effect of cognitive coupling on performance. *International Journal of Human-Computer Studies, 40*, 677–702. doi:10.1006/ijhc.1994.1031

Damasio, A. R. (1994). *Descartes' error: emotion, reason, and the human brain.* New York, NY: Putnam Publishing Group.

de Greef, H. P., & Neerincx, M. A. (1995). Cognitive support: Designing aiding to supplement human knowledge. *International Journal of Human-Computer Studies, 42*, 531–571. doi:10.1006/ijhc.1995.1023

Diaper, D. (2004). Understanding task analysis for human-computer interaction. In Diaper, D., & Stanton, N. A. (Eds.), *The handbook of task analysis for human-computer interaction.* Mahwah, NJ: Lawrence Erlbaum Associates.

Ekman, P. (1971). Constants across cultures in the face and emotion. *Journal of Personality and Social Psychology, 17*(2), 124–129. doi:10.1037/h0030377

Ekman, P. (1992). Are there basic emotions? *Psychological Review, 99*(3), 550–553. doi:10.1037/0033-295X.99.3.550

Ekman, P. (1993). Facial expression and emotion. *The American Psychologist, 48*(4), 384–392. doi:10.1037/0003-066X.48.4.384

Ekman, P. (1994). All emotions are basic. In Ekman, P., & Davidson, R. J. (Eds.), *The Nature of Emotions: Fundamental Questions* (pp. 7–19). New York: Oxford University Press.

Ekman, P. (1999). Basic Emotions. In Dalgleish, T., & Power, M. J. (Eds.), *Handbook of Cognition and Emotion* (pp. 43–60). Chichester: John Wiley & Sons.

Ellsworth, P. C., & Scherer, K. R. (2003). Appraisal processes in emotion. In Davidson, R. J., Scherer, K. R., & Goldsmith, H. H. (Eds.), *Handbook of Affective Sciences* (pp. 572–595). New York: Oxford University Press.

Fabri, M. (2008) The Virtual Messenger - Online Chat using Emotionally Expressive Avatars. In Christian Peter, Russell Beale, Elizabeth Crane, Lesley Axelrod, Gerred Blyth (Eds.) *Emotion in HCI: Joint Proceedings of the 2005, 2006, and 2007 Intl. Workshops.* Stuttgart: Fraunhofer IRB Verlag.

Fogg, B. J., & Nass, C. (1997). Silicon sycophans: The effects of computers that flatter. *International Journal of Human-Computer Studies, 46*, 551–561. doi:10.1006/ijhc.1996.0104

Forgas, J. P. (1999). On feeling good and being rude: Affective influences on language use and request formulations. *Journal of Personality and Social Psychology, 76*(6), 928–939. doi:10.1037/0022-3514.76.6.928

Försterling, F. (2001). *Attribution: An introduction to theories, research and applications. East Sussex.* Psychology Press.

Graf, C. (2005). Digital characters as affective interfaces. In Christian Peter, Russell Beale, Elizabeth Crane, Lesley Axelrod, Gerred Blyth (Eds.) *Emotion in HCI: Joint Proceedings of the 2005, 2006, and 2007 Intl. Workshops.* Stuttgart: Fraunhofer IRB Verlag.

Gross, J. J. (1999). Emotion and emotion regulation. In Pervin, L. A., & John, O. P. (Eds.), *Handbook of personality: Theory and research* (2nd ed., pp. 525–552). New York: Guilford.

Hartson, H. R. (1998). Human-computer interaction: interdisciplinary roots and trends. *Journal of Systems and Software*, *43*, 103–118. doi:10.1016/S0164-1212(98)10026-2

Hatipoglu, C. (2004). Do apologies in e-mails follow spoken or written norms?: Some examples from British English. *Studies About Languages*, *5*, 21–29.

Hone, K. (2006). Emphatic agents to reduce user frustration: The effects of varying agent characteristics. *Interacting with Computers*, *18*, 227–245. doi:10.1016/j.intcom.2005.05.003

Izard, C. E. (1992). Basic emotions, relations among emotions, and emotion- cognition relations. *Psychological Review*, *99*(3), 561–565. doi:10.1037/0033-295X.99.3.561

Izard, C. E. (1993). Four systems for emotion activation: cognitive and noncognitive processes. *Psychological Review*, *100*, 68–90. doi:10.1037/0033-295X.100.1.68

Izard, C. E. (2007). Basic emotions, natural kinds, emotion schemas, and a new paradigm. *Perspectives on Psychological Science*, *2*(3), 260–280. doi:10.1111/j.1745-6916.2007.00044.x

Izard, C. E. (2009). Emotion theory and research: highlights, unanswered questions, and emerging issues. *Annual Review of Psychology*, *60*, 1–25. doi:10.1146/annurev.psych.60.110707.163539

James, W. (1884). What is emotion? *Mind*, *4*, 188–204. doi:10.1093/mind/os-IX.34.188

Klein, J., Moon, Y., & Picard, R. W. (2002). This computer responds to user frustration: Theory, design and the results. *Interacting with Computers*, *14*, 119–140.

Kleinginna, P., & Kleinginna, A. (1981). A categorized list of emotion definitions, with suggestions for a consensual definition. *Motivation and Emotion*, *5*(4), 345–379. doi:10.1007/BF00992553

Kling, R., & Star, S. L. (1998). Human centered systems in the perspective of organizational and social informatics. *Computers & Society*, *28*(1), 22–29. doi:10.1145/277351.277356

Larsen, R. J., & Fredrickson, B. L. (1999). Measurement issues in emotion research. In Kahneman, D., Diener, E., & Schwarz, N. (Eds.), *Wellbeing: Foundations of hedonic psychology* (pp. 40–60). Russell Sage, New York.

Lazar, J., Jones, A., Hackley, M., & Shneiderman, B. (2005). Severity and impact of computer user frustration: A comparison of student and workplace users. *Interacting with Computers*, *18*, 187–207. doi:10.1016/j.intcom.2005.06.001

Lazarus, R. S. (1999). The cognition-emotion debate: A bit of history. In Dalgleish, T., & Power, M. J. (Eds.), *Handbook of Cognition and Emotion* (pp. 3–17). Chichester: John Wiley & Sons.

Leech, G. (1983). *Principles of pragmatics*. London: Longman.

Lewis, M. (1999). The role of the self in cognition and emotion. In Dalgleish, T., & Power, M. J. (Eds.), *Handbook of cognition and emotion* (pp. 125–142). Chichester: John Wiley & Sons.

Lewis, M. (2005). Bridging emotion theory and neurobiology through dynamic systems modeling. *The Behavioral and Brain Sciences*, *28*, 169–245. doi:10.1017/S0140525X0500004X

Lewis, M. D., & Granic, I. (1999). Self-organization of cognition-emotion interactions. In Dalgleish, T., & Power, M. J. (Eds.), *Handbook of Cognition and Emotion* (pp. 683–701). Chichester: John Wiley & Sons.

Lisetti, C.L., & Schiano, D.J. (2000). Automatic facial expression interpretation: Where human-computer interaction, artificial intelligence and cognitive science intersect. *Pragmatics and Cognition* [Special Issue on Facial Information Processing: A Multidisciplinary Perspective], *8(1)*, 185-235.

Liu, K., & Picard, R. W. (2005). Embedded empathy in continuous, interactive health assessment. In *CHI Workshop on HCI Challenges in Health Assessment*.

Mongrain, M., & Vettese, L. C. (2003). Conflict over Emotional Expression: Implications for Interpersonal Communication. *Personality and Social Psychology Bulletin*, *29*(4), 545–555. doi:10.1177/0146167202250924

Nass, C., & Moon, Y. (2000). Machines and mindlessness: Social Responses to Computers. *The Journal of Social Issues*, *56*(1), 81–103. doi:10.1111/0022-4537.00153

Nass, C., Steuer, J., & Tauber, E. R. (1994, April). *Computers are social actors*. Papers presented at the meeting of the Conference on Human Factors in Computing, Boston, Massachusetts.

Neese, R. M. (1990). Evolutionary explanations of emotions. *Human Nature (Hawthorne, N.Y.)*, *1*, 261–289. doi:10.1007/BF02733986

Nguyen, H., & Masthoff, J. (2009). Designing Empathic Computers: The Effect of Multimodal Empathic Feedback Using Animated Agent. In Persuasive '09: Proceedings of the 4th International Conference on Persuasive Technology, pp. 1-9. 2009, Claremont, California April 26 - 29, 2009

Nielsen, J. (1998). *Improving the Dreaded 404 Error Message*. Retrieved September 12, 2009, from http://www.useit.com/alertbox/404_improvement.html

Norman, D. A. (1980). Twelve issues for cognitive science. *Cognitive Science*, *4*, 1–32. doi:10.1207/s15516709cog0401_1

Norman, D. A. (2004). *Emotional Design: Why We Love (Or Hate) Everyday Things*. New York, NY: Basic Books.

Nussbaum, M. E. (2008). Collaborative discourse, argumentation, and learning: Preface and literature review. *Contemporary Educational Psychology*, *33*, 345–359. doi:10.1016/j.cedpsych.2008.06.001

O'Rorke, P., & Ortony, A. (1994). Explaining emotions. *Cognitive Science*, *18*, 283–323. doi:10.1207/s15516709cog1802_3

Ortony, A., Clore, G. L., & Collins, A. (1988). *Cognitive Structure of Emotions*. New York: Cambridge University Press.

Ortony, A., & Turner, T. J. (1990). What's basic about basic emotions? *Psychological Review*, *97*(3), 315–331. doi:10.1037/0033-295X.97.3.315

Panksepp, J. (2007). Neurologizing the psychology of affects: how appraisal-based constructivism and basic emotion theory can coexist. *Perspectives on Psychological Science*, *2*(3), 281–296. doi:10.1111/j.1745-6916.2007.00045.x

Papanikolaou, K. A., Mabbott, A., Bull, S., & Grigoriadou, M. (2006). Designing learner-controlled educational interactions based on learning/cognitive style and learner behavior. *Interacting with Computers*, *18*, 356–384. doi:10.1016/j.intcom.2005.11.003

Pelachaud, C. (2009). Studies on Gesture Expressivity for a Virtual Agent, *Speech Communication, special issue in honor of Björn Granstrom and Rolf Carlson, 51*, 630-639

Phelps, E. A. (2006). Emotion and cognition: insights from studies of the human amygdala. *Annual Review of Psychology*, *57*, 27–53. doi:10.1146/annurev.psych.56.091103.070234

Picard, R. W. (1997). Does HAL cry digital tears? Emotion and computers. In Stork, D. G. (Ed.), *HAL's Legacy: 2001's Computer as Dream and Reality* (pp. 279–303). Cambridge, MA: The MIT Press.

Picard, R. W. (2000). Toward computers that recognize and respond to user emotion. *IBM Systems Journal*, *39*, 705–719. doi:10.1147/sj.393.0705

Picard, R. W. (2010). Emotion research by the people, for the people. Accepted for publication in Emotion Review. Retrieved April 1, 2010, from http://affect.media.mit.edu/pdfs/10.Picard-ER-revised.pdf

Reeves, B., & Nass, C. (1996). *The media equation: How people treat computers, televisions, and new media like real people and places*. Cambridge: Cambridge University Press.

Russell, J. A. (2003). Core affect and the psychological construction of emotion. *Psychological Review*, *110*, 145–172. doi:10.1037/0033-295X.110.1.145

Scaife, M., & Rogers, Y. (1996). External cognition: how do graphical representations work? *International Journal of Human-Computer Studies*, *45*, 185–213. doi:10.1006/ijhc.1996.0048

Scherer, K. R. (2003). Introduction: Cognitive components of emotion. In Davidson, R. J., Scherand, K. R., & Goldsmith, H. H. (Eds.), *Handbook of affective sciences* (pp. 563–571). Oxford: Oxford University Press.

Schlenker, B. R., & Darby, B. W. (1981). The use of apologies in social predicaments. *Social Psychology Quarterly*, *44*(3), 271–278. doi:10.2307/3033840

Schweder, R. (1994). "You're not sick, you're just in love": Emotion as an interpretive system. In Ekman, P., & Davidson, R. (Eds.), *The nature of emotion* (pp. 32–44). New York: Oxford University Press.

Shneiderman, B. (1998). *Designing the user interface: Strategies for effective human-computer interaction*. Harlow: Addison-Wesley.

Shott, S. (1979). Emotion and Social Life: A Symbolic Interactionist Analysis. *American Journal of Sociology*, *84*(6), 1317–1334. doi:10.1086/226936

Suchman, L. (1987). Interactive artifacts. In Suchman (Ed.), *Plans and Situated Actions* (pp. 5-26). New York: Cambridge University Press.

Tajadura, A., & Vastfjall, D. (2006) Auditory-induced emotion-A neglected channel for communication in HCI. In Christian Peter, Russell Beale, Elizabeth Crane, Lesley Axelrod, Gerred Blyth (Eds.) *Emotion in HCI: Joint Proceedings of the 2005, 2006, and 2007 Intl. Workshops.* Stuttgart: Fraunhofer IRB Verlag

Tangney, J. P., Stuewig, J., & Mashek, D. J. (2007). Moral emotions and moral behavior. *Annual Review of Psychology*, *58*, 345–372. doi:10.1146/annurev.psych.56.091103.070145

Tooby, J., & Cosmides, L. (1990). The past explains the present: Emotional adaptations and the structure of ancestral environments. *Ethology and Sociobiology*, *11*, 407–424. doi:10.1016/0162-3095(90)90017-Z

Twidale, M. B. (2005). Over the Shoulder Learning: Supporting Brief Informal Learning. *Computer Supported Cooperative Work*, *14*, 505–547. doi:10.1007/s10606-005-9007-7

Tzeng, J. (2004). Toward a more civilized design: Studying the effects of computers that apologize. *International Journal of Human-Computer Studies*, *61*, 319–345. doi:10.1016/j.ijhcs.2004.01.002

Tzeng, J. (2006). Matching users' diverse social scripts with resonating humanized features to create a polite interface. *International Journal of Human-Computer Studies*, *64*, 1230–1242. doi:10.1016/j.ijhcs.2006.08.011

Voss, J. F., Wiley, J., & Carretero, M. (1995). Acquiring intellectual skills. *Annual Review of Psychology, 46*, 155–181. doi:10.1146/annurev. ps.46.020195.001103

Wierzbicka, A. (1992d). Talking about emotions: Semantics, culture and cognition. [Special issue on basic emotions]. *Cognition and Emotion, 6*(3/4), 285–319. doi:10.1080/02699939208411073

KEY TERMS AND DEFINITIONS

Human Computer Interaction (HCI): The discipline that investigates human physical, cognitive and affective activities that are enacted during the interaction with computers.

Human-Human-Computer Interaction (HHCI): A newly emerging field that examines the social interaction among individuals via technology, along with the interaction between the computer and individuals.

Emphatic Agent: An interactive agent with built-in active listening, empathy, and sympathy statements for feedback.

Chapter 15
Affect–Sensitive Computing and Autism

Karla Conn Welch
University of Louisville, USA

Uttama Lahiri
Vanderbilt University, USA

Nilanjan Sarkar
Vanderbilt University, USA

Zachary Warren
Vanderbilt University, USA

Wendy Stone
Vanderbilt University, USA

Changchun Liu
The MathWorks, USA

ABSTRACT

This chapter covers the application of affective computing using a physiological approach to children with Autism Spectrum Disorders (ASD) during human-computer interaction (HCI) and human-robot interaction (HRI). Investigation into technology-assisted intervention for children with ASD has gained momentum in recent years. Clinicians involved in interventions must overcome the communication impairments generally exhibited by children with ASD by adeptly inferring the affective cues of the children to adjust the intervention accordingly. Similarly, an intelligent system, such as a computer or robot, must also be able to understand the affective needs of these children - an ability that the current technology-assisted ASD intervention systems lack - to achieve effective interaction that addresses the role of affective states in HCI, HRI, and intervention practice.

DOI: 10.4018/978-1-61692-892-6.ch015

INTRODUCTION

Autism is a neurodevelopmental disorder characterized by core deficits in social interaction, social communication, and imagination (American Psychiatric Association, 2000). These characteristics often vary significantly in combination and severity, within and across individuals, as well as over time. Research suggests prevalence rates of autism has increased in the last 2 decades from 1 in 10000 to as high as approximately 1 in 110 for the broad autism spectrum (CDC, 2009). While, at present, there is no single universally accepted intervention, treatment, or known cure for Autism Spectrum Disorders (ASD) (NRC, 2001; Sherer and Schreibman, 2005); there is an increasing consensus that intensive behavioral and educational intervention programs can significantly improve long term outcomes for individuals and their families (Cohen et al., 2006; Rogers, 2000).

Affective cues are indicators, external or internal, of the manifestations of emotions and feelings experienced in a given environment. This research utilizes and merges recent technological advances in the areas of (i) robotics, (ii) virtual reality (VR), (iii) physiological signal processing, (iv) machine learning techniques, and (v) adaptive response technology in an attempt to create an intelligent system for understanding various physiological aspects of social communication in children with ASD. The individual, familial, and societal impact associated with the presumed core social impairments of children with ASD is enormous. Thus, there is a need to better understand the underlying mechanisms and processes associated with these deficits as well as develop intelligent systems that can be used to create optimal intervention strategies.

In response to this need, a growing number of studies have been investigating the application of advanced interactive technologies to address core deficits related to autism, namely computer technology (Bernard-Opitz et al., 2001; Moore et al., 2000; Swettenham, 1996), virtual reality

environments (Parsons et al., 2004; Strickland et al., 1996; Tartaro and Cassell, 2007), and robotic systems (Dautenhahn and Werry, 2004; Kozima et al., 2009; Michaud and Theberge-Turmel, 2002; Pioggia et al., 2005; Scassellati, 2005). Computer- and VR-based intervention may provide a simplified but exploratory interaction environment for children with ASD (Moore et al., 2000; Parsons et al., 2004; Strickland et al., 1996). Robots have been used to interact with children with ASD in common imitation tasks and can serve as social mediators to facilitate interaction with other children and caregivers (Dautenhahn and Werry, 2004; Kozima et al., 2009). In the rest of the chapter, the term "computer" is used to imply both computer- and robot-assisted ASD interventions.

Even though there is increasing research in technology-assisted autism intervention, there is a paucity of published studies that specifically address how to automatically detect and respond to affective cues of children with ASD. Such ability could be critical given the importance of human affective information in HCI (Picard, 1997; Prendinger et al., 2005) and HRI (Fong et al., 2003) and the significant impacts of the affective factors of children with ASD on the intervention practice (Ernsperger, 2003; Seip, 1996; Wieder and Greenspan, 2005). A computer that can detect the affective states of a child with ASD and interact with him/her based on such perception could have a wide range of potential impacts. Interesting activities likely to retain the child's attention could be chosen when a low level of engagement is detected. Complex social stimuli, sophisticated interactions, and unpredictable situations could be gradually, but automatically, introduced when the computer recognizes that the child is comfortable or not anxious at a certain level of interaction dynamics for a reasonably long period of time. A clinician could use the history of the child's affective information to analyze the effects of the intervention approach. With the record of the activities and the consequent emotional changes in a child, a computer could learn individual preferences and affective characteristics over time using machine-learning techniques and thus could alter the manner in which it responds to the needs of different children. This chapter presents the results of investigations which assess what effects there are on physiological response for children with ASD during performance-oriented and socially-oriented tasks. The ability to detect the physiological processes that are a part of impairments in social communication may prove an important tool for understanding the physiological mechanisms that underlie the presumed core impairments associated with ASD.

BACKGROUND

Physiology for Affect Recognition of Children with ASD

There are several modalities such as facial expression (Bartlett et al., 2003), vocal intonation (Lee and Narayanan, 2005), gestures and postures (Asha et al., 2005; Kleinsmith et al., 2005), and physiology (Kulic and Croft, 2007; Mandryk et al., 2006; Nasoz et al., 2004; Rani et al., 2004) that can be utilized to evaluate the affective states of individuals interacting with computer. This work evaluates affective states based on physiological data for several reasons. Children with ASD often have communicative impairments (both nonverbal and verbal), particularly regarding expression of affective states (American Psychiatric Association, 2000; Green et al., 2002; Schultz, 2005). These vulnerabilities place limits on computerized affective modeling based on traditional conversational and observational methodologies. For example, video has been used to teach children with ASD to recognize facial expressions and emotions of *others* (Stokes, 2000), but no published studies were found that used visual recognition through video to autonomously determine the affective states of people with ASD. A facial recognition algorithm could be designed to detect certain ex-

pressions but would have to accommodate when expressions are abnormal (e.g., smiling under mild pain, etc.) or lack variability (Schultz, 2005). Physiological signals, however, are continuously available and are not necessarily directly impacted by these difficulties (Ben Shalom et al., 2006; Groden et al., 2005; Toichi and Kamio, 2003). As such, physiological modeling may represent a methodology for gathering rich data despite the potential communicative impairments of children with ASD. In addition, physiological data may offer an avenue for recognizing aspects of affect that may be less obvious for humans but more suitable for computers by using signal processing and pattern recognition tools. Furthermore, there is evidence that the transition from one affective state to another state is accompanied by dynamic shifts in indicators of Autonomic Nervous System activity (Bradley, 2000). More than one physiological signal, judged as a favorable approach (Bethel et al., 2007), is examined in this research, and the set of signals consists of various cardiovascular, electrodermal, electromyographic, and skin temperature signals, all of which have been extensively investigated in psychophysiology literature (Bradley, 2000).

One of the prime challenges of this work is attaining reliable subjective reports. There have been reports that adolescents could be better sources of information than adults when it comes to measuring some psychiatric symptoms (Cantwell et al., 1997), but researchers are generally reluctant to trust the responses of adolescents on self-reports (Barkley, 1998). One should be especially wary of the dependability of self-reports from children with ASD, who may have deficits in processing (i.e., identifying and describing) their own emotions (Hill et al., 2004). While there have been some criticisms on the use of subjective report (i.e., self-assessment or the reports collected from observers) and its effect on possibly forcing the determination of emotions, the subjective report is by and large regarded as an effective way to evaluate affective responses. Due to the unresolved debate on the definition of emotion (e.g., objective entities or socially constructed labels), researchers in affective computing often face difficulties obtaining the ground truth to label the natural emotion data accordingly. As suggested by Cowie et al. (2001) and Pantic and Rothkrantz (2003), the immediate implication of such a controversy is that pragmatic choices (e.g., application and user-profiled choices) must be made to develop an automatic affect recognizer. As a result, subjective report is widely used for affective modeling and endowing a computer with the recognition abilities similar to those of the reporters (Picard, 1997; Silva et al., 2006).

An important question when estimating human affective response is how to operationalize the affective state. Although much existing research on affective modeling categorizes physiological signal data into "basic emotions," there is no consensus on a set of basic emotions among the researchers (Cowie et al., 2001). This fact implies that practical choices are required to select target affective states for a given application. Anxiety, engagement, and enjoyment/liking are chosen as the possible target affective states in our work. Anxiety is chosen for two primary reasons. First, anxiety plays an important role in various human-machine interaction tasks that can be related to task performance (Brown et al., 1997). Second, anxiety frequently co-occurs with ASD and plays an important role in the behavior difficulties of children with autism (Gillott et al., 2001). Engagement, meaning sustained attention to an activity or person (NRC, 2001), has been regarded as one of the key factors for children with ASD to make substantial gains in academic, communication, and social domains (Ruble and Robson, 2006). With playful activities during the intervention, the liking of the children (i.e., the enjoyment they experience when interacting with the computer) may create urges to explore and allow prolonged interaction for the children with ASD, who are susceptible to being withdrawn (Dautenhahn and Werry, 2004; Papert, 1993).

Literature in the human factors and psychophysiology fields provide a rich history in support of physiology methodologies for studying stress (Groden et al., 2005; Zhai et al., 2005), engagement (Pecchinenda and Smith, 1996), operator workload (Kramer et al., 1987), mental effort (Vicente et al., 1987), and other similar mental states based on physiological measures such as those derived from electromyogram (EMG), galvanic skin response (GSR; i.e., skin conductance), heart rate variability (HRV), and blink rates. Meehan et al. (2005) reported that changes in physiological activity are evoked by different amounts of presence in stressful VR environments. Prendinger et al. (2005) demonstrated that the measurement of GSR and EMG can be used to discriminate a user's instantaneous change in levels of anxiety due to sympathetic versus unconcerned reactions from a life-like virtual teacher. In general, it is expected that higher physiological activity levels can be associated with greater stress levels (Smith, 1989). Therefore, developing intelligent systems for exploration of physiological signals and the target affective states of anxiety, engagement, and enjoyment/liking that may be associated with core social deficits for children with ASD is both scientifically valid and technologically feasible.

Technology in the Treatment of ASD

Interventions often focus on social communication, including social-problem solving and social skills training, so that participants can gain experience and exposure to various situations representative of everyday living. The ultimate goal of such interventions is for some generalization of these skills to carry over into real-life situations. A growing number of studies have been exploring the application of interactive technologies for future use in interventions to address the social deficits of children with ASD. Initial results indicate that such technologies hold promise as a potential alternative intervention approach with broad accessibility. Various software packages and VR environments have been developed and applied to address specific deficits associated with autism, e.g., understanding of false belief (Swettenham, 1996), attention (Trepagnier et al., 2006), social problem-solving (Bernard-Opitz et al., 2001), and social conventions (Parsons et al., 2005). Research on applying robotics to ASD intervention has suggested that robots can allow simplified but embodied social interaction that is less intimidating or confusing for children with ASD (Robins et al., 2005). By employing HCI and HRI technologies, interactive intervention tools can partially automate the time-consuming, routine behavioral intervention sessions and may allow intensive intervention to be conducted at home (Dautenhahn and Werry, 2004). For the purpose of employing an affect-sensitive intelligent system, computers or robots could be the mode of technology for assisted ASD interventions.

Dautenhahn and colleagues have explored how a robot can become a playmate that might serve a therapeutic role for children with autism in the Aurora project. Dautenhahn et al. (2003) emphasize the importance of robot adaptability in autism rehabilitation. Research showed that children with ASD are engaged more with an autonomous robot in the "reactive" mode than with an inanimate toy or a robot showing rigid, repetitive, non-interactive behavior (Dautenhahn and Werry, 2004). Michaud and Theberge-Turmel (2002) investigated the impact of robot design on the interactions with children with ASD and pointed out that systems need to be versatile enough to adapt to the varying needs of different children. Pioggia et al. (2005) developed an interactive life-like facial display system for enhancing emotion recognition in people with ASD. Robotic technologies pose the advantage of furnishing robust systems that can support multimodal interaction and provide a repeatable, standardized stimulus while quantitatively recording and monitoring the performance progress of the children with ASD to facilitate autism intervention assessment and diagnosis (Scassellati, 2005).

There are numerous reasons why a VR-based intervention system may be particularly relevant for children with ASD. The strength of VR technology for ASD intervention includes malleability, controllability, reduced sensory stimuli, individualized approach, safety, and a reduction of human interaction during initial skill training (Strickland, 1997). VR does not necessarily include direct human-to-human interaction, which may work well for an initial intervention to remove the difficulties common in ASD related to mere human interaction that is part of a typical intervention setting involving a child and a clinician (Chen and Bernard-Opitz, 1993; Tartaro and Cassell, 2007). However, VR should not be considered an isolating agent, because dyadic communication accomplished between a child and a VR environment can lead into triadic communication including a clinician, caregiver, or peer and in due course potentially accomplish the intervention goals of developing social communication skills between the child with ASD and another person (Bernard-Opitz et al., 2001). Furthermore, the main sensory output of VR is auditory and visual, which may represent a reduction of information from a real-world setting but also represents a full description of a setting without need for imagined components (Sherman and Craig, 2003; Strickland, 1997). Individuals with ASD can improve their learning skills related to a situation if the proposed setting can be manifested in a physical or visual manner (Kerr and Durkin, 2004). Since VR mimics real environments in terms of imagery and contexts, it may allow for efficient generalization of skills from the VR environment to the real world (Cromby et al., 1996). However, since limited social insight and social cognition are vulnerabilities that are often part of the core deficits associated with ASD, individuals may lack the skills to envision abstract concepts or changes to situations on their own. Virtual environments can easily change the attributes of, add, or remove objects in ways that may not be possible in a real-world setting but could be valuable to teach abstract concepts. Therefore, VR can offer the benefit of representing abstract concepts through visual means (e.g., thought bubbles with text descriptions of a virtual character's thoughts) and seamlessly allows for changes to the environment (e.g., changing the color of a ball or making a table disappear) that may be difficult or even impossible to accomplish in a real-world setting (Sherman and Craig, 2003; Strickland, 1997). Furthermore, the highly variable nature autism in terms of individual symptoms means an individual approach is appropriate, and computers can accommodate individualized treatment (Strickland, 1997). The highly versatile VR environment can illustrate scenarios which can be changed to accommodate various situations that may not be feasible in a given therapeutic setting because of space limitations, resource deficits, safety concerns, etc. (Parsons and Mitchell, 2002). Therefore, VR represents a medium well-suited for creating interactive intervention paradigms for skill training in the core areas of impairment for children with ASD (i.e., social interaction, social communication, and imagination). However, to date the capability of VR technology has not been fully explored to examine the factors that lead to difficulties in impairments such as social communication, which could be critical in designing an efficient intervention plan.

Consensus statements from both the American Academy of Pediatrics (Myers et al., 2007) and the National Resource Council (NRC, 2001) underscore that effective intervention for children with ASD includes: provision of intensive intervention, individual instruction tailored to the qualities of the child, promotion of a generalization of skills, and incorporation of a high degree of structure/organization. Despite the urgent need and societal import of intensive treatment (Rutter, 2006), appropriate intervention resources for children with ASD and their families are often difficult to access and extremely costly when accessible (Jacobson et al., 1998; Sharpe and Baker, 2007;

Tarkan, 2002). Therefore, an important direction for research on ASD is the identification and development of intelligent systems that can make application of effective intensive treatment more readily accessible and cost effective (Parsons and Mitchell, 2002; Rogers, 2000). In addition, with trained professional resource limitations, there is potential for emerging technology to play a significant role in providing more accessible intensive individualized intervention (Goodwin, 2008). VR has shown the capacity to ease the burden, both time and effort, of trained clinicians in an intervention process as well as the potential to allow untrained personnel (e.g., parents or peers) to aid a participant in the intervention (Standen and Brown, 2005), thereby offering the facility of providing cost and time effective and readily accessible intervention. As such, the future creation of a VR-assisted affect-sensitive intelligent system, with a potential of individualized intervention, for autism intervention could meet all of the core components of effective intervention while at the same time increasing the ability of the intervention provider to systematically control and promote intervention related skills.

Affective cues are insights into the emotions and behaviors of children with ASD. The ability to utilize the power of these cues may permit a smooth, natural, and more productive interaction process (Gilleade et al., 2005; Kapoor et al., 2001; Picard, 1997; Prendinger et al., 2005), especially considering the core social and communicative vulnerabilities that limit individuals with ASD to accurately self-identify affective experiences (Hill et al., 2004). Common in autism intervention, clinicians who work with children with ASD intensively monitor affective cues of the children in order to make appropriate decisions about adaptations to their intervention and reinforcement strategies. For example, "likes and dislikes chart" is recommended to record the children's preferred activities and/or sensory stimuli during interventions that could be used as reinforcers and/

or "alternative behaviors" (Seip, 1996). Children with autism are particularly vulnerable to anxiety and intolerant of feelings of frustration, which requires a clinician to plan tasks at an appropriate level of difficulty (Ernsperger, 2003). The engagement of children with ASD is the ground basis for the "floor-time therapy" to help them develop relationships and improve their social skills (Wieder and Greenspan, 2005). Given the importance of affective cues in ASD intervention practice (Ernsperger, 2003; Seip, 1996; Wieder and Greenspan, 2005), using affective information as a means of implicit and bidirectional communication may be critical for allowing a computer to respond to a child's affective states. The design of affect-sensitive interaction, an area known as affective computing, is an increasingly important discipline within the HCI and HRI communities (Picard, 1997). However, to date little work has been done to explore this approach for technology-assisted intervention of individuals with ASD. Furthermore, *no existing technology specifically addresses how to autonomously detect and flexibly respond to affective cues of children with ASD within an intervention paradigm* (Bernard-Opitz et al., 2001; Dautenhahn and Werry, 2004; Kozima et al., 2009; Michaud and Theberge-Turmel, 2002; Mitchell et al., 2007; Parsons et al., 2005; Pioggia et al., 2005; Scassellati. 2005; Strickland, 1997; Swettenham, 1996; Tartaro and Cassell, 2007; Trepagnier et al., 2006). The primary contribution of the research covered in this chapter is to address this deficiency. The research develops HCI technologies capable of eliciting affective changes in individuals with ASD. We investigate how to augment HRI to be used in affect-sensitive interaction by endowing the technology with the ability to recognize and flexibly respond to the affective states of a child with ASD based on his/her physiological responses. The research also assesses the efficacy of measuring affect in VR.

COMPLETED RESEARCH ON AFFECT-SENSITIVE COMPUTING AND AUTISM

We briefly present our results to demonstrate the feasibility as well as the likelihood of success of applying affect-sensitive computing to individuals with ASD.

Affective Modeling and Closed-Loop Affect-Sensitive Interaction for Children with ASD During Non-Social Tasks

In Phase I of this study (Liu et al., 2008a) six participants (ages 13-16) with ASD completed two computer-based tasks (i.e., Anagram game, Pong) wherein changes in task difficulty evoked varying intensities of three target operationalized affective states: liking, anxiety, and engagement. Affective modeling based on initial simultaneous clinical observation, performance characteristic/evaluation, and physiological data produced affect-recognition capabilities with predictive accuracies averaging around 82.9% in future performance. In Phase II (Liu et al., 2008b), a robot-based basketball (RBB) task was designed wherein a robotic arm with a basketball hoop attached to its end-effector learned individual preferences based on the predicted liking level of children with ASD and selected an appropriate behavior in real-time. Each participant completed two sessions RBB1 (non-affect-sensitive) and RBB2 (affect-sensitive). The results showed that the three different behaviors of the robot had distinguishable impacts on the liking level of the children with ASD. To reduce the bias of validation, in RBB1 the robot selects behaviors randomly and the occurrence of each behavior is evenly distributed. Average labeled liking level for each behavior as reported by the therapist in RBB1 showed differences between behaviors and individual preferences of each child. The difference of the impact on liking of each robot behavior was significant for five of the six children and moderate for one child. By performing two-way ANOVA analysis on the behavior (i.e., most-preferred, moderately-preferred, and least-preferred behavior) and participant, it was found that the differences of reported liking for different behaviors were statistically significant ($p < 0.05$), whereas no significant effect due to different participants was observed.

Furthermore, it was also observed that different children with ASD may have different preferences for the robot's behaviors. These results demonstrated that it is important to have a robot learn the individual's preference and adapt to it automatically, which may allow a more tailored and affect-sensitive interaction between children with ASD and the robot. When a robot learns that a certain behavior is liked more by a particular child, it can choose that behavior as his/her "social feedback" or "reinforcer" in a robot-assisted individualized affect-sensitive autism intervention.

In the closed-loop affect-sensitive session, RBB2, the robot autonomously selected the desirable behavior based on interaction experiences (i.e., the consequent liking level of a participant predicted by the individual affective model developed in Phase I). To determine the effects of the session type and participant on the reported liking, a two-way ANOVA test was performed. The null hypothesis that there is no change in liking level between affect-sensitive sessions and non-affect-sensitive sessions could be rejected at the 99.5% confidence level. Additionally, no significant impact due to different participants was observed. This was an important result as the robot continued learning and utilizing the information regarding the probable liking level of children with ASD to adjust its behaviors. This ability enables the robot to adapt its behavior selection policy in real time and hence keeps the participant in a higher liking level. *These results suggest that endowing an affect-sensitive adaptive system with the ability to recognize and respond to the affective states of a child with ASD based* *on physiological information could be a viable means for autism intervention.*

Affective Reactions to Manipulation of Social Parameters in VR

This study examined affective and physiological variation in response to manipulated social parameters (e.g., eye gaze and social distance) during social interaction in VR for both children with ASD and typically developing (TD) children. Experiments have been completed for 7 pairs of children with ASD and TD (age 13-17 years) matched on age, gender, and reciprocal verbal ability. Social interactions were designed using VIZARD VR toolkit software to project virtual human characters (i.e., avatars) who displayed different eye gaze patterns and stood at different distances while telling personal stories to the participants. We measured physiological responses and collected reports from an observing therapist on the levels of affective states (i.e., anxiety and engagement) for each participant who completed two 1.5-hour sessions. The social parameters of interest, eye gaze and social distance, were examined in a 4x2 design, presented in a random order based on a Latin Squares design to account for sequencing and order effects. Four types of eye gaze dictated the percentage of time an avatar looked at the participant. These were tagged as *direct, averted, normal while speaking,* and *flip of normal* (Argyle and Cook, 1976; Colburn et al., 2000). Two types of social distance, termed *invasive* (1.5ft away) and *decorum* (4.5ft away), characterized the distance between the avatar and the participant (Schneiderman and Ewens, 1971). Figure 1 shows two examples of the avatars. Other social parameters, such as facial expression and vocal tone were kept as neutral as possible. Efforts were made to minimize reactions due solely to viewing an avatar by choosing the 10 most-neutral avatars based on a survey of 20 participants. Therefore, affective rating and physiological reactions during the experiment could

Figure 1. Snapshot of an avatar displaying straight gaze at the invasive distance (left) and an avatar standing at the decorum distance and looking to her right in an averted gaze (right)

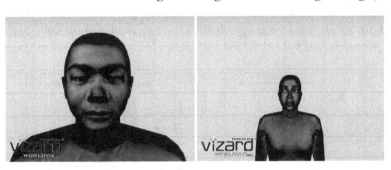

be reasonably expected to be related to change in eye gaze and/or social distance and not due to viewing the avatar alone.

Analysis of the subjective rating by the therapist revealed that manipulation of social parameters created affective changes in the participants (Table 1). The reported anxiety group mean was higher and the engagement group mean was lower for ASD than for the matched TD group, which is consistent with observations of social deficits of ASD children. The standard deviation (SD) for the ASD group was higher for both anxiety and engagement reports than that of the TD group. This result implied that the ASD group was more susceptible than the TD group to manipulation of social parameters in the VR trials. In addition, the range of subjective rating (9-point scale) was higher for the ASD group than the TD group on both affective states. *Thus, the results implied that our VR-based social interaction system was capable of creating affective changes among the participants.*

A set of 53 extracted physiological indices were analyzed to determine the extent of physi-

ological responses occurring during the VR-based social interaction. A detailed description of the sensor placement, signal processing, and routines used to extract the physiological indices from the raw signals can be found in our previous work (Liu et al., 2008a). Figure 2a.-d. shows a sample of results of physiological indices in response to effect of varying eye gaze with anxiety, and Figure 3a.-d.shows the same sample of physiological indices from effect of varying eye gaze with engagement. The variation of social interaction within the VR trials generated statistically significant physiological changes ($\geq 90\%$ confidence) in each of four major physiological categories – cardiovascular (ECG), electrodermal (EDA), skin temperature (ST), and electromyographic (EMG) – corresponding to both reported low anxiety (LA) and high anxiety (HA) states as well as low engagement (LE) and high engagement (HE) states. *Thus, the physiological indices are a viable means to differentiate among the ASD and TD groups.*

Table 1. Affective Intensity (full range [1-9]) Reported by Therapist

Group	Anxiety			Engagement		
	Mean	SD	Range	Mean	SD	Range
ASD (N=7)	4.9	1.7	8	4.7	1.6	8
TD (N=7)	4.4	1.4	6	5.1	1.4	7

Figure 2. Shown are the changes from baseline in physiological indices corresponding to Low Anxiety (LA) and High Anxiety (HA) states for the ASD and TD groups in response to variation of the avatar's eye gaze. Significant differences are evident between groups for physiological indices extracted from cardiovascular signals (a), electrodermal signals (b), skin temperature signals (c), and electomyographic signals (d)

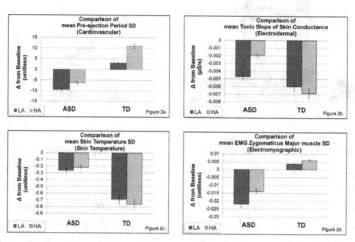

FUTURE RESEARCH DIRECTIONS

To address the core deficits of children with ASD in social communication in complex interactions, effective dynamic adjustment mechanisms would be demanded to incorporate multiple factors of interests such as affective and behavioral (e.g., attentive) cues, intervention goals, and task measures. As discussed earlier, expert therapists attempt to adeptly infer the affective cues ex-

Figure 3. Shown are the changes from baseline in physiological indices corresponding to Low Engagement (LE) and High Engagement (HE) states for the ASD and TD groups in response to variation of the avatar's eye gaze. Significant differences are evident between groups for physiological indices extracted from cardiovascular signals (a), electrodermal signals (b), skin temperature signals (c), and electomyographic signals (d)

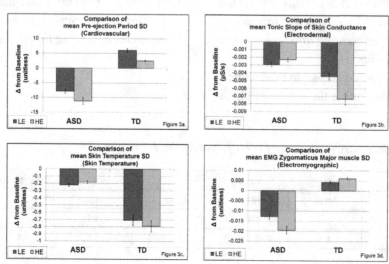

hibited by the children with ASD to adjust the intervention process (Ernsperger, 2003; Seip, 1996; Wieder and Greenspan, 2005). Therefore, a technology-assisted ASD intervention system must also be able to understand and respond to the affective needs of these children - an ability that the current ASD intervention systems lack - to achieve effective interaction leading to efficient intervention.

The physiology-based affect-sensitive technology described here could be employed to develop new intervention paradigms, which could promote interventions for individuals with ASD that are practical, widely available, and specific to the unique strengths and vulnerabilities of individuals with ASD. With further integration, a VR and physiological profiling system could be effective for use in developing and adapting controlled environments that help individuals explore social interaction dynamics gradually but automatically (i.e., introducing the aspects of social communication that are more challenging based on physiological data). Future work may include a reduction of the verbal components in the cognitive tasks which would allow application to the broader ASD population. Also, the research could benefit from exploring and merging other types of signals and features proven useful in affective computing, such as pupil diameter from eye-tracking data, with the current set of physiological signals. These ideas are currently being explored by researchers in our laboratory.

Note that the presented work requires physiological sensing that has its own limitations. For example, one needs to wear physiological sensors, and use of such sensors could be restrictive under certain circumstances. However, none of the participants in our studies had any objection in wearing the physiological sensors. Similar observations were achieved by Conati et al. (2003) that suggested concerns for intrusiveness of physiological sensors could be lessened for children in a game-like environment. Given the rapid progress in wearable computing with small, non-invasive

sensors and wireless communication, physiological sensors can be worn in a wireless manner such as in physiological sensing clothing and accessories (Picard, 1997; Wijesiriwardana et al., 2004), which could alleviate possible constraints on experimental design. Physiology-based affect recognition can be appropriate and useful for the application of interactive autism intervention and could be used conjunctively with other modalities (e.g., facial expression, vocal intonation, etc.) to allow flexible and robust affective modeling for children with ASD.

Future work may also involve designing socially-directed interaction experiments with embodied robots interacting with children with ASD. For example, the real-time affect recognition and response system described here could be integrated with a life-like android face developed by Hanson Robotics (hansonrobotics.com), which can produce accurate examples of common facial expressions that convey affective states. This affective information could be used as feedback for empathy exercises to help children with ASD recognize their own emotions.

CONCLUSION

There is increasing consensus that development of assistive therapeutic tools can make application of intensive intervention for children with ASD more readily accessible. In recent years, various applications of advanced interactive technologies have been investigated to facilitate and/or partially automate the existing behavioral intervention that addresses specific deficits associated with autism. However, the current technology-assisted therapeutic tools for children with ASD do not possess the ability of deciphering the affective cues of the children, which could be critical given that the affective factors of children with ASD have significant impacts on the intervention practice.

A physiology-based affective modeling framework for children with ASD was presented. The developed model could allow the recognition of affective states of the child with ASD from the physiological signals in real time and provide the basis for computer-based affect-sensitive interactive autism intervention. How to augment the interactive autism intervention was investigated by having a robot respond appropriately to the inferred level of a target affective state based on the affective model. VR-based intervention tools that address the social communication deficits of children with ASD were also developed and evaluated.

The impact of an intelligent system built on a computer-, robot-, or VR-based platform that can detect the affective states of a child with ASD and interact with him/her based on such perception could be transformative. Such a system could feasibly allow the manipulation and exacerbation of salient characteristics of interactions in a highly flexible environment that could potentially scaffold skills while minimizing potentially negative consequences. Thus, having a methodology that can objectively identify and predict social engagement as well optimal levels of affective arousal in a manner targeted to the specific child would represent a powerful intervention platform that addresses a serious potent barrier to the treatment of children with ASD.

Ultimately, continued exploration of this research could demonstrate the utility of affect-computing systems and physiologically-based affect recognition to address fundamental gaps in existing intervention paradigms designed to remediate clinically impairing social difficulties within an ASD population. Not only is the potential application of this technology particularly promising to this population, but demonstration of such a tool may hold even greater import in future extension of this methodology to individuals with ASD and other developmental disabilities wherein intellectual disabilities and communication limits are even more challenging.

REFERENCES

American Psychiatric Association. (2000). *Diagnostic and Statistical Manual of Mental Disorders: DSM-IV-TR* (4th ed.). Washington, DC: American Psychiatric Association.

Argyle, M., & Cook, M. (1976). *Gaze and Mutual Gaze*. Cambridge, MA: Cambridge University Press.

Asha, K., Ajay, K., Naznin, V., George, T., & Peter, D. (2005). *Gesture-based affective computing on motion capture data*. Paper presented at the International Conference on Affective Computing and Intelligent Interaction.

Barkley, R. A. (1998). *Attention Deficit Hyperactivity Disorder: A Handbook for Diagnosis and Treatment* (2nd ed.). New York: Guilford Press.

Bartlett, M. S., Littlewort, G., Fasel, I., & Movellan, J. R. (2003). *Real Time Face Detection and Facial Expression Recognition: Development and Applications to Human Computer Interaction*. Paper presented at the Conference on Computer Vision and Pattern Recognition Workshop.

Ben Shalom, D., Mostofsky, S. H., Hazlett, R. L., Goldberg, M. C., Landa, R. J., & Faran, Y. (2006). Normal physiological emotions but differences in expression of conscious feelings in children with high-functioning autism. *Journal of Autism and Developmental Disorders, 36*(3), 395–400. doi:10.1007/s10803-006-0077-2

Bernard-Opitz, V., Sriram, N., & Nakhoda-Sapuan, S. (2001). Enhancing social problem solving in children with autism and normal children through computer-assisted instruction. *Journal of Autism and Developmental Disorders, 31*(4), 377–384. doi:10.1023/A:1010660502130

Bethel, C., Salomon, K., Murphy, R., & Burke, J. (2007). *Survey of psychophysiology measurements applied to human-robot interaction.* Paper presented at the IEEE International Symposium on Robot and Human Interactive Communication, Jeju, Korea.

Bradley, M. M. (2000). Emotion and motivation. In Cacioppo, J. T., Tassinary, L. G., & Berntson, G. (Eds.), *Handbook of Psychophysiology* (pp. 602–642). New York: Cambridge University Press.

Brown, R. M., Hall, L. R., Holtzer, R., Brown, S. L., & Brown, N. L. (1997). Gender and video game performance. *Sex Roles, 36,* 793–812. doi:10.1023/A:1025631307585

Cantwell, D. P., Lewinsohn, P. M., Rohde, P., & Seeley, J. R. (1997). Correspondence between adolescent report and parent report of psychiatric diagnostic data. *Journal of the American Academy of Child and Adolescent Psychiatry, 36,* 610–619. doi:10.1097/00004583-199705000-00011

Centers for Disease Control and Prevention [CDC]. (2009). Prevalence of Autism Spectrum Disorders-ADDM Network, United States, 2006. *Morbidity and Mortality Weekly Report (MMWR) Surveillance Summaries, 58,* 1-20.

Chen, S. H., & Bernard-Opitz, V. (1993). Comparison of personal and computer-assisted instruction for children with autism. *Mental Retardation, 31*(6), 368–376.

Cohen, H., Amerine-Dickens, M., & Smith, T. (2006). Early intensive behavioral treatment: replication of the UCLA model in a community setting. Journal of Developmental & Behavioral Pediatrics, 27(2 Supplemental), S145-155.

Colburn, A., Drucker, S., & Cohen, M. (2000). The role of eye-gaze in avatar-mediated conversational interfaces. Paper presented at SIGGRAPH Sketches and Applications, New Orleans, Louisiana.

Conati, C., Chabbal, R., & Maclaren, H. (2003). *A study on using biometric sensors for detecting user emotions in educational games.* Paper presented at the Workshop on Assessing and Adapting to User Attitude and Affects: Why, When and How, Pittsburgh, Pennsylvania.

Cowie, R., Douglas-Cowie, E., Tsapatsoulis, N., Votsis, G., Kollias, S., Fellenz, W., & Taylor, J. G. (2001). Emotion recognition in human-computer interaction. *IEEE Signal Processing Magazine, 18*(1), 32–80. doi:10.1109/79.911197

Cromby, J. J., Standen, P. J., & Brown, D. J. (1996). The potentials of virtual environments in the education and training of people with learning disabilities. *Journal of Intellectual Disability Research, 40,* 489–501. doi:10.1111/j.1365-2788.1996. tb00659.x

Dautenhahn, K., & Werry, I. (2004). Towards interactive robots in autism therapy: Background, motivation and challenges. *Pragmatics & Cognition, 12,* 1–35. doi:10.1075/pc.12.1.03dau

Dautenhahn, K., Werry, I., Salter, T., & te Boekhorst, R. (2003). *Towards adaptive autonomous robots in autism therapy: Varieties of interactions.* Paper presented at the IEEE International Symposium on Computational Intelligence in Robotics and Automation, Kobe, Japan.

Ernsperger, L. (2003). *Keys to Success for Teaching Students with Autism.* Arlington, Texas: Future Horizons.

Fong, T., Nourbakhsh, I., & Dautenhahn, K. (2003). A survey of socially interactive robots. *Robotics and Autonomous Systems, 42*(3/4), 143–166. doi:10.1016/S0921-8890(02)00372-X

Gilleade, K., Dix, A., & Allanson, J. (2005). *Affective videogames and modes of affective gaming: Assist me, challenge me, emote me.* Paper presented at the Digital Games Research Association Conference.

Gillott, A., Furniss, F., & Walter, A. (2001). Anxiety in high-functioning children with autism. *Autism*, *5*(3), 277–286. doi:10.1177/1362361301005003005

Goodwin, M. S. (2008). Enhancing and accelerating the pace of Autism Research and Treatment: The promise of developing Innovative Technology. *Focus on Autism and Other Developmental Disabilities*, *23*, 125–128. doi:10.1177/1088357608316678

Green, D., Baird, G., Barnett, A. L., Henderson, L., Huber, J., & Henderson, S. E. (2002). The severity and nature of motor impairment in Asperger's syndrome: a comparison with specific developmental disorder of motor function. *Journal of Child Psychology and Psychiatry, and Allied Disciplines*, *43*(5), 655–668. doi:10.1111/1469-7610.00054

Groden, J., Goodwin, M. S., Baron, M. G., Groden, G., Velicer, W. F., & Lipsitt, L. P. (2005). Assessing cardiovascular responses to stressors in individuals with autism spectrum disorders. *Focus on Autism and Other Developmental Disabilities*, *20*(4), 244–252. doi:10.1177/10883576050200040601

Hill, E., Berthoz, S., & Frith, U. (2004). Brief report: cognitive processing of own emotions in individuals with autistic spectrum disorder and in their relatives. *Journal of Autism and Developmental Disabilities*, *34*(2). doi:10.1023/B:JADD.0000022613.41399.14

Jacobson, J. W., Mulick, J. A., & Green, G. (1998). Cost-benefit estimates for early intensive behavioral intervention for young children with autism – General model and single state case. *Behavioral Interventions*, *13*(4). doi:10.1002/(SICI)1099-078X(199811)13:4<201::AID-BIN17>3.0.CO;2-R

Kapoor, A., Mota, S., & Picard, R. W. (2001). *Towards a learning companion that recognizes affect*. Paper presented at Emotional and Intelligent II: The Tangled Knot of Social Cognition AAAI Fall Symposium.

Kerr, S., & Durkin, K. (2004). Understanding of thought bubbles as mental representations in children with autism: Implications for theory of mind. *Journal of Autism and Developmental Disorders*, *34*(6). doi:10.1007/s10803-004-5285-z

Kleinsmith, A., Ravindra De Silva, P., & Bianchi-Berthouze, N. (2005). *Recognizing emotion from postures: cross-cultural differences in user modeling*. Paper presented at User Modeling.

Kozima, H., Michalowski, M. P., & Nakagawa, C. (2009). Keepon: A playful robot for research, therapy, and entertainment. *International Journal of Social Robotics*, *1*(1), 3–18. doi:10.1007/s12369-008-0009-8

Kramer, A., Sirevaag, E., & Braune, R. (1987). A Psychophysiological Assessment of Operator Workload during Simulated Flight Missions. *Human Factors*, *29*(2), 145–160.

Kulic, D., & Croft, E. (2007). Physiological and subjective responses to articulated robot motion. *Robotica*, *25*, 13–27. doi:10.1017/S0263574706002955

Lee, C. M., & Narayanan, S. S. (2005). Toward detecting emotions in spoken dialogs. *IEEE Transactions on Speech and Audio Processing*, *13*(2), 293–303. doi:10.1109/TSA.2004.838534

Liu, C., Conn, K., Sarkar, N., & Stone, W. (2008a). Physiology-based affect recognition for computer-assisted intervention of children with autism spectrum disorder. *International Journal of Human-Computer Studies*, *66*(9), 662–677. doi:10.1016/j.ijhsc.2008.04.003

Liu, C., Conn, K., Sarkar, N., & Stone, W. (2008b). Online Affect Detection and Robot Behavior Adaptation for Intervention of Children with Autism. *IEEE Transactions on Robotics, 24*(4), 883–896. doi:10.1109/TRO.2008.2001362

Mandryk, R. L., Inkpen, K. M., & Calvert, T. W. (2006). Using physiological techniques to measure user experience with entertainment technologies. *International Journal of Human-Computer Studies, 25*(2), 141–158.

Meehan, M., Razzaque, S., Insko, B., Whitton, M., & Brooks, F. P. Jr. (2005). Review of four studies on the use of physiological reaction as a measure of presence in stressful virtual environments. *Applied Psychophysiology and Biofeedback, 30*(3), 239–258. doi:10.1007/s10484-005-6381-3

Michaud, F., & Theberge-Turmel, C. (2002). Mobile robotic toys and autism. In Dautenhahn, K., Bond, A. H., Canamero, L., & Edmonds, B. (Eds.), *Socially Intelligent Agents: Creating Relationships With Computers and Robots* (pp. 125–132). Norwell, MA: Kluwer.

Mitchell, P., Parsons, S., & Leonard, A. (2007). Using virtual environments for teaching social understanding to adolescents with autistic spectrum disorders. *Journal of Autism and Developmental Disorders, 37*, 589–600. doi:10.1007/s10803-006-0189-8

Moore, D. J., McGrath, P., & Thorpe, J. (2000). Computer aided learning for people with autism - A framework for research and development. *Innovations in Education and Training International, 37*(3), 218–228.

Myers, S. M., & Johnson, C. P., American Academy of Pediatrics, & Council on Children with Disabilities. (2007). Management of children with autism spectrum disorders. *Pediatrics, 120*(5), 1162–1182. doi:10.1542/peds.2007-2362

Nasoz, F., Alvarez, K., Lisetti, C., & Finkelstein, N. (2004). Emotion recognition from physiological signals using wireless sensors for presence technologies. *International Journal of Cognition, Technology, and Work – Special Issue on Presence, 6*(1), 4-14.

NRC (National Research Council). (2001). *Educating Children with Autism*. Washington, DC: National Academy Press.

Pantic, M., & Rothkrantz, L. J. M. (2003). Toward an affect-sensitive multimodal human–computer interaction. *Proceedings of the IEEE, 91*(9), 1370–1390. doi:10.1109/JPROC.2003.817122

Papert, S. (1993). *Mindstorms: Children, Computers, and Powerful Ideas* (2nd ed.). New York: Basic Books.

Parsons, S., & Mitchell, P. (2002). The potential of virtual reality in social skills training for people with autistic spectrum disorders. *Journal of Intellectual Disability Research, 46*, 430–443. doi:10.1046/j.1365-2788.2002.00425.x

Parsons, S., Mitchell, P., & Leonard, A. (2004). The use and understanding of virtual environments by adolescents with autistic spectrum disorders. *Journal of Autism and Developmental Disorders, 34*(4), 449–466. doi:10.1023/B:JADD.0000037421.98517.8d

Parsons, S., Mitchell, P., & Leonard, A. (2005). Do adolescents with autistic spectrum disorders adhere to social conventions in virtual environments? *Autism, 9*, 95–117. doi:10.1177/1362361305049032

Pecchinenda, A., & Smith, C. A. (1996). The affective significance of skin conductance activity during a difficult problem-solving task. *Cognition and Emotion, 10*(5), 481–504. doi:10.1080/026999396380123

Picard, R. W. (1997). *Affective Computing*. Cambridge, MA: MIT Press.

Pioggia, G., Igliozzi, R., Ferro, M., Ahluwalia, A., Muratori, F., & De Rossi, D. (2005). An android for enhancing social skills and emotion recognition in people with autism. *IEEE Transactions on Neural Systems and Rehabilitation Engineering, 13*(4), 507–515. doi:10.1109/TNSRE.2005.856076

Prendinger, H., Mori, J., & Ishizuka, M. (2005). Using human physiology to evaluate subtle expressivity of a virtual quizmaster in a mathematical game. *International Journal of Human-Computer Studies, 62*(2), 231–245. doi:10.1016/j.ijhcs.2004.11.009

Rani, P., Sarkar, N., Smith, C. A., & Kirby, L. D. (2004). Anxiety detecting robotic system – towards implicit human-robot collaboration. *Robotica, 22*, 85–95. doi:10.1017/S0263574703005319

Robins, B., Dickerson, P., & Dautenhahn, K. (2005). *Robots as embodied beings – Interactionally sensitive body movements in interactions among autistic children and a robot.* Paper presented at the IEEE International Workshop on Robot and Human Interactive Communication, Nashville, Tennessee.

Rogers, S. J. (2000). Interventions that facilitate socialization in children with autism. *Journal of Autism and Developmental Disorders, 30*(5), 399–409. doi:10.1023/A:1005543321840

Ruble, L. A., & Robson, D. M. (2006). Individual and environmental determinants of engagement in autism. *Journal of Autism and Developmental Disorders, 37*(8), 1457–1468. doi:10.1007/s10803-006-0222-y

Rutter, M. (2006). Autism: its recognition, early diagnosis, and service implications. *Journal of Developmental and Behavioral Pediatrics, 27*(Supplement 2), S54–S58.

Scassellati, B. (2005). *Quantitative metrics of social response for autism diagnosis.* Paper presented at the IEEE International Workshop on Robot and Human Interactive Communication, Nashville, Tennessee.

Schneiderman, M. H., & Ewens, W. L. (1971). The Cognitive Effects of Spatial Invasion. *Pacific Sociological Review, 14*(4), 469–486.

Schultz, R. T. (2005). Developmental deficits in social perception in autism: the role of the amygdala and fusiform face area. *International Journal of Developmental Neuroscience, 23*, 125–141. doi:10.1016/j.ijdevneu.2004.12.012

Seip, J. (1996). *Teaching the Autistic and Developmentally Delayed: A Guide for Staff Training and Development.* Delta, BC: Author.

Sharpe, D. L., & Baker, D. L. (2007). Financial issues associated with having a child with autism. *Journal of Family and Economic Issues, 28*, 247–264. doi:10.1007/s10834-007-9059-6

Sherer, M. R., & Schreibman, L. (2005). Individual behavioral profiles and predictors of treatment effectiveness for children with autism. *Journal of Consulting and Clinical Psychology, 73*(3), 525–538. doi:10.1037/0022-006X.73.3.525

Sherman, W. R., & Craig, A. B. (2003). *Understanding virtual reality: interface, application, and design.* Boston: Morgan Kaufmann Publishers.

Silva, P. R. D., Osano, M., Marasinghe, A., & Madurapperuma, A. P. (2006). A computational model for recognizing emotion with intensity for machine vision applications. *IEICE Transactions on Information and Systems. E (Norwalk, Conn.), 89-D*(7), 2171–2179.

Smith, C. A. (1989). Dimensions of appraisal and physiological response in emotion. *Journal of Personality and Social Psychology, 56*(3), 339–353. doi:10.1037/0022-3514.56.3.339

Standen, P. J., & Brown, D. J. (2005). Virtual reality in the rehabilitation of people with intellectual disabilities [review]. *Cyberpsychology & Behavior*, *8*(3), 272–282, discussion 283–288. doi:10.1089/cpb.2005.8.272

Stokes, S. (2000). *Assistive technology for children with autism*. Published under a CESA 7 contract funded by the Wisconsin Department of Public Instruction.

Strickland, D. (1997). Virtual reality for the treatment of autism. In Riva, G. (Ed.), *Virtual reality in neuropsycho-physiology* (pp. 81–86). Amsterdam: IOS Press.

Strickland, D., Marcus, L. M., Mesibov, G. B., & Hogan, K. (1996). Brief report: two case studies using virtual reality as a learning tool for autistic children. *Journal of Autism and Developmental Disorders*, *26*(6). doi:10.1007/BF02172354

Swettenham, J. (1996). Can children with autism be taught to understand false belief using computers? *Journal of Child Psychology and Psychiatry, and Allied Disciplines*, *37*(2), 157–165. doi:10.1111/j.1469-7610.1996.tb01387.x

Tarkan, L. (2002). Autism therapy is called effective, but rare. *New York Times*.

Tartaro, A., & Cassell, J. (2007). Using virtual peer technology as an intervention for children with autism. In Lazar, J. (Ed.), *Towards Universal Usability: Designing Computer Interfaces for Diverse User Populations*. Chichester, UK: John Wiley and Sons.

Toichi, M., & Kamio, Y. (2003). Paradoxical autonomic response to mental tasks in autism. *Journal of Autism and Developmental Disorders*, *33*(4), 417–426. doi:10.1023/A:1025062812374

Trepagnier, C. Y., Sebrechts, M. M., Finkelmeyer, A., Stewart, W., Woodford, J., & Coleman, M. (2006). Simulating social interaction to address deficits of autistic spectrum disorder in children. *Cyberpsychology & Behavior*, *9*(2), 213–217. doi:10.1089/cpb.2006.9.213

Vicente, K., Thornton, D., & Moray, N. (1987). Spectral-Analysis of Sinus Arrhythmia - a Measure of Mental Effort. *Human Factors*, *29*(2), 171–182.

Wieder, S., & Greenspan, S. (2005). Can children with autism master the core deficits and become empathetic, creative, and reflective? *The Journal of Developmental and Learning Disorders*, *9*, 1–29.

Wijesiriwardana, R., Mitcham, K., & Dias, T. (2004). *Fibre-meshed transducers based real time wearable physiological information monitoring system*. Paper presented at the International Symposium on Wearable Computers, Washington, DC.

Zhai, J., Barreto, A., Chin, C., & Li, C. (2005). User Stress Detection in Human-Computer Interactions. *Biomedical Sciences Instrumentation*, *41*, 277–286.

ADDITIONAL READING

Agrawal, P., Liu, C., & Sarkar, N. (2008). Interaction between human and robot: An affect-inspired approach. *Interaction Studies: Social Behaviour and Communication in Biological and Artificial Systems*, *9*(2), 230–257. doi:10.1075/is.9.2.05agr

Argyle, M., & Dean, J. (1965). Eye-contact, distance and Affiliation. *Sociometry*, *28*(3), 289–304. doi:10.2307/2786027

Bancroft, W. J. (1995). *Research in Nonverbal Communication and Its Relationship to Pedagogy and Suggestopedia*. ERIC.

Bellini, S., Peters, J. K., Benner, L., & Hopf, A. (2007). A Meta-Analysis of school-based social skills intervention for children with Autism Spectrum Disorders. *Journal of Remedial and Special Education*, *28*(3), 153–162. doi:10.1177/07419325070280030401

Bolte, S., Feineis-Matthews, S., & Poustka, F. (2008). Emotional processing in high-functioning autism – physiological reactivity and affective report. *Journal of Autism and Developmental Disorders*, *38*(4), 776–781. doi:10.1007/s10803-007-0443-8

Bradley, M. M. (1994). Emotional memory: a dimensional analysis. In Van Goozen, S., Van de Poll, N. E., & Sergeant, I. A. (Eds.), *Emotions: Essays on emotion theory* (pp. 97–134). Hillsdale, NJ: Erlbaum.

Burges, C. J. C. (1998). A tutorial on support vector machines for pattern recognition. *Data Mining and Knowledge Discovery*, *2*, 121–167. doi:10.1023/A:1009715923555

Cacioppo, J. T., Berntson, G. G., Larsen, J. T., Poehlmann, K. M., & Ito, T. A. (2000). The psychophysiology of emotion. In Lewis, M., & Haviland-Jones, J. M. (Eds.), *Handbook of Emotions* (pp. 173–191). New York: Guilford.

Cobb, S. V. G., Nichols, S., Ramsey, A., & Wilson, J. R. (1999). Virtual reality-induced symptoms and effects. *Presence (Cambridge, Mass.)*, *8*(2), 169–186. doi:10.1162/105474699566152

Conn, K., Liu, C., Sarkar, N., Stone, W., & Warren, Z. (2008). Towards Affect-sensitive Assistive Intervention Technologies for Children with Autism. In Or, J. (Ed.), *Affective Computing: Focus on Emotion Expression, Synthesis and Recognition* (pp. 365–390). Vienna, Austria: ARS/I-Tech Education and Publishing.

Eisenberg, N., Fabes, R., Murphy, B., Maszk, P., Smith, M., & Karbon, M. (1995). The role of emotionality and regulation in children's social functioning: a longitudinal study. *Child Development*, *66*, 1360–1384. doi:10.2307/1131652

Ekman, P. (1993). Facial expression and emotion. *The American Psychologist*, *48*, 384–392. doi:10.1037/0003-066X.48.4.384

Fombonne, E. (2003). Epidemiological surveys of autism and other pervasive developmental disorders: an update. *Journal of Autism and Developmental Disorders*, *33*, 365–382. doi:10.1023/A:1025054610557

Frijda, N. H. (1986). *The emotions*. New York: Cambridge University.

Frischen, A., Bayliss, A. P., & Tipper, S. P. (2007). Gaze cuing of Attention: Visual Attention, Social Cognition and Individual Differences. *Psychological Bulletin*, *133*, 694–724. doi:10.1037/0033-2909.133.4.694

Gresham, F. M., & MacMillan, D. L. (1997). Social competence and affective characteristics of students with mild disabilities. *Review of Educational Research*, *67*(4), 377–415.

Kanner, L. (1943). Autistic Disturbances of Affective Contact. *Nervous Child*, *2*, 217–250.

Klin, A., Jones, W., Schultz, R., Volkmar, F., & Cohen, D. (2002). Visual fixation patterns during viewing of naturalistic social situations as predictors of social competence in individuals with autism. *Archives of General Psychiatry*, *59*(9), 809–816. doi:10.1001/archpsyc.59.9.809

Lacey, J. I., & Lacey, B. C. (1958). Verification and extension of the principle of autonomic response-stereotypy. *The American Journal of Psychology*, *71*(1), 50–73. doi:10.2307/1419197

Mandryk, R. L., & Atkins, M. S. (2007). A fuzzy physiological approach for continuously modeling emotion during interaction with play technologies. *International Journal of Human-Computer Studies*, *65*(4), 329–347. doi:10.1016/j.ijhcs.2006.11.011

Neumann, S. A., & Waldstein, S. R. (2001). Similar patterns of cardiovascular response during emotion activation as a function of affective valence and arousal and gender. *Journal of Psychosomatic Research*, *50*, 245–253. doi:10.1016/S0022-3999(01)00198-2

Picard, R. W. (2009). Future Affective Technology for Autism and Emotion Communication. *Philosophical Transactions of the Royal Society B. Biological Sciences, 364*(1535), 3575–3584. doi:10.1098/rstb.2009.0143

Picard, R. W., Vyzas, E., & Healey, J. (2001). Toward machine emotional intelligence: analysis of affective physiological state. *IEEE Transactions on Pattern Analysis and Machine Intelligence, 23*(10), 1175–1191. doi:10.1109/34.954607

Robins, B., Dickerson, P., Stribling, P., & Dautenhahn, K. (2004). Robot-mediated joint attention in children with autism: A case study in robot–human interaction. *Interaction Studies: Social Behaviour and Communication in Biological and Artificial Systems, 5*(2), 161–198. doi:10.1075/is.5.2.02rob

Rogers, S. J. (1998). Empirically supported comprehensive treatments for young children with autism. *Journal of Clinical Child Psychology, 27*, 168–179. doi:10.1207/s15374424jccp2702_4

Vansteelandt, K., Van Mechelen, I., & Nezlek, J. (2005). The co-occurrence of emotions in daily life: a multilevel approach. *Journal of Research in Personality, 39*(3), 325–335. doi:10.1016/j.jrp.2004.05.006

Vapnik, V. N. (1998). *Statistical Learning Theory*. New York: Wiley-Interscience.

Watkins, C. J. C. H., & Dayan, P. (1992). Q-learning. *Machine Learning, 8*, 279–292. doi:10.1007/BF00992698

Werry, I., Dautenhahn, K., & Harwin, W. (2001). *Investigating a robot as a therapy partner for children with autism*. Paper presented at the 6th European conference for the advancement of assistive technology, Ljubljana, Slovenia.

Zhai, J., & Barreto, A. (2006). Stress Detection in Computer Users through Noninvasive Monitoring of Physiological Signals. *Biomedical Sciences Instrumentation, 42*, 495–500.

Chapter 16
Affective Games:
How iOpiates Elicit an Emotional Fix

Jonathan Sykes
Glasgow Caledonian University, Scotland

ABSTRACT

Video-games, like movies, music and storybooks are emotional artifacts. We buy media to alter our affective state. Through consumption they impact our physiology and thus alter our affective world. In this chapter the authors review the ways in which playing games can elicit emotion. This chapter will discuss the increased power of video-game technology to elicit affect, and show how the mash-up of traditional and interactive techniques have delivered a richness of emotion that competes with film and television. They then conclude by looking forward to a time when video-games become the dominant medium, and the preferred choice when seeking that emotional fix.

INTRODUCTION

As I sit here in my apartment and look around the room I feel surrounded. The mass of media has taken hold of my home - books overflow bookshelves, DVDs and CDs are barely contained by the racks, a giant screen TV hides the beautiful print that hangs on my wall, and hi-fi speakers dwarf the coffee table. I share my life with all this technology, all of this media, but what is it for? I know its purpose, the reason it exists is to entertain me - but to what end? What does it mean to

be entertained? It seems much more than simply passing the time. It is about changing the way I feel. Unhappy with my current affective state I am constantly looking to experience something outside my natural emotional repertoire. I need emotional stimulation. I want to experience fear, amusement, anger, sorrow. I am an emotion junky.

Being an emotion junky I am always looking for a supplier. Historically the largest dealer of affect altering product has been the film industry. Hollywood understands the monetary value of emotion, having peddled affective products for nearly 100 years. To maintain the flow of content to an addicted public, the film industry has

DOI: 10.4018/978-1-61692-892-6.ch016

developed many tools and techniques to elicit an emotional experience. They know the power of narrative, the importance of soundtrack, and the effect of aesthetic. But have we have reached the limits of traditional, linear technology? Although established media such as film and television might once have been the opiate of the people, there is evidence to suggest that interactive entertainment will soon eclipse linear media to become the *iOpiate* of the people. Video-games now outsell Hollywood box-office (Rosenberg, 2009), and traditional media struggles to hold attention as we multi-task between web-browsing, texting and watching television. This chapter will discuss the increased power of video-game technology to elicit affect, and show how the mash-up of traditional and interactive techniques have delivered a richness of emotion that competes with film and television. I will then finish by looking forward to a time when video-games will become the dominant medium for managing our affect. However, before I begin I shall define some of the terms used.

There is much debate concerning the terminology used in emotion research. Many researchers will use the terms 'affect', 'emotion' and 'mood' interchangeably, or like Norman (2002) stick to the term 'affect' to avoid making distinction between them. Here I will use the term 'emotion' to refer to a brief subjective feeling that is in response to some stimulus - such as the momentary feeling of fear we experience when watching a horror movie. I differentiate emotion from the term 'mood', which I use to represent longer episodes with no discernible stimulus - such as an extended bout of depression. I will use the term 'affect' as a general reference to our emotional experiences.

Of pornography, Supreme Court Justice Potter Steward once said "I shall not today attempt further to define [pornography]... but I know what it is when I see it". Most of us intuitively know what it means to 'play', but much like pornography, *defining* play turns out to be extraordinarily difficult. What appears playful in one context might seem very different in another. I find shop-

ping to be an excellent example. Making lists, choosing items, queuing to pay, trudging home with heavy bags - none of this strikes me as fun. But on a Saturday at the Farmers' Market I see couples happily choosing their evening meal; on the high street groups of young women seem to be at play as they enjoy the fellowship of clothes shopping with their closest friends. And what about a child running after a ball on the beach? They often seem much more at play than a professional soccer player lining up for a penalty kick. I will therefore follow Supreme Court Justice Potter's example and defer definition of play - as we all know what it is when we experience it. To those readers who would like to better understand the nature of play, I direct you to Huizinga (1938), Caillois (1958) and I also recommend Egendfelt Nielsen *et al.* (2008) for a superb review of play and game taxonomy.

EMOTIONAL ASPECTS OF PLAY

Which form of media do you believe delivers the greater emotional experience – film or video-games? I would guess that most of us are more likely to associate film with emotional engagement. We categorise films by the emotion they elicit - to experience fear visit the horror section; for amusement you need comedy; to raise your adrenaline levels check out the latest thriller. By contrast, video-games are organised by base mechanic - RPG, platform game, or first-person shooter. The reason many of us don't naturally associate gameplay with emotional experience is likely historical. The emotions evoked playing early video-games such as Pac Man or Space Invaders were mostly uni-dimensional, dominated by feelings of frustration and the occasional feeling of accomplishment - should we achieve entry into the high score table. In the following section I will review the kinds of feelings people experience with and through games and show how modern games offer a rich and varied emotional palette.

If you think back to the time when you last played a game, can you remember what you were feeling at the time? Were you laughing with your friends? Did you feel triumphant as you finished the boss-level? It is very likely that you remember the emotional component of your play experience. Indeed, neuroscientist and play researcher Jaak Panksepp (2004) argues that the two are inseparable owing to a neurological link where affective states are automatically activated during play. So important is this co-occurrence of play and affect, that his neurological definition of play explicitly *requires* concurrent firing of emotive behaviour patterns. It seems that without emotion, play cannot manifest.

The neurological evidence for co-presentation of play and affect would come as no surprise to play therapists, who have long argued that play is the language of children's feelings (Landreth & Homeyer, 1998). Without the verbal capacity of an adult, children have great difficulty expressing affect linguistically. Instead they use play to engage with their feelings. Sometimes the play can be expressive as in the knocking over towers of wooden blocks, other times it can be more symbolic as the child buries the 'bad man' in the sand pit and asks the toy animals to keep her safe. This concept of playing with emotion is borne out in adulthood also, where we control our fears in the play world as a means of dealing with the real world. During times of social stress, such as war, there is significant increase in the number of film and video-games released around the topic - giving us the chance to play with our emotions in a safe space.

Traditional thought on the evolutionary purpose of play is being re-examined, and the importance of emotion is coming to the fore. As highlighted by Sutton-Smith's examination of play rhetoric (2001), each scientific discipline tends to view play through its own specific lens. For example, Fagen (1976) was able to differentiate play behaviours in grizzly bears and found a positive correlation between play and survival.

Bears who play more, live longer - despite multiple disadvantages of play, such as increased attraction to predators, and the general risk of accident. For some, this supports their developmental view that play is a form of skill training preparing animals for later life. They argue that when play fighting, adolescents are actually developing the skills needed for hunting and defence - that this is the evolutionary importance of play. However, an experiment involving the deprivation of play in kittens did not result in an inability to hunt. Instead animals deprived of play appear to lack emotional intelligence - that is the ability to identify signals of emotion in others (see Brown, 2009, p60). The kittens could not determine the affective state of others, and as such failed to distinguish friend from foe. It seems that from an evolutionary perspective, the purpose of play is to develop the emotional intelligence necessary to live within a socially complex community. Through play we learn how to read emotion in others, we also learn to control our own emotions – whether play-fighting or losing at checkers.

Given that games are a sub-set of playful activity, and that play is an emotional pursuit, it is to be expected that video-games also elicit emotion. In his book, 21st Century Game Design, Chris Bateman (Bateman & Boon, 2005) details his review of the emotional episodes players report when playing video-games. He also lists the emotional experiences people seek when choosing a game. Based on over 1000 survey responses, where participants identified the principle emotion experienced when playing video-games and the extent to which they enhanced the experience, Bateman developed a Top 10 Video-game Emotion list (as shown in Table 1). It is interesting to note that the emotion people most look for in a game is amusement. Approximately 93% of respondents noted that 'amusement' was an emotion they seek when choosing video-game entertainment, and over 98% reported that they had experienced this emotion playing video-games previously. This maps onto other forms of entertainment, such

Table 1.Top 10 Emotions to Enhance Gameplay (Bateman & Boon, 2005)

Position	Emotion
1	Amusement
2	Contentment
3	Wonderment
4	Excitement
5	Curiosity
6	Fiero – the feeling we experience when triumphant against adversity
7	Surprise
8	Naches – the feeling of pride that comes from training others to play
9	Relief
10	Bliss

as film. In the UK, the largest grossing genre of 2008 was comedy, accounting for nearly 24% of box-office revenue (UK Film Council, 2009). It appears our lives are such that we need comedic relief when we turn to our media for emotional support.

Lazzaro (2008) has identified 4 high-level categories of enjoyment, which she calls the '4 Fun Keys'. In her original report (2004), the 4 categories were Hard Fun, Easy Fun, Altered States and People Factor (see Table 2 for an overview of each category). By 2008 the category 'Altered States' had been replaced by 'Serious Fun'. Lazzaro's most significant contribution comes from her attempt to match each of her 'fun' categories to a set of typical affective states, and the provision of example mechanics that might evoke them. For example she notes that fiero is more likely to co-occur with hard-fun, curiosity with easy-fun, amusement when playing with others, and relaxation when players were participating in serious-fun. Although each of Lazzaro's keys are associated with a principle emotion, they also open a further set of emotions. For example, fiero is the product of player's sense of achievement. Adventurers would have experienced this emotion upon reaching the North Pole, or completing their ascent of Everest. Others of us will have a similar experience when receiving good grades at school after expending great effort revising. But fiero is not the only emotion we experience when tasks are hard. We are likely to experience a feeling of hope at the outset as we plan for the challenge ahead, frustration and maybe anger as we deal with adversity, and relief when the task is complete. Indeed, the feeling of fiero is but one of a very varied palette of emotion.

One might expect the level of fiero evoked to correlate with size of achievement, such that the bigger the mountain we ascend, the greater the emotion we experience. However, I would argue instead that we all have our own mountains, however, they may appear as mere hills to others.

Table 2. Lazzaro's Four Fun Keys to Emotion (Lazzaro, 2008)

Key	Principle Emotion	Secondary Emotions	Mechanic Goal
Hard Fun	Fiero	Boredom Frustration Relief	Create challenge. Allow for strategy and mastery.
Easy Fun	Curiosity	Surprise Wonder Awe	Offer novelty, ambiguity, fantasy, and role-play.
People Fun	Amusement	Shadenfreude Naches Gratitude	Provide co=operation, competition, and socializing.
Serious Fun	Relaxation	Excitement Satisfaction	Self-challenge, learning or real work.

This is supported by Csikszentmihalyi's theory of Flow (1990). Flow is not tied to a specific set of emotions, but instead referred to as an optimal affective state. Flow is that feeling of being 'in the zone', where concepts of self, time, and the 'real word' subside and we feel at-one with our activity. It is an experience most of us will recognise, losing ourselves in a game to the point where hours have passed as though they were minutes. Activities that elicit Flow share a number of design features, too numerous to discuss here. However the most pertinent aspect of Flow is that it occurs when the activity is neither too easy, nor too hard. Tasks we find too easy rarely hold our attention for long periods, and those that we find too difficult also provide little engagement. As shown in Figure 1, when we develop skills, harder tasks become more engaging and activities once considered difficult will become too easy to hold our attention. For any task, different people have differing skill levels, and so my climbing a Monroe could elicit the same sensation of fiero as Hillary experienced when reaching the top of Everest.

Much less tangible than our emotional response to a video-game is the element Swink (2009) refers to as 'game feel' - the aesthetic sensation of control we experience when interacting with a video-game. Game feel is the melding of man and machine, where our cognition and motor-control are at one with the game, giving the sensation that our senses somehow extend into the game world. It can be likened to driving a car, where the mapping of cognition and car movement appears as one. We make a decision, and the car responds without conscious direction of our limbs. Our fine motor-control is no longer a perceptual barrier to the machine.

Swink argues that good design produces an intuitive interaction, where control feels natural. However, sometimes the design team fails to achieve that feeling, and instead the interaction might be described as too floaty or loose. Whenever we push a button or shake our wii remote the game responds. Mario might move left or right, he might jump or even double-jump. How the game responds, and in particular the timing of that response, will have distinct impact on how we perceive our level of control. When playing a video-game it will typically take a player 240 milliseconds (ms) to perceive, think, and then perform an action. Should the game take longer than 240 ms to respond to player input, the sensation of real-time interaction is lost. Responses of 0ms-100ms feel 'instant', whereas 150ms-240ms response would seem sluggish (Swink, 2009).

Much of our control sensation comes from the interaction envelope – that is the time it takes for Mario to reach maximum speed from button

Figure 1. Flow Channel (Csikszentmohalyi, 1990)

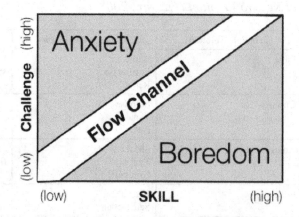

depression, and the time it takes for Mario to then stop moving on button release. Example envelopes are shown in Figures 2-4. In Figure 2 we see an interaction where Mario's acceleration increases exponentially when the button is pressed until a maximum speed is achieved, and then slowly ramps down when the button is released. This gives the perception of 'fluid and responsive' control. The envelope shown in Figure 3 is much more immediate, and as such the interaction feels 'stiff'. The interaction shown in Figure 4 offers little response upon button depression and a slow, gradual acceleration to maximum speed. Such an interaction would feel unresponsive, and the player might wonder if the controller was broken.

HOW GAMES ELICIT EMOTION

Game developers employ numerous techniques to generate emotion. Traditionally games elicit emotion through the game mechanics. However, in-line with the evolution of computing power, video-games can now generate rich visuals and dynamic audio in real-time and are able to borrow many techniques applied in film and animation. Modern video-games are a mash-up of different approaches, where emotions are evoked using a variety of media that now contribute to the video-

game experience. In the following section I shall introduce the fundamental structure of games, and then discuss ways in which we might elicit emotion through game mechanics, the game's aesthetic, narrative, and orchestral score to deliver a powerful experience comparable to film.

Game Mechanics and Emotion

The seminal work of Reeves and Nass (1996) where they substitute computers for humans in a number of social psychology experiments, show that our interaction with computers mirror many of our social and emotional interactions with humans. It seems that we approach interactions with artificial agents in much the same way as organic ones. Games such as Nintendogs, and the Petz series, and toys like Tamagotchi and Furby all exploit our natural tendency to humanize our relationship with artificial agents. Caretaking games/toys compel us to care for, and thus foster emotional attachment to virtual animals. Our emotional involvement with our virtual pets is such that we display examples of real emotional stress when away from our pet, and we mourn them when they 'die'. Artificial pets share a few simple mechanics that encourage owner attachment, such as appearing to be autonomous - in that the virtual pet appears to have free, rather than a programmed response to their owner; they are dependent on their owner for survival and/or

Figure 2. Fluid and responsive interaction (Swink, 2009)

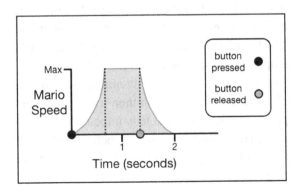

Figure 3. Stiff game-feel (Swink, 2009)

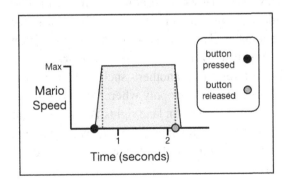

Figure 4. Unresponsive game-feel (Swink, 2009)

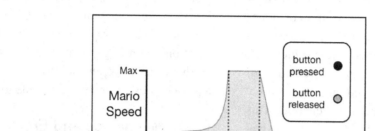

emotional health; and they reflect the accomplishment of the owner through positive or negative behaviours (Donath, 2004).

Through their MDA framework LeBlanc, Hunicke, and Zubek (2004) explain how game designers elicit emotion using game mechanics. MDA refers to game Mechanics, which affect player Dynamics, which then result in Aesthetic - or player feeling. Where houses use brick and cement in their construction, games use mechanics and resources. A game *mechanic* is a pattern of actions available to accomplish the player's game objectives. For example, to move our avatar in Monopoly we apply a 'roll-and-move' mechanic, which involves rolling dice and moving the number of squares identified.

Most game mechanics concern either the movement of resources (within the same play-space or between play-spaces), or the resolution of player conflict. The above roll-and-move mechanic is an example where the player moves within the same play-space. However, 'trading' is a mechanic that allows the movement of a resource from one space to another. This might be a private transaction where the player gives one set of resources to the bank in return for another - such as the purchase of property in Monopoly where the player gives currency in return for land rights. Alternatively, it might be accomplished openly between players, such as in Settlers of Catan where the actioned player initiates a trade of resource cards by

proclaiming a product they have available for trade and the items they require to complete the transaction. Should two or more players declare interest in the deal they enter into conflict for prized resources and an auction mechanic is implemented to bring about resolution - with the player offering the more valuable resources being the victor. In a video-game context a movement mechanic might be as simple as pressing left on the game pad to move Pac-Man three pixels to the left, or it might involve selecting an item and then pointing to its destination - such as in StarCraft. Like board-games, video-games also involve the movement of items from one play-space to another – for example, spawning characters in a first-person perspective shooting game (FPS) such as Unreal. For a comprehensive compilation of game mechanics, Bjork and Holopainen (2004) have done a superb job of describing most core game mechanics as a series of design patterns.

Game mechanics typically allow players to manage their own *resources*, and to challenge the management of their opponent's resources. The board-game Settlers of Catan, for example, employs traditional resources, such as brick, wheat, and wood. Players attempt to acquire sets of resources that they can then trade for victory points, while simultaneously impeding the progress on their opponent. Games such as Thebes and Space Dealer are less traditional, and use 'time' as a resource. Here specific actions have a temporal cost associated, and how you manage 'time' is key to winning the game. Video-games also concern resources although they are not always so salient. Tekken, for example, is a beat-em-up game where the goal is to deplete your opponent's health resource through the application of conflict resolution mechanics - such as punch, kick, etc.

We call the *function* of a mechanic its *dynamic* (LeBlanc *et al.*, 2004). 'The Downfall of Pompeii' is a board-game where players prepare for the impending eruption of Mount Vesuvius. The game includes a mechanic where the volcano erupts upon the drawing of the 2nd 'A.D.79' Omen card. In this way, the Omen deck is a mechanic that functions as a timer, informing the players of imminent disaster. LeBlanc *et al* (2004) make a distinction between the action (in this example, the mechanic of drawing Omen cards) from the function it performs (the countdown dynamic that results). Understanding how a series of game mechanics might elicit specific player dynamics is the dark art of game design. For example, the main mechanic of the board game Settlers of Catan involves the trade of resources between players. With player victory points being displayed openly, a common dynamic is for players to stop trading with the leading player – as this avoids feeding them the winning resources. Because of this, it is common for a further dynamic to appear where players avoid early lead position and instead make a late sprint to accumulate winning victory points. I am unsure whether Klaus Teuber, the designer of Settlers of Catan, initially meant for this dynamic to occur or whether this was a fortunate accident. Player dynamics are often hard to predict during the design process as they are influenced by a number of different factors - such as the state of the game, the strategies adopted by players, and the relationship between players.

The game's *aesthetic* is the subjective quality we experience as a direct consequence of the game's dynamic (LeBlanc et al., 2004). As such, the aesthetic does not refer to the overall play experience (including the graphics, sound, and narrative), but the experience of gameplay only. LeBlanc clearly identifies emotion evoked by mechanics and dynamics as being separate from affect generated by the game's audio, visual or haptic output. The emotional experience of aesthetic can be very powerful, despite the lack of multimedia support. Those of you who have experienced the dismay of losing good friends over a game of Diplomacy will, I am sure, concur.

Aesthetic Experience, Narrative and Emotion

In 1999 Ramachandran and Hirstein argued for a neurological theory of aesthetic experience, which academics have since built upon to describe the cognitive processes involved when we experience visual images. Leder et al (2004) present a cognitive model of how we process visual images – such as paintings, and Grodal's PECMA flow model (2009) offers a similar explanation of how film affects us emotionally. While there is some variation between the two models, they agree that our understanding of an image involves both conscious and subconscious processing.

Both authors agree that perception of an image involves subconscious processes necessary to identify visual forms, such as contour, colour, contrast, symmetry, order and grouping. Once processed, our implicit memory becomes activated (along with any emotional tags) as we attempt to find a match for the perceived image. Grodal (p149) gives the example where black and yellow lines are perceived and a matched association with 'tiger' is made. When the image is matched, related emotions are also activated, and in the tiger example can elicit a feeling of fear. Where difficulty exists matching form to memories (as can be the case with abstract paintings), the viewer might still experience a meaningful feeling of intense perceptual pleasure. This, claims Grodal, is because the brain is constantly looking for meaning, giving the sense of significance even where none is found.

Ramachandran and Hirstein (1999) found that we display aesthetic and affective preference for particular formations during the subconscious matching process. They report of a phenomenon where we naturally prefer images where defining features of a familiar image are amplified. They call this the peak-shift phenomenon. They found that the greater the amplification, the more typical the image becomes. For example, a caricature of Nixon may be considered more Nixon-like than a photograph of the ex-president. This suggests that affective preference for an image may increase with both familiarity and prototypicality (the extent to which the image represents a class of images). This is supported by Kunst-Wilson & Zajonc (1980) who found that familiarity, even where the image is degraded such that it is no longer recognizable, can still positively impact viewer preference.

In an attempt to comprehend the image, it is argued that we apply conscious processes. In the context of viewing a painting, this might involve drawing upon our knowledge of the artist, the historical importance of the painting, or what we might know of the subject depicted. In the context of film, the viewer attempts to align the image with the developing narrative, but will also draw upon their wider world knowledge. In this way the aesthetic experience is largely subjective and reliant upon our own personal connection. Subjective identification with art, whether aesthetic or narrative, is often key to our emotional engagement. In a bid to enhance the personal connection between media and consumer, authors and scriptwriters will apply techniques such as *imaginative elaboration* (Glassner, 2004, p98), where elements of the story are purposely ambiguous so as to facilitate audience self-projection. This then enhances the emotional tie between story and viewer. Applying this technique, writers provide only enough detail to make their characters believable, forcing the audience to breath their own personal experience into them. The result of this process is that

we then share personal, and potentially intimate connection with the character's story.

The first generation of video-games (going back to Pong) offered black and white graphics, simple beeps, and little narrative beyond a basic back-story. The primary avenue for emotion elicitation was the game's mechanics. As the machinery evolved, the software was able to exploit richer graphics, offer complex sounds, and provide a more involved story. Game developers typically applied narrative to provide emotional context for a player's actions (a notable exception being the text-based title 'Adventure', arguably the first interactive narrative and precursor to the MMORPG). Rescuing the kidnapped princess gives Mario a purpose, a reason to continue his ludic journey. Like our relationship with virtual pets, we find it hard to deny the pleas of the princess. The narrative hands us responsibility for her welfare, and makes it clear the princess is dependant upon us for survival. The story thus attempts to tie us emotionally to the outcome of the game, and gives added pertinence to our actions.

Traditionally stories are delivered linearly, with the medium dictating the pace and order of delivery. For example, films start at the beginning and then run at 24 frames per second until the last frame is shown. A film does not stop and wait for the audience to catch up should they miss the plot – it carries on regardless. Film does not allow the viewer to choose the direction of the story - this has been set by the production team and remains the same for each viewing. However, computer technology supports the possibility of interactive narrative, where the audience decides how the story will unfold, each and every time they play. Modern titles, such as Heavy Rain, have adjusted the gameplay/narrative balance and now play like interactive stories, and less like games. In Heavy Rain, for example, game mechanics are used to support the narrative, enhancing the perception of presence and increasing the viewer's sense of control over the character's fate.

It is thought that emotions generated through storytelling are potentially less potent than those that game mechanics elicit. This is because game mechanics affect you directly, whereas narrative generates 'fictional' emotion. It was philosopher Colin Radford (1975) who first promoted the paradox of fictional emotions. While watching a horror movie we see a 'monster', and although we know that the creature is a fiction and cannot truly harm us, we still feel an emotional reaction that seems much like fear. Feagin (1996) makes the case that fictional emotions are mostly sympathetic or empathic responses to the characters and their situation, and that this is subjectively different from feeling emotions first hand. In a laboratory setting, Mandryk & Inkpen (2004) compared the impact of both direct and fictional emotions. Using physiological indicators (both electrodermal and EMG) and subjective reports, arousal was measured when players were competing against both a computer-controlled opponent (fictional character) and a human opponent. As they hypothesised, player arousal increased significantly when competing against a human opponent, as did self-report measures. This suggests we have a different, and possibly less powerful emotional response to situations we know to be fictitious.

Music, Emotion, and Games

Music is a powerful tool for evoking human emotion. It has been used on battlefields to rouse and motivate soldiers, it was used in cinema to manipulate the tears of an audience long before talking movies existed, and is used daily to motivate exercise. There are a number of ways in which music might trigger an emotional response, one of which is the intrinsic structure of the piece. Sloboda (1991, 1992) has identified specific characteristics of music that are consistently found to elicit emotion, such as syncopations, enharmonic changes and melodic appoggiaturas. It appears to be that the structural changes within the piece influence our emotional experience of it. This

is accomplished through the disruption and/or maintenance of audience expectations.

It is not just the structure of music that leads to an emotional response. Music, like many sensory stimuli, can trigger strong memories of past emotional events. Upon retrieval of the memory we are prone to re-live the associated emotion. When we hear 'our song', our attention is drawn to the memory of that first dance with our loved one - and we re-live the positive affect experienced at that time. The difficulty of eliciting emotions via memory is that our life experiences are subjective. The music that triggers an emotional memory for me is unlikely to trigger a similar response in others. Therefore, for a game developer to elicit associated emotion through music, they must find culturally significant pieces - music that has a shared communal response. A good example of such is the soundtrack to Battlefield Vietnam where the music triggers iconic memories of life in the 60s - even for those of us too young to have experienced the era. The cultural importance of the 1960s - a decade which saw advances in the liberal political movement, change in popular music, space exploration leading to the moon landing, the death of JFK, and the Vietnam war - has resulted in extensive media exposure of the decade in the form of documentary, film, and television. The extensive media coverage has shaped our memories of the period to such an extent that we all share common emotions on which Battlefield Vietnam was able to capitalise.

The emotional power of audio in gameplay is best exemplified by work carried out at Sonic Studio in Sweden. They have developed Beowulf, a game for the iPhone that is primarily audio-based (Liljedahl, Papworth, & Lindberg, 2007). In the game you are blind, but for minor spatial visualisation that identifies the layout of rooms, thus avoiding the need for good spatial memory. As you move between locations you determine the terrain from subtle changes in the sound of your steps and ambient sounds such as the howling wind. The player must identify the content of a room, and combat against foe, based purely on the environment's soundscape - no narration is given. The game was not developed for the blind, but as an exploration of what can be accomplished when attention is shifted from the eyes to the ears. The studio reported that players found the game experience emotional, they became free to create their own mental imagery of the game world, allowing the designer to exploit the 'scary shadow syndrome' - a technique used in horror movies where a hint of what is off-screen has greater emotional impact than actually showing the monster.

Recent studies carried out within the eMotionLab at Glasgow Caledonian University have shown that our emotional relationship to music can impact our gaming behaviour (Cassidy & MacDonald, in press; Khan, Cassidy & Sykes, in press). Cassidy and MacDonald (2009) looked at driving performance while playing Project Gotham with (and without) music. The game comes with a number of modes, allowing players to race against time, race against an opponent, or navigate a course of cones. Under experimental conditions, Cassidy asked players to complete one of the cone navigation tasks while listening to player-selected music, or music that had been independently rated as having a highly arousing intrinsic structure. Interestingly, she found players were quicker and more accurate (i.e., hitting fewer cones) when they listened to their preferred music. A similar effect was found by Kahn *et al* (in press) when looking at music preference during exergaming. They found that music impacts the extent of effort exertion when participants jog on Nintendo's WiiFit. Music has long been known to encourage exercise, and songs with a high beat-per-minute are commonly used to increase exercise in the gym. However, Khan *et al* found listening to our preferred choice of music impacts exertion above and beyond the effect of the beats-per-minute measure.

Future iOpiates

So far we have discussed how current video-game technology might elicit emotion, showing how developers employ techniques used in game design, film production, music composition, and story telling. We will now consider the next evolutionary development of iOpiate - games that monitor our emotional engagement and dynamically tailor the experience accordingly.

During an emotional episode we undergo physiological changes such as increased heart-rate, changes in blood flow, and perspiration. We might also communicate our affect through facial gesture, intonation of voice, and/or body posture. To obtain an objective measure of emotion, psychologists employ a variety of techniques to record physiological changes. A widely used technique is the measurement of electro-dermal activity (EDA), where a small electrical current is passed across the surface of the skin. With increased arousal there is often an increase in perspiration, which will alter the resistance of the electrical current. Changes in the EDA measure will therefore indicate a possible autonomic change. Li & Chen (2006) have developed a system that can identify 22 features of our physiology and make an 85% accurate assessment of the discreet emotion experienced. An alternative approach to physiological measurement is to consider gesture. Ekman (1982) developed the Facial Action Coding System (FACS) as a means to determine discrete emotions through examination of facial gestures. This can be a laborious process of coding muscle activation to determine the emoted affect. To aid the coding of facial muscles there are now a number of software solutions which analyse video footage in real-time, such as Face Reader (published by Noldus).

In recent years researchers and private companies have made attempts to apply affective technology to video-games. In 2003, Sykes and Brown applied Clynes' (1978) work on sentics (the emotional aspect of touch) to investigate how arousal levels may be determined through measurement of gamepad button depression. A more complex solution is offered by Journey into the Wild Divine (JitWD), an off-the-shelf video-game that comes with bespoke technology to measure electrodermal activity and heart rate. Hazlett (2006) has also shown that we can track movement in facial muscles using electromyography to measure emotional valence of game players. More recently, in 2009 Emotiv released a headset for domestic use that can read EEG signals during gameplay. For a review of physiological devices that can measure emotion during gameplay see Mandryk, Inkpen, & Calvert (2006).

The reason why games have become the focus of affective technology is two-fold. Firstly, as explored earlier in this chapter, play is an emotionally rich experience. Video-games are a bridge between technology and the play experience, making them the ideal space for affective technologies. Secondly, video-games (unlike film, music or literature) are dynamic. They respond differently dependant upon the dialogue with their players. Repeated play does not provide the exact same experience, and we are not assured successful achievement of our goals every time we play. By allowing games to respond not merely to player intent but also player emotion, we have the opportunity to foster a richer ludic experience. As identified by Gilleade & Dix (2004), there are a number of different ways in which affective interaction could generate more satisfying experience. Games that detect the affective state of the player can provide bespoke gameplay where the challenge adapts relative to player stress. For example, the game Tetris involves rotation and placement of falling shapes. At the beginning the blocks fall slowly, making it easy for the player to perform the necessary actions. As players progress, the rate of descent increases making the game much more difficult, eventually becoming too hard for the player. By monitoring arousal levels, it would be possible to adjust the speed at which blocks fall to match the player's stress levels, thus maintaining

the optimal experience (i.e., flow). Alternatively, games might involve your affective state as part of a game mechanic. A good example of this can be found in JitWD's archery game. Here the player alters their state of arousal to aim the bow. To direct the aim down, the player must relax. However, as they begin to align the perfect shot the body naturally responds to the excitement of goal achievement and arousal increases, thus creating conflict between a player's intent and their affective response. It has also been suggested that affective gameplay could potentially allow for more realistic gameplay. In narrative driven games the non-player characters might react emotionally to affect expressed by the player (Hudlicka, 2009). If characters could respond to how we are feeling, the game-world would likely appear more believable, thus increasing the potential for enhanced emotional engagement.

CONCLUSION

Throughout the chapter we discussed how game technologies elicit affect, particularly through game mechanics, aesthetic, narrative and music. Although the emotion junky might not be satisfied by retro games such as Pong and Pac-Man, current iOpiates mash-up emotionally rich media offering an experience comparable to competing artifacts, such as TV or film. With the recent advancement in techniques to measure affect we will likely see greater emotional interaction, and can expect video-games to supersede linear media to become the emotion drug of choice for the next generation of junkies.

REFERENCES

Bateman, C., & Boon, R. (2005). *21st Century Game Design*. Hingham, MA: Charles River Media.

Bjork, S., & Holopainen, J. (2004). *Patterns in Game Design*. Hingham, MA: Charles River Media.

Brown, S. (2009). *Play: How it shapes the brain, opens the Imagination and invigorates the soul*. London: Penguin Books.

Caillois, R. (1958). *Man, Play and Games*. Chicago: University of Illinois Press.

Cassidy, G. G., & MacDonald, R. A. R. (2009, Fall). The effects of music choice on task performance: a study of the impact of self-selected and experimenter-selected music on driving game performance and experience. *Musicae Scientiae, 13*(2), 357–386.

Cassidy, G. G., & MacDonald, R. A. R. (in press). The effects of music on time perception and performance of a driving game. *Scandinavian Journal of Psychology*.

Clynes, M. (1978). *Sentics*. Garden City, NY: Anchor Press.

Csikszentmihalyi, M. (1990). *Flow: The psychology of optimal experience*. New York: Harper & Row.

Donath, J. (2004). Artificial pets: simple behaviors elicit complex attachments. In Bekoff, M. (Ed.), *The Encyclopedia of Animal Behavior. Santa Barbara*. Greenwood Press.

Egenfeldt Nielsen, S., Heide Smith, J., & Pajares Tosca, S. (2008). *Understanding Video Games*. London: Routledge Taylor and Francis Group.

Ekman, P. (1982). Methods for measuring facial action. In Scherer, K. R., & Ekman, P. (Eds.), *Handbook of methods in nonverbal behavior research*. Cambridge: Cambridge University Press.

Fagen, R. (1976). Modelling how and why play works. In J.S. Bruner, Alison Jolly & Kathy Sylva, (Eds.), *Play*, New York: Basic Books

Feagin, S. (1996). *Reading with Feeling*. New York: Cornell University Press.

Freeman, D. (2004). *Creating Emotion in Games*. London: New Riders.

Gillieade, K., & Dix, A. (2004). Using frustration in the design of adaptive videogames. *Proceedings of ACE 2004, Advances in Computer Entertainment Technology*, (pp 228-232). New York: Association for Computing Machinery

Glassner, A. (2004). *Interactive Storytelling Techniques for 21st Century Fiction*. Natick, MA: AK Peters.

Grodal, T. (2009). *Embodied Visions*. Oxford: Oxford University Press. doi:10.1093/acprof:oso/9780195371314.001.0001

Hazlett, R. L. (2006). *Measuring emotional valence during interactive experiences: Boys at video game play. CHI 2006 Proceedings* (pp. 22–27). New York: Association for Computing Machinery.

Hudlicka, E. (2009). Affective game engines: motivation and requirements. *Proceedings of the 4th International Conference On The Foundation Of Digital Games*. 299-306

Huizinga, J. (1938). *Homo Ludens*. London: Routledge.

Khan, R., & Cassidy, G. & Sykes. (in press). Impact of Music on Ergogenic and Psychophysical Outcomes of Exercise in a Gameplay Context. *International Journal of Computer Science in Sport*.

Khan, R., & Sykes, J. (2005). *Emotions evoked during collaborative and competitive play when players are co-located and spatially separated*. Paper presented at the Digital Games Research Association conference, Vancouver, Canada

Kunst-Wilson, W., & Zajonc, R. (1980). Affective discrimination of stimuli that cannot be recognized. *Science, 207,* 557–558. doi:10.1126/science.7352271

Landreth & Homeyer. (1998). Play as the language of children's feelings. In Fromberg, D., & Bergen, D. (Eds.), *Play from Birth to Twelve and Beyond: Contexts, Perspectives and Meanings* (pp. 193–196). London: Routledge.

Lazzaro, N. (2004). *Why we play games: Four keys to more emotion in player experiences*. Retrieved December 1st 2009 from www.xeodesign.com/xeodesign_whyweplaygames.pdf

Lazzaro, N. (2008). Why we play: Affect and the fun of games. In Sears, A., & Jacko, J. A. (Eds.), *The Human-Computer Interaction Handbook. Abingdon: Taylor and Francis Group.*

LeBlanc, M., Hunicke, R., & Zubek, R. (2004) *MDA: A formal approach to game design and game research*. Retrieved December 1st 2009, from www.cs.northwestern.edu/~hunicke/MDA.pdf

Leder, H., Belke, B., Oeberst, A., & Augustin, D. (2004). A model of aesthetic appreciation and aesthetic judgements. *The British Journal of Psychology, 95*, 489–508. doi:10.1348/0007126042369811

Li, L., & Chen, J. (2006). Emotion recognition using physiological signals. In Pan, Z. (Eds.), *Lecture Notes in Computer Science: Advances in Artificial Reality and Tele-existence* (pp. 437–446). Berlin: Springer-Verlag. doi:10.1007/11941354_44

Liljedahl, M., Papworth, N., & Lindberg, S. (2007). Beowolf - an Audio Mostly game. *Proceedings of the internationals conference on Advances in computer entertainment technology 2007* (ACE'07) (pp 200-203), New York: Association for Computing Machinery

Mandryk, R., & Inkpen, K. (2004). Physiological indicators for the evaluation of Co-located collaborative play. In *Proceedings of the ACM Conference on Computer Supported Cooperative Work (CSCW 2004)* (pp 102-111), New York: Association for Computing Machinery

Mandryk, R., Inkpen, K., & Calvert, T. (2006, March-April). Using Psychophysiological Techniques to Measure User Experience with Entertainment Technologies. [Special Issue on User Experience]. *Behaviour & Information Technology, 25*(2), 141–15. doi:10.1080/01449290500331156

Norman, D. (2002). Emotion and design: Attractive things work better. *Interaction, 9*(4), 36–42. doi:10.1145/543434.543435

Panksepp, J. (2004). *Affective Neuroscience*. Oxford: Oxford University Press.

Radford, C. (1975). 'How can we be moved by the fate of Anna Karenina?' *Proceedings of the Aristotelian Society*, supplementary vol. 49, 67-80

Ramachandran, V., & Hirstein, W. (1999). The Science of Art. *Journal of Consciousness Studies, 6*(6-7), 15–51.

Reeves, B., & Nass, C. (1996). *The Media Equation: how people treat computers, television and new media like real people and places*. New York: Cambridge University Press.

Rosenberg, D. (2009). Video games outsell movies in UK. *CNET*. Retrieved April 4th 2010 from http://news.cnet.com/8301-13846_3-10423150-62.html

Sloboda, J. A. (1991). Music structure and emotional response: Some empirical findings. *Psychology of Music, 19*, 110–120. doi:10.1177/0305735691192002

Sloboda, J. A. (1992). Empirical studies of emotional response to music. In Riess-Jones, M., & Holleran, S. (Eds.), *Cognitive basis of musical communication* (pp. 33–46). Washington, DC: American Psychological Society. doi:10.1037/10104-003

Sutton-Smith, B. (2001). *The Ambiguity of Play*. Cambridge, MA: Harvard University Press.

Swink, S. (2009). *Game Feel*. London: Morgan Kaufmann.

Sykes, J., & Brown, S. (2003). Affective gaming: measuring emotion through the gamepad. *Proceedings of Association for Computing Machinery (ACM) Special Interest Group on Computer-Human Interaction Conference (CHI)* (pp 732-733), New York: Association for Computing Machinery

UK Film Council. (2009). 09 Statistical Year Book, Retrieved 1st December 2009 from http://www.ukfilmcouncil.org/yearbook

ADDITIONAL READING

Frijda, N. (1986). *The Emotions*. Cambridge: Cambridge University Press.

Fullerton, T., Swain, C., & Hoffman, S. (2004). *Game design workshop*. Gilroy, CA: CMP Books.

Juslin, P. N., & Sloboda, J. A. (Eds.). (2009). *Handbook of Music and Emotion: Theory, Research, Applications*. Oxford: Oxford University Press.

Lewis, M., Haviland-Jones, J., & Barrett, L. (Eds.). (2008). *Handbook of Emotions*. London: Guildford Press.

Norman, D. (2004). *Emotional design*. New York: Basic Books.

Pellis, S., & Pellis, V. (2009). *The playful brain: Venturing to the limits of neuroscience*. Oxford: Oneworld Publishing.

Picard, R. (1998). *Affective Computing*. Cambridge, MA: MIT Press.

Plantinga, C., & Smith, G. M. (Eds.). (1999). *Passionate views: Film, cognition, and emotion*. Baltimore, MD: The John Hopkins University Press.

Salen, K., & Zimmerman, E. (2004). *Rules of play: Game design fundamentals*. Cambridge, MA: MIT Press.

Salen, K., & Zimmerman, E. (2006). *The game design reader: A rules of play anthology*. Cambridge, MA: MIT Press.

Epilogue
A Philosophical Perspective on Incorporating Emotions in Human Computer Interaction

Zeynep Başgöze
Middle East Technical University, Turkey

Ahmet Inam
Middle East Technical University, Turkey

Recently attempts are being made to enhance Human-Computer Interaction (HCI) in order to achieve a sound communication between humans and computers just as the way people communicate with each other. In order to succeed in doing so, human-like computers should be created. Creating a computer which understands and acts like a human being is considered as the best move for the intention of enhancing HCI.

THE NEED FOR AFFECTIVE COMMUNICATION

One of the issues that latest studies emphasize is the importance of inclusion of emotions in this interaction, since a real-life interaction does not seem to be provided without this aspect. Com-

puters emerged as a product of the human mind. However, if the aim is to make computers much more like human beings, then the fact that humans are not made up solely of the mind should be considered. Human beings possess substantial amount of abilities besides their thoughts. Emotions may not be perceived consciously, due to a multitude of things happening in the body which the mind—or the thoughts—cannot control. For example, emotions, physical responses of the bodies (reflexes, pains etc) as well as culture can be reckoned as such abilities. There are numerous factors which can ideologically and biologically influence humans outside of consciousness. As far as emotions are concerned, in order to act and respond like human beings, a human-like machine has to "infer" some affective features of humans such as mood and communicate accordingly.

On the other hand, from the human perspective, initially humans had difficulties in getting acquainted with the computer technology, since it seemed so distant and cold. Computers were perceived as mechanical, metallic and inorganic tools. Over time, everybody got used to utilizing these machines, but only as tools that facilitate their lives. Moreover, in reverse fashion, the facilitation of remote communication provided by these machines led people to become unsocial creatures who tend to stay at their homes in front of the computers. Alternatively, rather than humans just dictating whatever they want the computer to perform, a more active relationship which allows the computer to initiate/share affective communication could be constructed.

In order to succeed in constructing a proper HCI which can translate emotional reactions of users to the computer, we should first comprehend emotional reactions of human beings clearly. There exist some tools in order to measure physiological expressions of emotions such as skin conductance, heart rate, eye tracking ... etc. However, these tools' adequacy in measuring emotions is a questionable issue. Human beings are much more than the behaviors they show.

The existing technology of our times only allow for processing of measurements such as blood pressure, electrical pulsation, brain waves, and facial expressions which can be translated into the recognition of emotions. Although the helpfulness of these tools for observing the physical outputs of emotions is inarguable, it is almost impossible to identify and generalize an emotion in its entirety just by looking at these measures. People from different cultures may seem to understand and claim to perceive basic emotions, but what they really feel inside may be totally different. Moreover, different people and different cultures may have different emotional reactions.

Going back to computers, although they may be augmented with the aforementioned physiological technology, human-like machines will still be just "machines". This is because computers

exist in a world which cannot be considered as a phenomenal world, where human beings can touch, smell, see, hear and taste things, by utilizing the physical environment they live in. Humans are always in a continuous interaction with their outer world within which they can experience things. The reflections of their experiences, what they exactly feel, on the other hand, are in their brain. No one can define clearly and objectively someone else's feeling. In the very same way, computers, although they may "seem" to feel or process emotion-related information, they will not actually feel and define the exact meaning of the feelings of humans with which they interact.

This presents a huge problem both for philosophy and technology. Let's assume that human behaviors, actions and neural reactions can be measured somehow with electrical wirings or probes penetrating the skull (i.e. using EEG), and these outputs can also be reflected on a computer screen. The results on the screen may show that the person is excited. However, how that person feels and experiences that excitement may be considerably different than the reflections of this excitement outside the body. One's sensation of a specific feeling could conflict with another person's sensation of the same "physical" feeling. Can the machine experience the exact phenomena that humans experience, or not? This is a very crucial point to be addressed.

HUMAN-LIKE COMPUTERS

If scientists somehow achieve to create something which has the same neural networks as humans have, could we call it a "human being"? This also, is an important problem in philosophy. Philosophers diverge on the issue that a human being's identical twin or something similar to him/her could be created or not. Let's assume that the technical problems are solved with the help of genetic engineering and such a creature is created. If they clone someone at birth and provide the same external conditions for this clone while it is developing, would there be any differences with the original creature? Will this brand-new clone experience phenomenally? Will it feel intrinsically? Or will it play "being human", i.e. just imitate? What if some material is brought from somewhere else and a human body is constructed without missing any detail? Would this creature "feel" like a human being?

On another front, creating a complete human being with all its details seems impossible. This is because scientists induce while trying to congregate little parts in order to reach the sum or in other words, the whole picture. However, a human being is much more than the sum of its parts. There is a topological divergence here. One cannot assume that a human being can be created just by concatenating some cells together. As for the information or computer technologies, the whole is formed by gathering pieces together; but as for the human beings, when all pieces are brought together something more is obtained. Mystically, one can call it a soul or energy. It is so difficult to tell whether a machine can feel or not. Scientists can gather pieces together, but there will always be this extraneous piece which cannot be generated by technology.

However, if someone claims that there is a spot in the brain —an emotion center— which causes the emotional life to be impaired when it malfunctions, then we could project that technology to create a human-like machine. Still, to think of a body part as an independent organ, separate from all the others is a very simple approach. Every body part is connected with other parts of the body. The whole has always an influence on the functioning of any other body part. Hence, the parts influence the whole and the whole influences the parts, which is called double hermeneutics in philosophy. Therefore, although it may be the case that the malfunction of a single emotional spot causes emotional problems, actually the emotional problem may occur because of the failure of one

or more spots (neurons or neuron groups) which congregate the whole emotional system in the brain. It is doubtful that this type of complexity could be embodied within an algorithm.

Let's now move on to another example: Searle's Chinese Room argument (1980). In this thought experiment, Searle stands in a room without knowing any Chinese. He receives Chinese characters from the outside of the room and then uses an English book where he can find all information about the instructions of a computer program which provides him to respond properly to this Chinese input. Although Searle does not understand any word in Chinese, he can successfully "seem" to know Chinese, just by performing the written instructions appropriately. The view that a computer can 'understand' what it performs is known as Strong AI (Artificial Intelligence). Thus, assuming the existence of a computer program which is created without the knowledge of how the information between emotion and cognition flows is a similar trade to the Chinese room, making us argue of computers which can "feel". Therefore, believing that computers can 'feel' rather than just "seem" to feel is a strong AI argument.

On the other hand, it is not clear whether the human brain knows what is going on within itself or not. Perhaps the brain works like a Chinese room too. The brain may also be an organ which shows outputs depending on some chemical and electrical processes, but it may not know or understand anything about what it actually does. Moreover, what is going on amongst people may also be viewed as just an interaction. Thus, the world may be a huge hall with lots of Brain-ese rooms in it.

UNDERSTANDING THE HUMAN BRAIN

When considered as an organism, it is pretty much correct that whatever happens in the brain is a process with which we cannot intervene and which we do not comprehend very well. It is very similar to the nature, to the fact that we do not understand well the structure of a growing flower or spawning of ants ..., etc. It is self-contained. This is one of the problems that can be faced in simulating humans: The body has something very different than it is thought, it has an internal order. Could we find out about that order sometime? Contrary to what is called "the self", the body performs continuously by itself, without asking anything of the self. You may enter the room, your butt just finds the correct place to sit, when you get into the car, you can drive home without even thinking about it, the body rides a bike, it swims, talks, ... etc. Even sometimes one may talk without planning what to say, because the body is actually a tutor. It is wise; it is much more than every one of us. This is exactly why Eastern philosophies suggest building an excellent endearment with the body. Being a part of an academic world, a part of a culture, a part of the world, people always suppose that they are merely composed of thoughts. Moreover they see their bodies as their slaves which should obey them upon commands. On the contrary, the body is the master. People have to listen to their bodies, have to try to understand what it says, since their body is their advisor. In philosophy, this way of thinking actually began with Nietzsche. Usually, philosophers, and perhaps the computer engineers also, suppose themselves as pure reason, a program. This is the mark of rationalism. However, the tutor, the body has a very different way of reasoning.

Through neurology and physiology, we try to comprehend the body. But it is clear that humanity has a huge problem understanding the mind exclusively. As far as philosophers are concerned, since Plato, they have always tried to put the body out of the mind, claiming that the body is mischievous. It needs to pee, it gets hungry, and it is awful. 2500 years old Western way of thinking has always disregarded the body. Not only philosophy but religions have also made the same mistake. Religions ordered not to gratify the flesh cravings, they ordered to disregard what body wants and to fight it down, because people are composed of pure souls, the body does not mean anything. This is a big deception. The body is merged in the mind. If the mind does not get the wisdom of the body, then it is condemned to stay as incomplete.

THE MISSING LINK: INWARDNESS

Although we could develop a system which can communicate with people, producing emotional input and outputs which human beings can understand and interpret correctly, this system would still have no actual emotions, even if it can act as if it has emotions. Human beings have an inner world. Would this inner world be also copied when the outer world is copied? It seems it is not possible, because the ones who want to build this creature must first know about this inner world and build the human-like machine accordingly. In order to create such a computer, the creators must also consider thoughts and beliefs, as well as inwardness. Inwardness should be examined deeply, considering its relationship with the brain parts. Inwardness is a reality felt and lived by artists, mindful people, and scientists who ruminate while researching. Anybody who looks at the sky and senses the mystery and the wisdom hidden in it can also travel inward.

In conclusion, to see human beings from a dualistic point of view will absolutely create obstacles in the way of constructing human-like machines. The puzzle of the brain may seem to be solved biologically, however, thinking about simulating it just by gathering its cells together will stay a delusion. For a neurosurgeon, the brain may seem to be highly clear and understandable, since doctors know where the brain parts should be located. However, it is still unknown how those parts create consciousness or feelings and how the congruent or incongruent actions of people with respect to their feelings participate in daily interactions. Therefore, without understanding how exactly humans "work", no one may succeed in creating a computer which works like a human.

Compilation of References

Abboud, B., & Davoine, F. (2004) Appearance factorization based facial expression recognition and synthesis. In *IEEE International Conference on Pattern Recognition*, 958 – 965.

About.com. (2010). *Women's History: Maggie Kuhn Quotes*. Retrieved March 27, 2010 from http://womenshistory.about.com/cs/quotes/a/maggie_kuhn.htm

Adamo, S. A., & Hanlon, R. T. (1996). Do cuttlefish (cephalopoda) signal their intentions to conspecifics during agonistic encounters? *Animal Behaviour*, (52): 73–81. doi:10.1006/anbe.1996.0153

Adelmann, P. K., & Zajonc, R. B. (1989). Facial efference and the experience of emotion. *Annual Review of Psychology*, *40*, 249–280. doi:10.1146/annurev.ps.40.020189.001341

Adolphs, R., Tranel, D., Damasio, H., & Damasio, A. (1994). Impaired recognition of emotion in facial expressions following bilateral damage to the human amygdala. *Nature*, *372*(6507), 669–672. doi:10.1038/372669a0

Adolphs, R., Tranel, D., Hamann, S., Young, A. W., Calder, A. J., & Phelps, E. A. (1999). Recognition of facial emotion in nine individuals with bilateral amygdala damage. *Neuropsychologia*, *37*, 1111–1117. doi:10.1016/S0028-3932(99)00039-1

Adolphs, R. (2002). Recognizing emotion from facial expressions: Psychological and neurological mechanisms. *Behavioral and Cognitive Neuroscience Reviews*, *1*(1), 21–62. doi:10.1177/1534582302001001003

Adolphs, R., Gosselin, F., Buchanan, T. W., Tranel, D., Schyns, P., & Damasio, A. R. (2005). A Mechanism for Impaired Fear Recognition after Amygdala Damage. *Nature*, *433*, 68–72. doi:10.1038/nature03086

Adolphs, R., Tranel, D., & Damasio, A. R. (1998). The Human Amygdala in Social Judgment. *Nature*, *393*, 470–474. doi:10.1038/30982

Adolphs, R., Tranel, D., Damasio, H., & Damasio, A. R. (1995). Fear and the Human Amygdala. *The Journal of Neuroscience*, *15*, 5879–5891.

Adolphs, R., & Tranel, D. (2000). Emotion recognition and the human amygdala. In Aggleton, J. P. (Ed.), *The amygdala. A functional analysis* (pp. 587–630). New York: Oxford University Press.

Aftanas, L., & Golocheikine, S. A. (2001). Human anterior and frontal midline theta and lower alpha reflect emotionally positive state and internalized attention: high-resolution EEG investigation of meditation. *Neuroscience Letters*, *310*(1), 57–60. doi:10.1016/S0304-3940(01)02094-8

Afzal, S., Sezgin, T. M., Gao, Y., & Robinson, P. (2009). Perception of Emotional Expressions in Different Representations Using Facial Feature Points. *Proc. Int. Conf. Affective Computing and Intelligent Interaction*.

Aharon, I., Etcoff, N., Ariely, D., Chabris, C. F., O'Connor, E., & Breiter, H. C. (2001). Beautiful faces have variable reward value: Fmri and behavioral evidence. *Neuron*, *32*(3), 537–551. doi:10.1016/S0896-6273(01)00491-3

Ahern, G. L., & Schwartz, G. E. (1985). Differential lateralization for positive and negative emotion in the human brain: EEG spectral analysis. *Neuropsychologia, 23*, 745–755. doi:10.1016/0028-3932(85)90081-8

Akgun, M., Cagiltay, K., & Zeyrek, D. (in press). The Effect of Apologetic Error Messages and Mood States on Computer Users' Self-Appraisal of Performance. *Journal of Pragmatics.*

Albrecht, K. (2005). *Social intelligence: The new science of success.* New York: John Wiley & Sons Ltd.

Albrecht, I., Schröder, M., Haber, J., & Seidel, H.-P. (2005). Mixed feelings: expression of non-basic emotions in a muscle-based talking head. *Virtual Reality (Waltham Cross), 8*(4), 201–212. doi:10.1007/s10055-005-0153-5

Alexander, O., Rogers, M., Lambeth, W., Chiang, M., & Debevec, P. (2009), Creating a Photoreal Digital Actor: The Digital Emily Project, *IEEE European Conference on Visual Media Production* (CVMP).

Altemus, M., Deuster, P. A., Gallıven, E., Carter, C. S., & Gold, P. W. (1995). Suppression of hypothalmic-pituitary-adrenal axis responses to stress in lactating women. *The Journal of Clinical Endocrinology and Metabolism, 80*, 2954–2959. doi:10.1210/jc.80.10.2954

Alton, J. (1995). *Painting with Light.* Berkeley: University of California Press.

Alyüz, N., Gökberk, B., Dibeklioğlu, H., Savran, A., Salah, A. A., Akarun, L., & Sankur, B. (2008). 3D Face Recognition Benchmarks on the Bosphorus Database with Focus on Facial Expressions. *Proc. First European Workshop on Biometrics and Identity Management* (pp.62–71).

Amaral, D. G., Behniea, H., & Kelly, J. L. (2003). Topographic organization of projections from the amygdala to the visual cortex in the macaque monkey. *Neuroscience, 118*, 1099–1120. doi:10.1016/S0306-4522(02)01001-1

Amaral, D. G. (2002). The Primate Amygdala and the Neurobiology of Social Behavior: Implications for Understanding Social Anxiety. *Biological Psychiatry, 51*, 11–17. doi:10.1016/S0006-3223(01)01307-5

Ambady, N., Krabbenhoft, M., & Hogan, D. (2006). The 30-sec sale: Using thin-slice judgments to evaluate sales effectiveness. *Journal of Consumer Psychology, 16*(1), 4–13. doi:10.1207/s15327663jcp1601_2

Ambady, N., & Rosenthal, R. (1992). Thin slices of expressive behavior as predictors of interpersonal consequences: a meta-analysis. *Psychological Bulletin, 111*(2), 256–274. doi:10.1037/0033-2909.111.2.256

Ambady, N., Bernieri, F., & Richeson, J. (2000). Towards a histology of social behavior: judgmental accuracy from thin slices of behavior. In Zanna, M. (Ed.), *Advances in experimental social psychology* (pp. 201–272).

American Psychiatric Association. (2000). *Diagnostic and Statistical Manual of Mental Disorders: DSM-IV-TR* (4th ed.). Washington, DC: American Psychiatric Association.

Amir, N., Ron, S., & Laor, N. (2000). Analysis of an emotional speech corpus in Hebrew based on objective criteria. In *Proceedings of the ISCA Workshop on Speech & Emotion* (pp. 29-33).

Anders, S., Lotze, M., Erb, M., Grodd, W., & Birbaumer, N. (2004). Brain Activity Underlying Emotional Valence and Arousal: A Response-Related fMRI Study. *Human Brain Mapping, 23*, 200–209. doi:10.1002/hbm.20048

Ang, J., Dhillon, R., Krupski, A., Shriberg, E., & Stolcke, A. (2002). Prosody-based automatic detection of annoyance and frustration in human-computer dialog. In *Proceedings of ICSLP, 02*, 2037–2040.

Anolli, L. (2002). MaCHT—miscommunication as chance theory: toward a unitary theory of communication and miscommunication. In Anolli, L., Ciceri, R., & Riva, G. (Eds.), *Say not to say: new perspectives on miscommunication* (pp. 3–42). Amsterdam: IOS Press.

Antheunis, M. L., Valkenburg, P. M., & Peter, J. (2010). Getting acquainted through Social Network Sites: Testing a model of online uncertainty reduction and social attraction. *Computers in Human Behavior, 26*, 100–109. doi:10.1016/j.chb.2009.07.005

Anttonen, J., & Surakka, V. (2005). *Emotions and heart rate while sitting on a chair.* Paper presented at the CHI '05: Proceedings of the SIGCHI conference on Human factors in computing systems.

Arbib, M. A. (2005). From monkey-like action recognition to human language: An evolutionary framework for neurolinguistics. *The Behavioral and Brain Sciences, 28,* 105–167. doi:10.1017/S0140525X05000038

Argiolas, A. (1992). Oxytocin stimulation of penile erection. Pharmacology, site, and mechanism of action. *Annals of the New York Academy of Sciences, 652,* 194–203. doi:10.1111/j.1749-6632.1992.tb34355.x

Argyle, M., & Trower, P. (1979). *Person to person: ways of communicating.* HarperCollins Publishers.

Argyle, M., & Cook, M. (1976). *Gaze and Mutual Gaze.* Cambridge, MA: Cambridge University Press.

Aristotle,. (1967). *Poetics* (Else, G. F., Trans.). Ann Arbor: University of Michigan Press.

Armony, J. L., Servan-Schreiber, D., Cohen, J. D., & Ledoux, J. E. (1995). An anatomically constrained neural network model of fear conditioning. *Behavioral Neuroscience, 109,* 246–257. doi:10.1037/0735-7044.109.2.246

Asha, K., Ajay, K., Naznin, V., George, T., & Peter, D. (2005). *Gesture-based affective computing on motion capture data.* Paper presented at the International Conference on Affective Computing and Intelligent Interaction.

Averill, J. R. (1980). A constructivist view of emotion. In R. Plutchik & H. Kellerman (Eds.), *Emotion: Theory, research and experience: Vol. I. Theories of emotion* (pp. 305-339). New York: Academic.

Aziz-Zadeh, L., Sheng, T., & Gheytanchi, A. (2010). Common premotor regions for the perception and production of prosody and correlations with empathy and prosodic ability. *PLoS ONE, 5*(1), e8759. .doi:10.1371/journal.pone.0008759

Badler, N., & Platt, S. (1981). Animating facial expressions. *Computer Graphics,* 245–252.

Baid, C. E. (1973). *Drama.* New York: W. W. Norton & Company.

Balcı, K. (2004). Xface: MPEG-4 based open source toolkit for 3d facial animation. *Proc. Working Conference on Advanced Visual Interfaces,* (pp. 399-402).

Baldwin, D. A. (1995). Understanding the link between joint attention and language. In Moore, C., & Dunham, P. J. (Eds.), *Joint attention: Its origins and role in development* (pp. 131–158). Hillsdale, New Jersey: Erlbaum.

Bales, R. (1950). *Interaction process analysis: A method for the study of small groups.* Addison-Wesley.

Balleine, B., & Dickinson, A. (1991). Instrumental performance following reinforcer devaluation depends upon incentive learning. *Quarterly Journal of Experimental Psychology, Section B. Comparative Physiological Psychology, 43*(3), 279–296.

Balleine, B., & Dickinson, A. (1998). Consciousness: The interface between affect and cognition. In Cornwell, J. (Ed.), *Consciousness and Human Identity* (pp. 57–85). Oxford: Oxford University Press.

Bamberg, M., & Reilly, J. S. (1996). Emotion, narrative and affect. In Slobin, D. I., Gerhardt, J., Kyratzis, A., & Guo, J. (Eds.), *Social interaction, social context and language: Essays in honor of Susan Ervin-Tripp* (pp. 329–341). Norwood, New Jersey: Erlbaum.

Bandura, A. (1990). Self-efficacy mechanism in human agency. *The American Psychologist, 37,* 122–147. doi:10.1037/0003-066X.37.2.122

Banerjee, S., & Rudnicky, A. (2004). Using simple speech based features to detect the state of a meeting and the roles of the meeting participants. In *Proceedings of international conference on spoken language processing* (pp. 221-231).

Barbas, H. (2007). Flow of information for emotions through temporal and orbitofrontal pathways. *Journal of Anatomy, 211,* 237–249. doi:10.1111/j.1469-7580.2007.00777.x

Bargh, J. A., McKenna, K. Y., & Fitzsimons, G. M. (2002). Can you see the real me? Activation and expression of the "true self" on the Internet. *The Journal of Social Issues, 58*(1), 33–48. doi:10.1111/1540-4560.00247

Barkley, R. A. (1998). *Attention Deficit Hyperactivity Disorder: A Handbook for Diagnosis and Treatment* (2nd ed.). New York: Guilford Press.

Barrett, L. F. (2004). Feelings or Words? Understanding the Content in Self-Report Ratings of Experienced Emotion. *Journal of Personality and Social Psychology, 87*(2), 266–281. doi:10.1037/0022-3514.87.2.266

Barr-Zisowitz, C. (2000). "Sadness" - Is There Such a Thing? In Lewis, M., & Haviland-Jones, J. (Eds.), *Handbook of emotions* (pp. 607–622). New York: Guilford Press.

Bartlett, M. S., Littlewort, G., Frank, M., Lainscsek, C., Fasel, I., & Movellan, J. (2005). Recognizing Facial Expression: Machine Learning and Application to Spontaneous Behavior. *Proc. IEEE Int. Conf. Computer Vision and Pattern Recognition* (pp. 568–573).

Bartlett, M. S., Littlewort, G., Fasel, I., & Movellan, J. R. (2003). *Real Time Face Detection and Facial Expression Recognition: Development and Applications to Human Computer Interaction*. Paper presented at the Conference on Computer Vision and Pattern Recognition Workshop.

Barzilay, R., Collins, M., Hirschberg, J., & Whittaker, S. (2000). The rules behind the roles: identifying speaker roles in radio broadcasts. In *Proceedings of the 17th national conference on artificial intelligence* (pp. 679-684).

Bastiaansen, J. A. C. J., Thioux, M., & Keysers, C. (2009). Evidence for mirror systems in emotions. *Philosophical Transactions of the Royal Society B, 364*, 2391–2404. doi:10.1098/rstb.2009.0058

Bateman, C., & Boon, R. (2005). *21st Century Game Design*. Hingham, MA: Charles River Media.

Baumeister, R. F., Reis, H. T., & Delespaul, P. A. E. G. (1995). Subjective and experiential correlates of guilt in everyday life. *Personality and Social Psychology Bulletin, 21*, 1256–1268. doi:10.1177/01461672952112002

Baumeister, R. F., Stillwell, A. M., & Heatherton, T. F. (1994). Guilt: An interpersonal approach. *Psychological Bulletin, 115*, 243–267. doi:10.1037/0033-2909.115.2.243

Baumeister, R. F., Vohs, K. D., DeWall, C. N., & Zhang, L. (2007). How emotion shapes behavior: Feedback, anticipation, and reflection, rather than direct causation. *Personality and Social Psychology Review, 11*(2), 167–203. doi:10.1177/1088868307301033

Baumeister, R. F., Smart, L., & Boden, J. M. (1996). Relation of Threatened Egotism to Violence and Aggression: The Dark Side of High Self-Esteem. *Psychological Review, 103*, 5–33. doi:10.1037/0033-295X.103.1.5

Bechara, A., Damasio, H., & Damasio, A. R. (2000). Emotion, decision making and the orbitofrontal cortex. *Cerebral Cortex, 10*(3), 295–307. doi:10.1093/cercor/10.3.295

Beer, J., John, O. P., Scabini, D., & Knight, R. T. (2006). Orbitofrontal Cortex and Social Behavior: Integrating Self-Monitoring and Emotion-Cognition Interactions. *Journal of Cognitive Neuroscience, 18*, 871–879. doi:10.1162/jocn.2006.18.6.871

Ben Shalom, D., Mostofsky, S. H., Hazlett, R. L., Goldberg, M. C., Landa, R. J., & Faran, Y. (2006). Normal physiological emotions but differences in expression of conscious feelings in children with high-functioning autism. *Journal of Autism and Developmental Disorders, 36*(3), 395–400. doi:10.1007/s10803-006-0077-2

Ben-Ami, O., & Mioduser, D. (2004). The affective aspect of moderator's role conception and enactment by teachers in a-synchronous learning discussion groups. *Proceedings of World Conference on Educational Multimedia, Hypermedia and Telecommunications (ED-MEDIA) 2004*, 2831-2837.

Benedetti, R. (1994). *Actor at Work* (6th ed.). Englewood Cliffs, NJ: Prentice-Hall.

Berman, M. E., & Coccaro, E. F. (1998). Neurobiologic correlates of violence: relevance to criminal responsibility. *Behavioral Sciences & the Law, 16*(3), 303–318. doi:10.1002/(SICI)1099-0798(199822)16:3<303::AID-BSL309>3.0.CO;2-C

Bernard-Opitz, V., Sriram, N., & Nakhoda-Sapuan, S. (2001). Enhancing social problem solving in children with autism and normal children through computer-assisted instruction. *Journal of Autism and Developmental Disorders*, *31*(4), 377–384. doi:10.1023/A:1010660502130

Berridge, K. C. (2003). Pleasures of the brain. *Brain and Cognition*, *52*, 106–128. doi:10.1016/S0278-2626(03)00014-9

Berridge, K. C. (1996). Food reward: Brain substrates of wanting and liking. *Neuroscience and Biobehavioral Reviews*, *20*, 1–25. doi:10.1016/0149-7634(95)00033-B

Berridge, K. C. (2000). Measuring hedonic impact in animals and infants: microstructure of affective taste reactivity patterns. *Neuroscience and Biobehavioral Reviews*, *24*, 173–198. doi:10.1016/S0149-7634(99)00072-X

Berridge, K. C. (2004). Motivation concepts in behavioral neuroscience. *Physiology & Behavior*, *81*(2), 179–209. doi:10.1016/j.physbeh.2004.02.004

Bethel, C., Salomon, K., Murphy, R., & Burke, J. (2007). *Survey of psychophysiology measurements applied to human-robot interaction*. Paper presented at the IEEE International Symposium on Robot and Human Interactive Communication, Jeju, Korea.

Bharuthram, S. (2003). Politeness phenomena in the Hindu sector of the South African Indian English speaking community. *Journal of Pragmatics*, *35*, 1523–1544. doi:10.1016/S0378-2166(03)00047-X

Bhatti, M. W., Wang, Y., & Guan, L. (2004). A neural network approach for human emotion recognition in speech. In *Proceedings of the International Symposium on Circuits & Systems, ISCAS'04*, (Vol. 2, pp. II-181-4).

Bianchi-Berthouse, N., Cairns, P., Cox, A., Jennett, C., & Kim, W. W. (2006). On posture as a modality for expressing and recognizing emotions. In Christian Peter, Russell Beale, Elizabeth Crane, Lesley Axelrod, Gerred Blyth (Eds.) *Emotion in HCI: Joint Proceedings of the 2005, 2006, and 2007 Intl. Workshops*. Stuttgart: Fraunhofer IRB Verlag.

Bickmore, T., & Cassell, J. (2005). Social dialogue with embodied conversational agents. In van Kuppevelt, J., Dybkjaer, L., & Bernsen, N. (Eds.), *Advances in natural, multimodal, dialogue systems* (pp. 23–54). New York: Kluwer. doi:10.1007/1-4020-3933-6_2

Bickmore, T., & Schulman, D. (2007). Practical Approaches to Comforting Users with Relational Agents CHI 2007 April 28-May 3, 2007 • San Jose, CA, USA

Bilmes, J. (1988). The concept of preference in conversation analysis. *Language in Society*, *17*(2), 161–181. doi:10.1017/S0047404500012744

Birn, J. (Ed.). (2000). *Digital Lighting & Rendering*. Indianapolis: New Riders.

Bjork, S., & Holopainen, J. (2004). *Patterns in Game Design*. Hingham, MA: Charles River Media.

Blair, R. J. R., Morris, J. S., Frith, C. D., Perrett, D. I., & Dolan, R. J. (1999). Dissociable neural responses to facial expressions of sadness and anger. *Brain*, *122*, 883–893. doi:10.1093/brain/122.5.883

Blanz, V., & Vetter, T. (1999). A morphable model for the synthesis of 3D faces. *Proc. SIGGRAPH*, (pp. 187–194).

Block, B. (2001). *The Visual Story: Seeing the Structure of Film, TV, and New Media*. New York: Focal Press.

Blood, A. J., & Zatorre, R. J. (2001). Intensely pleasurable responses to music correlate with activity in brain regions implicated in reward and emotion. *Proceedings of the National Academy of Sciences of the United States of America*, *98*(20), 11818–11823. doi:10.1073/pnas.191355898

Bloom, L. (1998). Language development and emotional expression. *Pediatrics*, *102*(5), 1272–1277.

Bloom, L., & Beckwith, R. (1989). Talking with feeling: Integrating affective and linguistic expression in early language development. *Cognition and Emotion*, *3*, 315–342. doi:10.1080/02699938908412711

Bloom, L., & Tinker, E. (2001). The intentionality model and language acquisition: Engagement, effort, and the essential tension in development. *Monographs of the Society for Research in Child Development, 66*(4), i–viii, 1–91.

Blythe, M. A., & Hassenzahl, M. (2004). The Semantics of Fun: Differentiating Enjoyable Experiences. In Blythe, M. A., Overbeeke, K., Monk, A. F., & Wright, P. C. (Eds.), *Funology: From Usability to Enjoyment (Human-Computer Interaction Series)*. MA: Kulwer Academic Publishers.

Boal, A. (1979). *Theatre of the Oppressed*. New York, NY: Urizen Books.

Boal, A. (2002). *Games for Actors and Non-Actors* (2 ed.). London: Routledge.

Boehner, K., DePaula, R., Dourish, P., & Sengers, P. (2007). How emotion is made and measured. *International Journal of Human-Computer Studies, 65*, 275–291. doi:10.1016/j.ijhcs.2006.11.016

Bongers, K., & Dijksterhuis, A. (2008). Consciousness as a trouble shooting device? The role of consciousness in goal-pursuit. In Morsella, J. B. E., & Gollwitzer, P. (Eds.), *The Oxford Handbook of Human Action* (pp. 589–604). New York: Oxford University Press.

Boorstin, J. (1990). *Making Movies Work: Thinking Like a Filmmaker*. LA, CA: Silman-James Press.

Bornstein, R. F. (1992). Perception without Awareness: Retrospect and Prospect. In *Perception without Awareness: Cognitive, Clinical and Social Perspectives*. New York, New York: BoGuilford.

Bornstein, M. H., & Tamis-LeMonda, C. S. (1989). Maternal responsiveness and cognitive development in children. In Bornstein, M. H. (Ed.), *Maternal responsiveness: Characteristics and consequences. New directions for child development, no. 43* (pp. 49–61). San Francisco: Jossey-Bass.

Borod, J. C., Obler, L. K., Erhan, H. M., Grunwald, I. S., Cicero, B. A., & Welkowitz, J. (1998). Right hemisphere emotional perception: Evidence across multiple channels. *Neuropsychology, 12*, 446–458. doi:10.1037/0894-4105.12.3.446

Bos, N., Olson, J., Gergle, D., Olson, G., & Wright, Z. (2002). Effects of Four Computer-Mediated Communications Channels on Trust Development. *Proceedings of the SIGCHI* (pp. 135 – 140).

Boucsein, W. (1992). *Electrodermal Activity*. New York: Plenum Press.

Bousmalis, K., Mehu, M., & Pantic, M. (2009). Spotting agreement and disagreement: A survey of nonverbal audiovisual cues and tools. In *Proceedings of the international conference on affective computing and intelligent interaction* (Vol. II, pp. 121-129).

Bownds, D. M. (1999). *Biology of Mind - origins and structures of mind, brain, and consciousness*. Maryland: Fitzgerald Science Press.

Bozarth, M. A. (1994). Pleasure Systems in the Brain. In Warburton, D. M. (Ed.), *Pleasure: The politics and the reality* (pp. 5–14). New York: John Wiley & Sons.

Bradley, M. M., Hamby, S., Low, A., & Lang, P. J. (2007). Brain potentials in perception: picture complexity and emotional arousal. *Psychophysiology, 44*, 364–373. doi:10.1111/j.1469-8986.2007.00520.x

Bradley, M. M., Miccoli, L., Escrig, M. A., & Lang, P. J. (2008). The pupil as a measure of emotional arousal and autonomic activation. *Psychophysiology, 45*, 602–607. doi:10.1111/j.1469-8986.2008.00654.x

Bradley, M. M., & Lang, P. J. (2007). Emotion and motivation. In Cacioppo, J. T., Tassinary, L. G., & Berntson, G. G. (Eds.), *Handbook of Psychphysiology*. New York, NY: Cambridge University Press. doi:10.1017/CBO9780511546396.025

Bradley, M. M. (2000). Emotion and motivation. In Cacioppo, J. T., Tassinary, L. G., & Berntson, G. (Eds.), *Handbook of Psychophysiology* (pp. 602–642). New York: Cambridge University Press.

Bradley, M. M., & Lang, P. J. (1999). *Affective norms for English words (ANEW): Instruction manual and affective ratings*. Technical Report C-1. Gainesville, FL: The Center for Research in Psychophysiology, University of Florida.

Bradley, M. M., & Lang, P. J. (1999). *International affective digitized sounds (IADS): Stimuli, instruction manual and affective ratings*. Technical Report B-2. Gainesville, FL: Center for Research in Psychophysiology, University of Florida.

Braitenberg, V. (1984). *Vehicles: Experiments in synthetic psychology*. Cambridge, MA: The MIT Press.

Brand, R. J., Baldwin, D. A., & Ashburn, L. A. (2002). Evidence for 'motionese': Modifications in mothers' infant-directed action. *Developmental Science, 5*(1), 72–83. doi:10.1111/1467-7687.00211

Brass, M., & Heyes, C. (2005). Imitation: is cognitive neuroscience solving the correspondence problem? *Trends in Cognitive Sciences, 9*(10), 489–495. doi:10.1016/j.tics.2005.08.007

Brave, S., & Nass, C., & Hutchinson. (2005). Computers that care: Investigating the effects of orientation of emotion exhibited by an embodied computer agent. *International Journal of Human-Computer Studies, 62*, 161–178. doi:10.1016/j.ijhcs.2004.11.002

Brave, S., & Nass, C. (2008). Emotion in human-computer interaction. In Sears, A., & Jacko, J. (Eds.), *The human computer interaction handbook: Fundamentals, evolving technologies and emerging applications* (2nd ed., pp. 77–92). Hillsdale, NJ: Lawrence Erlbaum Associates.

Braver, T. S., Cohen, J. D., & Barch, D. M. (2002). The role of the prefrontal cortex in normal and disordered cognitive control: A cognitive neuroscience perspective. In Struss, D. T., & Knight, R. T. (Eds.), *Principles of frontal lobe function* (pp. 428–448). Oxford: Oxford University Press. doi:10.1093/acprof:oso/9780195134971.003.0027

Breazeal, C. (2002). *Designing Sociable Robots*. MIT Press.

Breazeal, C., Gray, J., & Berlin, M. (2009). An embodied cognition approach to mindreading skills for socially intelligent robots. *The International Journal of Robotics Research, 28*(5), 656–680. doi:10.1177/0278364909102796

Breazeal, C. (2001). Affective interaction between humans and robots. In Kelemen, J., & Sosík, P. (Eds.), *ECAL, Lecture Notes in Artificial Intelligence, 2159* (pp. 582–591).

Breiter, H. C., Gollub, R. L., Weisskoff, R. M., Kennedy, D. N., Makris, N., & Berke, J. D. (1997). Acute effects of cocaine on human brain activity and emotion. *Neuron, 19*(3), 591–611. doi:10.1016/S0896-6273(00)80374-8

Brown, J. D., Dutton, K. A., & Cook, K. E. (2001). From the top down: Self-esteem and self-evaluation. *Cognition and Emotion, 15*, 615–631.

Brown, B. (1996). *Motion Picture and Video Lighting*. Boston: Focal Press.

Brown, P., & Levinson, S. C. (1987). *Politeness: Some universals in language usage*. Cambridge: Cambridge University Press.

Brown, R. M., Hall, L. R., Holtzer, R., Brown, S. L., & Brown, N. L. (1997). Gender and video game performance. *Sex Roles, 36*, 793–812. doi:10.1023/A:1025631307585

Brown, S. (2009). *Play: How it shapes the brain, opens the Imagination and invigorates the soul*. London: Penguin Books.

Bruce, V., & Young, A. W. (1986). Understanding face recognition. *The British Journal of Psychology, 77*, 305–327.

Bruner, J. S. (1975). The ontogenesis of speech acts. *Journal of Child Language, 2*(1), 1–19. doi:10.1017/S0305000900000866

Bruner, J. S. (1983). *Child's talk: Learning to use language*. New York: Norton.

Buchanan, M. (2007). The science of subtle signals. Strategy+Business, 48, 68–77.

Buciu, I., Kotropoulos, C., & Pitas, I. (2003) ICA and Gabor representations for facial expression recognition. *IEEE International Conference on Image Processing (ICIP 2003)*, September 14-17,Barcelona, Spain, pp. 1054 – 1057.

Buck, R. (1980). Nonverbal behavior and the theory of emotion: The facial feedback hypothesis. *Journal of Personality and Social Psychology, 38*, 811–824. doi:10.1037/0022-3514.38.5.811

Bush, G., Luu, P., & Posner, M. I. (2000). Cognitive and emotional influences in anterior cingulate cortex. *Trends in Cognitive Sciences, 4*, 215–222. doi:10.1016/S1364-6613(00)01483-2

Bussey, T. J., Everitt, B. J., & Robbins, T. W. (1997). Dissociable effects of cingulate and medial frontal cortex lesions on stimulus reward learning using a novel Pavlovian autoshaping procedure for the rat: Implications for the neurobiology of emotion. *Behavioral Neuroscience, 111*(5), 908–919. doi:10.1037/0735-7044.111.5.908

Busso, C., Lee, S., & Narayanan, S. (2009). Analysis of emotionally salient aspects of fundamental frequency for emotion detection. *IEEE Transaction on Audio. Speech and Language Processing, 17*(4), 582–596. doi:10.1109/TASL.2008.2009578

Cabanac, M. (1971). Physiological role of pleasure. *Science, 173*(2), 1103–1107. doi:10.1126/science.173.4002.1103

Cabeza, R., & Nyberg, L. (2000). Imaging cognition II: An empirical review of 275 PET and fMRI studies. *Journal of Cognitive Neuroscience, 12*(1). doi:10.1162/08989290051137585

Cacioppo, J. T., Tassinary, L. G., & Berntson, G. G. (2007). *Handbook of Psychophysiology* (3rd ed.). Cambridge University Press. doi:10.1017/CBO9780511546396

Cahill, L., & McGaugh, J. L. (1998). Mechanisms of emotional arousal and lasting declarative memory. *Trends in Neurosciences, 21*(7), 273–313. doi:10.1016/S0166-2236(97)01214-9

Caillois, R. (1958). *Man, Play and Games*. Chicago: University of Illinois Press.

Calahan, S. (1996). *Storytelling through lighting: a computer graphics perspective.* Paper presented at the Siggraph Course Notes.

Calder, A. J., Burton, A. M., Miller, P., Young, A. W., & Akamatsu, S. (2001). A principal component analysis of facial expressions. *Vision Research, 41*(9), 1179–1208. doi:10.1016/S0042-6989(01)00002-5

Caldwell, J. D. (1992). Central oxytocin and female sexual behavior. *Annals of the New York Academy of Sciences, 652*, 166–179. doi:10.1111/j.1749-6632.1992.tb34353.x

Caldwell-Harris, C. L. (2008). Language research needs an "emotion revolution" AND distributed models of the lexicon. *Bilingualism: Language and Cognition, 11*(2), 169–171. doi:10.1017/S1366728908003301

Campbell, D. (1999). *Technical Theatre for Non-technical People*. New York City, NY: Allworth Press.

Campbell, J. (1972). *The Hero with a Thousand Faces*. New Jersey: Princeton University Press.

Cãnamero, D. (1997). Modeling motivations and emotions as a basis for intelligent behavior. In L. Johnson (Ed.), *Proceedings of the first international symposium on autonomous agents (agents'97)* (pp. 148–155). New York: ACM Press.

Cantwell, D. P., Lewinsohn, P. M., Rohde, P., & Seeley, J. R. (1997). Correspondence between adolescent report and parent report of psychiatric diagnostic data. *Journal of the American Academy of Child and Adolescent Psychiatry, 36*, 610–619. doi:10.1097/00004583-199705000-00011

Cardinal, R. N., Parkinson, J. A., Hall, J., & Everitt, B. J. (2002). Emotion and motivation: The role of the amygdala, ventral striatum, and prefrontal cortex. *Neuroscience and Biobehavioral Reviews, 26*, 321–352. doi:10.1016/S0149-7634(02)00007-6

Caridakis, G., Karpouzis, K., Wallace, M., Kessous, L., & Amir, N. (2010). Multimodal user's affective state analysis in naturalistic interaction. *Journal on Multimodal User Interfaces, 3*(1), 49–66. doi:10.1007/s12193-009-0030-8

Carletta, J. (2006). Announcing the AMI Meeting Corpus. *The ELRA Newsletter, 11*(1), 3–5.

Carmichael, M. S., Humbert, R., Dixen, J., Palmisano, G., Greenleaf, W., & Davidson, J. M. (1987). Plasma oxytocin increases in the human sexual response. *The Journal of Clinical Endocrinology and Metabolism, 64*, 27–31. doi:10.1210/jcem-64-1-27

Carr, L., Iacoboni, M., Dubeau, M.-C., Mazziotta, J. C., & Lenzi, G. L. (2003). Neural mechanisms of empathy in humans: A relay from neural systems for imitation to limbic areas. *Proceedings of the National Academy of Sciences of the United States of America, 100*(9), 5497–5502. doi:10.1073/pnas.0935845100

Carroll, J. M. (1997). Human-computer interaction: Psychology as a science of design. *International Journal of Human-Computer Studies, 46*, 501–522. doi:10.1006/ijhc.1996.0101

Carter, C. S. (1992). Oxytocin and sexual behavior. *Neuroscience and Biobehavioral Reviews, 16*, 131–144. doi:10.1016/S0149-7634(05)80176-9

Carver, C. S., & Scheier, M. F. (1998). *On the self-regulation of behavior*. New York: Cambridge University Press.

Carver, S. C., & Scheier, M. F. (1990). Principles of self-regulation: Action and emotion. In Higgins, E. T., & Sorrentino, R. M. (Eds.), *Handbook of motivation and cognition: Foundations of social behavior* (*Vol. 2*, pp. 3–52). New York: Guilford Press.

Cassell, J., Sullivan, J., Prevost, S., & Churchill, E. (Eds.). (2002). *Embodied Conversational Agents*. Cambridge, MA: MIT Press.

Cassidy, G. G., & MacDonald, R. A. R. (2009, Fall). The effects of music choice on task performance: a study of the impact of self-selected and experimenter-selected music on driving game performance and experience. *Musicae Scientiae, 13*(2), 357–386.

Cassidy, G. G., & MacDonald, R. A. R. (in press). The effects of music on time perception and performance of a driving game. *Scandinavian Journal of Psychology*.

Castelfranchi, C. (2005). Mind as an Anticipatory Device: For a Theory of Expectations. BVAI 2005 Brain, vision, and artificial intelligence (First international symposium, BVAI 2005, Naples, Italy, October 19-21, 2005) (proceedings). *Lecture Notes in Computer Science, 3704*, 258–276. doi:10.1007/11565123_26

Castelfranchi, C., & Miceli, M. (2009). The Cognitive-Motivational Compound of Emotional Experience. *Emotion Review, 1*(3), 221–228. doi:10.1177/1754073909103590

Castelfranchi, C. (1998). To believe and to feel: The case of "needs". In Canamero, D. (Ed.), *Emotional and Intelligent: The Tangled Knot of Cognition* (pp. 55–60). Menlo Park, CA: AAAI Press.

Castelfranchi, C., & Poggi, I. (1990). Blushing as a discourse: was Darwin wrong? In Crozier, R. (Ed.), *Shyness and Embarassement: Perspective from Social Psychology*. N. Y: Cambridge University Press. doi:10.1017/CBO9780511571183.009

Castelfranchi, C. (2000). Affective Appraisal vs. Cognitive Evaluation in Social Emotions and Interactions. In A. Paiva (ed.) *Affective Interactions. Towards a New Generation of Computer Interfaces*. Heidelbergh, Springer, LNAI 1814, 76-106.

Cato, M. A., Crosson, B., Gokcay, D., Soltysik, D., Wierenga, C., & Gopinath, K. (2004). Processing Words with Emotional Connotation: An fMRI Study of Time Course and Laterality in Rostral Frontal and Retrosplenial Cortices. *Journal of Cognitive Neuroscience, 16*(2), 167–177. doi:10.1162/089892904322984481

Cegarra, J., & Hoc, J. M. (2006). Cognitive styles as an explanation of experts' individual differences: A case study in computer-assisted troubleshooting diagnosis. *International Journal of Human-Computer Studies, 64*, 123–136. doi:10.1016/j.ijhcs.2005.06.003

Centers for Disease Control and Prevention [CDC]. (2009). Prevalence of Autism Spectrum Disorders-ADDM Network, United States, 2006. *Morbidity and Mortality Weekly Report (MMWR) Surveillance Summaries, 58*, 1-20.

Chaiken, S., & Trope, Y. (1999). *Dual-process theories in social psychology*. New York, NY: Guildford Press.

Chakrabarti, B., Bullmore, E., & Baron-Cohen, S. (2006). Empathizing with basic emotions: Common and discrete neural substrates. *Social Neuroscience, 1*(3-4), 364–384. doi:10.1080/17470910601041317

Chandrasiri, N. P., Barakonyi, I., Naemura, T., Ishizuka, M., & Harashima, H. (2002) Communication over the Internet using a 3D agent with real-time facial expression analysis, synthesis and text to speech capabilities. In *Proceeding of the 8th International Conference on Communication Systems*, 01, 480 – 484.

Chen, S. H., & Bernard-Opitz, V. (1993). Comparison of personal and computer-assisted instruction for children with autism. *Mental Retardation, 31*(6), 368–376.

Chen, S., & Chaiken, S. (1999). The heuristic-systematic model in its broader context. In Chaiken, S., & Trope, Y. (Eds.), *Dual-process theories in social psychology*. New York: Guildford Press.

Cheng, Y., O'Toole, A., & Abdi, H. (2001). Classifying adults' and children's faces by sex: Computational investigations of subcategorial feature encoding. *Cognitive Science, 25*, 819–838. doi:10.1207/s15516709cog2505_8

Chiappe, D., & MacDonald, K. (2005). The evolution of domain-general mechanisms in intelligence and learning. *132, 1*, 5-40.

Choi, S.-M., & Kim, Y.-G. (2005) An affective user interface based on facial expression recognition and eye–gaze tracking. *First International Conference on Affective Computing & Intelligent Interaction*, 3784, 907 – 914.

Chomsky, N. (1965). *Aspects of the theory of syntax*. Boston, MA: MIT Press.

Chomsky, N. (2000). *New horizons in the study of language and mind*. Cambridge: Cambridge University Press.

Chomsky, N. (2007). Biolinguistic explorations: Design, development, evolution. *Journal of Philosophical Studies, 15*(1), 1–21. doi:10.1080/09672550601143078

Chouchourelou, A., Matsuka, T., Harber, K., & Shiffrar, M., (2006). The visual analysis of emotional actions. *Social Neuroscience, 1*(1), 63-/74.

Christianson, S.-A. (1986). Effects of positive emotional events on memory. *Scandinavian Journal of Psychology, 27*, 287–299. doi:10.1111/j.1467-9450.1986.tb01207.x

Christianson, S.-A., & Loftus, E. F. (1987). Memory for traumatic events. *Applied Cognitive Psychology, 1*, 225–239. doi:10.1002/acp.2350010402

Clynes, M. (1978). *Sentics*. Garden City, NY: Anchor Press.

Coccaro, E. F., McCloskey, M. S., Fitzgerald, D. A., & Phan, K. L. (2007). (in press). Amygdala and Orbitofrontal Reactivity to Social Threat in Individuals with Impulsive Aggression. *Biological Psychiatry*. doi:10.1016/j.biopsych.2006.08.024

Cohen, I., Sebe, N., Garg, A., Chen, L. S., & Huang, T. S. (2003). Facial Expression Recognition from Video Sequences: Temporal and Static Modeling. *Computer Vision and Image Understanding, 91*(1-2), 160–187. doi:10.1016/S1077-3142(03)00081-X

Cohen, H., Amerine-Dickens, M., & Smith, T. (2006). Early intensive behavioral treatment: replication of the UCLA model in a community setting. Journal of Developmental & Behavioral Pediatrics, 27(2 Supplemental), S145-155.

Cohn, J., & Schmidt, K. (2004). The Timing of Facial Motion in Posed and Spontaneous Smiles. *International Journal of Wavelets, Multresolution, and Information Processing, 2*(2), 121–132. doi:10.1142/S021969130400041X

Cohn, J. (2006). Foundations of human computing: facial expression and emotion. In *Proceedings of the ACM international conference on multimodal interfaces* (pp. 233-238).

Cohn, J., Reed, L. I., Ambadar, Z., Xiao, J., & Moriyama, T. (2004). Automatic Analysis and Recognition of Brow Actions and Head Motion in Spontaneous Facial Behavior. Proc. *IEEE Int'l Conf. Systems, Man, and Cybernetics*, (pp. 610-616).

Colburn, A., Drucker, S., & Cohen, M. (2000). The role of eye-gaze in avatar-mediated conversational interfaces. Paper presented at SIGGRAPH Sketches and Applications, New Orleans, Louisiana.

Colley, A., & Todd, Z. (2002). Gender-linked differences in the style and content of e-mails to friends. *Journal of Language and Social Psychology, 21*, 380–392. doi:10.1177/026192702237955

Colley, A., Todd, Z., Bland, M., Holmes, M., Khanom, N., & Pike, H. (2004, September). Style and Content in E-Mails and Letters to Male and Female Friends. *Journal of Language and Social Psychology, 23*(3), 369–378. doi:10.1177/0261927X04266812

Conati, C., Chabbal, R., & Maclaren, H. (2003). *A study on using biometric sensors for detecting user emotions in educational games*. Paper presented at the Workshop on Assessing and Adapting to User Attitude and Affects: Why, When and How, Pittsburgh, Pennsylvania.

Constantin, C., Kalyanaraman, S., Stavrositu, C., & Wagoner, N. (2002). *To be or not to be emotional: Impression formation effects of emoticons in moderated chatrooms*. Paper presented at the communication technology and policy division at the 85th annual convention of the Association for Education in Journalism and Mass Communication (AEJMC). Miama, Fl.

Cootes, T. F., Edwards, G. J., & Taylor, C. J. (2001). Active appearance models. *IEEE Transactions on Pattern Analysis and Machine Intelligence, 23*(6), 681–685. doi:10.1109/34.927467

Corballis, M. C. (2002). *From hand to mouth. The origins of language*. Princeton, Oxford: Princeton University Press.

Corina, D. P., Bellugi, U., & Reilly, J. (1999). Neuropsychological studies in linguistic and affective facial expressions in deaf signers. *Language and Speech, 42*(2-3), 307–331. doi:10.1177/00238309990420020801

Cortes, J., & Gatti, F. (1965). Physique and self-description of temperament. *Journal of Consulting Psychology, 29*(5), 432–439. doi:10.1037/h0022504

Costa, M., Dinsbach, W., Manstead, A., & Bitti, P. (2001). Social presence, embarrassment, and nonverbal behavior. *Journal of Nonverbal Behavior, 25*(4), 225–240. doi:10.1023/A:1012544204986

Coulson, M. (2004). Attributing emotion to static body postures: Recognition accuracy, confusions, and viewpoint dependence. *Journal of Nonverbal Behavior, 28*(2), 117–139. doi:10.1023/B:JONB.0000023655.25550.be

Cowie, R., Douglas-Cowie, E., Tsapatsoulis, N., Votsis, G., Kollias, S., Fellenz, W., & Taylor, J. G. (2001). Emotion recognition in human-computer interaction. *IEEE Signal Processing Magazine, 18*(1), 32–80. doi:10.1109/79.911197

Craig, W. (1918). Appetites and aversions as constituents of instincts. *Biological Bulletin of Woods Hole, 34*, 91–107. doi:10.2307/1536346

Creed, C., & Beale, R. (2006). Multiple and extended interactions with affective embodied agents. In Christian Peter, Russell Beale, Elizabeth Crane, Lesley Axelrod, Gerred Blyth (Eds.) *Emotion in HCI: Joint Proceedings of the 2005, 2006, and 2007 Intl. Workshops*. Stuttgart: Fraunhofer IRB Verlag.

Critchley, H. D., Daly, E., Phillips, M., Brammer, M., Bullmore, E., & Williams, S. (2000). Explicit and implicit neural mechanisms for processing of social information from facial expressions: A functional magnetic resonance imaging study. *Human Brain Mapping, 9*, 93–105. doi:10.1002/(SICI)1097-0193(200002)9:2<93::AID-HBM4>3.0.CO;2-Z

Critchley, H. D., Mathias, C. J., & Dolan, R. J. (1995). Fear Conditioning in Humans: The Influence of Awareness and Autonomic Arousal on Functional Neuroanatomy. *The Journal of Neuroscience*, *15*(10), 6846–6855.

Crittenden, P. M. (1988). Relationships at risk. In Belsky, J., & Nezworski, T. (Eds.), *Clinical implications of attachment* (pp. 136–174). Hillsdale, NJ: Erlbaum.

Crittenden, P. M. (2004). *CARE-Index: Coding Manual.* Unpublished manuscript, Miami, FL.

Cromby, J. J., Standen, P. J., & Brown, D. J. (1996). The potentials of virtual environments in the education and training of people with learning disabilities. *Journal of Intellectual Disability Research*, *40*, 489–501. doi:10.1111/j.1365-2788.1996.tb00659.x

Crowley, J. L. (2006). Social Perception. *ACM Queue; Tomorrow's Computing Today*, *4*(6), 43–48. doi:10.1145/1147518.1147531

Crowther, B. (1989). *Film Noir: Reflections in a Dark Mirror.* New York: Continuum.

Crystal, D. (1969). *Prosodic systems and intonation in English.* Cambridge: Cambridge University Press.

Csikszentmihalyi, M. (1990). *Flow: The psychology of optimal experience.* New York: Harper & Row.

Culnan, M. J., & Markus, M. L. (1987). Information technologies. In Jablin, F. M., Putnam, L. L., & Roberts, K. H. (Eds.), *Handbook of organizational communication: an interdisciplinary perspective* (pp. 420–443). Newbury Park, CA: Sage.

Cunningham, M. R., Steinberg, J., & Grev, R. (1980). Wanting to and having to help: Separate motivations for positive mood and guiltinduced helping. *Journal of Personality and Social Psychology*, *38*, 181–192. doi:10.1037/0022-3514.38.2.181

Cunningham, D., Kleiner, M., Bültho, H., & Wallraven, C. (2004). The components of conversational facial expressions. *Proceedings of the Symposium on Applied Perception in Graphics and Visualization* (pp. 143-150).

Cuthbert, B. N., Schupp, H. T., Bradley, M. M., Birbaumer, N., & Lang, P. J. (2000). Brain potentials in affective picture processing: covariation with autonomic arousal and affective report. *Biological Psychology*, *52*, 95–111. doi:10.1016/S0301-0511(99)00044-7

Cutler, A. (1999). Prosodic structure and word recognition. In Friederici, A. D. (Ed.), *Language comprehension: A biological perspective* (pp. 41–70). Berlin, Heidelberg: Springer.

Cutler, A., Norris, D. G., & McQueen, Ja. M. (1996). Lexical access in continuous speech: Language-specific realisations of a universal model. In T. Otake and A. Cutler (Eds.), *Phonological structure and language processing: Cross-linguistic studies* (pp. 227-242). Berlin: Mouton de Gruyter.

Daft, R. L., & Lengel, R. H. (1984). Information richness: A new approach to managerial behavior and organization design. *Research in Organizational Behavior*, *6*, 191–233.

Dalal, N. P., & Casper, G. M. (1994). The design of joint cognitive systems: The effect of cognitive coupling on performance. *International Journal of Human-Computer Studies*, *40*, 677–702. doi:10.1006/ijhc.1994.1031

Damasio, A. R. (1994). *Descartes' error: emotion, reason, and the human brain.* New York: Grosset / Putnam.

Damasio, A. R. (1996). The somatic marker hypothesis and the possible functions of the prefrontal cortex. *Philosophical Transactions of the Royal Society of London. Series B, Biological Sciences*, *351*(1346), 1413–1420. doi:10.1098/rstb.1996.0125

Damasio, A. R. (1994) *Descartes' Error.* N.Y., Putnam's Sons, Frijda N. H. & Swagerman J. (1987) Can Computers Feel? Theory and Design of an Emotional System. *Cognition and Emotion, 1* (3) 235-57, 1987.

Dautenhahn, K., & Werry, I. (2004). Towards interactive robots in autism therapy: background, motivation and challenges. *Pragmatics & Cognition*, *12*(1), 1–35. doi:10.1075/pc.12.1.03dau

Dautenhahn, K., Werry, I., Salter, T., & te Boekhorst, R. (2003). *Towards adaptive autonomous robots in autism therapy: Varieties of interactions*. Paper presented at the IEEE International Symposium on Computational Intelligence in Robotics and Automation, Kobe, Japan.

Davidson, R. J. (2001). Towards a biology of personality and emotion. *Annals of the New York Academy of Sciences, 935*, 191–207. doi:10.1111/j.1749-6632.2001.tb03481.x

Davidson, R. J., Ekman, P., Saron, C. D., Senulis, J. A., & Friesen, W. V. (1990). Approach-withdrawal and cerebral asymmetry: emotional expression and brain physiology I. *Journal of Personality and Social Psychology, 58*, 330–341. doi:10.1037/0022-3514.58.2.330

Davidson, R. J., & Irwin, W. (1999). The functional neuroanatomy of emotion and affective style. *Trends in Cognitive Sciences, 3*, 11–21. doi:10.1016/S1364-6613(98)01265-0

Davidson, R. J., Jackson, D. C., & Kalin, N. H. (2000). Emotion, plasticity, context, and regulation: perspectives from affective neuroscience. *Psychological Bulletin, 126*(6), 890–909. doi:10.1037/0033-2909.126.6.890

Davidson, R. J. (2000). Cognitive neuroscience needs affective neuroscience (and vice versa). *Brain and Cognition, 42*(1), 89–92. doi:10.1006/brcg.1999.1170

Davidson, R. J., & Irwin, W. (1999). The functional neuroanatomy of emotion and affective style. *Trends in Cognitive Sciences, 3*(1), 11–21. doi:10.1016/S1364-6613(98)01265-0

Davidson, R. J. (1994). On emotion, mood, and related affective constructs. In (Ekman & Davidson, 1994) (pp. 56–58).

de Araujo, I. E., Kringelbach, M. L., Rolls, E. T., & Hobden, P. (2003). Representation of Umami taste in the human brain. *Journal of Neurophysiology, 90*(1), 313–319. doi:10.1152/jn.00669.2002

De Gelder, B., & Vroomen, J. (2000). Perceiving emotion by ear and by eye. *Cognition and Emotion, 14*(3), 289–311. doi:10.1080/026999300378824

de Greef, H. P., & Neerincx, M. A. (1995). Cognitive support: Designing aiding to supplement human knowledge. *International Journal of Human-Computer Studies, 42*, 531–571. doi:10.1006/ijhc.1995.1023

De Vignemont, F., & Singer, T. (2006). The empathic brain: how, when and why? *Trends in Cognitive Sciences, 10*(10), 435–441. doi:10.1016/j.tics.2006.08.008

Decety, J., & Ickes, W. (2009). *The social neuroscience of empathy*. Cambridge: MIT Press.

Decety, J., & Jackson, P. L. (2004). The functional architecture of human empathy. *Behavioral and Cognitive Neuroscience Reviews, 3*(2), 71–100. doi:10.1177/1534582304267187

Decety, J., & Jackson, P. L. (2006). A social-neuroscience perspective on empathy. *Current Directions in Psychological Science, 15*(2), 54–58. doi:10.1111/j.0963-7214.2006.00406.x

DeLancey, C. (2002). *Passionate engines: What emotions reveal about mind and artificial intelligence*. Oxford, UK: Oxford University Press.

Deng, Z., Neumann, U., Lewis, J. P., Kin, T.-Y., & Bulut, M. (2006). Expressive facial animation synthesis by learning speech coarticulation and expression spaces. *IEEE Transactions on Visualization and Computer Graphics, 12*(6), 1523–1534. doi:10.1109/TVCG.2006.90

Deng, Z., & Neumann, U. (2006) eFASE: expressive facial animation synthesis and editing with phoneme-isomap controls. *Proceedings of the 2006 ACM SIGGRAPH/Eurographics Symposium on Computer Animation* (LNCS, 251 – 260)., New York: Springer.

Depue, R. A., & Collins, P. F. (1999). Neurobiology of the structure of personality: Dopamine, facilitation of incentive motivation, and extraversion. *The Behavioral and Brain Sciences, 22*, 491–569. doi:10.1017/S0140525X99002046

Derks, D., Bos, A. E., & von Grumbkow, J. (2008). Emoticons and online message interpretation. *Social Science Computer Review, 26*, 379–388. doi:10.1177/0894439307311611

Derks, D., Fischer, A. H., & Bos, A. E. (2008). The role of emotion in computer-mediated communication: A review. *Computers in Human Behavior, 24*, 766–785. doi:10.1016/j.chb.2007.04.004

Desmet, P. M. A. (2003). Measuring emotion; development and application of an instrument to measure emotional responses to products. In Blythe, M. A., Overbeeke, K., Monk, A. F., & Wright, P. C. (Eds.), *Funology: from usability to enjoyment*. Dordrecht, Boston, London: Kluwer Academic Publishers.

Di Chiara, G., & Imperato, A. (1988). Drugs abused by humans preferentially increase synaptic dopamine concentrations in the mesolimbic system of freely moving rats. *Proceedings of the National Academy of Sciences of the United States of America, 85*, 5274–5278. doi:10.1073/pnas.85.14.5274

Diaper, D. (2004). Understanding task analysis for human-computer interaction. In Diaper, D., & Stanton, N. A. (Eds.), *The handbook of task analysis for human-computer interaction*. Mahwah, NJ: Lawrence Erlbaum Associates.

Dion, K., Berscheid, E., & Walster, E. (1972). What is beautiful is good. *Journal of Personality and Social Psychology, 24*(3), 285–290. doi:10.1037/h0033731

Domes, G., Heinrichs, M., Michel, A., Berger, C., & Herpertz, S. C. (2007). Oxytocin improves "mind-reading" in humans. *Biological Psychiatry, 61*, 731–733. doi:10.1016/j.biopsych.2006.07.015

Donath, J. (2004). Artificial pets: simple behaviors elicit complex attachments. In Bekoff, M. (Ed.), *The Encyclopedia of Animal Behavior. Santa Barbara*. Greenwood Press.

Dong, W., Lepri, B., Cappelletti, A., Pentland, A., Pianesi, F., & Zancanaro, M. (2007). Using the influence model to recognize functional roles in meetings. In *Proceedings of the 9th international conference on multimodal interfaces* (pp. 271-278).

Dove, G. (2009). Beyond perceptual symbols: A call for representational pluralism. *Cognition, 110*, 412–431. doi:10.1016/j.cognition.2008.11.016

Dovidio, J., & Ellyson, S. (1982). Decoding visual dominance: Attributions of power based on relative percentages of looking while speaking and looking while listening. *Social Psychology Quarterly, 45*(2), 106–113. doi:10.2307/3033933

Downer, J. L., & De, C. (1961). Changes in visual gnostic functions and emotional behavior following unilateral temporal pole damage in the "split-brain" monkey. *Nature, 191*, 50–51. doi:10.1038/191050a0

Drachen, A., & Heide-Smith, J. (2008). Player Talk - The functions of communication in multi-player Role Playing Games - Players and Media. *ACM Computers in Entertainment, 6*(3).

Drachen, A., Canossa, A., & Yannakakis, G. (2009). *Player Modeling using Self-Organization in Tomb Raider: Underworld*. Paper presented at the IEEE Computational Intelligence in Games (CIG).

Duchowski, A. T. (2007). *Eye tracking methodology: Theory and practice* (Second ed. ed.). Berlin: Springer.

Dumais, S., Cutrell, E., Cadiz, J. J., Jancke, G., Sarin, R., & Robbins, D. C. (2003). *Stuff I've seen: a system for personal information retrieval and re-use*. Proceedings of the 26th Annual International ACM SIGIR Conference on Research and Development in Information Retrieval (pp. 72-79).

Dyer, R., Green, R., Pitts, M., & Millward, G. (1995). What's the flaming problem? CMC - deindividuation or disinhibiting? In Kirby, M. A. R., Dix, A. J., & Finlay, J. E. (Eds.), *People and Computers, X*. Cambridge: Cambridge University Press.

Egenfeldt Nielsen, S., Heide Smith, J., & Pajares Tosca, S. (2008). *Understanding Video Games*. London: Routledge Taylor and Francis Group.

Ekman, P., & Davidson, R. J. (Eds.). (1994). *The nature of emotion: Fundamental questions*. New York: Oxford University Press.

Ekman, P., & Rosenberg, E. (2005). *What the face reveals: Basic and applied studies of spontaneous expression using the facial action coding system (facs)*. New York: Oxford University Press.

Ekman, P., & Friesen, W. V. (1978). *Facial action coding system: A technique for the measurement of facial movement*. Palo Alto, CA: Consulting Psychologists Press.

Ekman, P., & Rosenberg, E. (Eds.). (2005). *What the Face Reveals: Basic and Applied Studies of Spontaneous Expression Using the Facial Action Coding System (FACS)* (Revised 2nd Edition). New York, NY: Oxford University Press.

Ekman, P., & Friesen, W. V. (1978). *Facial Action Coding System. Consulting Psychologists Press*. Alto, CA: Palo.

Ekman, P., & Friesen, W. V. (1969). The repertoire of nonverbal behavior: Categories, origins, usage, and coding. *Semiotica*, *1*, 49–98.

Ekman, P. (1971). Constants across cultures in the face and emotion. *Journal of Personality and Social Psychology*, *17*(2), 124–129. doi:10.1037/h0030377

Ekman, P. (1992). Are there basic emotions? *Psychological Review*, *99*(3), 550–553. doi:10.1037/0033-295X.99.3.550

Ekman, P. (1993). Facial expression and emotion. *The American Psychologist*, *48*(4), 384–392. doi:10.1037/0003-066X.48.4.384

Ekman, P. (1999). Basic Emotions. In Dalgleish, T., & Power, M. J. (Eds.), *Handbook of Cognition and Emotion* (pp. 43–60). Chichester: John Wiley & Sons.

Ekman, P. (1994). All emotions are basic. In Ekman, P., & Davidson, R. J. (Eds.), *The Nature of Emotions: Fundamental Questions* (pp. 7–19). New York: Oxford University Press.

Ekman, P. (1982). Methods for measuring facial action. In Scherer, K. R., & Ekman, P. (Eds.), *Handbook of methods in nonverbal behavior research*. Cambridge: Cambridge University Press.

Ekman, P. (1992). An argument for basic emotions. In Stein, N. L., & Oatley, K. (Eds.), *Basic emotions: cognition & emotion* (pp. 169–200). Mahwah: Lawrence Erlbaum.

Ekman, P. (1994). Moods, emotions, and traits. In (Ekman & Davidson, 1994) (pp. 56–58).

Ekman, P., Friesen, W. V., & Hager, J. C.,(2002). *Facial Action Coding System*. The Manual.

El Kaliouby, R., Picard, R., & Baron-Cohen, S. (2006). Affective Computing and Autism. *Annals of the New York Academy of Sciences*, *1093*(1), 228–248. doi:10.1196/annals.1382.016

Elfenbein, H. A., & Ambady, N. (2002). On the universality and cultural specificity of emotion recognition: A meta-analysis. *Psychological Bulletin*, *128*, 203–235. doi:10.1037/0033-2909.128.2.203

Ellison, N., Rebecca, H., & Gibbs, J. (2006). Managing Impressions Online: Self-Presentation Processes in the Online Dating Environment. *Journal of Computer-Mediated Communication*, *11*(2), 415–441. doi:10.1111/j.1083-6101.2006.00020.x

Ellsworth, P. C., & Scherer, K. R. (2003). Appraisal processes in emotion. In Davidson, R. J., Scherer, K. R., & Goldsmith, H. H. (Eds.), *Handbook of Affective Sciences* (pp. 572–595). New York: Oxford University Press.

Elman, J., & Karmiloff-Smith, A. Bates, Elizabeth, Johnson, Mark, Parisi, Domenico, & Plunkett, Kim (1996). *Rethinking innateness. A connectionist perspective on development*. Cambridge, MA: MIT Press.

Elsabbagh, M., Hohenberger, A., Van Herwegen, J., Campos, R., Serres, J., de Schoenen, S., Aschersleben, G., & Karmiloff-Smith, A. (submitted). *Narrowing perceptual sensitivity to the native language in infancy: exogenous influences on developmental timing*.

Epstein, L. H., Truesdale, R., Wojcik, A., Paluch, R. A., & Raynor, H. A. (2003). Effects of deprivation on hedonics and reinforcing value of food. *Physiology & Behavior*, *78*, 221–227. doi:10.1016/S0031-9384(02)00978-2

Epstein, S. (1994). Integration of the cognitive and psychodynamic unconscious. *The American Psychologist, 49*, 709–724. doi:10.1037/0003-066X.49.8.709

Ernsperger, L. (2003). *Keys to Success for Teaching Students with Autism*. Arlington, Texas: Future Horizons.

Esslen, M., Pascual-Marqui, R. D., Hell, D., Kochi, K., & Lehmann, D. (2004). Brain areas and time course of emotional processing. *NeuroImage, 21*, 1189–1203. doi:10.1016/j.neuroimage.2003.10.001

Evans, J. St. B. T. (2003). In two minds: Dual process accounts of reasoning. *Trends in Cognitive Sciences, 7*, 454–459. doi:10.1016/j.tics.2003.08.012

Evans, J. St. B. T., & Over, D. E. (1996). *Rationality & Reasoning*. Hove: Psychology Press.

Evans, J. St. B. T. (2006). Dual system theories of cognition: Some issues. In R. Sun (Ed.), *Proceedings of 28th annual meeting of the cognitive science society.* (pp. 202-7). Mahwah, N.J.: Erlbaum.

Everitt, B. J. (1990). Sexual motivation: A neural and behavioural analysis of the mechanisms underlying appetitive and copulatory responses of male rats. *Neuroscience and Biobehavioral Reviews, 14*(2), 217–232. doi:10.1016/S0149-7634(05)80222-2

Fabri, M. (2008) The Virtual Messenger - Online Chat using Emotionally Expressive Avatars. In Christian Peter, Russell Beale, Elizabeth Crane, Lesley Axelrod, Gerred Blyth (Eds.) *Emotion in HCI: Joint Proceedings of the 2005, 2006, and 2007 Intl. Workshops.* Stuttgart: Fraunhofer IRB Verlag.

Fagen, R. (1976). Modelling how and why play works. In J.S. Bruner, Alison Jolly & Kathy Sylva, (Eds.), *Play*, New York: Basic Books

Faith, M., & Thayer, J. F. (2001). A dynamical systems interpretation of a dimensional model of emotion. *Scandinavian Journal of Psychology, 42*, 121–133. doi:10.1111/1467-9450.00221

Falck-Ytter, T., Gredebäck, G., & von Hofsten, C. (2006). Infants predict other people's action goals. *Nature Neuroscience, 9*(7), 878–879. doi:10.1038/nn1729

Fasel, B., & Luettin, J. (2003). Automatic facial expression analysis: Survey. *Pattern Recognition, 36*, 259–275. doi:10.1016/S0031-3203(02)00052-3

Favre, S., Dielmann, A., & Vinciarelli, A. (2009). Automatic role recognition in multiparty recordings using social networks and probabilistic sequential models. In *Proceedings of ACM international conference on multimedia.*

Feagin, S. (1996). *Reading with Feeling*. New York: Cornell University Press.

Fedoroff, J. P., Starkstein, S. E., & Forrester, A. W. (1992). Depression in patients with acute traumatic injury. *The American Journal of Psychiatry, 149*, 918–923.

Fencott, C. (1999). *Content and Creativity in Virtual Environment Design*. Paper presented at the 5th International Conference on Virtual Systems and Multimedia.

Ferguson, J. N., Aldag, J. M., Insel, T. R., & Young, L. J. (2001). Oxytocin in the medial amygdala is essential for social recognition in the mouse. *The Journal of Neuroscience, 21*(20), 8278–8285.

Ferguson, J. N., Young, L. J., & Insel, T. R. (2002). The neuroendocrine basis of social recognition. *Frontiers in Neuroendocrinology, 23*, 200–224. doi:10.1006/frne.2002.0229

Ferguson, E. (1982). *Motivation: An experimental approach*. Malabar, FL: Krueger Publishing Company.

Fernald, A. (1989). Intonation and communicative intent in mothers' speech to infants: is the melody the message? *Child Development, 60*(6), 1497–1510. doi:10.2307/1130938

Fernald, A. (1993). Approval and disapproval: Infant responsiveness to vocal affect in familiar and unfamiliar languages. *Child Development, 64*(3), 657–674. doi:10.2307/1131209

Firestone, L. L., Gyulai, F., Mintun, M., Adler, L. J., Urso, K., & Winter, P. M. (1996). Human brain activity response to fentanyl imaged by positron emission tomography. *Anesthesia and Analgesia, 82*(6), 1247–1251. doi:10.1097/00000539-199606000-00025

Fisher, C., & Sanderson, P. (1996). Exploratory Data Analysis: Exploring Continuous Observational Data. *Interaction, 3*, 25–34. doi:10.1145/227181.227185

Fitchen, J. (1961). *The Construction of Gothic Cathedrals: A Study of Medieval Vault Erection*. Oxford: Oxford University Press.

Fodor, E. M., Wick, D. P., & Hartsen, K. M. (2006). The power motive and affective response to assertiveness. *Journal of Research in Personality, 40*, 598–610. doi:10.1016/j.jrp.2005.06.001

Fodor, J. (1983). *The modularity of mind*. Cambridge, MA: MIT Press.

Fodor, J. A. (1975). *The language of thought*. New York: Crowell.

Fogassi, L., & Ferrari, Pier F. (2007). Mirror neurons and the evolution of embodied language. *Current Directions in Psychological Science, 16*(3), 136–141. doi:10.1111/j.1467-8721.2007.00491.x

Fogg, B. J., & Nass, C. (1997). Silicon sycophans: The effects of computers that flatter. *International Journal of Human-Computer Studies, 46*, 551–561. doi:10.1006/ijhc.1996.0104

Fong, T., Nourbakhsh, I., & Dautenhahn, K. (2003). A survey of socially interactive robots. *Robotics and Autonomous Systems, 42*(3/4), 143–166. doi:10.1016/S0921-8890(02)00372-X

Fontaine, J. R., Scherer, K. R., Roesch, E. B., & Ellsworth, P. C. (2007). The world of emotions is not two-dimensional. *Psychological Science, 18*, 1050–1057. doi:10.1111/j.1467-9280.2007.02024.x

Forgas, J. P. (2008). Affect and cognition. *Perspectives on Psychological Science, 3*(2), 94–101. doi:10.1111/j.1745-6916.2008.00067.x

Forgas, J. P. (1999). On feeling good and being rude: Affective influences on language use and request formulations. *Journal of Personality and Social Psychology, 76*(6), 928–939. doi:10.1037/0022-3514.76.6.928

Foroni, F., & Semin, G. R. (2009). Language that puts you in touch with your bodily feelings. The multimodal responsiveness of affective expressions. *Psychological Science, 20*(8), 974–980. doi:10.1111/j.1467-9280.2009.02400.x

Försterling, F. (2001). *Attribution: An introduction to theories, research and applications. East Sussex*. Psychology Press.

Forsyth, D., Arikan, O., Ikemoto, L., O'Brien, J., & Ramanan, D. (2006). Computational studies of human motion part 1: Tracking and motion synthesis. *Foundations and Trends in Computer Graphics and Vision, 1*(2), 77–254. doi:10.1561/0600000005

France, D. J., Shiavi, R. G., Silverman, S., Silverman, M., & Wilkes, D. M. (2000). Acoustical Properties of speech as indicators of depression and suicidal risk. *IEEE Transactions on Bio-Medical Engineering, 47*(7), 829–837. doi:10.1109/10.846676

Francis, S., Rolls, E. T., Bowtell, R., Mc-Glone, F., O'Doherty, J., & Browning, A. (1999). The representation of pleasant touch in the brain and its relationship with taste and olfactory areas. *Neuroreport, 10*, 453–459. doi:10.1097/00001756-199902250-00003

Franck, E., & De Raedt, R. (2007). (in press). Self-esteem reconsidered: Unstable self-esteem outperforms level of self-esteem as vulnerability marker for depression. [Corrected Proof.]. *Behaviour Research and Therapy*. doi:10.1016/j.brat.2007.01.003

Freeman, D. (2003). *Creating Emotions in Games*. IN: New Riders.

Freeman, D. (2004). *Creating Emotion in Games*. London: New Riders.

Fridlund, A. J., & Cacioppo, J. T. (1986). Guidelines for human electromyographic research. *Psychophysiology, 23*, 567–589. doi:10.1111/j.1469-8986.1986.tb00676.x

Friend, M. (2000). Developmental changes in sensitivity to vocal paralanguage. *Developmental Science, 3,* 148–162. doi:10.1111/1467-7687.00108

Friend, M. (2001). The transition from affective to linguistic meaning. *First Language, 21,* 219–243. doi:10.1177/014272370102106302

Friend, M. (2003). What should I do? Behavior regulation by language and paralanguage in early childhood. *Journal of Cognition and Development, 4*(2), 162–183. doi:10.1207/S15327647JCD0402_02

Frijda, N. H. (1994). Varieties of affect: Emotions and episodes, moods, and sentiments. In (Ekman & Davidson, 1994) (pp. 56–58).

Landreth & Homeyer. (1998). Play as the language of children's feelings. In Fromberg, D., & Bergen, D. (Eds.), *Play from Birth to Twelve and Beyond: Contexts, Perspectives and Meanings* (pp. 193–196). London: Routledge.

Fugelsang, J. A., & Dunbar, K. N. (2005). Brain-based mechanisms underlying complex causal thinking. *Neuropsychologia, 43,* 1204–1213. doi:10.1016/j.neuropsychologia.2004.10.012

Gadanho, S. C. (2003). Learning behavior-selection by emotions and cognition in a multi-goal robot task. *Journal of Machine Learning Research, 4*(Jul), 385–412. doi:10.1162/jmlr.2003.4.3.385

Gallese, V., Fadiga, L., Fogassi, L., & Rizzolatti, G. (1996). Action recognition in the premotor cortex. *Brain, 119,* 593–609. doi:10.1093/brain/119.2.593

Gallese, V. (2001). The "Shared Manifold" hypothesis: from mirror neurons to empathy. *Journal of Consciousness Studies, 8*(5-7), 33–50.

Gallese, V. (2008). Mirror neurons and the social nature of language: The neural exploitation hypothesis. *Social Neuroscience, 3*(3-4), 317–333.

Gallese, V., Fadiga, L., & Fogassi, L., & Rizzolatti, Giacomo. (1996). Action recognition in the premotor cortex. *Brain, 119*(2), 593–609. doi:10.1093/brain/119.2.593

Gallese, V., & Keysers, C., & Rizzolatti, Giacomo. (2004). A unifying view of the basis of social cognition. *Trends in Cognitive Sciences, 8*(9), 396–403. doi:10.1016/j.tics.2004.07.002

Galley, M., McKeown, K., Hirschberg, J., & Shriberg, E. (2004). Identifying agreement and disagreement in conversational speech: use of Bayesian Networks to model pragmatic dependencies. In *Proceedings of meeting of the association for computational linguistics* (pp. 669-676).

Garg, N., Favre, S., Salamin, H., Hakkani-Tur, D., & Vinciarelli, A. (2008). Role recognition for meeting participants: an approach based on lexical information and Social Network Analysis. In *Proceedings of the acm international conference on multimedia* (pp. 693-696).

Garrison, D. R., & Anderson, T. (2003). *E-Learning in the 21st Century: A Framework for Research and Practice.* London: Routledge Falmer.

Gaunt, N. (2002). Beyond the Fear of Cyber-strangers: Further Considerations for Domestic Online Safety. In Hosking, J. (Ed.), *Netsafe: Society* (pp. 107–118). Safety and the Internet.

Gauthier, I., Tarr, M. J., Aanderson, A., Skudlarski, P., & Gore, J. C. (1999). Activation of the middle fusiform 'face area' increases with expertise in recognizing novel objects. *Nature Neuroscience, 2,* 568–573. doi:10.1038/9224

Gazzaniga, M. (1985). *The social brain.* New York, NY: Basic Books.

Gazzola, V., Aziz-Zadeh, L., & Keysers, C. (2006). Empathy and the somatotopic auditory mirror system in humans. *Current Biology, 16*(18), 1824–1829. doi:10.1016/j.cub.2006.07.072

Ge, S. S., Wang, C., & Hang, C. C. (2008). A Facial Expression Imitation System in Human Robot Interaction, *The 17th IEEE International Symposium on Robot and Human Interactive Communication,* 213 – 218.

Geary, D. C., & Huffman, K. J. (2002). Brain and cognitive evolution: Forms of modularity and functions of mind. *Psychological Bulletin, 128,* 667–698. doi:10.1037/0033-2909.128.5.667

Ghent, J., & McDonald, J. (2005). Photo-realistic facial expression synthesis. *Image and Vision Computing, 23*(12), 1041–1050. doi:10.1016/j.imavis.2005.06.011

Gibbs, J. L., Ellison, N. B., & Heino, R. D. (2006). Self-presentation in online personals: The role of anticipated future interaction, self-disclosure, and perceived success in Internet dating. *Communication Research, 33*(2), 1–26. doi:10.1177/0093650205285368

Gibson, E. J., & Walk, R. D. (1960). The "Visual Cliff". *Scientific American, 202,* 67–71.

Gibson, J. J. (1979). *The Ecological Approach to Visual Perception.* New York, New York: Houghton Mifflin.

Gilleade, K., Dix, A., & Allanson, J. (2005). *Affective videogames and modes of affective gaming: Assist me, challenge me, emote me.* Paper presented at the Digital Games Research Association Conference.

Gillette, J. M. (1998). *Designing with Light* (3rd ed.). Mountain View, CA: Mayfield.

Gillieade, K., & Dix, A. (2004). Using frustration in the design of adaptive videogames. *Proceedings of ACE 2004, Advances in Computer Entertainment Technology,* (pp 228-232). New York: Association for Computing Machinery

Gillott, A., Furniss, F., & Walter, A. (2001). Anxiety in high-functioning children with autism. *Autism, 5*(3), 277–286. doi:10.1177/1362361301005003005

Gladwell, M. (2005). *Blink: The power of thinking without thinking.* New York: Little Brown & Company.

Glass, C., Merluzzi, T., Biever, J., & Larsen, K. (1982). Cognitive assessment of social anxiety: Development and validation of a self-statement questionnaire. *Cognitive Therapy and Research, 6*(1), 37–55. doi:10.1007/BF01185725

Glassner, A. (2004). *Interactive Storytelling Techniques for 21st Century Fiction.* Natick, MA: AK Peters.

Glenberg, A. M., & Robertson, D. A. (1999). Indexical understanding of instructions. *Discourse Processes, 28*(1), 1–26. doi:10.1080/01638539909545067

Glenberg, A. M., & Robertson, D. A. (2000). Symbol grounding and meaning: a comparison of high dimensional and embodied theories of meaning. *Journal of Memory and Language, 43*(3), 379–401. doi:10.1006/jmla.2000.2714

Gökçay, D., & Smith, M. A. (2008). TÜDADEN: Türkçede Duygusal ve Anlamsal Değerlendirmeli Norm Veri Tabanı. *Proceedings of Brain-Computer Workshop, 4.*

Goldin-Meadow, S. (2003). *The resilience of language. What gesture creation in deaf children can tell us about how all children learn language.* New York, Hove: Psychology Press (Taylor and Francis).

Goleman, D. (2005). *Emotional intelligence.* New York: Random House Publishing Group.

Goodwin, M. S. (2008). Enhancing and accelerating the pace of Autism Research and Treatment: The promise of developing Innovative Technology. *Focus on Autism and Other Developmental Disabilities, 23,* 125–128. doi:10.1177/1088357608316678

Graf, C. (2005). Digital characters as affective interfaces. In Christian Peter, Russell Beale, Elizabeth Crane, Lesley Axelrod, Gerred Blyth (Eds.) *Emotion in HCI: Joint Proceedings of the 2005, 2006, and 2007 Intl. Workshops.* Stuttgart: Fraunhofer IRB Verlag.

Grahe, J., & Bernieri, F. (1999). The importance of nonverbal cues in judging rapport. *Journal of Nonverbal Behavior, 23*(4), 253–269. doi:10.1023/A:1021698725361

Gratch, J., & Marsella, S. (2004). A domain-independent framework for modeling emotion. *Journal of Cognitive Systems Research, 5*(4), 269–306. doi:10.1016/j.cogsys.2004.02.002

Green, D., Baird, G., Barnett, A. L., Henderson, L., Huber, J., & Henderson, S. E. (2002). The severity and nature of motor impairment in Asperger's syndrome: a comparison with specific developmental disorder of motor function. *Journal of Child Psychology and Psychiatry, and Allied Disciplines, 43*(5), 655–668. doi:10.1111/1469-7610.00054

Greene, J. D., Nystrom, L. E., Engell, A. D., Darley, J. M., & Cohen, J. D. (2004). The neural bases of cognitive conflict and control in moral judgment. *Neuron*, *44*, 389–400. doi:10.1016/j.neuron.2004.09.027

Griffiths, P. (1997). *What emtions really are: The problem of psychological categories*. Chicago: Chicago University Press.

Grimm, S., Schmidt, C. F., Bermpohl, F., Heinzel, A., Dahlem, Y., & Wyss, M. (2006). Segregated neural representation of distinct emotion dimensions in the prefrontal cortex-an fMRI study. *NeuroImage*, *30*, 325–340. doi:10.1016/j.neuroimage.2005.09.006

Grodal, T. (2009). *Embodied Visions*. Oxford: Oxford University Press. doi:10.1093/acprof:oso/9780195371314.001.0001

Grodal, T. (2000). Video games and the pleasures of control. In I. Mahwah (Ed.), *D. Zillmann & P. Vorderer (Eds.), Media entertainment: The psychology of its appeal*. NJ: Lawrence Erlbaum Associates.

Groden, J., Goodwin, M. S., Baron, M. G., Groden, G., Velicer, W. F., & Lipsitt, L. P. (2005). Assessing cardiovascular responses to stressors in individuals with autism spectrum disorders. *Focus on Autism and Other Developmental Disabilities*, *20*(4), 244–252. doi:10.1177/10883576050200040601

Gross, R., Matthews, I., Cohn, J., Kanade, T., & Baker, S. (2010). Multi-PIE. *Image and Vision Computing*, *28*(5), 807–813. doi:10.1016/j.imavis.2009.08.002

Gross, J. J. (1999). Emotion and emotion regulation. In Pervin, L. A., & John, O. P. (Eds.), *Handbook of personality: Theory and research* (2nd ed., pp. 525–552). New York: Guilford.

Grossberg, S., & Schmajuk, N. (1987). Neural dynamics of attentionally-modulated pavlovian conditioning: Conditioned reinforcement, inhibition, and opponent processing. *Psychobiology*, *15*, 195–240.

Grossmann, T., & Johnson, M. H. (2007). The development of the social brain in human infancy. *The European Journal of Neuroscience*, *25*(4), 909–919. doi:10.1111/j.1460-9568.2007.05379.x

Grossmann, T., Striano, T., & Friederici, A. D. (2005). Infants' electric brain responses to emotional prosody. *Neuroreport*, *16*(16), 1825–1828. doi:10.1097/01.wnr.0000185964.34336.b1

Grossmann, T., Striano, T., & Friederici, A. D. (2006). Crossmodal integration of emotional information from face and voice in the infant brain. *Developmental Science*, *9*(3), 309–315. doi:10.1111/j.1467-7687.2006.00494.x

Guyton, A. C., & Hall, J. E. (2006). The Autonomic Nervous System and the Adrenal Medulla. In *Textbook of Medical Physiology* (11th ed., pp. 748–760). Philadelphia, Pennsylvania: Elsevier Inc.

Hagemann, D., Waldstein, S. R., & Thayera, J. F. (2003). Thayer Central and autonomic nervous system integration in emotion. *Brain and Cognition*, *52*, 79–87. doi:10.1016/S0278-2626(03)00011-3

Hall, E. (1959). *The silent language*. New York: Doubleday.

Hancock, J. T. (2007). Digital deception: Why, when and how people lie online. In Joinson, A. N., McKenna, K., Postmes, T., & Reips, U. (Eds.), *The Oxford Handbook of Internet Psychology* (pp. 289–301). Oxford: Oxford University Press.

Handy, C. (1995). Trust and the virtual organization. *Harvard Business Review*, *73*(3), 40–50.

Hanjalic, A., & Xu, L. Q. (2005). Affective video content representation and modeling. *IEEE Transactions on Multimedia*, *7*(1), 143–154. doi:10.1109/TMM.2004.840618

Hare, B. (2007). From nonhuman to human mind. What changed and why? *Current Directions in Psychological Science*, *16*(2), 60–64. doi:10.1111/j.1467-8721.2007.00476.x

Hare, B. (2007). From non-human to human mind. What changed and why? *Current Directions in Psychological Science, 16*(2), 60–64. doi:10.1111/j.1467-8721.2007.00476.x

Hare, B., & Tomasello, M. (2005). Human-like social skills in dogs? *Trends in Cognitive Sciences, 9*(9), 439–444. doi:10.1016/j.tics.2005.07.003

Harris, R. B., & Paradice, D. (2007). An investigation of the computer-mediated communication of emotion. *Journal of Applied Sciences Research, 3,* 2081–2090.

Harris, C. L., Berko Gleason, J., & Aycicegi, A. (2006). When is a first language more emotional? Psychophysiological evidence from bilingual speakers. In Pavlenko, A. (Ed.), *Bilingual minds. Emotional experience, expression and representation* (pp. 257–283). Clevedon: Multilingual Matters.

Harrison, N. A., & Critchley, H. D. (2007). Affective neuroscience and psychiatry. *The British Journal of Psychiatry, 191,* 192–194. doi:10.1192/bjp.bp.107.037077

Hartson, H. R. (1998). Human-computer interaction: interdisciplinary roots and trends. *Journal of Systems and Software, 43,* 103–118. doi:10.1016/S0164-1212(98)10026-2

Hasselmo, M. E., Rolls, E. T., & Baylis, G. C. (1989). The role of expression and identity in the face–selective responses of neurons in the temporal visual cortex of the monkey. *Behavioural Brain Research, 32,* 203–218. doi:10.1016/S0166-4328(89)80054-3

Hatipoglu, C. (2004). Do apologies in e-mails follow spoken or written norms?: Some examples from British English. *Studies About Languages, 5,* 21–29.

Hauk, O., Johnsrude, I., & Pulvermüller, F. (2005). Somatotopic representation of action words in human motor and premotor cortex. *Neuron, 41*(2), 301–307. doi:10.1016/S0896-6273(03)00838-9

Haxby, J. V., Hoffman, E. A., & Gobbini, M. I. (2000). The distributed human neural system for face perception. *Trends in Cognitive Sciences, 4,* 223–233. doi:10.1016/S1364-6613(00)01482-0

Hayes, M. H. (1996). *Statistical Digital Signal Processing and Modeling.* New York: Wiley.

Hazlett, R. L. (2006). *Measuring emotional valence during interactive experiences: Boys at video game play. CHI 2006 Proceedings* (pp. 22–27). New York: Association for Computing Machinery.

Hecht, M., De Vito, J., & Guerrero, L. (1999). Perspectives on nonverbal communication-codes, functions, and contexts. In L. Guerrero, J. De Vito, & M. Hecht (Eds.), *The nonverbal communication reader - classic and contemporary readings* (p. 3-18). Waveland Press.

Heinrichs, M., Baumgartner, T., Kirschbaum, C., & Ehlert, U. (2003). Social support and oxytocin interact to suppress cortisol and subjective responses to psychosocial stress. *Biological Psychiatry, 54,* 1389–1398. doi:10.1016/S0006-3223(03)00465-7

Hess, U., Blairy, S., & Kleck, R. E. (2000). The influence of facial emotion displays, gender, and ethnicity on judgments of dominance and affiliation. *Journal of Nonverbal Behavior, 24*(4), 265–283. doi:10.1023/A:1006623213355

Hill, E., Berthoz, S., & Frith, U. (2004). Brief report: cognitive processing of own emotions in individuals with autistic spectrum disorder and in their relatives. *Journal of Autism and Developmental Disabilities, 34*(2). doi:10.1023/B:JADD.0000022613.41399.14

Hillard, D., Ostendorf, M., & Shriberg, E. (2003). Detection of agreement vs. disagreement in meetings: Training with unlabeled data. In *Proceedings of the north American chapter of the association for computational linguistics - human language technologies conference.*

Hirshfield, L. M., Solovey, E. T., Girouard, A., Kebinger, J., Jacob, R. J. K., Sassaroli, A., et al. (2009). *Brain measurement for usability testing and adaptive interfaces: an example of uncovering syntactic workload with functional near infrared spectroscopy.* Paper presented at the In Proceedings of the 27th international conference on Human factors in computing systems (CHI).

Hoch, M., Fleischmann, G., & Girod, B. (1994). Modeling and animation of facial expressions based on B-splines. *The Visual Computer*, *11*, 87–95. doi:10.1007/BF01889979

Hofmann, H. A., & Schildberger, K. (2001). Assessment of strength and willingness to fight during aggressive encounters in crickets. *Animal Behaviour*, (62): 337–348. doi:10.1006/anbe.2001.1746

Hohenberger, A. (2004). S.Goldin-Meadow (2003). The resilience of language. What gesture creation in deaf children can tell us about how all children learn language. New York, Hove.: Psychology Press (Taylor and Francis). *Linguist List 15-683.*

Holland, P. C., & Gallagher, M. (2003). Double dissociation of the effects of lesions of basolateral and central amygdala on conditioned stimulus-potentiated feeding and Pavlovian-instrumental transfer. *The European Journal of Neuroscience*, *17*, 1680–1694. doi:10.1046/j.1460-9568.2003.02585.x

Holson, L. M. (2004, April 10). Out of Hollywood, rising fascination with video games. *The New York Times on the Web.*

Holstege, G., Georgiadis, J. R., Paans, A. M., Meiners, L. C., van der Graaf, F. H., & Reinders, A. A. (2003). Brain activation during human male ejaculation. *The Journal of Neuroscience*, *23*, 9185–9193.

Homer,. (1990). *The Iliad* (Fagles, R., Trans.). New York: Viking.

Hone, K. (2006). Emphatic agents to reduce user frustration: The effects of varying agent characteristics. *Interacting with Computers*, *18*, 227–245. doi:10.1016/j.intcom.2005.05.003

Horwitz, N. H. (1998). John F. Fulton (1899-1960). *Neurosurgery*, *43*(1), 178–184. doi:10.1097/00006123-199807000-00129

House, A., Dennis, M., Warlow, C., Hawton, K., & Moltneux, A. (1990). Mood disorders after stroke and their relation to lesion location. *Brain*, *113*, 1113–1129. doi:10.1093/brain/113.4.1113

Huang, L., & Su, C. (2006). Facial expression synthesis using manifold learning and belief propagation. *Soft Computing - A Fusion of Foundations. Methodologies and Applications*, *10*(12), 1193–1200.

Huber, D., Veinante, P., & Stop, R. (2005). Vasopressin and oxytocin excite distinct neuronal populations in the central amygdala. *Science*, *308*, 245–248. doi:10.1126/science.1105636

Hudlicka, E. (2009). Affective game engines: motivation and requirements. *Proceedings of the 4th International Conference On The Foundation Of Digital Games*. 299-306

Huizinga, J. (1938). *Homo Ludens*. London: Routledge.

Hyun, H. K., Kim, E. H., & Kwak, Y. K. (2005). Improvement of emotion recognition by Bayesian classifier using non-zero-pitch concept. *IEEE International Workshop on Robots and Human Interactive Communication*, ROMAN 2005, (pp. 312-316).

Iacoboni, M., Molnar-Szakacs, I., Gallese, V., Buccino, G., Mazziotta, J. C., & Rizzolatti, G. (2005). Grasping the intentions of others with one's own mirror neuron system. *PLoS Biology*, *3*(3), 529–535. doi:10.1371/journal.pbio.0030079

IJsselsteijn, W. A., Poels, K., & de Kort, Y. A. W. (2008). *The game experience questionnaire: Development of a self-report measure to assess player experiences of digital games.* Eindhoven, The Netherlands: FUGA technical report,TU Eindhoven.

Ikemoto, S., & Panksepp, J. (1999). The role of nucleus accumbens dopamine in motivated behavior: A unifying interpretation with special reference to reward-seeking. *Brain Research. Brain Research Reviews*, *31*(1), 6–41. doi:10.1016/S0165-0173(99)00023-5

Isbister, K., & Schaffer, N. (2008). *Game Usability: Advancing the Player Experience*. Morgan Kaufmann.

Ito, M., Okabe, D., & Matsuda, M. (Eds.). (2005). *Personal, portable, pedestrian: Mobile phones in Japanese life.* Cambridge, MA: MIT Press.

Izard, C. E. (2009). Emotion theory and research. *Annual Review of Psychology, 60,* 1–25. doi:10.1146/annurev.psych.60.110707.163539

Izard, C. E., Libero, D. Z., Putnam, P., & Haynes, O. M. (1993). Stability of emotion experiences and their relations to traits of personality. *Journal of Personality and Social Psychology, 64,* 847–860. doi:10.1037/0022-3514.64.5.847

Izard, C. E. (1992). Basic emotions, relations among emotions, and emotion- cognition relations. *Psychological Review, 99*(3), 561–565. doi:10.1037/0033-295X.99.3.561

Izard, C. E. (1993). Four systems for emotion activation: cognitive and noncognitive processes. *Psychological Review, 100,* 68–90. doi:10.1037/0033-295X.100.1.68

Izard, C. E. (2007). Basic emotions, natural kinds, emotion schemas, and a new paradigm. *Perspectives on Psychological Science, 2*(3), 260–280. doi:10.1111/j.1745-6916.2007.00044.x

Izard, C. E. (2009). Emotion theory and research: highlights, unanswered questions, and emerging issues. *Annual Review of Psychology, 60,* 1–25. doi:10.1146/annurev.psych.60.110707.163539

Jacobson, J. W., Mulick, J. A., & Green, G. (1998). Cost-benefit estimates for early intensive behavioral intervention for young children with autism – General model and single state case. *Behavioral Interventions, 13*(4). doi:10.1002/(SICI)1099-078X(199811)13:4<201::AID-BIN17>3.0.CO;2-R

James, W. (1884). What is emotion? *Mind, 4,* 188–204. doi:10.1093/mind/os-IX.34.188

Janis, I. L., & Mann, L. (1977). *Decision making: A psychological analysis of conflict, choice and commitment.* New York: Free Press.

Jayagopi, D., Hung, H., Yeo, C., & Gatica-Perez, D. (2009). Modeling dominance in group conversations from non-verbal activity cues. *IEEE Transactions on Audio. Speech and Language Processing, 17*(3), 501–513. doi:10.1109/TASL.2008.2008238

Ji, Q., Lan, P., & Looney, C. (2006). A probabilistic framework for modeling and real-time monitoring human fatigue. *IEEE Transactions on Systems, Man, and Cybernetics-A, 36*(5), 862–875. doi:10.1109/TSMCA.2005.855922

Jones, S. (2002). The Internet goes to college: How students are living in the future with today's technology. *Pew Internet and American Life Project.* Retrieved March 18, 2010 from http://www.pewinternet.org/~/media//Files/Reports/2002/PIP_College_Report.pdf.pdf.

Jones, S. (2009). *Generations online in 2009. Pew Internet and American Life Data Memo* [Online]. Retrieved March 16, 2010 from http://www.pewinternet.org/~/media//Files/Reports/2009/PIP_Generations_2009.pdf.

Jorge, R., & Robinson, R. G. (2002). Mood disorders following traumatic brain injury. *NeuroRehabilitation, 17,* 311–324.

Kahneman, D., & Frederick, S. (2002). Representativeness revisited: Attribute substitution in intuitive judgement. In Gilovich, T., Griffin, D., & Kahneman, D. (Eds.), *Heuristics and biases: The psychology of intuitive judgement* (pp. 49–81). Cambridge, UK: Cambridge University Press.

Kahneman, D., & Tversky, A. (1982). The simulation heuristic. In Kahneman, D., Slovic, P., & Tversky, A. (Eds.), *Judgment under uncertainty* (pp. 201–208). Cambridge, UK: Cambridge University Press.

Kalin, N. H., Shelton, S. E., & Davidson, R. J. (2004). The Role of the Central Nucleus of the Amygdala in Mediating Fear and Anxiety in the Primate. *The Journal of Neuroscience, 24,* 5506–5515. doi:10.1523/JNEUROSCI.0292-04.2004

Kanade, T., Cohn, J. F., & Tian, Y. (2000). Comprehensive database for facial expression analysis. *Proc. Fourth IEEE Int. Conf. on Automatic Face and Gesture Recognition* (pp. 46–53).

Kang, M., Kim, S., & Park, S. (2007). Developing an emotional presence scale for measuring students' involvement during e-learning process. *Proceedings of World Conference on Educational Multimedia, Hypermedia and Telecommunications (ED-MEDIA) 2007*, 2829-2831.

Kanwisher, N., McDermott, J., & Chun, M. M. (1997). The fusiform face area: A module in human extrastriate cortex specialized for face perception. *The Journal of Neuroscience, 17*, 4302–4311.

Kaplan, J. T., & Iacoboni, M. (2006). Getting a grip on other minds: Mirror neurons, intention understanding, and cognitive empathy. *Social Neuroscience, 1*(3-4), 175–183. doi:10.1080/17470910600985605

Kapoor, A., Mota, S., & Picard, R. W. (2001). *Towards a learning companion that recognizes affect*. Paper presented at Emotional and Intelligent II: The Tangled Knot of Social Cognition AAAI Fall Symposium.

Kapoor, A., Picard, R., & Ivanov, Y. (2004). Probabilistic combination of multiple modalities to detect interest. In *Proceedings of the international conference on pattern recognition* (pp. 969-972).

Karmiloff-Smith, A. (1979). Micro- and macrodevelopmental changes in language acquisition and other representational systems. *Cognitive Science, 3*(2), 91–118. doi:10.1207/s15516709cog0302_1

Karmiloff-Smith, A. (1986). From meta-processes to conscious access: Evidence from children's metalinguistic and repair data. *Cognition, 23*, 95–147. doi:10.1016/0010-0277(86)90040-5

Karmiloff-Smith, A. (1992). *Beyond modularity. A developmental perspective on cognitive science*. Cambridge, MA: MIT Press.

Kato, S., Kato, Y., Scott, D. J., & Akahori, K. (2008). Analysis of anger in mobile phone Emil communications in Japan. *Waseda Journal of Human Sciences, 21*(1), 29–39.

Kato, S., Kato, Y., & Tachino, T. (2007). Lesson practice which took in the lesson preliminary announcement using the mobile phone. *Poster-Proceedings of ICCE, 2007*, 21–22.

Kato, Y., & Akahori, K. (2006). Analysis of judgment of partners' emotions during e-mail and face-to-face communication. *Journal of Science Education in Japan, 29*(5), 354–365.

Kato, Y., Kato, S., & Akahori, K. (2007). Effects of emotional cues transmitted in e-mail communication on the emotions experienced by senders and receivers. *Computers in Human Behavior, 23*(4), 1894–1905. doi:10.1016/j.chb.2005.11.005

Kato, Y., Kato, S., & Scott, D. J. (2007). Misinterpretation of emotional cues and content in Japanese email, computer conferences, and mobile text messages. In Clausen, E. I. (Ed.), *Psychology of Anger* (pp. 145–176). Hauppauge, NY: Nova Science Publishers.

Kato, S., Kato, Y., & Akahori, K. (2006). Study on emotional transmissions in communication using bulletin board system. *Proceedings of World Conference on E-Learning in Corporate, Government, Healthcare, and Higher Education (E-Learn) 2006*, 2576-2584.

Kato, Y., Kato, S., Scott, D. J., & Sato, K. (2008). Emotional strategies in mobile phone email communication in Japan: focusing on four kinds of basic emotions. *Proceedings of World Conference on Educational Multimedia, Hypermedia and Telecommunications (ED-MEDIA) 2008*, 1058-1066.

Kato, Y., Kato, S., Scott, D. J., & Takeuchi, T. (2008). Relationships between the emotional transmissions in mobile phone email communication and the email contents in Japan. *Proceedings of World Conference on E-Learning in Corporate, Government, Healthcare, and Higher Education (E-Learn) 2008*, 2804-2811.

Kato, Y., Sugimura, K., & Akahori, K. (2001). An affective aspect of computer mediated communication: analysis of communications by E-mail. *Proceedings of ICCE/SchoolNetM*: 2 (pp. 636–642).

Keller, R. (1997). In what sense can explanations of language change be functional? In Gvozdanovic, J. (Ed.), *Language change and functional explanations* (pp. 9–19). Berlin: Mouton de Gruyter.

Kennedy, R. S., Lane, N. E., Berbaum, K. S., & Lilienthal, M. G. (1993). Simulator sickness questionnaire: an enhanced method for quantifying simulator sickness. *The International Journal of Aviation Psychology, 3*(3), 203–220. doi:10.1207/s15327108ijap0303_3

Kerns, J. C., Cohen, J. D., MacDonald, A. W. III, Cho, R. Y., Stenger, V. A., & Carter, C. S. (2004). Anterior cingulate conflict monitoring and adjustments in control. *Science, 303,* 1023–1026. doi:10.1126/science.1089910

Kerr, S., & Durkin, K. (2004). Understanding of thought bubbles as mental representations in children with autism: Implications for theory of mind. *Journal of Autism and Developmental Disorders, 34*(6). doi:10.1007/s10803-004-5285-z

Keysar, B., & Henly, A. S. (2002). Speakers' overestimation of their effectiveness. *Psychological Science, 13,* 207–212. doi:10.1111/1467-9280.00439

Keysers, C., & Gazzola, V. (2010). Social neuroscience: Mirror neurons recorded in humans. *Current Biology, 20*(8), R353–R354. doi:10.1016/j.cub.2010.03.013

Khan, R., & Cassidy, G. & Sykes. (in press). Impact of Music on Ergogenic and Psychophysical Outcomes of Exercise in a Gameplay Context. *International Journal of Computer Science in Sport.*

Khan, R., & Sykes, J. (2005). *Emotions evoked during collaborative and competitive play when players are co-located and spatially separated.* Paper presented at the Digital Games Research Association conference, Vancouver, Canada

Kiesler, S., Siegel, J., & McGuire, T. W. (1984). Social psychological aspects of computer-mediated communication. *The American Psychologist, 39,* 1123–1134. doi:10.1037/0003-066X.39.10.1123

Killcross, S., Robbins, T. W., & Everitt, B. J. (1997). Different types of fear-conditioned behaviour mediated by separate nuclei within amygdala. *Nature, 388*(6640), 377–380. doi:10.1038/41097

Kim, J. (2006). Emergence: Core ideas and issues. *Synthese, 151*(3), 547–559. doi:10.1007/s11229-006-9025-0

Kim, J. H., Gunn, D. V., Schuh, E., Phillips, B., Pagulayan, R. J., & Wixon, D. (2008). *Tracking real-time user experience (true): a comprehensive instrumentation solution for complex systems.* Paper presented at the Proceedings of twenty-sixth annual SIGCHI conference on Human factors in computing systems (CHI 2008).

Kito, T., & Lee, B. (2004). Interpersonal perception in Japanese and British observers. *Perception, 33,* 957–974. doi:10.1068/p3471

Klein, D. F., Skrobola, A. M., & Garfinkel, R. S. (1995). Preliminary look at the effects of pregnancy on the course of panic disorder. *Anxiety, 1,* 227–232.

Klein, J., Moon, Y., & Picard, R. W. (2002). This computer responds to user frustration: Theory, design and the results. *Interacting with Computers, 14,* 119–140.

Kleinginna, P., & Kleinginna, A. (1981). A categorized list of emotion definitions, with suggestions for a consensual definition. *Motivation and Emotion, 5*(4), 345–379. doi:10.1007/BF00992553

Kleinsmith, A., Ravindra De Silva, P., & Bianchi-Berthouze, N. (2005). *Recognizing emotion from postures: cross-cultural differences in user modeling.* Paper presented at User Modeling.

Kling, R., & Star, S. L. (1998). Human centered systems in the perspective of organizational and social informatics. *Computers & Society, 28*(1), 22–29. doi:10.1145/277351.277356

Klüver, H., & Bucy, P.C. (1939). Preliminary Analysis of Functions of the Temporal Lobes in Monkeys. *Archives of Neurology and Psychiatry, 42* (6), 979-1 000.

Knapp, M., & Hall, J. (1972). *Nonverbal communication in human interaction.* Harcourt Brace College Publishers.

Knoph, D. C. A. (1979). *The Book of Movie Photography.* London: Alfred Knopf.

Knutson, B., Fong, G. W., Adams, C. M., Varner, J. L., & Hommer, D. (2001). Dissociation of reward anticipation and outcome with event-related fMRI. *Neuroreport, 12,* 3683–3687. doi:10.1097/00001756-200112040-00016

Knutson, B., Wolkowitz, O. M., Cole, S. W., Chan, T., Moore, E. A., & Johnson, R. C. (1998). Selective alteration of personality and social behavior by serotonergic intervention. *The American Journal of Psychiatry, 155*(3), 373–379.

Koelstra, S., & Pantic, M. (2008). Non-rigid registration using free-form deformations for recognition of facial actions and their temporal dynamics. *Proc. IEEE Int. Conf. on Automatic Face and Gesture Recognition.*

Koepp, M. J., Gunn, R. N., Lawrence, A. D., Cunningham, V. J., Dagher, A., & Jones, T. (1998). Evidence for striatal dopamine release during a video game. *Nature, 393*(6682), 266–268. doi:10.1038/30498

Korsten, N. (2009). *Neural Architectures for an Appraisal Basis of Emotion.* PhD thesis, London:King's College.

Kosfeld, M., Heinrichs, M., Zak, P. J., Fischbacher, U., & Fehr, E. (2005). Oxytocin increases trust in humans. *Nature, 435*(7042), 673–676. doi:10.1038/nature03701

Kozima, H., Michalowski, M. P., & Nakagawa, C. (2009). Keepon: A playful robot for research, therapy, and entertainment. *International Journal of Social Robotics, 1*(1), 3–18. doi:10.1007/s12369-008-0009-8

Kramer, A., Sirevaag, E., & Braune, R. (1987). A Psychophysiological Assessment of Operator Workload during Simulated Flight Missions. *Human Factors, 29*(2), 145–160.

Krauss, R. M., & Fussell, S. R. (1996). Social Psychological models of interpersonal communication. In Higgins, E. T., & Kruglanski, A. W. (Eds.), *Social Psychology: Handbook of Basic Principles* (pp. 655–701). NY: The Guilford Press.

Kraut, R. E. (1978). Verbal and nonverbal cues in the perception of lying. *Journal of Personality and Social Psychology, 36*, 380–391. doi:10.1037/0022-3514.36.4.380

Kringelbach, M. L., O'Doherty, J., Rolls, E. T., & Andrews, C. (2003). Activation of the human orbitofrontal cortex to a liquid food stimulus is correlated with its subjective pleasantness. *Cerebral Cortex, 13*, 1064–1071. doi:10.1093/cercor/13.10.1064

Kringelbach, M. L. (2005). The orbitofrontal cortex: Linking reward to hedonic experience. *Nature Reviews. Neuroscience, 6*, 691–702. doi:10.1038/nrn1747

Kringelbach, M. L., & Rolls, E. T. (2004). The functional neuroanatomy of the human orbitofrontal cortex: evidence from neuroimaging and neuropsychology. *Progress in Neurobiology, 72*(5), 341–372. doi:10.1016/j.pneurobio.2004.03.006

Krinidis, S., & Pitas, I. (2006) Facial expression synthesis through facial expressions statistical analysis. In *Proc. 2006 European Signal Processing Conference.*

Krinidis, S., Buciu, I., & Pitas, I. (2003). *Facial expression analysis and synthesis: A survey.* Proceedings of HCI International, 10th Int. Conference on Human-Computer Interaction, pp. 1432 – 1433, June 22-27, Crete, Greece.

Kruger, J., Epley, N., Parker, P., & Ng, Z. (2005). Egocentrism over e-mail: Can we communicate as well as we think? *Journal of Personality and Social Psychology, 89*(6), 925–936. doi:10.1037/0022-3514.89.6.925

Kruger, J., Epley, N., Parker, P., & Ng, Z. (2005). Egocentrism over e-mail: Can we communicate as well as we think? *Journal of Personality and Social Psychology, 89*(6), 925–936. doi:10.1037/0022-3514.89.6.925

Kuhl, P. K. (1993). Early linguistic experience and phonetic perception: implications for theories of developmental speech perception. *Journal of Phonetics, 21*(1-2), 125–139.

Kuhl, P. K. (1994). Learning and representation in speech and language. *Current Opinion in Neurobiology, 4*(6), 812–822. doi:10.1016/0959-4388(94)90128-7

Kuhl, P. K. (2000). A new view of language acquisition. *Proceedings of the National Academy of Sciences of the United States of America, 97*(22), 11850–11857. doi:10.1073/pnas.97.22.11850

Kuhl, P. K. (2004). Early language acquisition: Cracking the speech code. *Nature Reviews. Neuroscience, 5*(11), 831–843. doi:10.1038/nrn1533

Kuhl, P. K. (2007). Is speech learning 'gated' by the social brain? *Developmental Science*, *10*(1), 110–120. doi:10.1111/j.1467-7687.2007.00572.x

Kuhl, P. K., Tsao, F.-M., & Liu, H.-M. (2003). Foreign-language experience in infancy: effects of short-term exposure and social interaction on phonetic learning. *Proceedings of the National Academy of Sciences of the United States of America*, *100*(15), 9096–9101. doi:10.1073/pnas.1532872100

Kulic, D., & Croft, E. (2007). Physiological and subjective responses to articulated robot motion. *Robotica*, *25*, 13–27. doi:10.1017/S0263574706002955

Kunda, Z. (1999). *Social cognition*. Boston: MIT Press.

Kuniavsky, M. (2003). *Observing the user experience. A practitioners guide to user research*. San Francisco: CA: Morgan Kauffman publishers.

Kunst-Wilson, W., & Zajonc, R. (1980). Affective discrimination of stimuli that cannot be recognized. *Science*, *207*, 557–558. doi:10.1126/science.7352271

Kuppens, P., & van Mechelen, I. (2007). Interactional appraisal models for the anger appraisals of threatened self-esteem, other-blame and frustration. *Cognition and Emotion*, *21*, 56–77. doi:10.1080/02699930600562193

Kwon, O. W., Chan, K., Hao, J., & Lee, T. W. (2003). Emotion Recognition by Speech Signals. In *Proceedings of International Conference EUROSPEECH* (pp. 125-128).

LaBar, K., & Phelps, E. (1998). Arousal-mediated memory consolidation: Role of the medial temporal lobe in humans. *Psychological Science*, *9*, 490–493. doi:10.1111/1467-9280.00090

Lagrange, M., Marchand, S., Raspaud, M., & Rault, J.-B. (2003). *Enhanced Partial Tracking Using Linear Prediction*. Paper presented at the DAFx, London.

Lahl, O., Göritz, A. S., Pietrowsky, R., & Rosenberg, J. (2009). Using the World-Wide Web to obtain large-scale word norms: 190,212 ratings on a set of 2,654 German nouns. *Behavior Research Methods*, *41*(1), 13–19. doi:10.3758/BRM.41.1.13

Lamm, C., Nusbaum, H. C., Meltzoff, A. N., & Decety, J. (2007). What are you feeling? Using functional magnetic resonance imaging to assess the modulation of sensory and affective responses during empathy for pain. *PLoS ONE*, *12*, e1292. .doi:10.1371/journal.pone.0001292

Landman, J., Vandewater, E. A., Stewart, A. J., & Malley, J. E. (1995). Missed opportunities: Psychological ramifications of counterfactual thought in midlife women. *Journal of Adult Development*, *2*, 87–97. doi:10.1007/BF02251257

Landry, S. H. (2008). The role of parents in early childhood learning. In R. E. Tremblay, R.G. Barr, R. de Peters, & M. Boivin (Eds.), *Encyclopedia on Early Childhood Development* [online] (pp. 1-6). Montreal Quebec: Centre of Excellence for Early Childhood Development. http://www.child-encyclopedia.com/documents/LandryANGxp.pdf. (Accessed 25/07/2010).

Lane, R. D., & Nadel, L. (2006). Facial Expression, Emotion, and Hemispheric Organization. In Kolb, B., & Taylor, L. (Eds.), *Cognitive Neuroscience of Emotion* (pp. 62–83). Oxford University Press.

Lang, P. J., & Bradley, M. M. (2010). Emotion and the motivational brain. *Biological Psychology*, *84*(3), 437–450. doi:10.1016/j.biopsycho.2009.10.007

Lang, P. J., Reenwald, M. K. C., Bradley, M. M., & Hamm, A. O. (1993). Looking at pictures: Affective, facial, visceral, and behavioral reactions. *Psychophysiotogy*, *30*, 261–273. doi:10.1111/j.1469-8986.1993.tb03352.x

Lang, P. J. (1995). The emotion probe: studies of motivation and attention. *The American Psychologist*, *50*, 372–385. doi:10.1037/0003-066X.50.5.372

Lang, P. J., Bradley, M. M., & Cuthbert, B. N. (2008). *International affective picture system (IAPS): Affective ratings of pictures and instruction manual*. Technical Report A-8. Gainesville, FL: University of Florida.

Larsen, R. J., & Fredrickson, B. L. (1999). Measurement issues in emotion research. In Kahneman, D., Diener, E., & Schwarz, N. (Eds.), *Well-being: Foundations of hedonic psychology* (pp. 40–60). Russell Sage, New York.

Laskowski, K., Ostendorf, M., & Schultz, T. (2008). Modeling vocal interaction for text independent participant characterization in multi-party conversation. In *Proceedings of the 9th isca/acl sigdial workshop on discourse and dialogue* (pp. 148-155).

Lawrence, L.L., & Fernald, Anne (1993). *When prosody and semantics conflict: infants' sensitivity to discrepancies between tone of voice and verbal content.* Poster session presented at the biennial meeting of the Society for Research in Child Development, New Orleans, LA.

Lazar, J., Jones, A., Hackley, M., & Shneiderman, B. (2005). Severity and impact of computer user frustration: A comparison of student and workplace users. *Interacting with Computers, 18*, 187–207. doi:10.1016/j.intcom.2005.06.001

Lazarus, R. S. (1999). The cognition-emotion debate: A bit of history. In Dalgleish, T., & Power, M. J. (Eds.), *Handbook of Cognition and Emotion* (pp. 3–17). Chichester: John Wiley & Sons.

Lazer, D., Pentland, A., Adamic, L., Aral, S., Barabasi, A., & Brewer, D. (2009). Computational social science. *Science, 323*, 721–723. doi:10.1126/science.1167742

Lazzaro, N. (2008). Why we play: Affect and the fun of games. In Sears, A., & Jacko, J. A. (Eds.), *The Human-Computer Interaction Handbook. Abingdon: Taylor and Francis Group.*

Lazzaro, N. (2004). *Why we play games: Four keys to more emotion in player experiences.* Retrieved December 1st 2009 from www.xeodesign.com/xeodesign_whyweplaygames.pdf

Lea, M., & Spears, R. (1995). Love at first byte? Building personal relationships over computer networks. In Wood, J. T., & Duck, S. (Eds.), *Understudied relationships: Off the beaten track* (pp. 197–233). Beverly Hills, CA: Sage.

Lea, M., O'Shea, T., Fung, P., & Spears, R. (1992). "Flaming" in computer-mediated communication: Observations, explanations, implications. In M. Lea (Ed.), *Contexts of Computer-Mediated Communication*, pp.89-112. NY: Harvester Wheasheaf.

LeBlanc, M., Hunicke, R., & Zubek, R. (2004) *MDA: A formal approach to game design and game research.* Retrieved December 1st 2009, from www.cs.northwestern.edu/~hunicke/MDA.pdf

Leder, H., Belke, B., Oeberst, A., & Augustin, D. (2004). A model of aesthetic appreciation and aesthetic judgements. *The British Journal of Psychology, 95*, 489–508. doi:10.1348/0007126042369811

Ledoux, J. E. (1992). Brain mechanisms of emotion and emotional learning. *Current Opinion in Neurobiology, 2*, 191–197. doi:10.1016/0959-4388(92)90011-9

LeDoux, J. (1995). Emotion: Clues from the brain. *Annual Review of Psychology, 46*, 209–235. doi:10.1146/annurev.ps.46.020195.001233

LeDoux, J. (2000). Emotion circuits in the brain. *Annual Review of Neuroscience, 23*, 155–184. doi:10.1146/annurev.neuro.23.1.155

LeDoux, J. (2007). The amygdala. *Current Biology, 17*(20), R868–R874. doi:10.1016/j.cub.2007.08.005

LeDoux, J. E. (2002). *The synaptic self.* New York, NY: Viking.

LeDoux, J. (1996). *The emotional brain.* New York: Simon & Schuster.

Lee, S. J., Park, K. R., & Kim, J. (2009). A comparative study of facial appearance modeling methods for active appearance models. *Pattern Recognition Letters, 30*(14), 1335–1346. doi:10.1016/j.patrec.2009.05.019

Lee, C. M., & Narayanan, S. S. (2005). Toward detecting emotions in spoken dialogs. *IEEE Transactions on Speech and Audio Processing, 13*(2), 293–303. doi:10.1109/TSA.2004.838534

Lee, A., & Bruckman, A. (2007). Judging You by the Company You Keep: Dating on Social Networking Sites. *Proceedings of the 2007 International ACM Conference on Supporting Group Work* (pp. 371-378).

Lee, C. M., Narayanan, S., & Pieraccini, R. (2001). Recognition of negative emotions from the speech signals. In *Proceedings of IEEE Workshop on Automatic Speech Recognition and Understanding* (pp. 240-243).

Lee, C.-S., & Elgammal, A. (2006) Nonlinear shape and appearance models for facial expression analysis and synthesis. *International Conference on Pattern Recognition, 1,* 497 – 502.

Leech, G. (1983). *Principles of pragmatics*. London: Longman.

Levelt, W. J. M. (1999). Models of word production. *Trends in Cognitive Sciences, 3*(6), 223–233. doi:10.1016/S1364-6613(99)01319-4

Levelt, W. J. M., Roelofs, A., & Meyer, A. S. (1999). A theory of lexical access in speech production. *The Behavioral and Brain Sciences, 22,* 1–75. doi:10.1017/S0140525X99001776

Levine, J., & Moreland, R. (1990). Progress in small roup research. *Annual Review of Psychology, 41,* 585–634. doi:10.1146/annurev.ps.41.020190.003101

Levine, J., & Moreland, R. (1998). Small groups. In Gilbert, D., & Lindzey, G. (Eds.), *The handbook of social psychology* (*Vol. 2*, pp. 415–469). New York: Oxford University Press.

Lewis, P. A., Critchley, H. D., Rotshtein, P., & Dolan, R. J. (2007). Neural Correlates of Processing Valence and Arousal in Affective Words. *Cerebral Cortex, 17,* 742–748. doi:10.1093/cercor/bhk024

Lewis, M. (2005). Bridging emotion theory and neurobiology through dynamic systems modeling. *The Behavioral and Brain Sciences, 28,* 169–245. doi:10.1017/S0140525X0500004X

Lewis, M. (1999). The role of the self in cognition and emotion. In Dalgleish, T., & Power, M. J. (Eds.), *Handbook of cognition and emotion* (pp. 125–142). Chichester: John Wiley & Sons.

Lewis, M. D., & Granic, I. (1999). Self-organization of cognition-emotion interactions. In Dalgleish, T., & Power, M. J. (Eds.), *Handbook of Cognition and Emotion* (pp. 683–701). Chichester: John Wiley & Sons.

Lewis, M. (2000). Self-Conscious Emotions: Embarrassment, Pride, Shame, and Guilt. In Lewis, M., & Haviland-Jones, J. (Eds.), *Handbook of emotions* (pp. 623–636). New York: Guilford Press, New York.

Lhermitte, F., Pillon, B., & Serdaru, M. (1986). Human anatomy and the frontal lobes. Part I: Imitation and utilization behavior: A neuropsychological study of 75 patients. *Annals of Neurology, 19,* 326–334. doi:10.1002/ana.410190404

Li, L., & Chen, J. (2006). Emotion recognition using physiological signals. In Pan, Z. (Eds.), *Lecture Notes in Computer Science: Advances in Artificial Reality and Tele-existence* (pp. 437–446). Berlin: Springer-Verlag. doi:10.1007/11941354_44

Li, X., Tao, J., Johanson, M. T., Soltis, J., Savage, A., Leong, K. M., & Newman, J. D. (2007). Stress and emotion classification using jitter and shimmer features. In *Proceedings of IEEE International Conference on Acoustics, Speech & Signal Processing, ICASSP2007* (Vol. 4, pp. IV-1081-4).

Liberman, A. M., & Mattingly, Ignatius G. (1985). The motor theory of speech perception revised. *Cognition, 21,* 1–36. doi:10.1016/0010-0277(85)90021-6

Liberman, A. M., & Whalen, D. H. (2000). On the relation of speech to language. *Trends in Cognitive Sciences, 4*(5), 187–196. doi:10.1016/S1364-6613(00)01471-6

Libkuman, T. M., Otani, H., Kern, R., Viger, S. G., & Novak, N. (2007). Multidimensional normative ratings for the International Affective Picture System. *Behavior Research Methods, 39,* 326–334.

Lieberman, M. D. (2007). Social cognitive neuroscience: A review of core processes. *Annual Review of Psychology, 58,* 259–289. doi:10.1146/annurev.psych.58.110405.085654

Lieberman, M. D. (2003). Reflective and reflexive judgment processes: A social cognitive neuroscience approach. In Forgas, J. P., Williams, K. R., & Hippel, W. v. (Eds.), *Social judgments: Implicit and explicit processes* (pp. 44–67). New York: Cambridge University Press.

Liebermann, P. (2000). *Human language and our reptilian brain: the subcortical bases of speech, syntax, and thought*. Cambridge, MA: Harvard University Press.

Liljedahl, M., Papworth, N., & Lindberg, S. (2007). Beowolf - an Audio Mostly game. *Proceedings of the internationals conference on Advances in computer entertainment technology 2007* (ACE'07) (pp 200-203), New York: Association for Computing Machinery

Lim, C. L., Rennie, C., Barry, R. J., Bahramali, H., & Lazzaro, I., manor, B., Gordon, E. (1997). Decompos-ing skin conductance into tonic and phasic measurements. *International Journal of Psychophysiology, 25*(2), 97–109. doi:10.1016/S0167-8760(96)00713-1

Linnoila, V. M. I., & Virkkunen, M. (1992). Aggression, suicidality, and serotonin. *The Journal of Clinical Psychiatry, 53*(supp. 10), 46–51.

Lisetti, C.L., & Schiano, D.J. (2000). Automatic facial expression interpretation: Where human- computer interaction, artificial intelligence and cognitive science intersect. *Pragmatics and Cognition* [Special Issue on Facial Information Processing: A Multidisciplinary Perspective], *8(1)*, 185-235.

Littlewort, G. C., Bartlett, M. S., & Lee, K. (2009). Automatic coding of facial expressions displayed during posed and genuine pain. *Image and Vision Computing, 27*(12), 1797–1803. doi:10.1016/j.imavis.2008.12.010

Liu, H.-M., Kuhl, Patricia K., & Tsao, F.-M. (2003). An association between mothers' speech clarity and infants' speech disrimination skills. *Developmental Science, 6,* F1–F10. doi:10.1111/1467-7687.00275

Liu, C., Conn, K., Sarkar, N., & Stone, W. (2008a). Physiology-based affect recognition for computer-assisted intervention of children with autism spectrum disorder. *International Journal of Human-Computer Studies, 66*(9), 662–677. doi:10.1016/j.ijhsc.2008.04.003

Liu, C., Conn, K., Sarkar, N., & Stone, W. (2008b). Online Affect Detection and Robot Behavior Adaptation for Intervention of Children with Autism. *IEEE Transactions on Robotics, 24*(4), 883–896. doi:10.1109/TRO.2008.2001362

Liu, K., & Picard, R. W. (2005). Embedded empathy in continuous, interactive health assessment. In *CHI Workshop on HCI Challenges in Health Assessment*.

Liu, Y. (2006). Initial study on automatic identication of speaker role in broadcast news speech. In *Proceedings of the human language technology conference of the naacl, companion volume: Short papers* (pp. 81-84).

Liu, Z., Shan, Y., & Zhang, Z. (2001). Expressive expression mapping with ratio images. *In International Conference on Computer Graphics and Interactive Techniques (SIGGRAPH)*, 271 – 276.

Lo, S. (2008). The nonverbal communication functions of emoticons in computer-mediated communication. *Cyberpsychology & Behavior, 11*(5), 595–597. doi:10.1089/cpb.2007.0132

Lorenz, K. (1977). *Aggressivitt: arterhaltende eigenschaft oder pathologische erscheinung?* Aggression und Toleranz.

Lorenz, K., & Leyhausen, P. (1973). *Motivation and animal behavior: An ethological view*. New York: Van Nostrand Co.

Lorini, E., & Castelfranchi, C. (2006). The Unexpected Aspects of Surprise. *IJPRAI, 20*(6), 817–834.

Lott, D., & Sommer, R. (1967). Seating arrangements and status. *Journal of Personality and Social Psychology, 7*(1), 90–95. doi:10.1037/h0024925

Lovallo, W. R., & Sollers, J. J. III. (2000). Autonomic nervous system. In Fink, G. (Ed.), *Encyclopedia of stress* (*Vol. 1*, pp. 275–284). San Diego: Academic Press.

Lugger, M., & Yang, B. (2006). *Classification of different speaking groups by means of voice quality parameters.* ITG-Sprach-Kommunikation.

Lugger, M., & Yang, B. (2008). Cascaded emotion classification via psychological emotions using a large set of voice quality parameters. In *Proceedings of IEEE International Conference on Acoustics, Speech & Signal Processing, ICASSP 2008* (pp. 4945-4948).

Luor, T., Wub, L., Lu, H., & Tao, Y. (2010). The effect of emoticons in simplex and complex task-oriented communication: An empirical study of instant messaging. *Computers in Human Behavior, 26*, 889–895. doi:10.1016/j.chb.2010.02.003

Luria, A. R. (1973). *The working brain. And introduction to neuropsychology.* New York: Basic Books.

Lyons, M. J., Budynek, J., & Akamatsu, S. (1999). Automatic Classification of Single Facial Images. *IEEE Transactions on Pattern Analysis and Machine Intelligence, 21*(12), 1357–1362. doi:10.1109/34.817413

MacDorman, K. F. (2006). Subjective ratings of robot video clips for human likeness, familiarity, and eeriness: An exploration of the uncanny valley. *Proceedings of the ICCS/CogSci-2006 Long Symposium: Toward Social Mechanisms of Android Science.*

Macedo, L., Cardoso, A., Reisenzein, R., Lorini, E., & Castelfranchi, C. (2009). Artificial Surprise. In Vallverdú, J., & Casacuberta, D. (Eds.), *Handbook of Research on Synthetic Emotions and Sociable Robotics: New Applications in Affective Computing and Artificial Intelligence.*

MacLennan, B. (1991). Synthetic ethology: An approach to the study of communication. In C. G. Langton, C. Taylor, J. D. Farmer, & S. Rasmussen (Eds.), *Artificial life II: Proceedings of the second workshop on artificial life* (pp. 631–658). Redwood City, Calif.: Addison-Wesley.

Mah, L., Arnold, M. J., & Grafman, J. (2004). Impairment of Social Perception Associated with Lesions of the Prefrontal Cortex. *The American Journal of Psychiatry, 161*, 1247–1255. doi:10.1176/appi.ajp.161.7.1247

Maksimova Y. (2005). *Deception and its Detection in Computer-mediated Communication.* Iowa State University Human Computer Interaction Technical Report, ISU-HCI-2005-006.

Malatesta, L., Raouzaiou, A., Karpouzis, K., & Kollias, S. (2006). MPEG-4 facial expression synthesis based on appraisal theory, *3rd IFIP Conference* on *Artificial Intelligence Applications and Innovations*, 378 – 384.

Mana, N., & Pianesi, F. (2006) HMM-based synthesis of emotional facial expressions during speech in synthetic talking heads. In Proc. International Conference on Multimodal Interfaces, 380 – 387.

Mandryk, R. L., Inkpen, K. M., & Calvert, T. W. (2006). Using physiological techniques to measure user experience with entertainment technologies. *International Journal of Human-Computer Studies, 25*(2), 141–158.

Mandryk, R., Inkpen, K., & Calvert, T. (2006, March-April). Using Psychophysiological Techniques to Measure User Experience with Entertainment Technologies. [Special Issue on User Experience]. *Behaviour & Information Technology, 25*(2), 141–15. doi:10.1080/01449290500331156

Mandryk, R. L., & Inkpen, K. M. (2004). *Physiological indicators for the evaluation of co-located collaborative play.* Paper presented at the CSCW.

Mandryk, R. L., Atkins, S. M., & Inkpen, K. M. (2006). *A continious and objective evaluation of emotional experience with interactive play environments.* Paper presented at the CHI 2006.

Mandryk, R., & Inkpen, K. (2004). Physiological indicators for the evaluation of Co-located collaborative play. In *Proceedings of the ACM Conference on Computer Supported Cooperative Work (CSCW 2004)* (pp 102-111), New York: Association for Computing Machinery

Manucia, G. K., Baumann, D. J., & Cialdini, R. B. (1984). Mood influences on helping: Direct effects or side effects? *Journal of Personality and Social Psychology, 46,* 357–364. doi:10.1037/0022-3514.46.2.357

Markman, K. D., Gavanski, I., Sherman, S. J., & McMullen, M. N. (1993). The mental simulation of better and worse possible worlds. *Journal of Experimental Social Psychology,* (29): 87–109. doi:10.1006/jesp.1993.1005

Markus, H., & Nurius, P. (1986). Possible selves. *The American Psychologist, 41,* 954–969. doi:10.1037/0003-066X.41.9.954

Marshall, C., & Rossman, G. B. (1999). *Designing Qualitative Research.* Thousand Oaks, CA: Sage.

Mast, M. (2002). Dominance as expressed and inferred through speaking time: A metaanalysis. *Human Communication Research, 28*(3), 420–450.

Mathew, R. J., Wilson, W. H., Coleman, R. E., Turkington, T. G., & DeGrado, T. R. (1997). Marijuana intoxication and brain activation in marijuana smokers. *Life Sciences, 60*(23), 2075–2089. doi:10.1016/S0024-3205(97)00195-1

Mathiak, K., & Weber, R. (2006). Toward brain correlates of natural behavior: fmri during violent video games. *Human Brain Mapping, 27*(12), 948–956. doi:10.1002/hbm.20234

Matsumoto, D. (1987). The role of facial response in the experience of emotion: More methodological problems and a meta-analysis. *Journal of Personality and Social Psychology, 52,* 759–768. doi:10.1037/0022-3514.52.4.769

Matsumoto, D., & Kudo, T. (1993). American-Japanese cultural differences in implicit theories of personality based on smile. *Journal of Nonverbal Behavior, 17*(4), 231–243. doi:10.1007/BF00987239

McAdams, D. P., & Bryant, F. B. (1987). Intimacy motivation and subjective mental health in a nationwide sample. *Journal of Personality, 55*(3), 395–413. doi:10.1111/j.1467-6494.1987.tb00444.x

McAdams, D. P., Jackson, J., & Kirshnit, C. (1984). Looking, laughing, and smiling in dyads as a function of intimacy motivation and reciprocity. *Journal of Personality, 52,* 261–273. doi:10.1111/j.1467-6494.1984.tb00881.x

McCarthy, M. M., McDonald, C. H., Brooks, P. J., & Goldman, D. (1996). An anxiolytic action of oxytocin is enhanced by estrogen in the mouse. *Physiology & Behavior, 60*(5), 1209–1215. doi:10.1016/S0031-9384(96)00212-0

McClelland, D. C. (1987). *Human motivation.* New York: Cambridge University Press.

McClelland, D. C., Koestner, R., & Weinberger, J. (1989). How do self-attributed and implicit motives differ? *Psychological Review, 96,* 690–702. doi:10.1037/0033-295X.96.4.690

McClelland, D. C. (1980). Motive dispositions. The merits of operant and respondent measures. In Wheeler, L. (Ed.), *Review of personality and social psychology* (*Vol. 1*, pp. 10–41). Beverly Hills, CA: Sage.

McCowan, I., Bengio, S., Gatica-Perez, D., Lathoud, G., Monay, F., Moore, D., et al. (2003). Modeling human interaction in meetings. In *Proceedings of IEEE international conference on acoustics, speech and signal processing* (pp. 748-751).

McFarland, D. (1981). *The oxford companion to animal behavior.* Oxford: Oxford University Press.

McGaugh, J. L. (2000). Memory—a century of consolidation. *Science, 287,* 248–251. doi:10.1126/science.287.5451.248

McGilloway, S., Cowie, R., & Douglas-Cowie, E. (2000). Approaching automatic recognition of emotion from voice: a rough benchmark. In *Proceedings of the ISCA Workshop on Speech and Emotion* (pp. 207-212).

McKenna, K. Y. A., & Bargh, J. A. (1999). Causes and consequences of social interaction on the Internet: A conceptual framework. *Media Psychology, 1,* 249–269. doi:10.1207/s1532785xmep0103_4

McKenna, K. Y. A., Green, A. S., & Glenson, M. E. J. (2002). Relationship formation on the Internet: What's the big attraction? *The Journal of Social Issues, 58*(1), 9–31. doi:10.1111/1540-4560.00246

Medlock, M., Wixon, D., Terrano, M., Romero, R. L., & Fulton, B. (2002). *Using the rite method to improve products: A definition and a case study.* Paper presented at the Proceedings of UPA Conference.

Medvec, V. H., Madey, S. F., & Gilovich, T. (1995). When less is more: Counterfactual thinking and satisfaction among Olympic medalists. *Journal of Personality and Social Psychology, 69,* 603–610. doi:10.1037/0022-3514.69.4.603

Meehan, M., Insko, B., Whitton, M., & Brooks, F. P. J. (2002). Physiological Measures of Presence in Stressful Virtual Environments. *ACM Transactions on Graphics, 21*(3), 645–652. doi:10.1145/566570.566630

Meehan, M., Razzaque, S., Insko, B., Whitton, M., & Brooks, F. P. Jr. (2005). Review of four studies on the use of physiological reaction as a measure of presence in stressful virtual environments. *Applied Psychophysiology and Biofeedback, 30*(3), 239–258. doi:10.1007/s10484-005-6381-3

Mehler, J., Jusczyk, P., Lambertz, G., Halsted, N., Bertoncini, J., & Amiel-Tison, C. (1988). A precursor of language acquisition in young infants. *Cognition, 29,* 143–178. doi:10.1016/0010-0277(88)90035-2

Mehrabian, A. (1968). Communication without words. *Psychology Today, 2*(4), 53–56.

Mehrabian, A. (1996). Pleasure-arousal-dominance: A general framework for describing and measuring individual differences in temperament. *Current Psychology (New Brunswick, N.J.), 14,* 261–292. doi:10.1007/BF02686918

Meltzoff, A., Kuhl, P., Movellan, J. R., & Sejnowski, T. (2009). Foundations for a New Science of Learning. *Science, 235*(5938), 284–288. doi:10.1126/science.1175626

Merkx, P. A. B., Truong, K. P., & Neerincx, M. A. (2007). *Inducing and measuring emotion through a multiplayer first-person shooter computer game.* Paper presented at the Proceedings of the Computer Games Workshop 2007.

Miceli, M., & Castelfranchi, C. (1997). Basic principles of psychic suffering: A preliminary account. *Theory & Psychology, 7,* 769–798. doi:10.1177/0959354397076003

Miceli, M., & Castelfranchi, C. (1998). How to Silence One's Conscience: Cognitive Defences Against the Feeling of Guilt. *Journal for the Theory of Social Behaviour, 28*(3), 287–318. doi:10.1111/1468-5914.00076

Miceli, M., & Castelfranchi, C. (2000). The role of evaluation in cognition and social interaction. In Dautenhahn, K. (Ed.), *Human cognition and agent technology* (pp. 225–261). Amsterdam: Benjamins.

Miceli, M. e Castelfranchi, C. (2002). The mind and the future: The (negative) power of expectations. *Theory & Psychology, 12* (3), 335-.366

Miceli, M., Castelfranchi, C. (2005) Anxiety as an epistemic emotion: An uncertainty theory of anxiety, *ANXIETY STRESS AND COPING* (09957J0), 18,291-319.

Michaud, F., & Theberge-Turmel, C. (2002). Mobile robotic toys and autism. In Dautenhahn, K., Bond, A. H., Canamero, L., & Edmonds, B. (Eds.), *Socially Intelligent Agents: Creating Relationships With Computers and Robots* (pp. 125–132). Norwell, MA: Kluwer.

Mikels, J. A., Fredrickson, B. L., Larkin, G. R., Lindberg, C. M., & Reuter-Lorenz, P. A. (2005). Emotional category data on images from the International Affective Picture System. *Behavior Research Methods, 37*(4), 626–630.

Milborrow, S., & Nicolls, F. (2008). Locating Facial Features with an Extended Active Shape Model. *Proc. European Conference on Computer Vision, 4,* (pp. 504-513).

Miller, E. K., & Cohen, J. D. (2001). An integrative theory of prefrontal cortex function. *Annual Review of Neuroscience, 24,* 167–202. doi:10.1146/annurev.neuro.24.1.167

Millet, M. S. (1996). *Light Revealing Architecture.* New York: Wiley.

Miltner, W. H. R., & Braun, C.Arnold. M., Witte, H., Taub, E. Coherence of gamma-band EEF activity as a basis for associative learning. *Nature, 397*, 434–436. doi:10.1038/17126

Ministry of Internal Affairs and Communications. Japan (2006). *White Paper 2006: Information and Communications in Japan*. [Online]. Retrieved June 1, 2007 from http://www.johotsusintokei.soumu.go.jp/whitepaper/eng/WP2006/2006-index.html

Mischel, W., Ebbesen, E. B., & Zeiss, A. R. (1973). Selective attention to the self: Situational and dispositional determinants. *Journal of Personality and Social Psychology, 27*, 129–142. doi:10.1037/h0034490

Mitchell, P., Parsons, S., & Leonard, A. (2007). Using virtual environments for teaching social understanding to adolescents with autistic spectrum disorders. *Journal of Autism and Developmental Disorders, 37*, 589–600. doi:10.1007/s10803-006-0189-8

Mitra, S., & Acharya, T. (2007). Gesture recognition: A survey. *IEEE Transactions on Systems, Man and Cybernetics. Part C, Applications and Reviews, 37*(3), 311–324. doi:10.1109/TSMCC.2007.893280

Mogenson, G. J., Jones, D. L., & Yim, C. Y. (1980). From motivation to action: Functional interface between the limbic system and the motor system. *Progress in Neurobiology, 14*, 69–97. doi:10.1016/0301-0082(80)90018-0

Moll, H., & Tomasello, M. (2007). Co-operation and human cognition: The Vygotskian intelligence hypothesis. *Philosophical Transactions of the Royal Society, 362*, 639–648. doi:10.1098/rstb.2006.2000

Mongrain, M., & Vettese, L. C. (2003). Conflict over Emotional Expression: Implications for Interpersonal Communication. *Personality and Social Psychology Bulletin, 29*(4), 545–555. doi:10.1177/0146167202250924

Monsell, S., & Driver, J. (2000). *Control of cognitive processes*. Cambridge, MA: MIT Press.

Moor, P. J., Heuvelman, A. & Verleura, R. (2010) Flaming on YouTube. Computers *in Human Behavior*. Article in Press for June 2010.

Moore, D. J., McGrath, P., & Thorpe, J. (2000). Computer aided learning for people with autism - A framework for research and development. *Innovations in Education and Training International, 37*(3), 218–228.

Morahan-Martin, J. (2007). Internet use and abuse and psychological problems. n A. N. Joinson, K. McKenna, T. Postmes, & U. Reips (Eds.), *The Oxford Handbook of Internet Psychology*, pp. 331-345. Oxford: Oxford University Press.

Morie, J. F., Tortell, R., & Williams, J. (2007). Would You Like To Play a Game? Experience and in Game-based Learning. In Perez, H. O. R. (Ed.), *Computer Games and Team and Individual Learning* (pp. 269–286). Oxford, UK: Elsevier Press.

Morie, J. F., Williams, J., Dozois, A., & Luigi, D.-P. (2005). The Fidelity of Feel: Emotional Affordance in Virtual Environments. *Proceedings of the 11th International Conference on Human-Computer Interaction*.

Morie, J., Iyer, K., Valanejad, K., Sadek, R., Miraglia, D., Milam, D., et al. (2003). *Sensory design for virtual environments*. Paper presented at the SIGGRAPH Conference 2003.

Morris, J.S., Frith, C.D., Perrett, D.I., Rowland, D., Young, A.W., Calder, A.J., & Dolan, R.J. (1996). A differential neural response in the human amygdala to fearful and happy facial expressions. *Nature, 31*, 383(6603), 812-815.

Morrison, D., Wang, R., & De Silva, L. C. (2007). Ensemble methods for spoken emotion recognition in call-centres. *Speech Communication, 49*, 98–112. doi:10.1016/j.specom.2006.11.004

Mower, O. (1960). *Learning Theory and Behavior*. New York: J. Wiley and Sons. doi:10.1037/10802-000

Mozziconacci, S. J. L., & Hermes, D. J. (1995). A study of intonation patterns in speech expressing emotion or attitude: production and perception. In *Proceedings of 13th International Congress of Phonetic Sciences (ICPh'95)* (Vol. 3, pp. 178-181).

Mpiperis, I., Malassiotis, S., & Strintzis, M. G. (2008). Bilinear models for 3-D face and facial expression recognition. *IEEE Transactions on Information Forensics and Security, 3*(3), 498–511. doi:10.1109/TIFS.2008.924598

Mukamel, R., Ekstrom, A. D., Kaplan, J., Iacoboni, M., & Fried, I. (2010). Single-neuron responses in humans during execution and observation of actions. *Current Biology, 10*(8), 750–756. doi:10.1016/j.cub.2010.02.045

Murphy, M. R., Checkley, S. A., Seckl, J. R., & Lightman, S. L. (1990). Naloxone inhibits oxytocin release at orgasm in man. *The Journal of Clinical Endocrinology and Metabolism, 71*, 1056–1058. doi:10.1210/jcem-71-4-1056

Murphy, R. R., Lisetti, C., Tardif, R., Irish, L., & Gage, A. (2002). Emotion-based control of cooperating heterogeneous mobile robots. *IEEE Transactions on Robotics and Automation, 18*(5), 744–757. doi:10.1109/TRA.2002.804503

Murphy, E. (2004). Recognizing and promoting collaboration in an online asynchronous discussion. *British Journal of Educational Technology, 35*(4), 421–431. doi:10.1111/j.0007-1013.2004.00401.x

Murphy-Chutorian, E., & Trivedi, M. (2009). Head pose estimation in computer vision: A survey. *IEEE Transactions on Pattern Analysis and Machine Intelligence, 31*(4), 607–626. doi:10.1109/TPAMI.2008.106

Murray-Smith, R. (2009). (to appear). Empowering people rather than connecting them. *International Journal of Mobile HCI.*

Myers, S. M., & Johnson, C. P., American Academy of Pediatrics, & Council on Children with Disabilities. (2007). Management of children with autism spectrum disorders. *Pediatrics, 120*(5), 1162–1182. doi:10.1542/peds.2007-2362

Nacke, L. E. (2009). *Affective Ludology. Scientific Measurement of User Experience in Interactive Entertainment.* Sweden: Bleking Technical University.

Nacke, L., Lindley, C., & Stellmach, S. (2008). *Log who's playing: psychophysiological game analysis made easy through event logging.* Paper presented at the Proceedings of Fun and Games, Second International Conference.

Naqvi, N., Shiv, B., & Bechara, A. (2006). The role of emotion in decision making. *Current Directions in Psychological Science, 15*(5), 260–264. doi:10.1111/j.1467-8721.2006.00448.x

Nasoz, F., Alvarez, K., Lisetti, C., & Finkelstein, N. (2004). Emotion recognition from physiological signals using wireless sensors for presence technologies. *International Journal of Cognition, Technology, and Work – Special Issue on Presence, 6*(1), 4-14.

Nass, C., & Brave, S. (2005). *Wired for speech: How voice activates and advances the Human-Computer relationship.* Boston: The MIT Press.

Nass, C., & Moon, Y. (2000). Machines and mindlessness: Social Responses to Computers. *The Journal of Social Issues, 56*(1), 81–103. doi:10.1111/0022-4537.00153

Nass, C., Steuer, J., & Tauber, E. R. (1994, April). *Computers are social actors.* Papers presented at the meeting of the Conference on Human Factors in Computing, Boston, Massachusetts.

Nazzi, T., Bertoncini, J., & Mehler, J. (1998). Language discrimination by newborns: Towards an understanding of the role of rhythm. *Journal of Experimental Psychology. Human Perception and Performance, 24*(3), 756–766. doi:10.1037/0096-1523.24.3.756

Nazzi, T., & Ramus, F. (2003). Perception and acquisition of linguistic rhythm by infants. *Speech Communication, 41*(1-2), 233–243. doi:10.1016/S0167-6393(02)00106-1

Neese, R. M. (1990). Evolutionary explanations of emotions. *Human Nature (Hawthorne, N.Y.), 1*, 261–289. doi:10.1007/BF02733986

Neumann, I. D., Kromer, S. A., Toschi, N., & Ebner, K. (2000). Brain oxytocin inhibits the (re)activity of the hypothalamo–pituitary–adrenal axis in male rats: Involvement of hypothalamic and limbic brain regions. *Regulatory Peptides*, *96*, 31–38. doi:10.1016/S0167-0115(00)00197-X

Nguyen, H., & Masthoff, J. (2009). Designing Empathic Computers: The Effect of Multimodal Empathic Feedback Using Animated Agent. In Persuasive '09: Proceedings of the 4th International Conference on Persuasive Technology, pp. 1-9. 2009, Claremont, California April 26 - 29, 2009

Nicholson, J., Takahashi, K., & Nakatsu, R. (1999). Emotion recognition in speech using neural networks. In *Proceedings of ICONIP '99, 6th International Conference on Neural Information Processing* (Vol. 2, pp. 495-501).

Niedenthal, P. M. (2007). Embodying emotion. *Science*, *316*(5827), 1002–1005. doi:10.1126/science.1136930

Nielsen, J. (1998). *Improving the Dreaded 404 Error Message*. Retrieved September 12, 2009, from http://www.useit.com/alertbox/404_improvement.html

Niewiadomski, R., Bevacqua, E., Maurizio, M., & Pelachaud, C., (2009c) Greta: an interactive expressive ECA system. *AAMAS* (2), pp. 1399-1400

Niewiadomski, R., Hyniewska, S., & Pelachaud, C. (2009a) Modeling emotional expressions as sequences of Behaviors, International conference on Intelligent virtual agents IVA'09, Amsterdam.

Niewiadomski, R., Hyniewska, S., & Pelachaud, C. (2009b) Evaluation of Multimodal Sequential Expressions of Emotions in ECA, International conference on Affective Computing & Intelligent Interaction ACII'09, Amsterdam.

Nisbett, R., & Wilson, T. (1977). Telling more than we can know: Verbal reports on mental processes. *Psychological Review*, *84*(3), 231–259. doi:10.1037/0033-295X.84.3.231

Norman, D. A. (1980). Twelve issues for cognitive science. *Cognitive Science*, *4*, 1–32. doi:10.1207/s15516709cog0401_1

Norman, D. A. (2004). *Emotional Design: Why We Love (Or Hate) Everyday Things*. New York, NY: Basic Books.

Norman, D. (2002). Emotion and design: Attractive things work better. *Interaction*, *9*(4), 36–42. doi:10.1145/543434.543435

NRC (National Research Council). (2001). *Educating Children with Autism*. Washington, DC: National Academy Press.

Nussbaum, M. E. (2008). Collaborative discourse, argumentation, and learning: Preface and literature review. *Contemporary Educational Psychology*, *33*, 345–359. doi:10.1016/j.cedpsych.2008.06.001

Nusseck, M., Cunningham, D. W., Wallraven, C., & Bülthoff, H. H. (2008). The contribution of different facial regions to the recognition of conversational expressions. *Journal of Vision (Charlottesville, Va.)*, *8*(8), 1–23. doi:10.1167/8.8.1

Nwe, T. L., Foo, S. W., & De Silva, L. C. (2003). Speech emotion recognition using hidden Markov models. *Speech Communication*, *41*, 603–623. doi:10.1016/S0167-6393(03)00099-2

Nwe, T. L., Wei, F. S., & De Silva, L. C. (2001). Speech based emotion classification. In *Proceedings of IEEE Region 10 International Conference on Electrical &. Electron Technology*, *1*, 291–301.

O'Doherty, J. P. (2004). Reward representations and reward-related learning in the human brain: insights from neuroimaging. *Current Opinion in Neurobiology*, *14*, 769–776. doi:10.1016/j.conb.2004.10.016

O'Donnell, M., Creamer, M., Elliott, P., & Bryant, R. (2007). Tonic and Phasic Heart Rate as Predictors of Psttraumatic Stress Disorder. *Psychosomatic Medicine*, *69*, 256–261. doi:10.1097/PSY.0b013e3180417d04

O'Rorke, P., & Ortony, A. (1994). Explaining emotions. *Cognitive Science*, *18*, 283–323. doi:10.1207/s15516709cog1802_3

Oatley, K., & Jenkins, J. M. (1996). *Understanding emotion*. Cambridge, MA: Blackwell.

Oatley, K., Keltner, D., & Jenkins, J. M. (2006). *Understanding Emotions*. Wiley-Blackwell Publishers.

Ochsner, K. N., Bunge, S. A., Gross, J. J., & Gabrieli, J. D. (2002). Rethinking feelings: An fmri study of the cognitive regulation of emotion. *Journal of Cognitive Neuroscience*, *14*(8), 1215–1229. doi:10.1162/089892902760807212

Ochsner, K., & Barrett, L. F. (2001). The neurscience of emotion. In Mayne, T., & Bonnano, G. (Eds.), *Emotion: Current Issues and Future Directions* (pp. 38–81). New York: Guilford.

Okabe, D., & Ito, M. (2006). Keitai in public transportation. In Ito, M., Okabe, D., & Matsuda, M. (Eds.), *Personal, Portable, Pedestrian: Mobile Phones in Japanese Life* (pp. 205–217). Cambridge, MA: MIT Press.

Okun, M. S., Bowers, D., Springer, U., Shapira, N. A., Malone, D., & Rezai, A. R. (2004). What's in a 'smile?' Intra-operative observations of contralateral smiles induced by deep brain stimulation. *Neurocase*, *10*, 271–279. doi:10.1080/13554790490507632

Olds, J., & Milner, P. (1954). Positive reinforcement produced by electrical stimulation of septal area and other regions of rat brain. *Journal of Comparative and Physiological Psychology*, *47*, 418–427. doi:10.1037/h0058775

Olguin Olguin, D., Waber, B., Kim, T., Mohan, A., Koji, A., & Pentland, A. (2009). Sensible organizations: technology and methodology for automatically measuring organizational behavior. *IEEE Transactions on Systems, Man abd Cybernetics – Part B*, *39* (1), 43-55.

Olofsson, J. K., Nordin, S., Sequeira, H., & Polich, J. (2008). Affective picture processing: An integrative review of ERP findings. *Biological Psychology*, *77*, 247–265. doi:10.1016/j.biopsycho.2007.11.006

O'Reilly, R. C., David, C., Noelle, D., Braver, T. S., & Cohen, J. D. (2002). Prefrontal cortex in dynamic categorization tasks: Representational organization and neuromodulatory control. *Cerebral Cortex*, *12*, 246–257. doi:10.1093/cercor/12.3.246

Ortony, A., & Turner, T. (1990). What's basic about basic emotions? *Psychological Review*, *97*, 315–331. doi:10.1037/0033-295X.97.3.315

Ortony, A., Clore, G. L., & Collins, A. (1988). *Cognitive Structure of Emotions*. New York: Cambridge University Press.

Ortony, A., & Turner, T. J. (1990). What's basic about basic emotions? *Psychological Review*, *97*(3), 315–331. doi:10.1037/0033-295X.97.3.315

Ortony, A. (1987) Is Guilt an Emotion? *Cognition and Emotion*, I, 1, 283-98, 1987.

Osgood, C. E., May, W. E., & Miron, M. S. (1975). *Cross cultural univrsals of affective meaning*. University of Illinois Press.

Osgood, C. E., Suci, G. J., & Tannenbaum, P. H. (1957). *The measurement of meaning*. University of Illinois Press.

Otsuka, K., Takemae, Y., & Yamato, J. (2005). A probabilistic inference of multiparty conversation structure based on Markov-switching models of gaze patterns, head directions, and utterances. In *Proceedings of ACM international conference on multimodal interfaces* (pp. 191-198).

Oudeyer, P. Y. (2003). The production and recognition of emotions in speech: features and algorithms. *International Journal of Human-Computer Studies*, *59*, 157–183. doi:10.1016/S1071-5819(02)00141-6

Oyserman, D. (2001). Self-concept and identity. In Tesser, A., & Schwarz, N. (Eds.), *The Blackwell Handbook of Social Psychology* (pp. 499–517). Malden, MA: Blackwell.

Özbay, H. (2000). *Introduction to feedback control theory*. London: CRC Press.

Oztop, E., & Kawato, M., & Arbib, Michael. (2006). Mirror neurons and imitation: A computationally guided review. *Neural Networks*, *19*(3), 254–271. doi:10.1016/j.neunet.2006.02.002

Öztürk, Ö., Eraslan, D., & Kayahan, B. (2005). Emosyon ve temel insan davranışlarının evrimsel gelişimi. *Yeni Symposium, 43* (1), 14-19.

Paavola, L. (2006). Maternal sensitive responsiveness, characteristics and relations to child early communicative and linguistic development. *ACTA UNIVERSITATIS OULUENSIS B Humaniora* 73. Doctoral dissertation, University of Oulu, Finland.

Padoa-Schioppa, C., & Assad, J. A. (2006). Neurons in the orbitofrontal cortex encode economic value. *Nature*, *441*(7090), 223–226. doi:10.1038/nature04676

Pagulayan, R., Keeker, K., Wixon, D., Romero, R. L., & Fuller, T. (2003). User-centered design in games. In *The human-computer interaction handbook: fundamentals, evolving technologies and emerging applications*. L. Erlbaum Associates Inc.

Panksepp, J. (2005). On the embodied neural nature of core emotional affects. *Journal of Consciousness Studies*, *12*, 8–10, 158–184.

Panksepp, J. (1998). *Affective neuroscience-the foundations of human and animal emotions*. Oxford: Oxford University Press.

Panksepp, J. (1982). Toward a General Psychobiological Theory of Emotions. *The Behavioral and Brain Sciences*, *5*, 407–467. doi:10.1017/S0140525X00012759

Panksepp, J. (2007). Neurologizing the psychology of affects: how appraisal-based constructivism and basic emotion theory can coexist. *Perspectives on Psychological Science*, *2*(3), 281–296. doi:10.1111/j.1745-6916.2007.00045.x

Panksepp, J. (2004). *Affective Neuroscience*. Oxford: Oxford University Press.

Panksepp, J. (1999). The Preconscious Substrates of Consciousness: Affective States and the Evolutionary Origins of the Self. In Gallagher, S., & Shear, J. (Eds.), *Models of the Self* (pp. 113–130). Exeter, UK: Imprint Academic.

Panksepp, J. (1992). A critical role for 'affective neuroscience' in resolving what is basic about emotions. *Psychological Review*.

Pantic, M., Nijholt, A., Pentland, A., & Huang, T. (2008). Human-Centred Intelligent Human-Computer Interaction (HCI2): how far are we from attaining it? *International Journal of Autonomous and Adaptive Communications Systems*, *1*(2), 168–187. doi:10.1504/IJAACS.2008.019799

Pantic, M., Pentland, A., Nijholt, A., & Huang, T. (2007). Human computing and machine understanding of human behavior: A survey. In *Lecture notes in articial intelligence* (*Vol. 4451*, pp. 47–71). New York: Springer Verlag.

Pantic, M., & Rothkrantz, L. J. M. (2003). Toward an affect-sensitive multimodal human–computer interaction. *Proceedings of the IEEE*, *91*(9), 1370–1390. doi:10.1109/JPROC.2003.817122

Papanikolaou, K. A., Mabbott, A., Bull, S., & Grigoriadou, M. (2006). Designing learner-controlled educational interactions based on learning/cognitive style and learner behavior. *Interacting with Computers*, *18*, 356–384. doi:10.1016/j.intcom.2005.11.003

Papert, S. (1993). *Mindstorms: Children, Computers, and Powerful Ideas* (2nd ed.). New York: Basic Books.

Papez, J. W. (1937). A proposed mechanism of emotion. *Archives of Neurology and Psychiatry, 38*, 725–743.

Papoušek, M. (1989). Determinants of responsiveness to infant vocal expression of emotional state. *Infant Behavior and Development*, *12*, 505–522. doi:10.1016/0163-6383(89)90030-1

Papoušek, M. (1992). Early ontogeny of vocal communication in parent-infant interactions. In H. Papoušek, Uwe Jürgens, & Mechthild Papoušek (Eds.), *Nonverbal vocal communication. Comparative and developmental approaches* (pp. 230-261). Cambridge: CUP and Paris: Edition de la Maison des Sciences de l'Homme.

Park, C. H., Lee, D. W., & Sim, K. B. (2002). Emotion recognition of speech based on RNN. In *Proceedings of International Conference on Machine Learning & Cybernetics(ICMLC'02)* (Vol. 4, pp.2210-2213).

Parsons, S., & Mitchell, P. (2002). The potential of virtual reality in social skills training for people with autistic spectrum disorders. *Journal of Intellectual Disability Research, 46*, 430–443. doi:10.1046/j.1365-2788.2002.00425.x

Parsons, S., Mitchell, P., & Leonard, A. (2004). The use and understanding of virtual environments by adolescents with autistic spectrum disorders. *Journal of Autism and Developmental Disorders, 34*(4), 449–466. doi:10.1023/B:JADD.0000037421.98517.8d

Parsons, S., Mitchell, P., & Leonard, A. (2005). Do adolescents with autistic spectrum disorders adhere to social conventions in virtual environments? *Autism, 9*, 95–117. doi:10.1177/1362361305049032

Pater, J., Stager, C., & Werker, J. (2004). The perceptual acquisition of phonological contrasts. *Language, 80*(3), 361–379. doi:10.1353/lan.2004.0141

Patterson, M. L. (1994). Strategic functions of nonverbal exchange. In Daly, J. A., & Wiemann, J. M. (Eds.), *Strategic Interpersonal Communication* (pp. 273–293). Hillsdale, NJ: Erlbaum.

Pavlidis, I., Dowdall, J., Sun, N., Puri, C., Fei, J., & Garbey, M. (2007). Interacting with human physiology. *Computer Vision and Image Understanding, 108*(1-2), 150–170. doi:10.1016/j.cviu.2006.11.018

Pecchinenda, A., & Smith, C. A. (1996). The affective significance of skin conductance activity during a difficult problem-solving task. *Cognition and Emotion, 10*(5), 481–504. doi:10.1080/026999396380123

Pecina, S., Cagniard, B., Berridge, K. C., Aldridge, J. W., & Zhuang, X. (2003). *Hyperdopaminergic mutant mice have higher "wanting" but not "liking" for sweet rewards. Journal of Neuroscience, 23(28), 9395-9402. Reber, A. S. (1993). Implicit learning and tacit knowledge.* Oxford: Oxford University Press.

Peciña, S., & Berridge, K. C. (2000). Opioid eating site in accumbens shell mediates food intake and hedonic 'liking': Map based on microinjection Fos plumes. *Brain Research, 863*, 71–86. doi:10.1016/S0006-8993(00)02102-8

Pedersen, C. A. (1997). Oxytocin control of maternal behavior. Regulation by sex steroids and offspring stimuli. *Annals of the New York Academy of Sciences, 807*, 126–145. doi:10.1111/j.1749-6632.1997.tb51916.x

Pedersen, C. A., Vadlamudi, S. V., Boccia, M. L., & Amico, J. A. (2006). Maternal behavior deficits in nulliparous oxytocin knockout mice. *Genes Brain & Behavior, 5*(3), 274–281. doi:10.1111/j.1601-183X.2005.00162.x

Pelachaud, C. (2009). Studies on Gesture Expressivity for a Virtual Agent, *Speech Communication, special issue in honor of Björn Granstrom and Rolf Carlson, 51,* 630-639

Pelachaud, C., (2009) Modelling Multimodal Expression of Emotion in a Virtual Agent, *Philosophical Transactions of Royal Society B Biological Science,* B, 364, pp. 3539-3548.

Pentland, A. (2008). *Honest signals: how they shape our world.* Cambridge, MA: MIT Press.

Perconti, P. (2002). Context-dependence in human and animal communication. *Foundations of Science, 7*, 341–362. doi:10.1023/A:1019613210814

Pessoa, L. (2008). On the relationship between emotion and cognition. *Nature Reviews. Neuroscience, 9*, 148–158. doi:10.1038/nrn2317

Petitto, L. A. (1987). On the autonomy of language and gesture: Evidence from the acquisition of personal pronouns in American Sign Language. *Cognition, 27*, 1–52. doi:10.1016/0010-0277(87)90034-5

Pezzulo, G., Butz, M. V., Castelfranchi, C., & Falcone, R. (2008). Anticipation in Natural and Artificial Cognition. In Pezzulo, G., Butz, M.V., Castelfranchi, C. & Falcone, R. (Eds.), *The Challenge of Anticipation: A Unifying Framework for the Analysis and Design of Artificial Cognitive Systems* (LNAI 5225, pp. 3-22). New York: Springer.

Pfeifer, R. (1988). Artificial intelligence models of emotion. In V. Hamilton, G. H. Bower, & N. H. Frijda (Eds.), *Cognitive perspectives on emotion and motivation, volume 44 of series d: Behavioural and social sciences* (p. 287-320). Netherlands: Kluwer Academic Publishers.

Pfurtscheller, G., Zalaudek, K., & Neuper, C. (1998). Event-related beta synchronization after wrist, finger and thumb movement. *Electroencephalography and Clinical Neurophysiology, 109*, 154–160. doi:10.1016/S0924-980X(97)00070-2

Phelps, E. A. (2006). Emotion and Cognition: Insights from Studies of the Human Amygdala. *Annual Review of Psychology, 57*, 27–53. doi:10.1146/annurev.psych.56.091103.070234

Phillips, M. L., Drevets, W. C., Rauch, S. L., & Lane, R. (2003). Neurobiology of Emotion Perception I: The Neural Basis of Normal Emotion Perception. *Biological Psychiatry, 54*, 504–514. doi:10.1016/S0006-3223(03)00168-9

Picard, R. (1997). *Affective computing*. Cambridge, Mass, London, England: MIT Press.

Picard, R. (2000). *Affective computing*. Cambridge, MA: The MIT Press.

Picard, R. W. (2000). Toward computers that recognize and respond to user emotion. *IBM Systems Journal, 39*, 705–719. doi:10.1147/sj.393.0705

Picard, R. W. (1997). *Affective Computing*. Cambridge, MA: MIT Press.

Picard, R. (1997). *Does HAL cry digital tears? Emotion and computers;* HAL's Legacy: 2001's Computer as Dream and Reality, Cambridge, 279-303.

Picard, R. W. (2010). Emotion research by the people, for the people. Accepted for publication in Emotion Review. Retrieved April 1, 2010, from http://affect.media.mit.edu/pdfs/10.Picard-ER-revised.pdf

Pickering, M., & Garrod, S. (2007). Do people use language production to make predictions during comprehension? *Trends in Cognitive Sciences, 11*(3), 105–110. doi:10.1016/j.tics.2006.12.002

Pighin, F., Szeliski, R., & Salesin, D., H. (2002). Modeling and animating realistic faces from images. *International Journal of Computer Vision, 50*(2), 143–169. doi:10.1023/A:1020393915769

Pioggia, G., Igliozzi, R., Ferro, M., Ahluwalia, A., Muratori, F., & De Rossi, D. (2005). An android for enhancing social skills and emotion recognition in people with autism. *IEEE Transactions on Neural Systems and Rehabilitation Engineering, 13*(4), 507–515. doi:10.1109/TNSRE.2005.856076

Pitkanen, A., Savander, V., & LeDoux, J. E. (1997). Organization of intra-amygdaloid circuitries in the rat: an emerging framework for understanding functions of amygdala. *Trends in Neurosciences, 20*, 517–523. doi:10.1016/S0166-2236(97)01125-9

Plutchik, R. (2001). The Nature of Emotions. *American Scientist, 89*, 344.

Poels, K., Kort, Y. d., & IJsselsteijn, W. (2007). *It is always a lot of fun!: exploring dimensions of digital game experience using focus group methodology.* Proceedings of the 2007 conference on Future Play.

Poggi, I. (2007). *Mind, hands, face and body: A goal and belief view of multimodal communication.* Weidler Buchverlag Berlin.

Poizner, H., Bellugi, U., & Klima, E. S. (1990). Biological foundations of language: Clues from sign language. *Annual Review of Neuroscience, 13*, 283–307. doi:10.1146/annurev.ne.13.030190.001435

Pollak, S. D., Messner, M., Kistler, D. J., & Cohn, J. F. (2009). Development of perceptual expertise in emotion recognition. *Cognition*, *110*(2), 242–247. doi:10.1016/j.cognition.2008.10.010

Pollick, F. E., Paterson, H. M., Bruderlin, A., & Sanford, A. J. (2001). Perceiving affect from arm movement. *Cognition*, *82*, B51–B61. doi:10.1016/S0010-0277(01)00147-0

Polzin, T. S., & Waibel, A. (2000). Emotion-sensetive human-computer interfaces. In *Proceedings of the ISCA Workshop on Speech and Emotion* (pp. 201-206).

Pourtois, G., Debatisse, D., Despland, P., & de Gelder, B. (2002). Facial expressions modulate the time course of long latency auditory brain potentials. *Brain Research. Cognitive Brain Research*, *14*(1), 99–105. doi:10.1016/S0926-6410(02)00064-2

Prendinger, H., Mori, J., & Ishizuka, M. (2005). Using human physiology to evaluate subtle expressivity of a virtual quizmaster in a mathematical game. *International Journal of Human-Computer Studies*, *62*(2), 231–245. doi:10.1016/j.ijhcs.2004.11.009

Preston, S., D., & de Waal, F. B. M. (2002). Empathy: It's ultimate and proximate bases. *The Behavioral and Brain Sciences*, *25*, 1–72.

Prinz, W. (1997). Perception and action planning. *The European Journal of Cognitive Psychology*, *9*(2), 129–154. doi:10.1080/713752551

Propp, V., Wagner, L. A., & Scott, L. (1968). *Morphology of the Folktale (American Folklore Society Publications)*. Austin, TX: University of Texas Press.

Proulx, T., & Heine, S. J. (2009). Connections from Kafka: Exposure to schema threats improves implicit learning of an artificial grammar. *Psychological Science*, *20*, 1125–1131. doi:10.1111/j.1467-9280.2009.02414.x

Proust, M. (1971). *The Past Recaptured* (Mayor, A., Trans.). New York: Random House.

Pulvermüller, F. (2005). Brain mechanisms linking language and action. *Nature Reviews. Neuroscience*, *6*(7), 576–582. doi:10.1038/nrn1706

Pulvermüller, F., Härle, M., & Hummel, F. (2000). Neurophysiological distinction of semantic verb categories. *Neuroreport*, *11*(12), 2789–2793. doi:10.1097/00001756-200008210-00036

Radford, C. (1975). 'How can we be moved by the fate of Anna Karenina?' *Proceedings of the Aristotelian Society*, supplementary vol. 49, 67-80

Raento, M., Oulasvirta, A., & Eagle, N. (2009). Smartphones: an emerging tool for social scientists. *Sociological Methods & Research*, *37*(3), 426. doi:10.1177/0049124108330005

Ramachandran, V., & Hirstein, W. (1999). The Science of Art. *Journal of Consciousness Studies*, *6*(6-7), 15–51.

Rani, P., Sims, J., Brackin, R., & Sarkar, N. (2002). Online Stress Detection using Psychophysiological Signal for Implicit Human - Robot Cooperation. *Robotica*, *20*, 673–686. doi:10.1017/S0263574702004484

Rani, P., Sarkar, N., Smith, C. A., & Kirby, L. D. (2004). Anxiety detecting robotic system – towards implicit human-robot collaboration. *Robotica*, *22*, 85–95. doi:10.1017/S0263574703005319

Raos, V., Evangeliou, M. N., & Savaki, H. E. (2004). Observation of action: grasping with the mind's hand. *NeuroImage*, *23*, 193–201. doi:10.1016/j.neuroimage.2004.04.024

Raos, V., Evangeliou, M. N., & Savaki, H. E. (2007). Mental simulation of action in the service of action perception. *The Journal of Neuroscience*, *27*, 12675–12683. doi:10.1523/JNEUROSCI.2988-07.2007

Raouzaiou, A., Tsapatsoulis, N., Karpouzis, K., & Kollias, S. (2002). Parameterized Facial Expression Synthesis Based on MPEG-4. *EURASIP Journal on Applied Signal Processing*, (10): 1021–1038. doi:10.1155/S1110865702206149

Ravaja, N. (2004). Contributions of psychophysiology to media research: Review and recommendations. *Media Psychology*, *6*, 193–235. doi:10.1207/s1532785xmep0602_4

Ravaja, N., Saari, T., Salminen, M., Laarni, J., & Kallinen, K. (2006). Phasic emotional reactions to video game events: A psychophysiological investigation. *Media Psychology, 8*, 343–367. doi:10.1207/s1532785xmep0804_2

Ravaja, N., & Kivikangas, J. M. (2008). *Psychophysiology of digital game playing: The relationship of self-reported emotions with phasic physiological responses.* Paper presented at the Proceedings of Measuring Behavior 2008.

Ray, W. J., & Cole, H. (1985). EEG alpha activity reflects attentional demands, and beta activity reflects emotional and cognitive processes. *Science, 228*(4700), 750–752. doi:10.1126/science.3992243

Redondo, J., Fraga, I., Padrón, I., & Comesaña, M. (2007). The Spanish adaptation of ANEW (Affective Norms for English Words). *Behavior Research Methods, 39*(3), 600–605.

Redondo, J., Fraga, I., Padrón, I., & Piñeiro, A. (2008). Affective ratings of sound stimuli. *Behavior Research Methods, 40*(3), 784–790. doi:10.3758/BRM.40.3.784

Reeves, B., & Nass, C. (1996). *The media equation: How people treat computers, television, and new media like real people and places. New York (USA).* NY, USA: Cambridge University Press New York.

Reeves, B., & Nass, C. (1996). *The media equation: How people treat computers, televisions, and new media like real people and places.* Cambridge: Cambridge University Press.

Reeves, B., & Nass, C. (1996). *The Media Equation: how people treat computers, television and new media like real people and places.* New York: Cambridge University Press.

Reilly, J. S., & McIntire, M. L. (1991). *WHERE SHOE: The acquisition of wh-questions in ASL. Papers and Reports in Child Language Development* (pp. 104–111). Stanford University, Department of Linguistics.

Reilly, J. S., & Seibert, L. (2003). Language and emotion. In Davidson, R., Scherer, K., & Goldsmith, H. (Eds.), *Handbook of affective sciences* (pp. 535–559). New York: Oxford University Press.

Reisenzein, R. (2009). Emotional Experience in the Computational Belief–Desire Theory of Emotion. *Emotion Review, 1*(3), 214–222. doi:10.1177/1754073909103589

Rezabek, L. L., & Cochenour, J. J. (1998). Visual cues in computer-mediated communication: Supplementing text with emotions. *Journal of Visual Literacy, 18*, 210–215.

Richmond, V., & McCroskey, J. (1995). *Nonverbal behaviors in interpersonal relations.* Allyn and Bacon.

Rienks, R., & Heylen, D. (2006). Dominance Detection in Meetings Using Easily Obtainable Features. [). New York: Springer.]. *Lecture Notes in Computer Science, 3869*, 76–86. doi:10.1007/11677482_7

Rienks, R., Zhang, D., & Gatica-Perez, D. (2006). Detection and application of in fluence rankings in small group meetings. In *Proceedings of the international conference on multimodal interfaces* (pp. 257-264).

Rifkin, J. (2009). *The empathic civilization. The race to global consciousness in a world in crisis.* Cambridge: Polity Press.

Riva, G. (2002). The sociocognitive psychology of computer-mediated communication: the present and future of technology-based interactions. *Cyberpsychology & Behavior, 5*(6), 581–598. doi:10.1089/109493102321018222

Rizzolatti, G., Fadiga, L., Fogassi, L., & Gallese, V. (1996). Premotor cortex and the recognition of motor actions. *Brain Research. Cognitive Brain Research, 3*, 131–141. doi:10.1016/0926-6410(95)00038-0

Rizzolatti, G., & Arbib, M. (1998). Language within our grasp. *Trends in Neurosciences, 21*(5), 188–194. doi:10.1016/S0166-2236(98)01260-0

Rizzolatti, G., & Craighero, L. (2004). The mirror-neuron system. *Annual Review of Neuroscience, 27*, 169–192. doi:10.1146/annurev.neuro.27.070203.144230

Robins, B., Dickerson, P., & Dautenhahn, K. (2005). *Robots as embodied beings – Interactionally sensitive body movements in interactions among autistic children and a robot.* Paper presented at the IEEE International Workshop on Robot and Human Interactive Communication, Nashville, Tennessee.

Robinson, R. G., Kubos, K. L., Starr, L. B., Rao, K., & Price, T. R. (1984). Mood disorders in stroke patients. Importance of location of lesion. *Brain, 107,* 81–93. doi:10.1093/brain/107.1.81

Robinson, T. E., & Berridge, K. C. (2000)... *Addiction (Abingdon, England), 95*(Supplement 2), S91–S117.

Rocco, E. (1998). Trust breaks down in electronic contexts but can be repaired by some initial face-to-face contact. *Proceedings CHI '98 (Los Angeles CA, 1998) ACM Press* (pp. 496-502).

Roese, N. J. (1997). Counterfactual thinking. *Psychological Bulletin, 121,* 133–148. doi:10.1037/0033-2909.121.1.133

Roese, N. J., & Olson, J. M. (1995). *What might have been: The social psychology of counterfactual thinking.* Mahwah, NJ: Lawrence Erlbaum.

Rogers, S. J. (2000). Interventions that facilitate socialization in children with autism. *Journal of Autism and Developmental Disorders, 30*(5), 399–409. doi:10.1023/A:1005543321840

Rolls, E. T. (2000). The orbitofrontal cortex and reward. *Cerebral Cortex, 10*(3), 284–294. doi:10.1093/cercor/10.3.284

Rolls, E. T., Kringelbach, M. L., & de Araujo, I. E. (2003a). Different representations of pleasant and unpleasant odours in the human brain. *The European Journal of Neuroscience, 18,* 695–703. doi:10.1046/j.1460-9568.2003.02779.x

Rolls, E. T., O'Doherty, J., Kringelbach, M. L., Francis, S., Bowtell, R., & McGlone, F. (2003b). Representations of pleasant and painful touch in the human orbitofrontal and cingulate cortices. *Cerebral Cortex, 13,* 308–317. doi:10.1093/cercor/13.3.308

Rolls, E. T. (1999). *The brain and emotion.* Oxford: Oxford University Press.

Rolls, E. T. (2000). The orbitofrontal cortex and reward. *Cerebral Cortex, 10*(3), 284–294. doi:10.1093/cercor/10.3.284

Rolls, E. T. (2004). The functions of the orbitofrontal cortex. *Brain and Cognition, 55*(1), 11–29. doi:10.1016/S0278-2626(03)00277-X

Rolls, E. T., O'Doherty, J., Kringelbach, M. L., Francis, S., Bowtell, R., & McGlone, F. (2003). Representations of pleasant and painful touch in the human orbitofrontal and cingulate cortices. *Cerebral Cortex, 13,* 308–317. doi:10.1093/cercor/13.3.308

Rong, J., Li, G., & Chen, Y. P. (2009). Acoustic feature selection for automatic emotion recognition from speech. *Information Processing & Management, 45,* 315–328. doi:10.1016/j.ipm.2008.09.003

Rosenberg, D. (2009). Video games outsell movies in UK. *CNET.* Retrieved April 4th 2010 from http://news.cnet.com/8301-13846_3-10423150-62.html

Ross, C., Orr, S. O., Sisic, M., Arseneault, J. M., Simmering, M. G., & Orr, R. R. (2009). Personality and motivations associated with Facebook use. *Computers in Human Behavior, 25,* 578–586. doi:10.1016/j.chb.2008.12.024

Rowe, D. W., Sibert, J., & Irwin, D. (1998). *Heart Rate Variability: Indicator of User State as an Aid to Human - Computer Interaction.* Paper presented at the Conference on Human Factors in Computing Systems.

Rozenkrants, B., & Polich, J. (2008). Affective ERP Processing in a Visual Oddball Task: Arousal, Valence, and Gender. *Clinical Neurophysiology, 119*(10), 2260–2265. doi:10.1016/j.clinph.2008.07.213

Rubin, D. C., & Talarico, J. M. (2009). A comparison of dimensional models of emotion: Evidence from emotions, prototypical events, autobiographical memories, and words. *Memory (Hove, England), 17*(8), 802–808. doi:10.1080/09658210903130764

Rubin, D. L., & Greene, K. (1992). Gender typical style in written language. *Research in the Teaching of English, 26*, 7–40.

Ruble, L. A., & Robson, D. M. (2006). Individual and environmental determinants of engagement in autism. *Journal of Autism and Developmental Disorders, 37*(8), 1457–1468. doi:10.1007/s10803-006-0222-y

Russel, J. A. (1980). A circumplex model of affect. *Journal of Personality and Social Psychology, 39*(6), 1161–1178. doi:10.1037/h0077714

Russell, J. A., & Barrett, L. F. (1999). Core affect, prototypical emotional episodes, and other things called emotion: dissecting the elephant. *Journal of Personality and Social Psychology, 76*, 805–819. doi:10.1037/0022-3514.76.5.805

Russell, J. A. (1980). A circumplex model of affect. *Journal of Personality and Social Psychology, 39*(6), 1161–1178. doi:10.1037/h0077714

Russell, J. A., & Fernández–Dols, J. M. (Eds.). (1997). *The Psychology of Facial Expression*. Cambridge, UK: Cambridge University Press. doi:10.1017/CBO9780511659911

Russell, J. A. (1980). A circumplex model of affect. *Journal of Personality and Social Psychology, 39*(6), 1161–1178. doi:10.1037/h0077714

Russell, J. A. (2003). Core affect and the psychological construction of emotion. *Psychological Review, 110*, 145–172. doi:10.1037/0033-295X.110.1.145

Rutter, M. (2006). Autism: its recognition, early diagnosis, and service implications. *Journal of Developmental and Behavioral Pediatrics, 27*(Supplement 2), S54–S58.

Ruttkay, Z., & Pelachaud, C. (Eds.). (2004). *From Brows till Trust: Evaluating Embodied Conversational Agents*. Kluwer.

Sackeim, H. A., Greenberg, M. S., Weiman, A. L., Gur, R. C., Hungerbuhler, J. P., & Geschwind, N. (1982). Hemispheric asymmetry in the expression of positive and negative emotions. Neurologic evidence. *Archives of Neurology, 39*, 210–218.

Salah, A. A., Çınar, H., Akarun, L., & Sankur, B. (2007). Robust Facial Landmarking for Registration. *Annales des Télécommunications, 62*(1-2), 1608–1633.

Salamin, H., Favre, S., & Vinciarelli, A. (2009). Automatic role recognition in multiparty recordings: Using social aliation networks for feature extraction. *IEEE Transactions on Multimedia, 11*(7), 1373–1380. doi:10.1109/TMM.2009.2030740

Salamone, J. D. (1994). The involvement of nucleus accumbens dopamine in appetitive and aversive motivation. *Behavioural Brain Research, 61*, 117–133. doi:10.1016/0166-4328(94)90153-8

Salter, T. (2009). A Need for Flexible Robotic Devices. *AMD Newsletter, 6*(1), 3.

Samsonovic, A. V., & Ascoli, G. A. (2010). Principal Semantic Components of Language and the Measurement of Meaning. *PLoS ONE, 5*(6), e10921. doi:10.1371/journal.pone.0010921

Sánchez-Navarro, P. J., Martínez-Selva, J. M., Torrente, G., & Román, F. (2008). Psychophysiological, Behavioral, and Cognitive Indices of the Emotional Response: A Factor-Analytic Study. *The Spanish Journal of Psychology, 11*(1), 16–25.

Sander, D., Grafman, J., & Zalla, T. (2003). The human amygdala: an evolved system for relevance detection. *Reviews in the Neurosciences, 14*, 303–316.

Sander, D., Grandjean, D., & Scherer, K. R. (2005). A systems approach to appraisal mechanisms in emotion. *Neural Networks, 18*, 317–352. doi:10.1016/j.neunet.2005.03.001

Sander, D., Grandjean, D., & Scherer, K. R. (2005). *A systems approach to appraisal mechanisms in emotion, Neural Networks*. Elsevier.

Sandler, W., & Lillo-Martin, D. (2006). *Sign language and linguistic universals.* Cambridge: Cambridge University Press.

Sato, W., Yoshikawa, S., Kochiyama, T., & Matsumura, M. (2004). The amygdala processes the emotional significance of facial expressions: an fMRI investigation using the interaction between expression and face direction. *NeuroImage, 22,* 1006–1013. doi:10.1016/j.neuroimage.2004.02.030

Sato, K. (2007). Impact of social presence in computer-mediated communication to effective discussion on bulletin board system. *Proceedings of World Conference on Educational Multimedia, Hypermedia and Telecommunications (ED-MEDIA) 2007,* 722-731.

Sauter, D. A., Eisner, F., Calder, A. J., & Scott, S. K. (2006). Perceptual cues in nonverbal vocal expressions of emotion. *Quarterly Journal of Experimental Psychology, 63,* 2251–2272. doi:10.1080/17470211003721642

Scaife, M., & Rogers, Y. (1996). External cognition: how do graphical representations work? *International Journal of Human-Computer Studies, 45,* 185–213. doi:10.1006/ijhc.1996.0048

Scassellati, B. (2005). *Quantitative metrics of social response for autism diagnosis.* Paper presented at the IEEE International Workshop on Robot and Human Interactive Communication, Nashville, Tennessee.

Schau, H. J., & Gilly, M. C. (2003). We are what we post? Self-presentation in personal web space. *The Journal of Consumer Research, 30*(3), 385–404. doi:10.1086/378616

Scheflen, A. (1964). The significance of posture in communication systems. *Psychiatry, 27,* 316–331.

Schegloff, E. (1987). Single episodes of interaction: an exercise in conversation analysis. *Social Psychology Quarterly, 50*(2), 101–114. doi:10.2307/2786745

Scherer, K. R., Schorr, A., & Johnstone, T. (2001). *Appraisal Processes in Emotion: Theory, Methods, Research.* New York: Oxford University Press.

Scherer, K. (1979). *Personality markers in speech.* Cambridge, MA: Cambridge University Press.

Scherer, K. (2003). Vocal communication of emotion: a review of research paradigms. *Speech Communication, 40,* 227–256. doi:10.1016/S0167-6393(02)00084-5

Scherer, K. R. (2003). Introduction: Cognitive components of emotion. In Davidson, R. J., Scherand, K. R., & Goldsmith, H. H. (Eds.), *Handbook of affective sciences* (pp. 563–571). Oxford: Oxford University Press.

Scherer, K. R. (2001) Appraisal considered as a process of multilevel sequential checking. In Scherer, K.R., Schorr, A., & Johnstone, T., (Eds) *Appraisal Processes in Emotion: Theory Methods,* Research. Oxford, New York: Oxford University Press, 92-129.

Schermerhorn, P., & Scheutz, M. (2005, June). The effect of environmental structure on the utility of communication in hive-based swarms. In *Ieee swarm intelligence symposium 2005* (pp. 440–443). IEEE Computer Society Press. doi:10.1109/SIS.2005.1501661

Schermerhorn, P., & Scheutz, M. (2007a). Investigating the adaptiveness of communication in multi-agent behavior coordination. *Adaptive Behavior, 15*(4), 423–445. doi:10.1177/1059712307084690

Schermerhorn, P., & Scheutz, M. (2003). Implicit cooperation in conflict resolution for simple agents. In *Agent 2003.* Chicago, IL: University of Chicago.

Schermerhorn, P., & Scheutz, M. (2006, May). Social coordination without communication in multi-agent territory exploration tasks. In *Proceedings of the fifth international joint conference on autonomous agents and multiagent systems (AAMAS-06)* (pp. 654–661). Hakodate, Japan.

Schermerhorn, P., & Scheutz, M. (2007b, April). Social, physical, and computational tradeoffs in collaborative multi-agent territory exploration tasks. In *Proceedings of the first ieee symposium on artificial life* (pp. 295–302).

Schermerhorn, P., & Scheutz, M. (2009, March/April). The impact of communication and memory in hive-based foraging agents. In *Proceedings of the 2009 IEEE symposium on artificial life* (pp. 29–36).

Scheutz, M. (2004d). On the utility of adaptation vs. signalling action tendencies in the competition for resources. In *Proceedings of aamas 2004* (pp. 1378–1379). New York: ACM Press.

Scheutz, M. (2004e). Useful roles of emotions in artificial agents: A case study from artificial life. In [New York: AAAI Press.]. *Proceedings of AAAI, 2004*, 31–40.

Scheutz, M., & Schermerhorn, P. (2004a). The more radical, the better: Investigating the utility of aggression in the competition among different agent kinds. In *Proceedings of sab 2004* (pp. 445–454). Cambridge, MA: MIT Press.

Scheutz, M., & Schermerhorn, P. (2004b). The role of signaling action tendencies in conflict resolution. *Journal of Artificial Societies and Social Simulation, 1*(7).

Scheutz, M., & Schermerhorn, P. (2005a). (in press). Many is more: The utility of simple reactive agents with predictive mechanisms in multiagent object collection tasks. *Web Intelligence and Agent Systems, 3*(1), 97–116.

Scheutz, M., & Schermerhorn, P. (2005b, June). Predicting population dynamics and evolutionary trajectories based on performance evaluations in alife simulations. In *Proceedings of gecco 2005* (pp. 35–42). New York: ACM Press. doi:10.1145/1068009.1068015

Scheutz, M., Sloman, A., & Logan, B. (2000). Emotional states and realistic agent behaviour. In Geril, P. (Ed.), *Proceedings of gameon 2000, imperial college london* (pp. 81–88). Delft: Society for Computer Simulation.

Scheutz, M. (2002b). The evolution of affective states and social control. In Hemelrijk, C. K. (Ed.), *Proceedings of international workshop on self-organisation and evolution of social behaviour* (pp. 358–367). Monte Verità, Switzerland.

Scheutz, M., & Sloman, A. (2001). Affect and agent control: Experiments with simple affective states. In Zhong, N., Liu, J., Ohsuga, S., & Bradshaw, J. (Eds.), *Intelligent agent technology: Research and development* (pp. 200–209). New Jersey: World Scientific Publisher.

Scheutz, M. (2000). Surviving in a hostile multiagent environment: How simple affective states can aid in the competition for resources. In H. J. Hamilton (Ed.), *Advances in artificial intelligence, 13th biennial conference of the canadian society for computational studies of intelligence, ai 2000, montréal, quebec, canada, may 14-17, 2000, proceedings* (Vol. 1822, pp. 389–399). Springer.

Scheutz, M. (2001). The evolution of simple affective states in multi-agent environments. In D. Cañamero (Ed.), *Proceedings of AAAI fall symposium* (pp. 123–128). Falmouth, MA: AAAI Press.

Scheutz, M. (2002a). Agents with or without emotions? In R. Weber (Ed.), *Proceedings of the 15th international flairs conference* (pp. 89–94). AAAI Press.

Scheutz, M. (2004a). An artificial life approach to the study of basic emotions. In *Proceedings of cognitive science 2004.*

Scheutz, M. (2004b). A framework for evaluating affective control. In *Proceedings of the ace 2004 symposium at the 17th european meeting on cybernetics and systems research* (p. 645-650).

Scheutz, M. (2004c). How to determine the utility of emotions. In *Proceedings of AAAI spring symposium 2004* (p. 122-127).

Scheutz, M. (2006, June). Cross-level interactions between conflict resolution and survival games. In *Proceedings of artificial life x* (pp. 459–465).

Scheutz, M., & Logan, B. (2001). Affective versus deliberative agent control. In S. Colton (Ed.), *Proceedings of the aisb '01 symposium on emotion, cognition and affective computing* (pp. 1–10). York: Society for the Study of Artificial Intelligence and the Simulation of Behaviour.

Scheutz, M., & Schermerhorn, P. (2002). Steps towards a theory of possible trajectories from reactive to deliberative control systems. In R. Standish (Ed.), *Proceedings of the 8th conference of artificial life* (pp. 283–292). Cambridge, MA: MIT Press.

Scheutz, M., & Schermerhorn, P. (2003, October). Many is more but not too many: Dimensions of cooperation of agents with and without predictive capabilities. In Proceedings of ieee/wic iat-2003 (pp. 378–384). Washington, DC: IEEE Computer Society Press. doi:10.1109/IAT.2003.1241105doi:10.1109/IAT.2003.1241105

Scheutz, M., & Schermerhorn, P. (2008, August). The limited utility of communication in simple organisms. In *Proceedings of artificial life xi* (pp. 521–528).

Schirmer, A., & Kotz, S. (2003). ERP evidence for a sex-specific Stroop effect in emotional speech. *Journal of Cognitive Neuroscience, 15*(8), 1135–1148. doi:10.1162/089892903322598102

Schlenker, B. R., & Darby, B. W. (1981). The use of apologies in social predicaments. *Social Psychology Quarterly, 44*(3), 271–278. doi:10.2307/3033840

Schmidt, L. A., & Fox, N. A. (1999). Conceptual, biological, and behavioral distinctions among different categories of shy children. In Schmidt, L. A., & Schulkin, J. (Eds.), *Extreme fear, shyness and social phobia* (pp. 47–66). Oxford: Oxford University Press.

Schneider, W., & Shiffrin, R. M. (1977). Controlled and automatic human information processing I: Detection, search and attention. *Psychological Review, 84*, 1–66. doi:10.1037/0033-295X.84.1.1

Schneiderman, M. H., & Ewens, W. L. (1971). The Cognitive Effects of Spatial Invasion. *Pacific Sociological Review, 14*(4), 469–486.

Schoenbaum, G., & Roesch, M. (2005). Orbitofrontal cortex, associative learning, and expectancies. *Neuron, 47*, 633–636. doi:10.1016/j.neuron.2005.07.018

Schouten, J. W. (1991). Selves in transition: Symbolic consumption in personal rites of passage and identity re-construction. *The Journal of Consumer Research, 17*, 412–425. doi:10.1086/208567

Schuller, B., Reiter, S., Muller, R., Al-Hames, M., Lang, M., & Rigoll, G. (2005). Speaker independent speech emotion recognition by ensemble classification. In *Proceedings of IEEE International Conference on Multimedia & Expo (ICME'05)*.

Schultheiss, O. C. (Ed.). (2001). *An information processing account of implicit motive arousal* (*Vol. 12*). Greenwich, CT: JAI Press.

Schultheiss, O. C., & Brunstein, J. C. (2001). Assessing implicit motives with a research version of the TAT: Picture profiles, gender differences, and relations to other personality measures. *Journal of Personality Assessment, 77*(1), 71–86. doi:10.1207/S15327752JPA7701_05

Schultheiss, O. C., Rösch, A. G., Rawolle, M., Kordik, A., & Graham, S. (in press). *Implicit motives: Current research and future directions. To appear in Urdan, T* (Karabenick, S., & Pajares, F., Eds.). *Vol. 16*). Advances in Motivation and Achievement.

Schultheiss, O. C. (2008). Implicit motives. In O. P. John, R. W. Robins & L. A. Pervin (Eds.), *Handbook of Personality: Theory and Research* (3 ed., pp. 603-33). New York: Guilford.

Schultheiss, O. C., & Wirth, M. M. (2008). Biopsychological aspects of motivation. In J. Heckhausen & H. Heckhausen (Eds.), *Moivation and Action* (2 ed., pp. 247-71). New York: Cambridge University Press.

Schultz, W. (2000). Multiple reward signals in the brain. *Nature Reviews. Neuroscience, 1*(3), 199–207. doi:10.1038/35044563

Schultz, W., Dayan, P., & Montague, P. R. (1997). A neural substrate of prediction and reward. *Science, 275*, 1593–1599. doi:10.1126/science.275.5306.1593

Schultz, R. T. (2005). Developmental deficits in social perception in autism: the role of the amygdala and fusiform face area. *International Journal of Developmental Neuroscience, 23*, 125–141. doi:10.1016/j.ijdevneu.2004.12.012

Schwarz, N., & Clore, G. L. (1996). Feelings and phenomenal experiences. In Higgins, E. T., & Kruglanski, A. (Eds.), *Social psychology: Handbook of basic principles* (pp. 433–465). New York: Guilford.

Schweder, R. (1994). "You're not sick, you're just in love": Emotion as an interpretive system. In Ekman, P., & Davidson, R. (Eds.), *The nature of emotion* (pp. 32–44). New York: Oxford University Press.

Scott, D. J. (2008). Gender Differences in Japanese College Students' Participation in a Qualitative Study. [Association for the Advancement of Computing in Education]. *AACE Journal, 16*(4), 385–404.

Scott, D. J., Coursaris, C. K., Kato, Y., & Kato, S. (2009). The Exchange of Emotional Content in Business Communications: A Comparison of PC and Mobile E-mail Users. In M. Head and E. Li (Eds.) *Advances in Electronic Business: Vol. 4 - Mobile and Ubiquitous Commerce.* Hershey PA: IGI Global Publishing. pp. 201-219.

Sebe, N., Cohen, I., & Huang, T. S. (2005). Multimodal emotion recognition. In *Handbook of Pattern Recognition and Computer Vision.* World Scientific. doi:10.1142/9789812775320_0021

Seip, J. (1996). *Teaching the Autistic and Developmentally Delayed: A Guide for Staff Training and Development.* Delta, BC: Author.

Sennersten, C. (2008). *Gameplay (3D Game Engine + Ray Tracing = Visual Attention through Eye Tracking).* Blekinge Tekniska Högskola.

Shah, J. Y. (2005). The automatic pursuit and management of goals. *Current Directions in Psychological Science, 14*(1), 10–13. doi:10.1111/j.0963-7214.2005.00325.x

Shami, M. T., & Verhelst, W. (2007). An evaluation of the robustness of existing supervised machine learning approaches to the classification of emotions in speech. *Speech Communication, 49,* 201–212. doi:10.1016/j.specom.2007.01.006

Shami, M. T., & Kamel, M. S. (2005). Segment-based approach to the recognition of emotions in speech. *IEEE International Conference on Multimedia & Expo (ICME'05),* Amsterdam, The Netherlands.

Sharpe, D. L., & Baker, D. L. (2007). Financial issues associated with having a child with autism. *Journal of Family and Economic Issues, 28,* 247–264. doi:10.1007/s10834-007-9059-6

Sherer, M. R., & Schreibman, L. (2005). Individual behavioral profiles and predictors of treatment effectiveness for children with autism. *Journal of Consulting and Clinical Psychology, 73*(3), 525–538. doi:10.1037/0022-006X.73.3.525

Sherman, W. R., & Craig, A. B. (2003). *Understanding virtual reality: interface, application, and design.* Boston: Morgan Kaufmann Publishers.

Shneiderman, B. (1998). *Designing the user interface: Strategies for effective human-computer interaction.* Harlow: Addison-Wesley.

Short, J., Williams, E., & Christie, B. (1976). *The Social Psychology of Telecommunications.* NY: John Wiley.

Shott, S. (1979). Emotion and Social Life: A Symbolic Interactionist Analysis. *American Journal of Sociology, 84*(6), 1317–1334. doi:10.1086/226936

Siegel, J., Dubrovsky, V., Kiesler, S., & McGuire, T. W. (1986). Group process and computer-mediated communication. *Organizational Behavior and Human Decision Processes, 37,* 157–187. doi:10.1016/0749-5978(86)90050-6

Siegel, J., Dubrovsky, V., Kiesler, S., & McGuire, T. W. (1986). Group processes in computer-mediated communication. *Organizational Behavior and Human Decision Processes, 37,* 157–187. doi:10.1016/0749-5978(86)90050-6

Silva, P. R. D., Osano, M., Marasinghe, A., & Madurapperuma, A. P. (2006). A computational model for recognizing emotion with intensity for machine vision applications. *IEICE Transactions on Information and Systems. E (Norwalk, Conn.), 89-D*(7), 2171–2179.

Simon, H. (1967). Motivational and emotional controls of cognition. *Psychological Review, 74*, 29–39. doi:10.1037/h0024127

Singer, T., Seymour, B., O'Doherty, J., Kaube, H., Dolan, R. J., & Frith, C. D. (2004). Empathy for pain involves the affective but not sensory components of pain. *Science, 303*(5661), 1157–1162. doi:10.1126/science.1093535

Skinner, B. (1953). *Science and Human Behavior*. New York: Macmillan.

Skuse, D., Morris, J., & Lawrence, K. (2003). The Amygdala and Development of the Social Brain. *Annals of the New York Academy of Sciences, 1008*, 91–101. doi:10.1196/annals.1301.010

Sloboda, J. A. (1991). Music structure and emotional response: Some empirical findings. *Psychology of Music, 19*, 110–120. doi:10.1177/0305735691192002

Sloboda, J. A. (1992). Empirical studies of emotional response to music. In Riess-Jones, M., & Holleran, S. (Eds.), *Cognitive basis of musical communication* (pp. 33–46). Washington, DC: American Psychological Society. doi:10.1037/10104-003

Sloman, S. A. (1996). The empirical case for two systems of reasoning. *Psychological Bulletin, 119*, 3–22. doi:10.1037/0033-2909.119.1.3

Sloman, A., Chrisley, R., & Scheutz, M. (2005). The architectural basis of affective states and processes. In Fellous, J., & Arbib, M. (Eds.), *Who needs emotions? the brain meets the machine*. New York: Oxford University Press.

Sloman, A. (1992). Prolegomena to a theory of communication and affect. In Ortony, A., Slack, J., & Stock, O. (Eds.), *Communication from an artificial intelligence perspective: Theoretical and applied issues* (pp. 229–260). Heidelberg, Germany: Springer.

Sloman, A. (2000). Models of models of mind, in *Proceedings Symposium on How to Design a Functioning Mind* AISB'00, Birmingham, April 2000. In (pp. 1–9).

Sloman, A., & Croucher, M. (1981) Why robots will have emotions. In Proceedings of *IJCAI'81*, Vancouver, Canada, 1981, p. 197

Smith, E. E., & Kossyln, S. M. (2006). *Cognitive psychology: Mind and Brain*. Upper Saddle River, NJ: Prentice Hall.

Smith, E. R., & DeCoster, J. (2000). Dual-process models in social and cognitive psychology: Conceptual integration and links to underlying memory systems. *Personality and Social Psychology Review, 4*(2), 108–131. doi:10.1207/S15327957PSPR0402_01

Smith, E. E., & Kosslyn, S. M. (2007). *Cognitive psychology. Mind and brain*. New Jersey: Prentice Hall.

Smith, C. A. (1989). Dimensions of appraisal and physiological response in emotion. *Journal of Personality and Social Psychology, 56*(3), 339–353. doi:10.1037/0022-3514.56.3.339

Smith, K. S., Mahler, S. V., Pecina, S., & Berridge, K. C. (2009). Hedonic Hotspots: Generating Sensory Pleasure in the Brain. (capital letters?). In Kringelbach, M. L., & Berridge, K. C. (Eds.), *Pleasures of the Brain* (pp. 1–35). New York: Oxford University Press.

Smolensky, P. (1988). On the proper treatment of connectionism. *The Behavioral and Brain Sciences, 11*, 1–74. doi:10.1017/S0140525X00052432

Song, M., Wang, H., Bu, J., Chen, C., & Liu, Z. (2006) Subtle facial expression modeling with vector field decomposition. In *IEEE International Conference on Image Processing*, 2101 – 2104.

Soyel, H., & Demirel, H. (2007). Facial expression recognition using 3D facial feature distances. *Lecture Notes in Computer Science, 4633*, 831–843. doi:10.1007/978-3-540-74260-9_74

Spangler, W. D. (1992). Validity of questionnaire and TAT measures of need for achievement: Two meta-analyses. *Psychological Bulletin*, (112): 140–154. doi:10.1037/0033-2909.112.1.140

Sproull, L., & Kiesler, S. (1991). *Connections: new ways of working in the networked organizations.* Cambridge, MA: MIT Press.

Squire, M., & Zola, S. M. (1996). Memory, memory impairment, and the medial temporal lobe. *Cold Spring Harbor Symposia on Quantitative Biology, 61,* 185–195.

Staats, A. (1990). The Paradigmatic Behaviorism Theory of Emotions: Basis for Unification. *Clinical Psychology Review, 10,* 539–566. doi:10.1016/0272-7358(90)90096-S

Standen, P. J., & Brown, D. J. (2005). Virtual reality in the rehabilitation of people with intellectual disabilities [review]. *Cyberpsychology & Behavior, 8*(3), 272–282, discussion 283–288. doi:10.1089/cpb.2005.8.272

Stanovich, K. E. (1999). *Who is Rational? Studies of Individual Differences in Reasoning.* Mahway, NJ: Lawrence Elrbaum Associates.

Stanton, S. J., Hall, J. L., & Schultheiss, O. C. (In press). Properties of motive-specific incentives. In Schultheiss, O. C., & Brunstein, J. C. (Eds.), *Implicit motives.* New York: Oxford University Press.

Stegmann, M. B. (2002). *Analysis and segmentation of face images using point annotations and linear subspace techniques.* Technical Report, Informatics and Mathematical Modelling, Technical University of Denmark (DTU). Retrieved 19 September 2009, from http://www2.imm.dtu.dk/~aam/.

Steiner, J. E., Glaser, D., Hawilo, M. E., & Berridge, K. C. (2001). Comparative expression of hedonic impact: affective reactions to taste by human infants and other primates. *Neuroscience and Biobehavioral Reviews, 25,* 53–74. doi:10.1016/S0149-7634(00)00051-8

Stephan, A. (2006). The dual role of 'emergence' in the philosophy of mind and in cognitive science. *Synthese, 151*(3), 485–498. doi:10.1007/s11229-006-9019-y

Stern, K., & McClintock, M. K. (1998). Regulation of ovulation by human pheromones. *Nature, 392*(6672), 177–179. doi:10.1038/32408

Stern, R. M., Ray, W. J., & Quigley, K. S. (2001). *Psychophysiological Recording.* New York: Oxford University Press.

Stevenson, R. A., & James, T. W. (2008). Affective auditory stimuli: Characterization of the International Affective Digitized Sounds (IADS) by discrete emotional categories. *Behavior Research Methods, 40*(1), 315–321. doi:10.3758/BRM.40.1.315

Stokes, S. (2000). *Assistive technology for children with autism.* Published under a CESA 7 contract funded by the Wisconsin Department of Public Instruction.

Strickland, D., Marcus, L. M., Mesibov, G. B., & Hogan, K. (1996). Brief report: two case studies using virtual reality as a learning tool for autistic children. *Journal of Autism and Developmental Disorders, 26*(6). doi:10.1007/BF02172354

Strickland, D. (1997). Virtual reality for the treatment of autism. In Riva, G. (Ed.), *Virtual reality in neuropsychophysiology* (pp. 81–86). Amsterdam: IOS Press.

Styan, J. L. (1960). *The Elements of Drama.* Cambridge: Cambridge University Press.

Suchman, L. (1987). Interactive artifacts. In Suchman (Ed.), *Plans and Situated Actions* (pp. 5-26). New York: Cambridge University Press.

Sucontphunt, T., Mo, Z., Neumann, U., & Deng, Z. (2008) Interactive 3D facial expression posing through 2D portrait manipulation. *Proceeding of Graphics Interface, 71*(10 – 12), 177 – 184.

Suddendorf, T., & Corballis, M. C. (2007). The evolution of foresight: What is mental time travel and is it unique to humans? *The Behavioral and Brain Sciences, 30,* 299–313. doi:10.1017/S0140525X07001975

Sun, Y., & Yin, L. (2009). Evaluation of spatio-temporal regional features for 3D face analysis. *Proc. IEEE Computer Society Conf. on Computer Vision and Pattern Recognition Workshops.*

Surawski, M., & Osso, E. (2006). The eects of physical and vocal attractiveness on impression formation of politicians. *Current Psychology (New Brunswick, N.J.)*, *25*(1), 15–27. doi:10.1007/s12144-006-1013-5

Suri, R. E., & Schultz, W. (1999). A neural network model with dopamine-like reinforcement signal that learns a spatial delayed response task. *Neuroscience*, *91*, 871–890. doi:10.1016/S0306-4522(98)00697-6

Susskind, J. M., Littlewort, G., Bartlett, M. S., Movellan, J. R., & Anderson, A. K. (2007). Human and computer recognition of facial expressions of emotion. *Neuropsychologia*, *45*(1), 152–162. doi:10.1016/j.neuropsychologia.2006.05.001

Susskind, J. M., Hinton, G. E., Movellan, J. R., & Anderson, A. K. (2008). Generating Facial Expressions with Deep Belief Nets. In Kordic, V. (Ed.), *Affective Computing, Emotion Modelling, Synthesis and Recognition*. ARS Publishers.

Sutton-Smith, B. (2001). *The Ambiguity of Play*. Cambridge, MA: Harvard University Press.

Swettenham, J. (1996). Can children with autism be taught to understand false belief using computers? *Journal of Child Psychology and Psychiatry, and Allied Disciplines*, *37*(2), 157–165. doi:10.1111/j.1469-7610.1996.tb01387.x

Swickert, R. J., Hittner, J. B., Harris, J. L., & Herring, J. A. (2002). Relationships among Internet use, personality and social support. *Computers in Human Behavior*, *18*, 437–451. doi:10.1016/S0747-5632(01)00054-1

Swink, S. (2009). *Game Feel*. London: Morgan Kaufmann.

Sykes, J., & Brown, S. (2003). Affective gaming: measuring emotion through the gamepad. *Proceedings of Association for Computing Machinery (ACM) Special Interest Group on Computer-Human Interaction Conference (CHI)* (pp 732-733), New York: Association for Computing Machinery

Tachino, T., Kato, Y., & Kato, S. (2007). An approach to utilize ubiquitous device for game-based learning environment. *Proceedings of DIGITEL*, *2007*, 209–211.

Tajadura, A., & Vastfjall, D. (2006) Auditory-induced emotion-A neglected channel for communication in HCI. In Christian Peter, Russell Beale, Elizabeth Crane, Lesley Axelrod, Gerred Blyth (Eds.) *Emotion in HCI: Joint Proceedings of the 2005, 2006, and 2007 Intl. Workshops.* Stuttgart: Fraunhofer IRB Verlag

Tamis-LeMonda, C. S., Bornstein, M. H., & Baumwell, L. (2001). Maternal responsiveness and children's achievement of language milestones. *Child Development*, *72*(3), 748–767. doi:10.1111/1467-8624.00313

Tamis-LeMonda, C. S., & Rodriguez, E. T. (2008). Parents' role in fostering young children's learning and language development. In R.E. Tremblay, R.G. Barr, R. de Peters, and M. Boivin (Eds.), *Encyclopedia on Early Childhood Development* [online] (pp. 1-10). Montreal Quebec: Centre of Excellence for Early Childhood Development. http://www.ccl-cca.ca/pdfs/ECLKC/encyclopedia/TamisLemondaRodriguezANGxpCSAJELanguage.pdf. Accessed 25/07/2010.

Tang, H., & Huang, T. S. (2008). 3D facial expression recognition based on automatically selected features. *Proc. IEEE Computer Society Conf. on Computer Vision and Pattern Recognition Workshops.*

Tangney, J. P., Miller, R. S., Flicker, L., & Barlow, D. H. (1996). Are shame, guilt, and embarrassment distinct emotions? *Journal of Personality and Social Psychology*, *70*, 1256–1269. doi:10.1037/0022-3514.70.6.1256

Tangney, J. P., Stuewig, J., & Mashek, D. J. (2007). Moral emotions and moral behavior. *Annual Review of Psychology*, *58*, 345–372. doi:10.1146/annurev.psych.56.091103.070145

Tanji, J., & Hoshi, E. (2008). Role of the lateral prefrontal cortex in executive behavioral control. *Physiological Reviews*, *88*, 37–57. doi:10.1152/physrev.00014.2007

Tarkan, L. (2002). Autism therapy is called effective, but rare. *New York Times*.

Tartaro, A., & Cassell, J. (2007). Using virtual peer technology as an intervention for children with autism. In Lazar, J. (Ed.), *Towards Universal Usability: Designing Computer Interfaces for Diverse User Populations*. Chichester, UK: John Wiley and Sons.

Terracciano, A., McCrae, R. R., Hagemann, D., & Costa, P. T. Jr. (2003). Individual Difference Variables, Affective Differentiation, and the Structures of Affect. *Journal of Personality, 71*(5), 669–703. doi:10.1111/1467-6494.7105001

Terzopoulos, D., & Waters, K. (1990). Physically-based facial modeling and animation. *Journal of Visualization and Computer Animation, 1*(4), 73–80.

Tewes, A., Würtz, R. P., & Von der Malsburg (2005) A flexible object model for recognising and synthesising facial expressions. In Takeo Kanade, Nalini Ratha, & Anil Jain (eds.), *Proceedings of the International Conference on Audio- and Video-based Biometric Person Authentication*,(LNCS, 81-90) Springer.

Thomas, F., & Johnston, O. (1981). *The Illusions of Life: Disney Animation*. New York: Abbeville Press Publishers.

Thompsen, P. A., & Foulger, D. A. (1996). Effects of pictographs and quoting on flaming in electronic mail. *Computers in Human Behavior, 12*(2), 225–243. doi:10.1016/0747-5632(96)00004-0

Thompson, D. B. K. (2001). *Film Art: An Introduction* (6th ed.). New York: Mc Graw Hill.

Thrash, T. M., & Elliot, A. J. (2002). Implicit and self-attributed achievement motives: concordance and predictive validity. *Journal of Personality, 70*(5), 729–755. doi:10.1111/1467-6494.05022

Tian, Y., Kanade, T., & Cohn, J. F. (2001). Recognizing action units for facial expression analysis. *IEEE Transactions on Pattern Analysis and Machine Intelligence, 23*(2), 97–115. doi:10.1109/34.908962

Tice, D. M., Bratslavsky, E., & Baumeister, R. F. (2001). Emotional distress regulation takes precedence over impulse control: If you feel bad, do it! *Journal of Personality and Social Psychology, 80*, 53–67. doi:10.1037/0022-3514.80.1.53

Tischler, H. (1990). *Introduction to sociology*. Harcourt Brace College Publishers.

Toichi, M., & Kamio, Y. (2003). Paradoxical autonomic response to mental tasks in autism. *Journal of Autism and Developmental Disorders, 33*(4), 417–426. doi:10.1023/A:1025062812374

Tomasello, M. (1999). *The cultural origins of human cognition*. Cambridge, MA: Harvard University Press.

Tomasello, M., & Carpenter, M. (2007). Shared intentionality. *Developmental Science, 10*(1), 121–125. doi:10.1111/j.1467-7687.2007.00573.x

Tomasello, M., & Rakoczy, H. (2003). What makes human cognition unique? From individual to shared to collective intentionality. *Mind & Language, 18*(2), 121–147. doi:10.1111/1468-0017.00217

Tomasello, M. (2003). *Constructing a language: A usage-based theory of language acquisition*. Cambridge, MA: Harvard University Press.

Tomasello, M. (2008). *Origins of human communication*. Cambridge, MA: MIT Press.

Tong, Y., Liao, W., & Ji, Q. (2007). Facial action unit recognition by exploiting their dynamic and semantic relationships. *IEEE Transactions on Pattern Analysis and Machine Intelligence, 29*(10), 1683–1699. doi:10.1109/TPAMI.2007.1094

Tooby, J., & Cosmides, L. (1990). The past explains the present: Emotional adaptations and the structure of ancestral environments. *Ethology and Sociobiology, 11*, 407–424. doi:10.1016/0162-3095(90)90017-Z

Tracy, J. L., & Robins, R. W. (2007). The psychological structure of pride: A tale of two facets. *Journal of Personality and Social Psychology, 92*, 506–525. doi:10.1037/0022-3514.92.3.506

Tranter, S., & Reynolds, D. (2006). An overview of automatic speaker diarization systems. *IEEE Transactions on Audio, Speech, and Language Processing, 14*(5), 1557–1565. doi:10.1109/TASL.2006.878256

Trappl, R., Petta, P., & Payr, S. (Eds.). (2001). *Emotions in humans and artifacts*. Cambridge, MA: MIT Press.

Trepagnier, C. Y., Sebrechts, M. M., Finkelmeyer, A., Stewart, W., Woodford, J., & Coleman, M. (2006). Simulating social interaction to address deficits of autistic spectrum disorder in children. *Cyberpsychology & Behavior, 9*(2), 213–217. doi:10.1089/cpb.2006.9.213

Truong, K., & Van Leeuwen, D. (2007). Automatic discrimination between laughter and speech. *Speech Communication, 49*(2), 144–158. doi:10.1016/j.specom.2007.01.001

Tulving, E. (2002). Episodic memory: From mind to brain. *Annual Review of Psychology, 53*, 11–25. doi:10.1146/annurev.psych.53.100901.135114

Tummolini, L., Castelfranchi, C., Ricci, A., Viroli, M., & Omicini, A. (2004) What I See is What You Say: Coordination in a Shared Environment with Behavioral Implicit Communication. In G. Vouros (Ed.) *ECAI 04 Proceedings of the Workshop on Coordination in Emergent Societies* (CEAS 2004).

Turner, R. A., Altemus, M., Enos, T., Cooper, B., & McGuinness, T. (1999). Preliminary research on plasma oxytocin in normal cycling women: investigating emotion and interpersonal distress. *Psychiatry, 62*(2), 97–113.

Twidale, M. B. (2005). Over the Shoulder Learning: Supporting Brief Informal Learning. *Computer Supported Cooperative Work, 14*, 505–547. doi:10.1007/s10606-005-9007-7

Tzeng, J. (2004). Toward a more civilized design: Studying the effects of computers that apologize. *International Journal of Human-Computer Studies, 61*, 319–345. doi:10.1016/j.ijhcs.2004.01.002

Tzeng, J. (2006). Matching users' diverse social scripts with resonating humanized features to create a polite interface. *International Journal of Human-Computer Studies, 64*, 1230–1242. doi:10.1016/j.ijhcs.2006.08.011

Tzourio-Mazoyer, N., de Schonen, S., Crivello, F., Reutter, B., Aujard, Y., & Mazoyer, B. (2002). Neural correlates of woman face processing by 2-month-old infants. *NeuroImage, 15*(2), 454–461. doi:10.1006/nimg.2001.0979

UK Film Council. (2009). 09 Statistical Year Book, Retrieved 1st December 2009 from http:// www.ukfilmcouncil.org/yearbook

Underwood, B., Moore, B. S., & Rosenhan, D. L. (1973). Affect and self-gratification. *Developmental Psychology, 8*, 209–214. doi:10.1037/h0034158

Valstar, M. F., Güneş, H., & Pantic, M. (2007). How to Distinguish Posed from Spontaneous Smiles Using Geometric Features. *Proc. ACM International Conference Multimodal Interfaces*, (pp. 38-45).

Valstar, M., & Pantic, M. (2006). Fully automatic facial action unit detection and temporal analysis. *Proc. Computer Vision and Pattern Recognition Workshop*.

Van den Stock, J., Righart, R., & de Gelder, B. (2007). Body expressions influence recognition of emotions in the face and voice. *Emotion (Washington, D.C.), 7*(3), 487–494. doi:10.1037/1528-3542.7.3.487

van Ijzendoorn, M. H., Dijkstra, J., & Bus, A. G. (1995). Attachment, intelligence, and language: A meta-analysis. *Social Development, 4*(2), 115–128. doi:10.1111/j.1467-9507.1995.tb00055.x

van Veen, V., & Carter, C. S. (2002). The timing of action-monitoring processing in the anterior cingulate cortex. *Journal of Cognitive Neuroscience, 14*, 593–602. doi:10.1162/08989290260045837

van Veen, V., & Carter, C. S. (2006). Conflict and cognitive control in the brain. *Current Directions in Psychological Science, 15*(5), 237–240. doi:10.1111/j.1467-8721.2006.00443.x

Ververidis, D., & Kotropoulos, C. (2006). Emotional speech recognition: resources, features, and methods. *Speech Communication, 48,* 1162–1181. doi:10.1016/j.specom.2006.04.003

Ververidis, D., Kotropoulos, C., & Pitas, I. (2004). Automatic emotional speech classification. In *proceedings of IEEE International Conference on Acoustics, Speech &. Signal Processing, 1,* I-593–I-596.

Vicente, K., Thornton, D., & Moray, N. (1987). Spectral-Analysis of Sinus Arrhythmia - a Measure of Mental Effort. *Human Factors, 29*(2), 171–182.

Vinciarelli, A. (2007). Speakers role recognition in multiparty audio recordings using social network analysis and duration distribution modeling. *IEEE Transactions on Multimedia, 9*(9), 1215–1226. doi:10.1109/TMM.2007.902882

Vinciarelli, A. (2009). Capturing order in social interactions. *IEEE Signal Processing Magazine, 26*(5), 133–137. doi:10.1109/MSP.2009.933382

Vinciarelli, A., Pantic, M., & Bourlard, H. (2009). Social Signal Processing: Survey of an Emerging Domain. *Image and Vision Computing, 27*(12), 1743–1759. doi:10.1016/j.imavis.2008.11.007

Vinciarelli, A., Pantic, M., Bourlard, H., & Pentland, A. (2008). Social Signal Processing: State-of-the-art and future perspectives of an emerging domain. In *Proceedings of the ACM international conference on multimedia* (pp. 1061-1070).

Viola, P., & Jones, M. J. (2004). Robust real-time face detection. *International Journal of Computer Vision, 57*(2), 137–154. doi:10.1023/B:VISI.0000013087.49260.fb

Võ, M. L.-H., Conrad, M., Kuchinke, L., Urton, K., Hofmann, M. J., & Jacobs, A. M. (2009). The Berlin Affective Word List Reloaded (BAWL-R). *Behavior Research Methods, 41,* 534–538. doi:10.3758/BRM.41.2.534

Vogiatzis, D., Spyropoulos, C., Konstantopoulos, S., Karkaletsis, V., Kasap, Z., Matheson, C., & Deroo, O. (2008) An affective robot guide to museums. *In Proc. 4th International Workshop on Human-Computer Conversation.*

Voss, J. F., Wiley, J., & Carretero, M. (1995). Acquiring intellectual skills. *Annual Review of Psychology, 46,* 155–181. doi:10.1146/annurev.ps.46.020195.001103

Vuilleumier, P., Richardson, M. P., Armony, J. L., Driver, J., & Dolan, R. J. (2004). Distant influences of amygdala lesion on visual cortical activation during emotional face processing. *Nature Neuroscience, 7*(11), 1271–1278. doi:10.1038/nn1341

Vural, E., Çetin, M., Erçil, A., Littlewort, G., Bartlett, M., & Movellan, J. (2007). Drowsy driver detection through facial movement analysis. *Lecture Notes in Computer Science, 4796,* 6–19. doi:10.1007/978-3-540-75773-3_2

Vygotsky, L. S. (1962). *Thought and language.* Cambridge, MA: MIT Press. doi:10.1037/11193-000

Waibel, A., Schultz, T., Bett, M., Denecke, M., Malkin, R., Rogina, I., & Stiefelhagen, R. (2003). SMaRT: the Smart Meeting Room task at ISL. In *Proceedings of IEEE international conference on acoustics, speech, and signal processing* (pp. 752-755).

Walker-Andrews, A. S. (1997). Infants' perception of expressive behaviors: differentiation of multimodal information. *Psychological Bulletin, 121,* 1–20. doi:10.1037/0033-2909.121.3.437

Walker-Andrews, A. S., & Grolnick, W. (1983). Discrimination of vocal expression by young infants. *Infant Behavior and Development, 6,* 491–498. doi:10.1016/S0163-6383(83)90331-4

Wallis, J. D., & Miller, E. K. (2003). Neuronal activity in primate dorsolateral and orbital prefrontal cortex during performance of a reward preference task. *The European Journal of Neuroscience, 18,* 2069–2081. doi:10.1046/j.1460-9568.2003.02922.x

Walther, J. B. (1992). Interpersonal effects in computer mediated interaction: a relational perspective. *Communication Research, 19,* 52–90. doi:10.1177/009365092019001003

Walther, J. B., & Burgoon, J. K. (1992). Relational communication in computer-mediated interaction. *Human Communication Research, 19,* 50–88. doi:10.1111/j.1468-2958.1992.tb00295.x

Walther, J. B., & D'Addario, P. (2001). The impacts of emoticons on message interpretation in computer-mediated communication. *Social Science Computer Review, 19,* 324–347. doi:10.1177/089443930101900307

Wang, H. & Wang, K. (2008) Affective interaction based on person independent facial expression space. *Neurocomputing, Special Issue for Vision Research, 71*(10 – 12), 1889 – 1901.

Wang, H., & Ahuja, N. (2003) Facial expression decomposition. In *IEEE International Conference on Computer Vision,* 958 – 965.

Ward, R. D., & Marsden, P. H. (2003). Physiological responses to different WEB page designs. *International Journal of Human-Computer Studies, 59*(1-2), 199–212. doi:10.1016/S1071-5819(03)00019-3

Waters, K. (1987). A muscle model for animating three – dimensional facial expression. *Computer Graphics, 22*(4), 17–24. doi:10.1145/37402.37405

Watson, D., Wiese, D., Vaidya, J., & Tellegen, A. (1999). The Two General Activation Systems of Affect: Structural Findings, Evolutionary Considerations, and Psychobiological Evidence. *Journal of Personality and Social Psychology, 76*(5), 820–838. doi:10.1037/0022-3514.76.5.820

Watzlawick, P., Beavin, J., & Jackson, D. (1967). *The pragmatics of human communication.* New York: Norton.

Wedekind, C., Seebeck, T., Bettens, F., & Paepke, A. J. (1995). MHC-dependent mate preferences in humans. *Proceedings. Biological Sciences, 260*(1359), 245–249. doi:10.1098/rspb.1995.0087

Weinberger, J., & McClelland, D. C. (1990). Cognitive versus traditional motivational models: Irreconcilable or complementary? In Higgins, E. T., & Sorrentino, R. M. (Eds.), *Implicit motives 45, Handbook of motivation and cognition: Foundations of social behavior* (Vol. 2, pp. 562–597). New York, NY: Guilford Press.

Werker, J. F., & Tees, R. C. (1984). Cross-language speech perception: Evidence for perceptual reorganization during the first year of life. *Infant Behavior and Development, 7,* 49–63. doi:10.1016/S0163-6383(84)80022-3

Werker, J. F. (1993). Developmental changes in cross-language speech perception: implications for cognitive models of speech processing. In G. Altman and R. Shillock (Eds.), *Cognitive models of speech processing. The second Sperlonga Meeting* (pp. 57-78). Hillsdale, NJ: Erlbaum.

Whalen, P., Rauch, S. L., Etcoff, N. L., McInerney, S. C., Lee, M. B., & Jenike, M. A. (1998). Masked presentations of emotional facial expressions modulate amygdala activity without explicit knowledge. *The Journal of Neuroscience, 18,* 411–418.

Whalen, P. J., Kagan, J., Cook, R. G., Davis, F. C., Kim, H., Polis, S., McLaren, D. G., Somerville, L. H., McLean, A. A., Maxwell, J. S., & Johnstone, T. (2004). Human amygdala responsivity to masked fearful eye whites. *Science, 17,* 306 (5704), 2061.

Whitehill, J., Littlewort, G., Fasel, I., Bartlett, M., & Movellan, J. (2009). Towards Practical Smile Detection. *IEEE Transactions on Pattern Analysis and Machine Intelligence, 31*(11), 2106–2111. doi:10.1109/TPAMI.2009.42

Whitty, M. T. (2008). Revealing the 'real' me, searching for the 'actual' you: Presentations of self on an internet dating site. *Computers in Human Behavior, 24*(4), 1707–1723. doi:10.1016/j.chb.2007.07.002

Wicker, B., Keysers, C., Plailly, J., Royet, J. P., Gallese, V., & Rizzolatti, G. (2003). Both of us disgusted in My insula: the common neural basis of seeing and feeling disgust. *Neuron, 40,* 655–664. doi:10.1016/S0896-6273(03)00679-2

Wieder, S., & Greenspan, S. (2005). Can children with autism master the core deficits and become empathetic, creative, and reflective? *The Journal of Developmental and Learning Disorders*, *9*, 1–29.

Wierzbicka, A. (1992d). Talking about emotions: Semantics, culture and cognition. [Special issue on basic emotions]. *Cognition and Emotion*, *6*(3/4), 285–319. doi:10.1080/02699939208411073

Wijesiriwardana, R., Mitcham, K., & Dias, T. (2004). *Fibre-meshed transducers based real time wearable physiological information monitoring system*. Paper presented at the International Symposium on Wearable Computers, Washington, DC.

Williams, J. R., Carter, C. S., & Insel, T. (1992). Partner preference development in female prairie voles is facilitated by mating or the central infusion of oxytocin. *Annals of the New York Academy of Sciences*, *652*, 487–489. doi:10.1111/j.1749-6632.1992.tb34393.x

Williams, J. R., Insel, T. R., Harbaugh, C. R., & Carter, C. S. (1994). Oxytocin administered centrally facilitates formation of a partner preference in female prairie voles (Microtus ochrogaster). *Journal of Neuroendocrinology*, *6*(3), 247–250. doi:10.1111/j.1365-2826.1994.tb00579.x

Williams, A. (2003). Facial expression of pain: An evolutionary account. *The Behavioral and Brain Sciences*, *25*(4), 439–455.

Wilson, J. M., Straus, S. G., & McEvily, B. (2006). All in due Time: Development of Trust in Computer-mediated and Face-toFace Teams. *Organizational Behavior and Human Decision Processes*, *99*, 16–33. doi:10.1016/j.obhdp.2005.08.001

Winkielman, P., Berridge, K. C., & Wilbarger, J. (2005). Unconscious affective reactions to masked happy versus angry faces influence consumption behavior and judgments of value. *Personality and Social Psychology Bulletin*, *31*, 121–135. doi:10.1177/0146167204271309

Winter, D. G. (1996). *Personality: Analysis and interpretation of lives*. New York: McGraw-Hill.

Witmer, B. G., & Singer, M. J. (1998). Measuring Presence in Virtual Environments: A Presence Questionnaire. *Presence (Cambridge, Mass.)*, *7*(3), 225–240. doi:10.1162/105474698565686

Womack, B., & Hansen, J. L. H. (1996). Classification of speech under stress using target driven features. *Speech Communication*, *20*, 131–150. doi:10.1016/S0167-6393(96)00049-0

Wood, W., Quinn, J., & Kashy, D. (2002). Habits in everyday life: Thought, emotion, and action. *Journal of Personality and Social Psychology*, *83*, 1281–1297. doi:10.1037/0022-3514.83.6.1281

Wrangham, R., & Peterson, D. (1996). *Demonic Males: Apes and the Origins of Human Violence*. Boston, MA: Houghton Mifflin.

Yamamoto, M., & Akahori, K. (2005). Development of an e-learning system for higher education using the mobile phone. *Proceedings of World Conference on Educational Multimedia, Hypermedia and Telecommunications (ED-MEDIA) 2005*, 4169-4172.

Yang, B., & Lugger, M. (2009). Emotion recognition from speech signals using new harmony features. Article in Press. *Signal Processing*, 1–9.

Yang, M., Kriegman, D., & Ahuja, N. (2002). Detecting faces in images: a survey. *IEEE Transactions on Pattern Analysis and Machine Intelligence*, *24*(1), 34–58. doi:10.1109/34.982883

Yang, M. H., & Ahuja, N. (2001). *Face Detection and Gesture Recognition for Human – Computer Interaction*. New York: Kluwer Academic Publishers.

Yang, M. H., Kriegman, D., & Ahuja, N. (2002). Detecting Faces in Images: A Survey. *IEEE Transactions on Pattern Analysis and Machine Intelligence*, *24*(1), 34–58. doi:10.1109/34.982883

Yin, L., Basu, A., Bernögger, S., & Pinz, A. (2001). Synthesizing realistic facial animations using energy minimization for model-based coding. *Pattern Recognition*, *34*(11), 2201–2213. doi:10.1016/S0031-3203(00)00139-4

Yin, L., Chen, X., Sun, Y., Worm, T., & Reale, M. (2008). A High-Resolution 3D Dynamic Facial Expression Database. *Proc. 8th Int. Conf. on Automatic Face and Gesture Recognition.*

Yin, L., Wei, X., Sun, Y., Wang, J., & Rosato, M. J. (2006). A 3D facial expression database for facial behavior research. *Proc. Int. Conf. on Automatic Face and Gesture Recognition,* (pp.211–216).

Yongmian, Z. Q. J. Z. Z. B. Y. (2008). Dynamic Facial Expression Analysis and Synthesis With MPEG-4 Facial Animation Parameters. *IEEE Trans. on Circuits and Systems for Video Technology, 18*(10), 1383–1396. doi:10.1109/TCSVT.2008.928887

Young, A. W., Hellawell, D. J., Van De Wal, C., & Johnson, M. (1996). Facial expression processing after amygdalotomy. *Neuropsychologia, 34*(1), 31–39. doi:10.1016/0028-3932(95)00062-3

Young, P. (1959). The role of affective processes in learning and motivation. *Psychological Review, 66*, 104–125. doi:10.1037/h0045997

Yurchisin, J., Watchravesringkan, K., & McCabe, D. B. (2005). An Exploration of Identity Re-creation in the Context of Internet Dating. *Social Behavior and Personality, 33*(8), 735–750. doi:10.2224/sbp.2005.33.8.735

Zahm, D. S. (2000). An integrative neuroanatomical perspective on some subcortical substrates of adaptive responding with emphasis on the nucleus accumbens. *Neuroscience and Biobehavioral Reviews, 24*(1), 85–105. doi:10.1016/S0149-7634(99)00065-2

Zald, D. H. (2003). The human amygdala and the emotional evaluation of sensory stimuli. *Brain Research. Brain Research Reviews, 41*, 88–123. doi:10.1016/S0165-0173(02)00248-5

Zancanaro, M., Lepri, B., & Pianesi, F. (2006). Automatic detection of group functional roles in face to face interactions. In *Proceedings of international conference on multimodal interfaces* (pp. 47-54).

Zelazo, P. D., Chandler, M., & Crone, Eveline (Eds) (2009). *Developmental social cognitive neuroscience.* New York, Hove: Psychology Press.

Zeng, Z., Pantic, M., Roisman, G. I., & Huang, T. S. (2009). A Survey of Affect Recognition Methods: Audio, Visual, and Spontaneous Expressions. *IEEE Transactions on Pattern Analysis and Machine Intelligence, 31*(1), 39–58. doi:10.1109/TPAMI.2008.52

Zhai, J., Barreto, A., Chin, C., & Li, C. (2005). User Stress Detection in Human-Computer Interactions. *Biomedical Sciences Instrumentation, 41*, 277–286.

Zhang, Y., & Ji, Q. (2005). Active and dynamic information fusion for facial expression understanding from image sequences. *IEEE Transactions on Pattern Analysis and Machine Intelligence, 27*(5), 699–714. doi:10.1109/TPAMI.2005.93

Zhang, Q., Liu, Z., Guo, B., Terzopoulos, D., & Shum, H.-Y. (2006). Geometry – driven photorealistic facial expression shyntesis. *IEEE Trans. on Visualization and Computer Graphics, 12*(1), 48–60. doi:10.1109/TVCG.2006.9

Zhang, Y., & Prakash, E., C., & Sung, E. (2002). Constructing a realistic face model of an individual for expression animation. *International Journal of Information Technology, 8*(2), 10–25.

Zhang, S., Wu, Z., Meng, H. M., & Cai, L. (2007) Facial expression synthesis using PAD emotional parameters for a chinese expressive avatar. *In Proceedings of the 2nd International Conference on Affective Computing and Intelligent Interaction, 4738*, 24 – 35.

Zhao, S., Grasmuck, S., & Martin, J. (2008). Identity construction on Facebook: Digital empowerment in anchored relationships. *Computers in Human Behavior, 24*, 1816–1836. doi:10.1016/j.chb.2008.02.012

Zhou, G., Hansen, J. H. L., & Kaiser, J. F. (2001). Nonlinear feature based classification of speech under stress. *IEEE Transactions on Speech and Audio Processing, 9*(3), 201–216. doi:10.1109/89.905995

Zimbardo, P. G. (1970). The Human Choice: Individuation, Reason, and Order versus Deindividuation, Impulse and Chaos. In A. WJ. Levine (Eds), *Nebraska Symposium on Motivation* (pp. 237-307). Lincoln: University of Nebraska press.

Zinck, A. (2008). Self-referential emotions. *Consciousness and Cognition, 17*, 496–505. doi:10.1016/j.concog.2008.03.014

About the Contributors

Didem Gökçay received her BS and MS degrees in the Department of Electrical and Electronics Engineering at Middle East Technical University. She finished her PhD in the Department of Computer Science at University of Florida as a Fulbright scholar. She worked as a research assistant in the Cognitive Neuropsychology Laboratory of the University of Florida Brain Institute for 6 years developing tasks with emotional stimuli and programs for the analysis of psychophysiology and fMRI measurements. Her postdoctoral fellowship was mutually funded by the Salk Institute and University of California San Diego, while she worked at the Research Center for the Neuroscience of Autism on morphology and function of neuroanatomical structures. Currently she is an Assistant Professor at the Informatics Institute of Middle East Technical University. She also directs the METUNEURO Laboratory which specializes in MRI and fMRI postprocessing. Her main interest is the interplay between emotion and cognition, and more specifically key anatomical structures such as the anterior cingulate which participate in the underlying emotional processes.

Gülsen Yıldırım received her BS degree in the department of Electrical and Electronics Engineering at Middle East Technical University in 2001. She continued her graduate studies in the field of Robotics at the same department. Her research focused on the development and the control of modular exoskeleton robots as well as pattern recognition, machine learning and intelligent control. In the meanwhile, she worked as a research assistant at the Computer Engineering Department of Atılım University. Since 2004, she has been working as an IT professional specialized in software engineering, software management, project management & coordination. Her main expertise areas are mobile game development, online multiplayer games and enterprise systems. Currently, she is project manager and coordinator of Turkish e-Government Gateway Project and she continues her graduate studies in the Cognitive Science Department of Informatics Institute of Middle East Technical University. Her current research includes affective computing, affective interactions, face recognition in both humans and machines, pattern recognition, and human-computer interaction.

***

Mahir Akgun earned his BS degree in Computer Education and Instructional Technology and MS degree in Cognitive Sciences Program of the Middle East Technical University. His research focuses on social, cultural and emotional aspects of usability issues, technology integration in learning environments and higher-order thinking skills. He currently pursues his PhD Degree in Instructional Systems Program at the Pennsylvania State University.

Goknur Kaplan Akıllı completed her major in Mathematics Education at Hacettepe University, Turkey in 2001 and ranked first in graduating class of the Faculty of Education. In 2004, she was conferred her M.S. degree by the Department of Computer Education and Instructional Technology, Middle East Technical University (METU), Turkey, with her thesis entitled "A Proposal of Instructional Design/Development Model for Game-like Learning Environments: The FIDGE Model," which has been nominated for many national and international awards. She was named an "Academic All-Star" by Microsoft Research and the Serious Games Summit in 2005 and 2006. She is the author of several internationally recognized publications. Currently, she is a Ph.D. candidate at the Pennsylvania State University and is working on her dissertation examining 'learning through argumentation' in an online fantasy sports community.

Zeynep Başgöze was born in 1982, Ankara. She graduated from Bogazici University Philosophy Department in 2005 at the 2nd rank. She graduated from the department Cognitive Science at Middle East Technical University in 2008 with the MS degree. She received an institutional best thesis award with her MSc thesis 'Emotional Conflict Resolution in Healthy and Depressed Population'. She is currently a PhD student in Cognitive Science Department and she works as research and teaching assistant for both Cognitive Science and Information Systems Departments of Informatics Institute, in METU. In her PhD thesis she is working on fMRI experiments on the healthy and depressed populations.

Ioan Buciu received the Diploma of Electrical Engineering in 1996 and the Master of Science degree in microwaves in 1997, both from the University of Oradea. From 1997 to 2000, he served as a Teaching Assistant with the Department of Applied Electronics, University of Oradea. During 2001 - 2005, he was a researcher and a PhD student at the Artificial Intelligence and Information Analysis Lab, Department of Informatics, Aristotle University of Thessaloniki, Greece. He received the Ph.D. degrees in Electrical and Computer Engineering in 2008 from the "Politehnica" University of Timisoara, Romania. Currently he is with the Department of Electronics, Electrical Engineering and Information Technology, University of Oradea. He has co-authored 3 book chapters, 9 journal papers and over 35 conference papers. He currently serves as Associate Executive Editor for the International Journal of Computers, Communications & Control (IJCCC). His current research interests lie in the area of human-computer interaction (HCI), image processing, pattern recognition, machine learning, and artificial intelligence, subspace image decomposition, temporal information retrieval and dimensionality reduction. His area of expertise also includes face analysis, support vector machines, and image representation.

Cristiano Castelfranchi: Full professor of "Cognitive Sciences", University of Siena; director of the Institute of Cognitive Sciences and Technologies ISTC-CNR, Roma. Cognitive scientist, with a background in linguistics and psychology; active in the Multi-Agent Systems, Social Simulation, and Psychology and Cognitive Science communities. Co-chair of the First AAMAS-2002 and AAMAS-2009; chair of several international workshops in these fields; advisory member of several international conferences and societies (like Cognitive Science; IFMAS); member of the editorial board of international journals. Invited speaker at IJCAI'97 (and many other conferences and workshops in AI, logic, philosophy, linguistics, psychology, economics). Award as "fellows" of ECCAI for "pioneering work in the field"; "Mind and Brain" 2008 award Univ. of Torino. Research fields of interest include: social cognition and emotions; cognitive approach to communication and interaction; cognitive agent architecture; multi-agent systems; agent-based social simulation; cognitive foundations of complex social phenomena (dependence, power, cooperation, norms, organization, social functions, etc.).

Kürşat Çagıltay is Associate Professor of the Department of Instructional Technology at the Middle East Technical University (METU), Ankara, Turkey. He earned his BS in Mathematics and MS in Computer Engineering from Middle East Technical University. He holds a double Ph.D. in Cognitive Science and Instructional Systems Technology from Indiana University, USA. His research focuses on Human Computer Interaction, Instructional Technology, Social and cognitive issues of electronic games, socio-cultural aspects of technology, distance learning, Human Performance Technologies.

Anders Drachen is an independent consultant and games-user research specialist. His work focuses on developing methods for evaluating user behavior and user experience in digital games, for research purposes as well as for improving user-oriented testing in the game- and creative industries.

Magy Seif El-Nasr is an assistant Professor in the School of Interactive Arts and Technology at Simon Fraser University, where she directs the Engage Me In Interactive Experiences (EMIIE) Lab. She earned her Ph.D. degree from Northwestern University in Computer Science. Dr. Seif El-Nasr received several awards and recognition within the games and interactive narrative communities, including Best Paper Award at the International Conference of Virtual Storytelling 2003 and several notable citations in industry books and magazines. She is on the editorial board of the International Journal of Intelligent Games and Simulation, and ACM Computers in Entertainment. Her research work includes designing and developing tools that enhance the engagement of interactive environments used for training, education, and entertainment. She has collaborated and has on-going relationships with several game companies, including Electronic Arts, Bardel Entertainment, RedHill Studios, and Radical Entertainment. http://www.sfu.ca/~magy.

Ayşen Erdem received M.D. degree from the University of Hacettepe, Faculty of Medicine, Ankara, Turkey, in 1992, and the specialist degree in Physiology from the University of Hacettepe, Faculty of Medicine, Ankara, Turkey, in 1997. She is currently an Associate Professor in the Department of Physiology at the University of Hacettepe, Faculty of Medicine.

Cornelia Emilia Gordan received the Diploma on Electronics Engineering in 1986 at Politehnica University of Timisoara, Romania, and PhD Degree in Electrical Engineering in 1999 at the University of Oradea, Romania. She currently holds the positions of Professor at University of Oradea and Chief of Applied Electronics Department, in the same academic institution. She is IEEE Senior Member since 1998. She is author or co-author of over 70 papers, published in national or international journals or Conference proceedings, and managed projects with leading Romanian or European companies or governmental organizations. Prof. Gordan's present research interests include digital signal processing, adaptive signal processing, time-frequency analysis of non-stationary signals. She is currently member of the Editorial board of the Journal of Electrical and Electronics Engineering from Oradea, BDI recognized. She was reviewer for several international conferences and journals.

Theo Gevers is an Associate Professor of Computer Science at the University of Amsterdam, The Netherlands and an ICREA Research Professor at the Computer Vision Center (UAB), Barcelona, Spain. At the University of Amsterdam he is a teaching director of the MSc of Artificial Intelligence. He currently holds a VICI-award (for excellent researchers) from the Dutch Organisation for Scientific

Research. His main research interests are in the fundamentals of content-based image retrieval, colour image processing and computer vision. He chaired numerous workshops and conferences, and served as the guest editor of special issues for International Journal of Computer Vision and Computer Vision and Image Understanding. He has published over 100 papers on colour image processing, image retrieval and computer vision. He is program committee member of a various number of conferences, and an invited speaker at major conferences. He is a lecturer of post-doctoral courses given at various major conferences (CVPR, ICPR, SPIE, CGIV). He is member of the IEEE.

Hatice Gunes received her PhD degree in computing sciences from University of Technology Sydney (UTS), Australia, in 2007. Until 2008, she was a postdoctoral research associate at UTS, where she worked on an Australian research council–funded Linkage Project for UTS and iOmniscient Pty Ltd. She is currently a postdoctoral research associate with the Intelligent Behaviour Understanding Group (iBUG) at Imperial College London, U.K. working on a European Commission (EC-FP7) project, and is also an honorary associate of UTS. Gunes has published over 35 technical papers in the areas of video analysis and pattern recognition, with applications to video surveillance, human-computer interaction, emotion recognition and affective computing. She is a member of the IEEE and the ACM.

Annette Hohenberger received her diploma in psychology and her MA and PhD in linguistics from the University of Frankfurt, Germany, between 1987 and 1997. She was working in the Linguistics Department of the University of Frankfurt, at the Max Planck Institute for Human Cognitive and Brain Sciences in Munich, and is now an Assist. Prof. in the Department of Cognitive Science at Middle East Technical University, Ankara, Turkey. Her research interests can broadly be specified as: cognitive development (early understanding of human goal-directed action, imitation, Theory of Mind), psycholinguistics (language development, language production, evidentiality, syntactic priming), and sign language (slips of the hand, working memory, Turkish and German Sign Language). She proactively participates in studies of climate change and sustainability (cognitive aspects of understanding and acting on the global challenge of climate change).

Ahmet İnam was born in 1947. He graduated from METU Electrical Engineering in 1971. In 1980, he graduated from Istanbul University Faculty of Arts Philosophy Department with a PhD degree, where his major area was Systematic Philosophy and Logic; his minor area was Ancient Greek Literature. The title of his PhD thesis was: Logic In Edmund Husserl's Philosophy. He first became a research assistant in METU, Human Sciences in 1980, where in 1983 he became an Associate Professor. He was appointed as a Professor at the same university in 1989. He was the head of the METU Philosophy department between 1994-2000, as well as at the present, since 2003. He continues to study on logic, philosophy of science, epistemology, history of philosophy, philosophy of culture and ethics. He has published over thirty books of poetry, essay and commentaries and over 600 articles.

Serkan Karaismailoğlu received M.S. degree in Physiology from the University of Hacettepe, Faculty of Medicine, Ankara, Turkey, in 2008. He is currently working toward the Ph.D. degree in Physiology at the University of Hacettepe, Faculty of Medicine. He was awarded with Young Scientist Award in 2009 in 35th National Physiology Congress of Turkish Physiological Sciences.

Shogo Kato is an Assistant Professor in the School of Arts and Sciences, Tokyo Woman's Christian University in Japan and a part-time instructor in the Faculty of Economics, Dokkyo University in Japan. He earned a Ph.D. from Tokyo Institute of Technology in 2005. His general research interests include educational technology; the application of behavior science, psychology, and information and communication technology (ICT) to educational scenes. Dr. Kato is particularly interested in the emotional aspects in virtual community, such as Internet bullying.

Yuuki Kato is an Assistant Professor in the School of Education at Tokyo University of Social Welfare in Japan. He earned a Ph.D. from Tokyo Institute of Technology in 2005. His general research interests include educational technology; the application of behavior science, psychology, and information and communication technology (ICT) to educational scenes. Dr. Kato is particularly interested in the emotional aspects in technology-mediated human communications.

Uttama Lahiri is a research assistant in the Robotics and Autonomous Systems Laboratory (RASL), Vanderbilt University. She received the M.Tech. degree in electrical engineering in 2004 from Indian Institute of Technology, Kharagpur, India. She is currently working toward the Ph.D. degree in mechanical engineering at Vanderbilt. From 2004 to 2007 she worked for Tata Steel, Jamshedpur in plant automation. Her current research interests include machine learning, adaptive response systems, signal processing, human-computer interaction, and robotics.

Changchun Liu received the B.E. degree in mechanical engineering from Tsinghua University, Beijing, China, in 1999, and the M.S. degree in mechtronics from Shenyang Automation Institute, Chinese Academy of Sciences, Shenyang, China, in 2002. In 2009 he received the Ph.D. degree in electrical engineering and computer science at Vanderbilt University. He then joined The MathWorks as a Senior Software Engineer. His research interests include human–machine interaction, affective computing, pattern recognition, machine learning, robotics, and signal processing.

Cindy Mason has a unique interdisciplinary background with a Ph.D. in AI and a California state certification in Oriental Medicine. She has completed training as a fellow at the Stanford School of Medicine and at the Berkeley Primary Care. Since 2001, Cindy is a research associate at Stanford's Computer Science Department. Prior to her work with Stanford she was a research engineer at U.C. Berkeley EECS Department. She is a computer scientist linking the seemingly disparate fields of distributed systems and artificial intelligence with Chinese philosophy and medicine. Her work on EOP draws on her experience with mental patients at Berkeley Primary Care and in critical care at Stanford Hospital. Her main computational interests are bridging ideas on mental state from medical disciplines and philosophies to affective computing and applications involving big data and distributed systems. She has made innovative contributions to the field of artificial intelligence, psychoneuroimmunology and rehabilitative medicine. Her work on haptic medicine, a field she founded, is used in over 5 countries. She holds a number of awards and was recently named in the 2009 Cambridge International Top 2000 Scientists.

Gelareh Mohammadi was born in Tehran, Iran; she received her B.Sc. in Bioelectrical Engineering from Tehran Polytechnic in 2003 and her M.Sc. in Electrical Engineering from Sharif University of Technology in 2006. From 2008 to 2009 she was with Signal Processing Laboratories of EPFL (École Polytechnique Fédérale de Lausanne) as a research assistant working in Computer Vision field and from

2009 she has started her PhD at EPFL Laboratory of Idiap Research Institute (L'Idiap). Her research area is Social Signal Processing and currently she is working on nonverbal vocal communication. Her Research interests include Signal and Image Processing, Feature Extraction, Pattern Recognition, Machine Learning, Computer Vision and Compressive sensing.

Jacquelyn Ford Morie has been at the forefront of immersive world technology since 1990, working on affective and meaningful implementations of virtual environments. She received her PhD in this topic from the University of East London's SmartLab in 2008. She has developed multi-sensory techniques for virtual reality (VR) that can predictably elicit emotional responses from participants within simulated environments, for example inventing a scent collar that can be used to deliver scents to a participant in a VR scenario. She is also active in online 3D virtual worlds and has been bringing her VR techniques to these more social worlds. Her other research interests include topics such as space, identity and play in virtual worlds, and she has presented extensively on these topics at conferences worldwide.

Ioan Nafornita received the M.Sc. and Ph.D. degrees in Electrical and Computer Engineering in 1968 and 1981, respectively, from the "Politehnica" University of Timisoara, Romania, where he currently holds the position of Professor and leads the Signal Processing Group. He is a member of IEEE and a corresponding member of the Romanian Academy of Technical Sciences, section of Information Technology and Communications, Computers and Telecommunications. He supervised more than 25 Ph.D. students and is author or co-author of over 100 papers, published in national or international journals or Conference proceedings. He managed projects with leading Romanian or international companies or governmental organizations. Dr. Nafornita's current research interests include digital signal processing, adaptive signal processing, statistical signal processing, time-frequency representations and analysis and synthesis of circuits. He currently serves as Editor-in-Chief for the Scientific Bulletin of the "Politehnica" Timisoara, Transactions on Electronics and Telecommunications and served as a reviewer for international conferences and journals.

Albert Ali Salah received his PhD from Boğaziçi University, Dept. of Computer Engineering in 2007. Between 2008-2009 he worked as a BRICKS/BSIK scholar at the Center of Mathematics and Computer Science (CWI) in Amsterdam, and joined the Informatics Institute of University of Amsterdam in 2009. His research interests include computer vision, pattern recognition, machine learning, with applications to human-computer interaction and biometrics. He has over 50 scholarly publications in these areas. He is the inaugural recipient of the European Biometrics Award (2006). He is a member of IEEE, IAPR, and EuroCogII.

Nilanjan Sarkar received his Ph.D. from the University of Pennsylvania, Philadelphia, Pennsylvania in 1993. He joined Queen's University, Canada as a Postdoctoral fellow and then went to the University of Hawaii as an Assistant Professor. In 2000 he joined Vanderbilt University as Director of the RASL. Currently he is an Associate Professor of mechanical engineering and computer engineering. His research focuses on human–robot interaction, affective computing, dynamics, and control.

Matthias Scheutz received degrees in philosophy (M.A. 1989, Ph.D. 1995) and formal logic (M.S. 1993) from the University of Vienna and in computer engineering (M.S. 1993) from the Vienna University of Technology (1993) in Austria. He also received the joint Ph.D. in cognitive science and computer science from Indiana University in 1999. Matthias is currently an associate professor of computer and cognitive science in the Department of Computer Science at Tufts University. He has over 100 peer-reviewed publications in artificial intelligence, artificial life, agent-based computing, natural language processing, cognitive modeling, robotics, human-robot interaction and foundations of cognitive science. His current research and teaching interests include multi-scale agent-based models of social behavior and complex cognitive and affective robots with natural language capabilities for natural human-robot interaction.

Douglass Scott is a Professor at Waseda University's School of Human Sciences in the Human Informatics and Cognitive Sciences Department. Dr. Scott's academic background includes an M.A. in Japanese culture and society (University of Michigan, 1987) and a Ph.D. in educational foundations and policy (University of Michigan, 1997). Dr. Scott's research interests include gender and intercultural differences in the use of communication technologies, particularly mobile telephones. His current research projects include emotional transfer in Japanese young people's text messages and the comparative study of Japanese and American young people's use of communication technologies.

Nicu Sebe is an associate professor in the Department of Information Engineering and Computer Science, University of Trento, where he is leading the research in the areas of multimedia information retrieval and human-computer interaction in computer vision applications. Until Spring 2009, he was with the University of Amsterdam, the Netherlands. He is the author of two monographs and was involved in the organization of the major conferences and workshops addressing the computer vision and human-centered aspects of multimedia information retrieval and human behaviour understanding. He has served as the guest editor for several special issues in IEEE Computer, Computer Vision and Image Understanding, Image and Vision Computing, Multimedia Systems, ACM TOMCCAP, and IEEE Transactions on Multimedia. He is the co-chair of the IEEE Computer Society Task Force on Human-centered Computing and is an associate editor of IEEE Transactions on Multimedia, Machine Vision and Applications, Image and Vision Computing, Electronic Imaging and of Journal of Multimedia.

Mark Ashton Smith has obtained his PhD from the Center for the Neural Basis of Cognition (CNBC), University of Pittsburgh and Carnegie Mellon University, Pittsburgh, in 1998. He is formerly affiliated with University of Cambridge, UK. Currently he is the Head of the Department of Psychology in Girne American University in North Cyprus, developing a Cognitive Program. His research interests include the philosophy of psychology, theory of mind, joint attention, normativity and – more generally - human unique cognition in an evolutionary context. His laboratory research investigates working memory interventions, and their effect on executive control, intelligence and cognitive biases.

Wendy Stone received the Ph.D. degree in clinical psychology from the University of Miami, Coral Gables, FL, in 1981. In 1988, she joined Vanderbilt University, Nashville, TN, where she is currently a Professor in the Department of Pediatrics and the Department of Psychology and Human Development. She is also the Director of the Treatment and Research Institute for Autism Spectrum Disorders (TRIAD) and the Marino Autism Research Institute (MARI), Vanderbilt Kennedy Center, Nashville. Her current research interests include early identification and intervention for children with autism spectrum disorders.

Jonathan Sykes is a senior play researcher at Glasgow Caledonian University. He is director of eMotionLab, a premier research facility which offers both consultancy and development services in the area of game production and play-testing. Skilled in the design and evaluation of the play experience, the focus of Jonathan's research is the application of emotional play technologies to pursued uptake of positive behaviour, primarily in regard to health and wellbeing, and lifelong education. Both a psychologist and usability engineer, Jonathan's work is very much player-centred, and focused on the player experience. He has worked with Microsoft's Game User Research group to develop player-centred approaches to game design and evaluation, and written academic papers and text-book chapters on the subject. He also works as a senior lecturer at Glasgow Caledonian University where he delivers undergraduate courses in both player-centred game design, and emotional game design.

John Taylor is presently European Editor-in-Chief of the journal Neural Networks and was President of the International Neural Network Society (1995) and the European Neural Network Society (1993/4). He is Emeritus Professor of Mathematics at King's College, London, after 25 years there as Professor of Mathematics, and is Director of the Centre for Neural Networks at King's College. He has published over 500 scientific papers (in theoretical physics, astronomy, particle physics, pure mathematics, neural networks, higher cognitive processes, brain imaging, consciousness) since he started scientific research in 1953, authored 12 books, edited 13 others, including the titles, Artificial Neural Networks (ed, North-Holland, 1992), The Promise of Neural Networks (Springer,1993), Mathematical Approaches to Neural Networks (ed, Elsevier,1994), Neural Networks (ed, A Waller,1995) and The Race for Consciousness (MIT Press, 1999). His latest book is 'The Mind: A User's Manual', published in 2006 by Wiley. His most recent award was the IEEE CIS Pioneer Award in 2009 for 'contributions to neural network models of the brain.

Alessandro Vinciarelli is Lecturer at the University of Glasgow (UK) and Senior Researcher at the Idiap Research Institute (Switzerland). His main research interest is Social Signal Processing (SSP), the new domain aimed at bridging the social intelligence gap between people and computers. Alessandro is the coordinator of the Social Signal Processing Network (www.sspnet.eu), a large European collaboration aimed at providing access to SSP related resources (benchmarks and software tools) to the scientific community, and he is PI or co-PI of several national and international projects. Alessandro is author and co-author of around 50 publications, including 17 journal papers, one authored book and one edited book. Alessandro is also Associate Editor for the social sciences column of the IEEE Signal Processing Magazine and co-founder of Klewel (www.klewel.com), a multimedia analysis company recognized through several national (Swiss) and international awards.

Zachary Warren received his Ph.D. in clinical psychology from the University of Miami, Miami, Florida in 2005. He joined the Division of Genetics and Developmental Pediatrics at the Medical University of South Carolina as a Postdoctoral fellow. In 2006 he joined Vanderbilt University as Director of the Parent Support and Education Program for the Treatment and Research Institute for Autism Spectrum Disorders (TRIAD). Currently he is an Assistant Professor of clinical psychiatry and clinical pediatrics. His research focuses on early childhood development and intervention for children with autism spectrum disorders.

Karla Conn Welch received her Ph.D. in 2009 from Vanderbilt University, Nashville, Tennessee. In 2005 she was awarded a National Science Foundation Graduate Research Fellowship. In 2010 she joined the University of Louisville as an Assistant Professor of electrical and computer engineering. Her current research interests include machine learning, adaptive response systems, and robotics.

Index

Symbols

A